Discovery and Explanation in Biology and Medicine

SCIENCE AND ITS CONCEPTUAL FOUNDATIONS
David L. Hull, Editor

Discovery and Explanation in Biology and Medicine

Kenneth F. Schaffner

THE UNIVERSITY OF CHICAGO PRESS   *Chicago & London*

KENNETH F. SCHAFFNER is University Professor of Medical Humanities at the George Washington University. He received his Ph.D. in philosophy from Columbia University and his M.D. from the University of Pittsburgh.

The University of Chicago Press, Chicago 60637
The University of Chicago Press, Ltd., London
© 1993 by the University of Chicago
All rights reserved. Published 1993
Printed in the United States of America
02 01 00 99 98 97 96 95 94 93   5 4 3 2 1

ISBN (cloth): 0-226-73591-5
ISBN (paper): 0-226-73592-3

Library of Congress Cataloging-in-Publication Data

Schaffner, Kenneth F.
    Discovery and explanation in biology and medicine / Kenneth F. Schaffner
        p.   cm. — (Science and its conceptual foundations)
    Includes bibliographical references and index
    ISBN 0-226-73591-5. — ISBN 0-226-73592-3 (pbk.)
    1. Medicine—Research—Philosophy. 2. Biology—Research—Philosophy. I. Title. II. Series.
    R852.S32   1993
    610′ .72—dc20   93-21826
                                                              CIP

This book has been printed from camera-ready copy prepared by the author.

To Jeanette
for her patience, love, and encouragement

.

Summary of Contents

List of Illustrations   xix
Preface   xxiii
Acknowledgments   xxv

ONE   Introduction: The Scope and Aim of This Book   1

TWO   Discovery in the Biomedical Sciences: Logic or Intuitive Genius (or Both)?   8

THREE   Theories and "Laws" in Biology and Medicine   64

FOUR   The Logic and Methodology of Empirical Testing in Biology and Medicine   129

FIVE   Evaluation: Local and Global Approaches   169

SIX   Explanation and Causation in Biology and Medicine: General Considerations   261

SEVEN   Historicity, Historical Explanations, and Evolutionary Theory   325

EIGHT   Functional Analysis and Teleological Explanation   362

NINE   Reduction and Reductionism in Biology and Medicine   411

Ten   Conclusion and Research Issues
for the Future   517

Notes   525
Bibliography   569
Index   607

Contents

List of Illustrations xix
Preface xxiii
Acknowledgments xxv

ONE   Introduction: The Scope and Aim of This Book 1

1.1 Introduction 1
1.2 Discovery, Evaluation, and Theory Structure 1
1.3 The Complexity of Explanation and Reduction in Biology and Medicine 4

TWO   Discovery in the Biomedical Sciences: Logic or Intuitive Genius (or Both)? 8

2.1 Introduction 8
2.2 Hanson on a Logic of Scientific Discovery 11
2.3 The Natural Selection Theory of Antibody Formation 13
2.4 Criticism of the Retroductive Model 16
2.5 The Logic of Generation 19
2.6 The Double Aspect of the Logic of Discovery 21
2.7 An Example of the Logics of Generation and Evaluation in Clinical Diagnosis 31
2.8 The Clonal Selection Theory 37
2.9 Simon's Theory of Selective Forgetting in Discovery 44
2.10 Hempel's Objections to a Logic of Scientific Discovery 48
2.11 Problems, Disciplinary Matrices, BACON, and Analogy 50

THREE   Theories and "Laws" in Biology and Medicine 64

3.1 Introduction 64

3.2 General Approaches to Analyzing Theory
      Structure in Biology and Medicine 65

3.3 Some Recent Debates Concerning Theory
      Structure in Biology 67

3.4 Examples of Representative Theories in Biology
      and Medicine 74

    3.4.1 The Theory of the Genetic Code 74

    3.4.2 The Operon Theory 76

    3.4.3 The Clonal Selection Theory 82

    3.4.4 The Two-Component Theory of the Immune
            Response 84

    3.4.5 The Theory of Evolution and Population Ge-
            netics 89

            The Metatheoretical Function of Evolutionary
            Theory 90

            The Unrepresentativeness of Evolutionary
            Theory 90

            The Complexity of More Realistic Evolution-
            ary Theories of Population Genetics 94

3.5 "Middle-Range" Theories as Overlapping
      Interlevel Temporal Models 97

3.6 The Semantic Approach to Scientific Theories 99

    3.6.1 The State Space Approach 101

    3.6.2 The Set-Theoretic Approach (in Generalized
            Form) 105

3.7 The Frame System Approach to Scientific
      Theories 107

    3.7.1 Rosch and Putnam on Prototypes and Stereo-
            types 107

    3.7.2 The Frame Concept 109

    3.7.3 Frames and Nonmonotonicity 112

    3.7.4 Object-Oriented Programming
            Approaches 114

3.8 Additional Problems with Simple Axiomatiza-
      tions in Biology and Medicine 117

3.9 A Proposal Regarding Current Debates on Theory Structure, Universality, and Biological Generalizations 119

3.10 Summary 125

Appendix 126

FOUR The Logic and Methodology of Empirical Testing in Biology and Medicine 129

4.1 Epistemological Considerations: Generalized Empiricism 130

4.2 Interpretative Sentences and Antecedent Theoretical Meaning 131

4.3 An Introduction to the Logic of Experimental Testing 133

4.3.1 Deduction: A Syntactic Approach to Testing 133

4.3.2 The Nossal-Lederberg Experiment 133

4.4 Observation in Biology and Medicine — The Issue of Relevant Observations 137

4.5 The Special Nature of Initial Conditions in Biology and Medicine: Auxiliary Hypotheses 139

4.6 The Methods of Experimental Inquiry 142

4.6.1 Mill's Methods 143

4.6.2 Bernard's Method of Comparative Experimentation and Its Relation to Mill's Views 145

4.6.3 The Deductive Method 153

4.6.4 The Hypothetical Method 154

4.7 Direct versus Indirect Evidence: Arguments for a Continuum 156

4.8 Glymour's Analysis of Relevant Evidence 165

4.9 Summary 167

FIVE Evaluation: Local and Global Approaches 169

PART I: LOCAL EVALUATION AND STATISTICAL HYPOTHESIS TESTING 169

5.1 Introduction 169

5.2 Can Evaluations of Hypotheses and Theories Be Represented by Probabilities? 170

5.3 Classical Approaches 173

    5.3.1 The Fisherian Approach 173

    5.3.2 The Neyman-Pearson Theory of Testing 173

5.4 The Bayesian Approach to Probability and Statistics 177

    5.4.1 Bayes's Theorem 178

    5.4.2 Bayesian Conditionalization *179*

    5.4.3 Bayes's Theorem and Novel Predictions 181

    5.4.4 The Old Evidence Problem 183

    5.4.5 Bayes's Theorem and the Convergence of Personal Probabilities 186

5.5 Bayesian Hypothesis Testing 187

5.6 Some Additional Arguments Favoring Bayesianism 188

PART II: GLOBAL EVALUATION AND EXTENDED THEORIES 193

5.7 Transition to More Global Approaches 193

5.8 Scientific Fallibilism and Conditionalized Realism 194

    5.8.1 Lessons from the History of Science 194

    5.8.2 Current Debates Concerning Realism in Science 195

    5.8.3 Conditionalized Realism 197

    5.8.4 Social Constructivism 199

5.9 The Problem of Commensurability 200

    5.9.1 The Theory-ladenness of Criteria 201

    5.9.2 The Theory-ladenness of Scientific Terms 201

    5.9.3 The Theory-ladenness of Observations 202

    5.9.4 Responses to the Problem of Incommensurability 202

5.10 Metascientific Units of Global Evaluation: Paradigms, Research Programs, and Research Traditions 205

5.11 The Extended Theory as the Appropriate Metascientific Unit of Global Evaluation in the Biomedical Sciences 211

5.11.1 Centrality 211

5.11.2 Generality 212

5.11.3 Change of Central Hypotheses 213

5.11.4 Factoring the Extended Theory into Components 213

5.11.5 The Semantic Conception of an Extended Theory 214

5.12 A Bayesian Logic of Global Evaluation 215

5.13 The Clonal Selection Theory as an Extended Theory 220

5.13.1 The Form of the Clonal Selection Theory, 1957–1959 222

5.13.2 The Main Competitor of the CST: The Extended Instructive Theory 224

5.13.3 Arguments between Proponents of the CST and Proponents of the IT 225

5.14 Types of Factors Involved in the CST-IT Debate 231

5.14.1 Simplicity 232

5.14.2 Theoretical Context Sufficiency 236

5.14.3 Empirical Adequacy 238

5.14.4 Ad Hoc Hypotheses and Global Evaluation 241

5.14.5 Hypothesis Centrality, ad Hoc Theory Modifications, and Theory Integrity 246

5.14.6 General Bayesian Comparative Considerations 247

5.14.7 Where Might the Numbers Come from in a Bayesian Approach to Global Evaluation? 248

5.15 Conclusion 250

Appendix 1: A Mendelian Example Illustrating the Concepts of "Significance" and "Power" 252

Appendix 2: A Mendelian Example Employing a Bayesian Approach 256

SIX Explanation and Causation in Biology and Medicine: General Considerations 261

6.1 Introduction 261

6.2   General Models of Explanation in Science 265

6.2.1 The Deductive-Nomological Model 265

6.2.2 Deductive Statistical and Inductive Statistical Models 267

6.2.3 The Statistical Relevance Model 269

6.3   Recent Debates Concerning Explanation: The Role of Causal Explanation 270

6.3.1 Hempel's Analysis 271

6.3.2 Brody's and van Fraassen's (Initial) Aristotelian Approach 272

6.3.3 Salmon's Later Emphasis on the Role of Causal Explanations in the S-R Model   274

6.4   Short-Term and Long-Term Learning in *Aplysia* 276

6.4.1 Sensitization and Short-Term Memory   277

6.4.2 Long-term Memory in *Aplysia* 280

6.4.3 Additional Complexity and Parallel Processing 281

6.5   What Does this Example Tell Us about Explanation in Neurobiology?   284

6.5.1 Causal Generalizations of Varying Scope Are Prevalent in Neurobiology   284

6.5.2 Causal versus Perspectival Sequences   290

6.6   What Does this Example Tell Us about Scientific Explanation in General?   291

6.7   Causality and Causal Explanation 296

6.7.1 Hume on Causation   297

6.7.2 The Heterogeneous Character of Causation 298

The Conditional Component 299

The Epistemological Component 302

The Ontic Component and Process Metaphysics 305

6.8   Probabilistic Extensions of Causal Explanation 307

6.9   Unification and Pragmatic Approaches to Explanation 312

6.9.1 Kitcher on Unification 312

6.9.2 Van Fraassen's Analysis of Explanations as Answers to "Why-Questions" 313

6.9.3 Railton's Concept of the"Ideal Explanatory Text" 318

6.9.4 The Meshing of Different Levels of Detail in the Ideal Explanatory Text 319

6.10 Summary and Conclusion 322

SEVEN   Historicity, Historical Explanations, and Evolutionary Theory 325

7.1 Introduction 325

7.2 Models of Historical Explanation in Biology 328

7.2.1 Gallie's Account 329

7.2.2 Goudge's Integrating and Narrative Explanations 331

7.2.3 Gallie and Goudge Redux 333

7.2.4 Beckner's Genetic Analyses and Genetic Explanations 337

7.3 A Historical Explanation of the Frequency of the Sickle-Cell Gene in African-Americans 339

7.3.1 Sickle-Cell Trait and Sickle-Cell Disease 339

7.3.2 Evolutionary Theory and Population Genetics 340

7.3.3 Wright's Model 341

7.3.4 A Standard Account of Balanced Polymorphism 343

7.3.5 Allison's and Livingstone's Research on the Sickle-Cell Gene 347

7.4 Evolutionary and Embryological Historical Explanations as Data-deficient Causal Sequence Explanations 351

7.4.1 Mechanistic Historical Explanations 351

7.4.2 From Scriven to Sober, Horan, and Brandon on Evolutionary Explanation 353

Scriven 353

Sober 354

Horan 354

Brandon 355

7.4.3 Evaluation and Explanation 356

7.4.4 Conclusion 359

Appendix: The Hierarchical Turn in Evolutionary Theorizing and New Techniques for Obtaining Data on Evolution 360

EIGHT Functional Analysis and Teleological Explanation 362

8.1 Introduction 362

8.2 Intentional Analysis of Teleology 364

8.3 Cybernetic or Systems Analyses of Goal-Directed Systems 365

8.4 Nagel's Account of Functional Analysis 368

8.5 Evolutionary Analyses of Functional Explanation 370

8.5.1 The Canfield, Ruse, and Brandon Analyses 371

8.5.2 The Ateleological Character of Evolutionary Theory: The Views of Stebbins and Lewontin 373

8.5.3 Aptation, Adaptation, and Exaptation 380

8.5.4 The "Cloner" Example 383

8.5.5 Functional Ascriptions Appear To Be Licensed by a "Vulgar" Form of Evolutionary Theory 384

8.5.6 Miller's Discovery of the Immunological Function of the Thymus 385

8.5.7 Two Senses of "Function" 388

8.5.8 Why Goal Postulation Is Explanatory: A Heuristic Approach 390

8.6 Anthropomorphic Accounts of Functional Analysis 392

8.6.1 Hempel's Analysis 392

8.6.2 Wimsatt's Analysis 394

8.6.3 Wright's Analysis 396

The Etiological Translation Schema 396

Criticisms of Wright's Analysis 397

8.6.4 Cummins's Containment Account 399

8.6.5 Rosenberg's Intentional Account of Complex Teleological Language 401

8.7 Teleological and Functional Explanations 405

8.7.1 The Relation of Goal-Directed Behavior to Functional Analysis 405

8.7.2 Explanation in Functional Analysis and Goal-Directed Behavior 406

NINE Reduction and Reductionism in Biology and Medicine 411

9.1 Introduction 411

9.2 Arguments for In-Principle Emergentism 414

9.2.1 Structural Arguments 415

9.2.2 Evolutionary Arguments 420

9.3 Intertheoretic and Branch Reduction 423

9.3.1 The Nagel Model 423

9.3.2 The Kemeny-Oppenheim Model 425

9.3.3 The Suppes-Adams (Semantic) Model 425

9.3.4 The General Reduction Model 426

9.3.5 The General Reduction-Replacement Model 427

9.4 Criticisms and Elaborations of Intertheoretic Reduction Models 432

9.4.1 Theory Structure Issues: Are "Laws" Relevant? 433

9.4.2 Connectability Problems 437

Connectability of Natural Kinds 437

Problems Posed by Construing Connectability Assumptions as Synthetic Identities 466

9.4.3 Derivability Problems 477

Kitcher on Derivational Reduction 478

The Problem of Analogy in Reduction 481

9.5 Multiple Levels, Causes, and the Possibility of an Alternative Causal/Mechanical Model of Reduction 487

9.5.1 Multiple Levels of Analysis in Reduction 487

9.5.2 Might a Fully Causal/Mechanical Approach of Reduction Be Possible? 490

9.5.3 The Relation between the Causal/Mechanical Account of Reduction and the GRR Model and Two Versions of the GRR Model—Simple and Complex 493

9.6 Arguments against In-Principle Emergentism 500

9.6.1 Polanyi Reconsidered 501

9.6.2 Structural versus Ultimate Reductionism 503

9.6.3 Bohr, Elsasser, and Generalized Quantum Complementarity 505

9.7 The Peripherality of Reductionism as a Research Program and the Need for Research Methodologies of the Middle Range 509

9.7.1 The Peripherality of Reductionism Thesis 508

9.7.2 Watson-Crick Replication and the Peripherality Thesis 509

9.7.3 The Operon Theory Revisited—Again 511

9.8 Suggestion for a Bayesian Explication of the Peripherality Thesis 513

9.9 Conclusion 515

TEN Conclusion and Research Issues for the Future 517

10.1 Introduction 517

10.2 Discovery, Evaluation, and the Experimental Testing of Hypotheses and Theories 517

10.3 Evaluation and Theory Structure 519

10.4 Explanation and Reduction in Biology and Medicine 521

Notes 525
Bibliography 569
Index 607

List of Illustrations

FIGURES

2.1 Diagram of a contemporary version of the clonal selection theory 38

3.1A, 3.1B *lac* enzyme regulation and mutations 78, 79

3.2 Variations of o^c mutations 81

3.3 The two-component theory of the immune response 86

3.4 Relations among some of the components in evolutionary population biology theory 96

3.5 Simple frames for the concepts of "gene," "regulator gene," and "I$^+$ gene" 109

3-6 Inheritance relations in genetics 112

3.7 Overlapping features of operon models 118

4.1 Average lymphocyte : polymorph ratio of mice thymectomized in the neonatal period compared to sham-thymectomized controls 151

4.2 The *lac* operon model in 1961 159

5.1 Haurowitz's 1967 instructional theory 221

5.2 Distribution of p under H_0 and H_1 with selected critical region 254

5.3 Two possible choices for the initial (prior) distribution of p 257

5.4 Final distributions for p based on a sample of n = 100 using the two initial distributions given in 5.3 above 258

6.1 *Aplysia californica*, the sea hare, as viewed from the side and from above, with the parapodia retracted in order to show mantle, gill, and siphon 276

6.2 Short- and long-term sensitization of the withdrawal reflex in *Aplysia*. A: Timecourse of sensitization after a single strong electric shock to the tail or neck of *Aplysia* (arrow). B: Sensitization in groups of animals receiving varied amounts of stimulation 278

6.3 Simplified diagram of the gill component of the withdrawal reflexes in *Aplysia* 279

6.4 Molecular model of short-term sensitization 281

6.5 A speculative model of how long-term memory may operate in "parallel" 282

6.6 The gill- and siphon-withdrawal reflex circuit showing the sites found to be modified by sensitizing stimuli 284

6.7 A full adder 289

6.8 Developmental stages of color coat genes in the mouse 321

7.1 Stable equilibrium point of the sickle cell allele 346

8.1 The "cloner" 382

9.1 DNA Cloning in Plasmids 454

9.2 DNA Sequencing by the Maxam and Gilbert Method 456

9.3 Restriction maps of cloned color-normal and mutant red and green pigment genes 458

9.4 Fodor's schematic representation of the proposed relation between the reduced and reducing science on a revised account of the unity of science 460

9.5 The *lac* operator and promotor sequences 464

9.6 Enzyme kinetic graph representing the results of the "Pajama" experiment, Cross II 484

9.7 Replication of DNA 502

TABLES

2.1 Types and phases of scientific inference 20

2.2, 2.3, 2.4 Evoking strength, frequency, and import in INTERNIST-1 26–27

3.1 The genetic code 75

3.2 Immune deficiency diseases 88

7.1 General fitness table 344

7.2 Sickle-cell fitness table 345

9.1 Reductionistic and antireductionist approaches in biology and medicine 412

9.2 CM and GRR approaches in different states of completion of reductions 496

Preface

THE CONCEPT OF THIS BOOK had its inception in 1971, stimulated by my reading and teaching Claude Bernard's (1957 [1865]) *An Introduction to the Study of Experimental Medicine* to my students at the University of Chicago. Work in the philosophy of biology was in its comparative infancy at that time but was growing rapidly, particularly in the Chicago discussion group on the subject I attended along with David Hull, Dick Lewontin, Dick Levins, Stu Kauffman, Arnold Ravin, Dudley Shapere, Leigh van Valen, and Bill Wimsatt. The kindred field of philosophy of medicine was at best in its embryonic stage during that period. Specific research on this book commenced in 1974 while I was on a Guggenheim Fellowship and proceeded at a varying pace during my stay at the University of Pittsburgh until 1981. Along the way this research resulted in some of the preliminary publications cited in the Acknowledgments section following this Preface.

In 1981, with the encouragement of Jack Myers, M.D., University Professor of Medicine, I became a regular student at the University of Pittsburgh's School of Medicine in order to pursue a more in-depth knowledge of the biomedical sciences in both basic science and clinical contexts; I received the M.D. in 1986. I am indebted to the University of Pittsburgh's Department of History and Philosophy of Science, and in particular to Peter Machamer and Clark Glymour, then serving as Department Chairmen, and to my students, for tolerating with extremely good humor my extensively juggled schedule during those years that I studied medicine. I am also most grateful to former President Posvar, to then Deans Drew, Leon, Pounds, and Rosenberg, and to Mrs. Barris for administratively facilitating this endeavor.

From 1986 through 1991 and into 1992, I extensively revamped this book in the light of that educational experience. The stimulating environment of the University of Pittsburgh's philosophy of science community afforded me many opportunities for conversations on topics in philosophy with John Earman, Clark Glymour, Adolf Grünbaum, Peter Hempel, Jim Lennox, Peter Machamer, Ted McGuire, Merrilee Salmon, Wes Salmon, and the late Wilfrid Sellars. Discussions with David Evans, Jay

Kadane, Teddy Seidenfeld, and Herb Simon from nearby CMU have also been of great assistance.

For earlier discussions and comments on materials that have been brought together in this book I am indebted to Bill Bechtel, Bruce Buchanan, Art Caplan, Pat Churchland, Paul Churchland, Lindley Darden, Tris Engelhardt, Ron Giere, Marjorie Grene, David Hull, Philip Kitcher, Dick Lewontin, Ed Manier, Tom Nickles, Ed Pellegrino, Michael Ruse, Dudley Shapere, Mark Siegler, Arthur Silverstein, Jack Smart, Fred Suppe, and especially to Bill Wimsatt. Readers will also note that many of the points of departure (as well as of criticism) in this book are occasioned by Alex Rosenberg's work. I have drawn on important insights and contributions by John Beatty, Mort Beckner, Bob Brandon, Dick Burian, Tom Kuhn, Larry Laudan, Liz Lloyd, Ernst Mayr, Ron Munson, Eliot Sober, Paul Thompson, and Wim van der Steen. I have received occasional (and most valuable) scientific advice over the years from Mel Cohn, Francis Crick, Neils Jerne, Eric Kandel, Joshua Lederberg, Richard Levins, Jacques Monod before his untimely death in 1976, and Bruce Rabin, though none should be considered responsible for any scientific errors in this text. I am also indebted to two anonymous referees for very helpful comments, and in particular to David Hull for his careful review of the manuscript. My research assistants Andrea Woody and Michelle Sforza were most helpful in improving the readability and grammar of the manuscript. It has been a pleasure to work with the University of Chicago Press and to have the painstaking editorial assitance of Ronnie Hawkins, M.D., as copy editor. I am also grateful to Dean Peter F.M. Koehler at the University of Pittsburgh and to Vice-President Roderick S. French at the George Washington University for research support as the manuscript entered its final stage.

My greatest intellectual debt is to the late Ernest Nagel, who was my teacher and dissertation director at Columbia and from whom I learned a respect for scientific detail as well as the importance of a critical methodology. I also had the good fortune to meet and spend much time with Imre Lakatos at a point when many of the ideas in this book were in the process of gestation. Above all, I want to thank my wife, Jeanette, to whom this book is dedicated, for long-standing encouragement and support as it wound its way to completion.

Acknowledgments

I WANT TO THANK the following publishers for permission to adapt material from my previously published articles for use in this book:

Parts of the material in chapter 2 appeared in "Discovery in the Biomedical Sciences: Logic or Irrational Intuition," *in Scientific Discovery: Case Studies*, ed. T. Nickles, 171–205 (Copyright © 1980 by D. Reidel Publishing Company, Dordrecht, the Netherlands). Other parts of that chapter are adapted from my introduction to *Logic of Discovery and Diagnosis in Medicine*, ed. K. Schaffner (copyright © 1985 by the University of California Press, Berkeley).

Chapter 3 is a considerably expanded version of material that appeared in "Theory Structure in the Biomedical Sciences," *The Journal of Medicine and Philosophy*: 57–95 (copyright © 1980 by the Society for Health and Human Values. This chapter also draws on some material that appeared in "Computerized Implementation of Biomedical Theory Structures: An Artificial Intelligence Approach," *PSA – 1986*, vol. 2, ed. A. Fine and P. Machamer, 17–32 (copyright © 1987 by the Philosophy of Science Association, East Lansing, Mich.).

Chapter 4 adapts some of the ideas initially presented in "Correspondence Rules" *Philosophy of Science* 36:280–90. (copyright © 1969 by the Philosophy of Science Association, East Lansing, Mich.). It also contains some material that was presented in "Clinical Trials: The Validation of Theory and Therapy" in *Physics, Philosophy, and Psychoanalysis*, ed. R. S. Cohen and L. Laudan, 191-208 (copyright © 1983 by D. Reidel Publishing Company, Dordrecht, the Netherlands).

A much-condensed version of some of the material in chapter 5 was presented in "Theory Change in Immunology: The Clonal Selection Theory, Part I: Theory Change and Scientific Progress; Part II: The Clonal Selection Theory" *Theoretical Medicine* 13 (no. 2): 191–216 (copyright © 1992 by Kluwer Academic Publishers, Dordrecht, the Netherlands). This chapter also uses some ideas developed in "Einstein Versus Lorentz: Research Programmes and the Logic of Comparative Theory Evaluation,"

British Journal for the Philosophy of Science 25:45–78 (copyright ©
1974 by the British Society for the Philosophy of Science, London).

Portions of chapter 6 appeared in "Philosophy of Medicine,"
in *Introduction to the Philosophy of Science*, ed. M. Salmon, 310–345
(copyright © 1992 by Prentice-Hall, Englewood Cliffs, N.J.). Parts
of this chapter also are adapted from "Explanation and Causation in the Biomedical Sciences," in *Mind and Medicine*, ed. L.
Laudan, 79–124 (copyright © 1983 by the University of California
Press, Berkeley).

Chapter 9 draws on some of the material developed in "Approaches to Reduction," *Philosophy of Science* 34:137–147 (copyright © 1967 by the Philosophy of Science Association, East
Lansing, Mich.). The section on the general reduction-replacement model includes material adapted from "Reduction, Reductionism, Values and Progress in the Biomedical Sciences,"
appearing in *Logic, Laws and Life*, vol. 6 of the University of Pittsburgh Series in the Philosophy of Science, ed R. Colodny, 143–171
(copyright © 1977 by the University of Pittsburgh Press, Pittsburgh). In addition, the section "The Problem of Analogy in Reduction" contains material from "Logic of Discovery and
Justification in Regulatory Genetics," *Studies in the History and
Philosophy of Science* 4:349–385 (copyright © 1974 by Pergamon
Press). This chapter also draws on some material from "The
Peripherality of Reductionism in the Development of Molecular
Biology," *Journal of the History of Biology* 7:111–139 (copyright ©
1974 by D. Reidel Publishing Company, Dordrecht, the Netherlands).

As noted in the Preface, preliminary work on the materials
in this book began with the support of the John Simon Guggenheim Memorial Foundation. These early investigations were also
facilitated by the granting of library privileges by Northwestern
University Medical Center, the University of Chicago, and the
American Medical Association. I am also grateful to the History
and Philosophy of Science program at the National Science
Foundation and to the National Endowment for the Humanities
for support of my research on the philosophy of biology and the
philosophy of medicine.

Any opinions, findings, and conclusions or recommendations expressed in this publication are those of the author and do
not necessarily reflect the views of any of the supporting institutions or agencies acknowledged above.

CHAPTER ONE

Introduction: The Scope and Aim of This Book

1.1 Introduction

THIS BOOK IS AN INQUIRY INTO PHILOSOPHICAL ISSUES in biology and medicine. One of its themes is that what have traditionally been seen as medical sciences, including immunology, human genetics, the neurosciences, and internal medicine, can provide salutary examples for the philosophy of science. Taken in conjunction with the recent vigorous growth and advances in the philosophy of biology as more traditionally conceived, I view medical and biological examples as synergistically relatable both to each other and to philosophy of science. Such examples serve in this book both as illustrations of general philosophical theses and as tests of the clarity and adequacy of our philosophical conceptions. In addition, I believe that the philosophy of biology has more in common with general philosophy of science than a number of philosophers of biology seem to think, and I have attempted to develop and utilize those linkages throughout this book.

1.2 Discovery, Evaluation, and Theory Structure

The title of this book is *Discovery and Explanation in Biology and Medicine*. In chapter 2 I review some aspects of the tortuous history of the legitimacy of scientific discovery as a philosophical topic. I divide scientific practice in this domain into the phases of generation, preliminary evaluation, and justification of new hypotheses (and theories) and point out that some of the traditional work (including Hanson's writings) has conflated the first two phases. I argue that frequently rational analysis and reconstruction of both the generation and preliminary evaluation phases

1

can be accomplished, and I provide examples of such analysis and reconstruction from immunology and from internal medicine. I draw on the recent philosophical, cognitive science, and artificial intelligence literature to support my claims. The analysis of scientific discovery immediately raises questions about the nature of scientific theories and their representation, as well as about the boundaries of scientific fields, and these questions are subsequently pursued in the form of detailed answers in later chapters of the book.

The first of these questions, concerning the nature of scientific theories in biology and medicine and how best to represent them, is the subject of chapter 3 and is reexamined in chapters 5, on local and global evaluation, and 9, on reduction. Chapter 3, on theories and laws in biology and medicine, proposes (or rather reproposes, since I first urged many of the views discussed in that chapter in my 1980 essay) that many of the theories we encounter in the biomedical sciences are different from the standard type of theory we see in physics. In the medically related biological sciences such as molecular genetics, immunology, physiology, embryology, and the neurosciences, we find "theories of the middle range," theories in a sense midway between the universal mechanisms of biochemistry and the universal generalizations of neo-Darwinian evolution.[1] The problem of "generalizations" in biology and medicine is a complex one and it has been addressed in several different contexts over the past nearly thirty years. Smart first raised the question whether there were any "laws" in biology, and the discussion has been joined by Ruse (1973), Wimsatt (1976b), Beatty (1981), Kitcher (1984), Rosenberg (1985), the U.S. National Academy of Sciences (Morowitz 1985), Lloyd (1988), van der Steen and Kamminga (1990), and Beatty (1992). I maintain that further analysis of the senses of "universal" within the framework of theories of the middle range provides a solution to this issue. I also suggest that the semantic approach to scientific theories, which has attracted considerable interest on the part of philosophers of biology in the 1980s, is a natural context in which to give added structure to these theories of the middle range. In my examination of the semantic approach, I generalize the set-theoretic characterization from previous accounts (such as Lloyd's [1988] and Thompson's [1989]), and I also respond to some criticisms posed by Suppe in his recent (1989) book.

Chapter 4, on the logic and methodology of empirical testing in biology and medicine, discusses the way in which the notion of a theory as analyzed in this book makes contact with the empirical world. This discussion reanalyzes the logical empiricists' concept of a "correspondence rule" and indicates, with the help of an important experiment in immunology, how empirical control is exerted over theories. I use the term "generalized empiricism" to characterize the position I formulate in this and subsequent chapters. I also discuss the issue of "direct evidence," considered in physics by Shapere (1982) and Galison (1987), and later in the chapter examine the concept in regard to molecular biology. The discussion then proceeds to a consideration of Mill's methods and Claude Bernard's criticism of them. The importance of Mill's "method of difference" and its relationship to his little-analyzed "deductive method" and to Bernard's "method of comparative experimentation" are examined, and then illustrated using a key set of experiments from recent molecular biology: the isolation and characterization of the "repressor" of the *lac* operon.

Though chapter 4 represents a preliminary discussion of the ways that empirical findings exercise control over theory, a fuller account requires both an analysis of "evaluation" in science and attention to the historical dimension of scientific theories. These topics are the subject of chapter 5, which presents a Bayesian approach to local and global evaluation. I briefly characterize the "received" classical or frequentist view of statistical hypothesis testing, so widespread in both the basic biological and the clinical sciences, and then go on to defend a Bayesian position. This Bayesian position can accommodate (in a translated and reconceptualized way) traditional statistical testing, and it can also be used as a general framework within which to develop a more "global" notion of intertheoretic comparison and evaluation. However, first some underbrush needs to be cleared away, and as part of an effort to do so I criticize the relativistic positions of Kuhn and Feyerabend as well as the "constructivist program" of Latour and Woolgar (1979) and Knorr-Cetina (1981) for misunderstanding and mislocating the nature of experimental control of models and theories in biology. Then the concept of a "theory of the middle range," introduced in chapter 3, is generalized to take into account changes of the theory over time. The generalized notion of a theory so produced I call a "temporally extended theory." I discuss this generalized notion of theory, describe some of its features, and show how it raises and answers interesting questions related to the largely ignored problem of theory individuation. In this chapter I also show how other important evaluational concepts, such as simplicity, the freedom from ad hoc hypotheses, and the effect of the theoretical context, can be brought together within the Bayesian framework. I apply these ideas to a quite detailed historical example drawn from immunology: the competition between the instructive theory and the clonal selection theory of the immune response in the decade 1957–1967. I close this chapter by summarizing what I believe are the strengths and weaknesses of the Bayesian approach in contrast with other approaches that might be taken to theory evaluation, including some comments on Glymour's (1980) bootstrapping account of confirmation.

1.3 The Complexity of Explanation and Reduction in Biology and Medicine

In chapter 6, on explanation in biology and medicine, I begin to develop what will emerge as a lengthy account of scientific explanation, with applications to the neurosciences, Mendelian genetics, molecular genetics, and population genetics. This part of the book draws on the notion of a temporally extended middle-range theory as well as on the Bayesian perspective developed in the early chapters. The key notion of explanation elaborated in chapter 6 is one that appeals to (possibly probabilistic) causal model systems instantiating (interlevel) generalizations of both broad and narrow scope. A six-component model, involving semantic, causal, unificatory, logical (deductive), comparative-evaluational inductive, and ideal explanatory text background components, is developed and applied to a complex recent example from the neurosciences: simple learning in the sea snail *(Aplysia)*. This work draws on seminal writings in scientific explanation from Hempel, Salmon, van Fraassen, Railton, and Kitcher, among others. The chapter also includes an in-depth analysis of causation, utilizing some of Mackie's (1974) suggestions, but develops them in the context of a broader framework of contributions from Collingwood and from Hart and Honoré. This analysis combines theses about how we learn our primitive causal concepts with what I conceive of as a necessary metaphysical component in causation. The relation between probabilistic and nonprobabilistic approaches to causation is also explored.

This account of explanation developed in chapter 6 is then further elaborated in the context of some issues in scientific explanation that are usually conceived of as specific to the biological and medical sciences. In chapter 7 I resurrect the old debate over historical explanation, present it in a new light, and show that, though the explanations provided by evolutionary theory are indeed "explanations," they are extraordinarily weak and conjectural ones. I support this by using a detailed illustration — the sickle-cell trait and sickle-cell disease example, drawing on the work of Allison and Livingstone — to show just how many empirically *un*substantiated assumptions need to be made in order to construct even the strongest examples of historical explanation in biology and medicine. I also compare my position with that recently developed by Brandon (1990). The view developed in this chapter goes against the generally accepted view in biology, medicine, and philosophy of biology, which holds that evolutionary theory can provide us with prototypes for explanatory paradigms.

In chapter 8 I consider the role of "functional" statements and "teleological" explanations in biology and medicine. My main thesis here is that the most common interpretation of functional statements (and their "explanatory" force) is licensed by a "vulgar" understanding of evolution that lacks scientific support, but that such functional language *is* heuristically important as well as irreducible to efficient causal language. I develop this thesis in the context of a comprehensive review of what I term intentional, cybernetic, evolutionary, and anthropomorphic accounts of function and teleology, covering the views of Nagel, Ruse, Brandon, Hempel, Wimsatt, and Wright, among others. I also furnish a "translation schema" for functional language explicitly providing for the irreducibility of such locutions to efficient causal language. The discovery of "the function" of the thymus is used to illustrate these views.

These analyses of historical explanation and of functional and teleological explanation clear the ground for a detailed analysis of reduction in biology and medicine, which is the subject of chapter 9. In this chapter I briefly review some of the claims that have been made by biologists about the nonreducible character of biology and then turn to an in-depth analysis of intertheoretic reduction. This is a subject about which there have been a large number of papers and books written in the past forty years. I provide a lengthy historical and philosophical overview of this literature, analyzing it under the topics of the various models proposed and treating the problems of the connectability of different levels of analysis (e.g., "gene" and "DNA") and the appropriateness of conceptualizing reduction along deductive versus causal lines. The subject is pursued with attention to the relation between Mendelian and molecular genetics, and the important critiques of Hull, Wimsatt, Fodor, the Churchlands, Rosenberg, and Kitcher, as well as their positive views, are considered. My general conclusion in this chapter is that a fairly complex model, which I call the general reduction-replacement model, is the most plausible one, but that it has two subforms: one "simple" application to "unilevel" theories and one "complex" characterization for application to theories of the middle range, discussed in chapters 3 and 5. This "complex" GRR model is related to methodological rules regarding changes in temporally extended theories, and to the reduction–replacement distinction. The chapter concludes with attention to a Bayesian application to reductionistically oriented research which I term the "peripherality thesis."

In the final chapter, I draw together the various themes of the book in a summary fashion intended to demonstrate the unity of the book as well as to point the way toward a number of unresolved problems. It should be noted that this volume is both narrower and broader than most of the recent general introductions to the philosophy of biology. Recent philosophy of biology has been dominated by the philosophical issues of evolution, and though evolutionary theory is treated in chapters 3, 7, and 9, I do not attempt to offer a fully comprehensive account of it. Readers interested in these areas may want to supplement this book with Rosenberg's (1985) introduction to philosophy of biology and also parts of Sober's (1984b and 1988), Lloyd's (1988), Thompson's (1989), and Brandon's (1990) monographs on evolution. This book carries the philosophy of science into medical contexts, introducing many examples from immunology, which is largely unexplored territory for most philosophers of biology.

Though many of my examples are drawn from the medical sciences, I have not in this book addressed normative or ethical issues, other than those naturally arising in the context of inductive logic. The advances in genetics and in the neurosciences discussed in this volume raise difficult and profound ethical issues concerning control over life and over the mind itself, but one additional chapter would have been inadequate to cover them, and more would have made this already long volume far too long; these issues will be deferred to another time.

CHAPTER TWO

Discovery in the Biomedical Sciences: Logic or Intuitive Genius (or Both)?

2.1 Introduction

THE THESIS THAT THE PROCESS of scientific discovery involves logically analyzable procedures, as opposed to intuitive leaps of genius, has generally not been a popular one in this century. Since the advent of logical empiricism in the early twentieth century, the logic of science has been generally understood to be a logic of *justification*. Scientific discovery has been considered to be of interest to historians, psychologists, and sociologists, but has until fairly recently usually been barred from the list of topics that demand logical analysis by philosophers.

This situation has not always been the case; historically, in point of fact, the logic of scientific discovery and the logic of scientific justification have more than once traded prince and pauper status in the philosophy of science. With some historical support, let us initially understand a logic of scientific discovery to be a set of well-characterized and applicable rules for *generating new scientific hypotheses*, and a logic of scientific justification to be a set of rules for *assessing* or *evaluating* the merits of proffered claims about the world in the light of their purportedly supportive evidence. (These rules may either be presented in the scientific literature per se, or be given in a rational reconstruction, as in the work of philosophers of science.) If this is accepted as a viable characterization of two actual aspects of science, then it is not too difficult to understand why a believer in a logic of scientific discovery might well not see the utility of a separate logic of justification, for a *logic* of justification might appear to him or her to be only the tool of an uncreative critic, while a *logic* of discovery itself could be said to provide sufficient justification for its own progeny. On the other hand, if it is thought that there is no such thing as a logic of discovery and that all scientific conjectures, regardless of their source, must be subjected to rigorous critical evaluation, perhaps with the aid of principles collated and systematized as a logic of justification, then a logic of justification becomes of paramount importance in understanding science. Views representing these different extremes, as well as some less extreme positions, can be found both in the historical and in the contemporary literature of the philosophy of science.

In his *Rules for the Direction of the Mind*, René Descartes (1960 [1701]) believed he was proposing a method for arriving at new knowledge that possessed demonstrative force. Francis Bacon in *Novum Organum* (1960 [1620]) similarly expounded a logic of scientific discovery that would have denied any distinction, except perhaps a temporal one, between a logic of scientific discovery and a logic of justification. In the nineteenth century, John Stuart Mill (1959 [1843]) recommended various methods of experimental inquiry that can be viewed as methods for the discovery of new scientific knowledge, and he was severely criticized by his contemporary, William Whewell, for so doing. Whewell argued that Mill's methods, which bore a close resemblance to Bacon's "prerogatives of instances," begged the question of the existence of a set of rules for scientific discovery by taking "for granted the very thing which is most difficult to discover, the reduction of the phenomena to formulae as are here [in Mill's *Logic*] presented to us" (1968 [1849], 286). Whewell succinctly expressed his own view as follows:

> The conceptions by which facts are bound together are suggested by the sagacity of discoverers. This sagacity cannot be taught. It commonly succeeds by guessing; and this success seems to consist in framing several *tentative* hypotheses and selecting the right one. But a supply of appropriate hypotheses cannot be constructed by rule, nor without inventive talent. (1968 [1849], 286)

The debate has continued into the twentieth century and into our own day. In 1917 F. C. S. Schiller introduced his well-known distinction between the logic of *proof* and the logic of scientific *discovery* but recommended somewhat vaguely that science "proclaim a logic of its own," different from traditional demonstrative logic but a "logic" nonetheless (Schiller 1917, 273). What is needed, Schiller wrote, is not a logic which describes only the static relations of an unchanging system of knowledge, but one which is open to perceive motion, and willing to accept the dynamic process of a knowledge that never ceases to grow and is never really stereotyped into a system. (1917, 273)

Schiller wrote in the pragmatic tradition, but with the rise of logical empiricism the existence of a significant logical component in the discovery process of science was again denied by influential thinkers. For example, Hans Reichenbach, who introduced the distinction, analogous to Schiller's, between the "context of discovery" and the "context of justification," wrote:

The mystical interpretation of the hypothetico-deductive method as an irrational guessing springs from a confusion of *context of discovery* and *context of justification*. The act of discovery escapes logical analysis; there are no logical rules in terms of which a "discovery machine" could be constructed that would take over the creative function of the genius. But it is not the logician's task to account for scientific discoveries; all he can do is to analyze the relation between given facts and a theory presented to him with the claim that it explains these facts. In other words, logic is concerned only with the context of justification. And the justification of a theory in terms of observational data is the subject of the theory of induction. (1958, 231)[1]

Sir Karl Popper, who stands at the opposite pole from Reichenbach on a number of issues in the philosophy of science, contended in his enormously influential book *The Logic of Scientific Discovery* — the translation of the German title *Logik der Forschung* is most misleading — that:

The initial stage, the act of conceiving or inventing a theory, seems to me neither to call for logical analysis nor to be susceptible of it. The question how it happens that a new idea occurs to a man — whether it is a musical theme, a dramatic conflict, or a scientific theory — may be of great interest to empirical psychology; but it is irrelevant to the logical analysis of scientific knowledge. This latter is concerned not with *questions of fact* . . . but only with questions of *justification or validity*. . . .

Accordingly I shall distinguish sharply between the process of conceiving a new idea, and the methods and results of examining it logically. (1959, 31–32)

For Popper, as for Reichenbach, the logical analysis of science is restricted to an examination of the structures of already given scientific theories and of the testing and post-discovery evaluative procedures of scientists.

2.2 Hanson on a Logic of Scientific Discovery

Beginning in the late 1950s, the writings of N. R. Hanson (1958, 1961, 1963, 1967) slowly began to direct the attention of philosophers of science back toward the discovery process in science. Hanson argued that the "philosophical flavor" of the analyses of such notions as theory, hypothesis, law, evidence, observation, and the like, as developed by philosophers of science, was at great variance with the concepts as employed by creative scientists. The reason, Hanson claimed, was that inquiry into an area that was still problematic, and that required "theory-*finding*" thinking, analyzed science quite differently from that type of inquiry whose task was to "rearrange old facts and explanations into more elegant formal patterns" (1958, 2–3). As part of his approach, Hanson contended that what he termed the hypothetico-deductive, or H-D, account of science was rather misleading. Hanson maintained:

Physicists do not start from hypotheses; they start from data. By the time a law has been fixed into an H-D system, really original physical thinking is over. The pedestrian process of deducing observation statements from hypotheses comes only after the physicist sees that the hypothesis will at least explain the initial data requiring explanation. This H-D account is helpful only when discussing the argument of a finished research report, or for understanding how the experimentalist or the engineer develops the theoretical physicist's hypotheses; the analysis leaves undiscussed the reasoning which often points to the first tentative proposals of laws. . . .

. . . the initial suggestion of an hypothesis is very often a reasonable affair. It is not so often affected by intuition, insight, hunches, or other imponderables as biographers or scientists suggest. Disciples of the H-D account often

dismiss the dawning of an hypothesis as being of psychological interest only, or else claim it to be the province
solely of genius and not of logic. They are wrong. If
establishing an hypothesis through its predictions has a
logic, so has the conceiving of an hypothesis. (1958, 70–71)

Hanson later (1967) argued that the process of scientific discovery could be analyzed conceptually, at least partially. Discovery was Janus-faced: it had philosophically relevant aspects just
as it had philosophically irrelevant aspects. Hanson maintained
that "verification" and "confirmation" of scientific theories were
also Janus-faced, and that one could analyze them not only in
terms of scientists' *behavior* but also with respect to the *ideas* of
"verification" and "confirmation," a task which represented the
research program of the logical empiricists such as Reichenbach
and Carnap. For Hanson, it was irresponsible to turn over *all*
analysis of discovery to the psychologists, historians, and sociologists, who would only analyze the behavioral aspect largely
as fact-gatherers. Hanson wrote that "settling on the meaning of
'discovery' is too important to our understanding of science to be
abandoned to scientific discoverers or to psychologists or to sociologists or to historians of science" (1967, 323). For Hanson, "the
idea of discovery" was "conceptually too complex for any 'average' historical, psychological, or sociological analysis," and
ought to be done by "conceptual analysts" — namely by philosophers of science (1967, 324).

Hanson's analysis was presented in several of his writings in
slightly different forms, ranging from an analysis of the logic of
discovery to a typology of scientific discoveries. He tended to focus, erroneously I shall argue, on the concept of *retroductive inference*. On this matter, Hanson contended he was largely following
and developing the suggestions of Aristotle and C. S. Peirce in
proposing that there is a kind of inference, termed "retroductive
inference," that captures the type of reasoning implicit in creative scientific discoveries. Like Peirce, Hanson stressed that
retroductive reasoning was quite different from both inductive
and deductive reasoning. In his most developed article on this
logic, titled "Is there a Logic of Scientific Discovery?" (1961) Hanson proposed the following schematic form for retroductive reasoning:

(1) Some surprising, astonishing phenomena p_1, p_2,
p_3 . . . are encountered.

(2) But p_1, p_2, p_3 . . . would not be surprising were a hypothesis of H's type to obtain. They would follow as a matter of course from something like H and would be explained by it.

(3) Therefore there is good reason for elaborating a hypothesis of the type of H; for proposing it as a possible hypothesis from whose assumption p_1, p_2, p_3 . . . might be explained.

In an important footnote to (1), Hanson added that

The astonishment may consist in the fact that p is at variance with accepted theories — for example, the discovery of discontinuous emission of radiation by hot black bodies, or the photoelectric effect, the Compton effect, and the continuous-ray spectrum, or the orbital aberrations of Mercury, the refrangibility of white light, and the high velocities of Mars at 90 degrees. What is important here is *that* the phenomena are encountered as anomalous, not *why* they are so regarded. (1961, 33)

Other than for Hanson's emphasis that retroductive inference leads to a *type* of hypothesis rather than to a detailed or specific hypothesis, this schema for retroductive reasoning or retroductive inference seems to be identical with Peirce's characterization of retroduction or "abduction." That a form of logical *inference* is intended is supportable by citing another footnote to (3) above, in which Hanson quotes Peirce approvingly:

This is a free development of remarks in Aristotle . . . and Peirce . . . . Peirce amplifies: "It must be remembered that retroduction, although it is very little hampered by logical rules, nevertheless, is logical inference, asserting its conclusion only problematically, or conjecturally, it is true, but nevertheless having a perfectly definite logical form." (1961, 33)

It will be helpful to illustrate what Hanson refers to as retroductive inference by means of an example.

2.3 The Natural Selection Theory of Antibody Formation

In March 1954, Niels Kaj Jerne, an immunologist then working at the Danish State Serum Institute and a recent Nobel Laureate, was walking home through Copenhagen. Jerne had been conducting research on antibody "avidity" — that property of an antibody that determines the rate at which it reacts with antigen.

In 1954, the extant theories of antibody generation were all species of an "instructive" theory. Antibodies are crucially important macromolecules which vertebrates (including humans) manufacture to protect them against disease, and antigens are those molecular aspects of invading bacteria, viruses, fungi, and toxins which stimulate (or generate) antibody synthesis. Antigens fit like highly specific *keys* into the antibody *locks* (the combining sites on the antibody), thus initiating (unlocking) the immune response that destroys the antigens.[2] A component hypothesis of all *instructive* theories of antibody formation is that *antigens convey structural information* to the immune system, which then uses this information, like a template, on which to construct the complementarily fitting antibody.[3]

Prior to his discovery of the natural selection theory of antibody formation, Jerne had been injecting rabbits with diphtheria toxin and antitoxin and had been examining the sera of horses for antibodies to bacteriophage at various stages in the development of the equine immune response. He had been struck by, and puzzled by, the existence of a large variety of different types of antibody — present at very low levels of concentration — in the sera of the horses.

Jerne recalls that walk through Copenhagen in March 1954 in the following terms, which is worth quoting *in extenso*:

> Can the truth (*the capability to synthesize an antibody*) be learned? If so, it must be assumed not to pre-exist; to be learned, it must be acquired. We are thus confronted with the difficulty to which Socrates calls attention in *Meno* (Socrates, 375 B.C.), namely that it makes as little sense to search for what one does not know as to search for what one knows; what one knows one cannot search for, since one knows it already, and what one does not know one cannot search for, since one does not even know what to search for. Socrates resolves this difficulty by postulating that learning is nothing but recollection. The truth (*the capability to synthesize an antibody*) cannot be brought in, but was already inherent.

> The above paragraph is a translation of the first lines of Søren Kierkegaard's "Philosophical Bits or a Bit of Philoso-

phy" (Kierkegaard 1844). By replacing the word "truth" by the italicized words, the statement can be made to present the logical basis of the selective theories of antibody formation. Or, in the parlance of Molecular Biology: synthetic potentialities cannot be imposed upon nucleic acid, but must pre-exist.

I do not know whether reverberations of Kierkegaard contributed to the idea of a selective mechanism of antibody formation that occurred to me one evening in March, 1954, as I was walking home in Copenhagen from the Danish State Serum Institute to Amaliegade. The train of thought went like this: the only property that all antigens share is that they can attach to the combining site of an appropriate antibody molecule; this attachment must, therefore, be a crucial step in the sequences of events by which the introduction of an antigen into an animal leads to antibody formation; a million structurally different antibody-combining sites would suffice to explain serological specificity; if all 10^{17} gamma-globulin molecules per ml of blood are antibodies, they must include a vast number of different combining sites, because otherwise normal serum would show a high titer against all usual antigens; three mechanisms must be assumed: (1) a random mechanism for ensuring the limited synthesis of antibody molecules possessing all possible combining sites, in the absence of antigen, (2) a purging mechanism for repressing the synthesis of such antibody molecules that happen to fit to auto-[or anti-self-]antigens, and (3) a selective mechanism for promoting the synthesis of those antibody molecules that make the best fit to any antigen entering the animal. The framework of the theory was complete before I had crossed Knippelsbridge. I decided to let it mature and to preserve it for a first discussion with Max Delbruck on our freighter trip to the U.S.A., planned for that summer. (1969, 301)

The "selective mechanism" cited in (3) above was somewhat more elaborated by Jerne in his first publication on the theory in 1955. There he suggested that the antibody or globulin molecules that make the best fit to an antigen entering the animal "may then be engulfed by a phagocytic cell. When the globulin molecules thus brought into a cell have been dissociated from the surface of the antigen, the antigen has accomplished its role and can be eliminated." Jerne added that "the introduction of the selected molecules into a cell or the transfer of these molecules into another cell is the signal for the synthesis or reproduction of molecules identical to those introduced, i.e., of specific antibodies" (1955, 849–850).

We can reformulate Jerne's inference to (1)–(3) above in the retroductive pattern as follows:

(1) (a)The presence of a large variety of types of antibody at low levels of concentration detectable by combining with various antigens is a puzzling phenomenon. (It is puzzling in the light of the then current instructive theories of antibody formation.)
(b)The only property that all these antigens share is that they combine with antibody molecules, therefore this must be an essential property in antibody generation.

(2) But (a) and (b) in (1) above would not be surprising were a selective type of theory to obtain. Such a theory would have to have as component hypotheses: (i) "a random mechanism for ensuring the limited synthesis of antibody molecules possessing all possible combining sites, in the absence of antigen," (ii) "a purging mechanism for repressing the synthesis of such antibody molecules that happen to fit to auto-antigens," and (iii) "a selective mechanism for promoting the synthesis of those antibody molecules that make the best fit to any antigen entering the animal."

(3) Therefore there is good reason for elaborating a selective type of theory, on the basis of which 1(a) and 1(b) would be explained.

2.4   Criticism of the Retroductive Model

The above example illustrates the retroductive mode of inference, but it also raises some serious questions about its completeness and its distinction from what Hanson castigated as the H-D approach. Hanson's analysis has been criticized both directly (Achinstein 1970, 1971, 1987) and indirectly (Harman 1965, 1968). These authors make some valid points against the simple retroductive model outlined and illustrated above; I believe, however, that they do not go far enough in their criticism, and also that they are not sufficiently sensitive to an important distinction in the logic of scientific discovery between (1) a logic of *generation* and (2) a logic of *preliminary evaluation*. In the following pages I shall attempt to develop these points.

Achinstein has argued that Hanson (and Peirce) neglect the "*background* of theory which the scientist often has to begin with, and which may provide at least part of and in some cases the entire basis for an inference to a law." That this is not completely accurate is seen from the quotation given earlier (p. 13) from Hanson, specifically, his footnote cited there. It is, however, worth stressing that not only the perception of an anomaly but also the inference to a new theory may be based on a background. It must be added, though, that it is not only background *theory* but also various experimental results and (low-level) generalizations which may not yet be systematized into any theory nor be part of any *one* specific theory, that serve as parts of a premise set from which an inference to a new theory or hypothesis is made. The statement that antigens possess the property of combining with antibody is an example of such a generalization. The variety of types of antibody found in horse sera is an example of an experimental result in the premise set.

Another difficulty that is raised by the simple retroductive model is that it licenses peculiar inferences. Both Harman and Achinstein have maintained that an inference to a new theory or hypothesis is legitimate only if the new theory is a *better explanation* of the anomalous facts, p_1, p_2, p_3 . . . in Hanson's notation, than any other *competing* theory or hypothesis. (Harman terms such an explanation the "best explanation.") Otherwise *any* sort of theory could be inferred from p_1, p_2, p_3, and so on. As Harman notes:

> In general, there will be several hypotheses which might explain the evidence, so one must be able to reject all such alternative hypotheses before one is warranted in making the inference. Thus one infers from the premise that a given hypothesis would provide a "better" explanation for the evidence than would any hypothesis, to the conclusion that the given hypothesis is true. (1965, 89)

I believe that this conclusion—to the truth of the hypothesis—is too strong, and following Hanson I would want rather to argue to the plausibility or probability of the hypothesis. With that exception, however, I think Harman is making an important but incomplete point.

In my view, the notion of *inference* in *reasoning to* a hypothesis is obscure both in Hanson and in his critics. Hanson, in his far-ranging writings on retroduction, never distinguished clearly between (1) a *logic of generation*, by which a new hypothesis is first articulated, and (2) a *logic of preliminary evaluation*, in terms of which a hypothesis is assessed for its plausibility. Neither is the distinction clear in Achinstein's and Harman's accounts of retroductive logic nor in my early attempt (1974) to develop an identity thesis between the logics of discovery and of justification. In the writings of the more recent commentators on the logic of discovery, the distinction becomes clearer, though often complex. Laudan (1980) seems to wish to freight discovery methods with the probitive force assignable, in my view, to preliminary justificatory contexts. Nickles (1985) provides an overview of some of these recent analyses. The clearest distinctions tend to appear in the writings in the artificial intelligence area. Herbert Simon is one contributor to this area (as well as to the philosophy of science), and he has over the past twenty-five years developed in great detail a theory of scientific discovery that draws on his own and others' artificial intelligence research.

Simon's approach to the logic of discovery is best situated in the context of an information-processing theory of problem-solving behavior, whether this behavior be ascribed to humans or to computer programs. Simon (1977, 266) succinctly stated his central thesis concerning scientific discovery: "Scientific discovery is a form of problem solving, and . . . the processes whereby science is carried on can be explained in the terms that have been used to explain the processes of problem solving."

In his early work with Newell in 1958 (published in Newell, Shaw, and Simon 1962), Simon began from the important generation-evaluation distinction noted above. Newell and Simon (1962, 149) note that, in examining human problem solving, "one useful distinction differentiates processes for finding possible solutions (*generating* members of P [a set of elements] that may belong to S [a subset of P having specified properties]), from processes for determining whether a solution proposal is in fact a solution (verifying that an element of P that has been generated does belong to S)." This first set of processes are termed *solution-generating* processes and are distinguished from the second class of *verifying processes*. Newell and Simon go on to outline the difficulties associated with a geometrically increasing "problem maze" in which, for example, each choice point bifurcates into two (or more) possible actions on the way toward a solution point. Trial and error searches through such a maze quickly become impossibly time-consuming (and expensive). Successful problem solving accordingly requires principles, termed *heuristics* after Polya (1957), that serve as guides through such mazes. Newell, Shaw, and Simon "use the term heuristic to denote any principle or device that contributes to the reduction in the average search to solution" (1962, 152). Such heuristics permit the problem solver to explore only a very small part of the maze. One example of such a heuristic is "means end analysis," in which (a) "the present situation is compared with the desired situation (problem goal) and one or more *differences* between them noticed . . . (b) Memory is searched for an *operator* or operators associated with one of the differences that has been detected. Then (c) such an operator is used to change the present situation" (Simon 1977, 278–279). Another heuristic which Simon suggests is "factoring a problem into subproblems and tackling first the subproblems containing the smallest number of unknowns" (1977, 279–280).

To Simon, a creative scientific discoverer's work, in contrast to that scientist's contemporaries' more pedestrian efforts, can possibly be explained by varying combinations of (1) more luck, (2) harder work, and (3) more powerful selective heuristics. Simon maintains that his information-processing, problem-solving approach can account for putative "illuminationist" accounts given by scientists, about which we shall have more to say later in our discussion of a detailed example. I shall also discuss heuristics in more detail further below, however, first we need to examine more carefully the nature of a logic of generation.

2.5 The Logic of Generation

Let us understand the task of a logic of generation as the production of new hypotheses—its function is to articulate heretofore unasserted conclusions. (To be more accurate, we should say unasserted conclusions of which the investigator — or computer — is unaware or which are not in the retrievable memory.) These heretofore unasserted conclusions may range from the strikingly original through the moderately novel, as when standard ideas are put together in new ways to solve a problem, to the trivial. A logic of generation need not per se distinguish among and assess the quality of originality of its progeny.[4] Moreover, as a logic of *generation* per se, it need not assess the plausibility of its products; that is a task for a logic of preliminary evaluation. Such preliminary assessors may, however, be built into a hypothesis generator.

TABLE 2.1

Types and phases of scientific inference

	Type of Inference → / Phase of Inference ↓		Nondemonstrative Inference (induction, analogue, and retroduction)		Demonstrative Inference (essentially deductive)	
Author's proposal for the domain of scientific discovery	Generative:	Weak:	Retroduction, and/or analogical reasoning	Weak:	Mathematical heuristics	Traditional context of scientific discovery
		Strong:	Traditional naive Baconian induction and enumerative induction, "evocation" in the logic of diagnosis	Strong:	Well-established algorithms for generating solutions	
	Evaluative:	Weak:	Retroduction, logic of comparative theory evaluation, Bayesian "private" logic of nonstatistical hypothesis testing	Weak:	Proofs by approximation	
. . . and the domain of scientific justification		Strong:	Eliminative Induction, statistical hypothesis testing (Neyman-Pearson, Fisherean, and Bayesian methods), "public" statistical distributions	Strong:	Standard checking of logic/mathematical theorems. (Certain inductive logics also belong here such as Carnap's.)	Traditional context of scientific justification

These "new" hypotheses can fall either into the demonstrative area, such as a new conjecture or new theorem in mathematics, or into the nondemonstrative area, involving an empirical discovery. I take demonstrative reasoning to involve reasoning to *necessarily* true conclusions from true premises and nondemonstrative reasoning to cover all other forms of reasoning. The point about the demonstrative-nondemonstrative distinction is to stress that it is not synonymous with the generative-evaluative distinction; rather it is orthogonal to it.

The logic of evaluation (or logic of justification, to employ a phrase with roughly equivalent meaning) involves *assessing* proffered claims of support or of entailment. It can appear in weak or strong forms and can be employed in nondemonstrative and demonstrative areas. I have summarized in an incomplete way some examples of this reasoning under the different rubrics in table 2.1. The distinction between "type" and "phase" shown in the table is to assist the reader in the discussion that follows. The reader will note that I have listed retroduction both in the weak generative nondemonstrative category and in the weak evaluative nondemonstrative class. I did this because of the ambiguity I believe we find in Hanson, Achinstein, and Harman, among others, as into which class retroductive inference falls.

2.6 The Double Aspect of the Logic of Discovery

The inquiry to be pursued here is both descriptive and normative. Descriptive research from human problem solving and the results of computer-simulated problem solving in the areas of clinical diagnostics and scientific discovery will be examined. In addition, I will explore in depth an actual historical case of scientific discovery — Burnet's account of the genesis of the clonal selection theory. This information will be utilized, together with material from the philosophy of science, to formulate the outlines of a normative theory of scientific discovery. The normative aspects of science and the relation of these to the philosophy of science will not be examined in depth in these pages, but interested readers can refer to my position as developed in my 1977 and 1982 essays.

The thesis that will be urged in this chapter is that *both* aspects of discovery — generation and weak evaluation — are important parts of a logic of discovery. It is, on this view, crucial to make the generative-evaluative distinction for two reasons. The first is that a *fully* developed logic of discovery requires both a logic of generation and a logic of weak evaluation. The second reason is that, in the opinion of this author, there are significant aspects of the "discovery process," constituted by the logic of preliminary or weak evaluation, that need articulation. It is a component of the thesis to be urged here that both aspects of the discovery process are, at least partially, amenable to logical and philosophical analysis and that such analysis is needed to fully understand the complexities of scientific inquiry. In the remaining sections of this essay, I shall elaborate on both points. We begin with a discussion of some current inquiry into a logic of generation.

Contemporary investigation into a *generative* logic for hypotheses and theories is in its infancy. Much of it comes from artificial intelligence (AI) research in problem solving by computers, and references to this work will be provided below. The logic of generation is currently restricted to essentially nonnovel solutions, though as will be noted below, there are areas in which nonoriginal hypotheses, when taken in combination, are nonetheless difficult for even experienced scientists to generate.

I will comment briefly on one example of generative logic developed in the chemistry of molecular structures and more extensively on an example drawn from the logic of clinical diagnosis in internal medicine. These examples will both enable us to see the distinction between generation and weak evaluation more clearly and indicate more specifically the current limitations of a generative logic of scientific discovery.

Joshua Lederberg, a geneticist and Nobel Laureate, and Edward Feigenbaum, a computer scientist, began working in the mid-1960s at Stanford University to develop a computer program that would discover the chemical structure of molecules on the basis of the molecule's mass spectrum and, if available, the nuclear magnetic resonance spectrum. They were soon joined by Bruce Buchanan, a philosopher turned computer scientist, and by the early 1970s had developed the program known as DENDRAL (Buchanan and Shortliffe 1984, 8).[5] DENDRAL contains the following basic elements, according to its originators:

1. Conceptualizing organic chemistry in terms of topological graph theory, that is, a general theory of ways of combining atoms.

2. Embodying this approach in an exhaustive hypothesis generator. This is a program which is capable, in principle, of "imagining" every conceivable molecular structure.

3. Organizing the generator so that it avoids duplication and irrelevancy, and moves from structure to structure in an orderly and predictable way. The key concept is that induction becomes a process of efficient selection from the domain of all possible structures. Heuristic search and evaluation are used to implement this efficient selection. (Feigenbaum, Buchanan, and Lederberg 1971, 168)

Note in item (3) above that even at this early stage (of generation) some principles of preliminary evaluation are required in the logic of discovery and in point of fact are embedded in the hypothesis generator.

In this book, which focuses on biology and medicine, I will not be able to discuss the DENDRAL program in any additional detail. I have considered it in my 1980b and my 1985, and detailed treatments can be found in Lindsay et al. 1980 and in Buchanan 1985. It may be of interest to note that the program has been developed into a successor program known as Meta-DENDRAL (again see Lindsay et al. 1980 and Buchanan 1985 for detailed information), which has generated most impressive results. Concerning this discovery program, Buchanan states:

The Meta-DENDRAL program is capable of rationalizing the mass-spectral fragmentations of sets of molecules in terms of substructural features of the molecules. On known test cases, aliphatic amines and estrogenic steroids, the Meta-DENDRAL program rediscovered the well-characterized fragmentation processes reported in the literature. On the three classes of ketoandrostanes for which no general class rules have been reported, the mono-, di, and triketoandrostanes, the program found general rules describing the mass spectrometric behavior of those classes . . . . This is the first instance we know of in which general symbolic laws have been discovered by a computer program and published in a scientific journal as new results. (1985, 107)

A set of distinctions similar to the generation-weak-evaluation-strong-evaluation differences appears in AI research on the logic of clinical diagnosis. Our example here is taken from the investigations of Drs. Jack D. Myers, Harry Pople, Jr., and Randolph Miller at the University of Pittsburgh. They have programmed into a computer characteristics of about 75% of all diseases known to contemporary internal medicine. This data base is then used as background for a discovery program, originally known as DIALOG (*dia*gnostic *log*ic), later as INTERNIST-1, and now in two variants as CADUCEUS and QMR.[6] (Because the AI and diagnostic logic literature still refers to the program as INTERNIST-1, I shall also do so.) INTERNIST-1 can take "new" cases, such as of the Massachusetts General Hospital patients presented weekly in the pages of the *New England Journal of Medicine*, and provide a diagnosis of the patients' illnesses which often result from diseases joined together in unique and complicated ways.

The INTERNIST-1 program's logic is illustrative of a logic of discovery in that it incorporates a number of the distinctions made above and in addition develops the phase of preliminary evaluation by further breaking it down into several subphases. This example thus confirms the general thesis I have advanced above, that the logic of discovery has a generative aspect and also one or more important preliminary evaluative aspects. Under the generative aspect of INTERNIST-1's program, signs and symptoms of a disease *evoke* disease models. These models, which are potential explanations of the signs and symptoms, are then processed in the preliminary evaluation phase, consisting of several subphases. The first of these is a weighing subphase of preliminary evaluation, to be described in more detail below. Second is a subphase where the program then uses a heuristic that further partitions the disease models by employing a concept of dominance. The partitioning cuts the set of evoked models down to a short list of highly plausible alternative candidates, termed a "considered" list. This list may then be tested in an interrogative interaction involving several further preliminary evaluation subphases, during which the computer requests additional data in an attempt to reach a conclusive diagnosis. The program will proceed in a broad *ruleout* subphase if five or more plausible disease models are being considered, or will enter a narrower *discriminate* subphase if the "considered" list contains two to four models. In either case, questions are asked of the physician, adding more information to the computer's data, which might count heavily for one disease model and strongly against another. If there is sufficient information to warrant detailed testing of only *one* model, an activity wherein I characterize the program as performing "strong evaluation," the program enters what Myers et al. call a *pursuing* phase,[7] which may terminate in a *conclusion*—the final diagnosis. (In any of its subphases, the program may indicate which data it is temporarily *disregarding*. These are data not explained by the top-ranked model.) If the detailed testing does not yield a strongly supported conclusion that excludes significant alternative diseases, the program reverts to the discriminate (interrogative) subphase for further investigation. It would take us beyond the scope of this chapter to provide the full and complex details of the INTERNIST-1 program. (The program is constantly evolving and a growing literature on some of these developments should be consulted by the interested reader.)[8] Some additional detail and a specific example largely based on the earlier research with INTERNIST-1 will, however, be introduced to illustrate the points at which the logic of generation and the logic of preliminary evaluation function as the two main components of a logic of discovery in the biomedical sciences.

Before I commence with a specific example of INTERNIST-1, it might be useful to point out a fundamental weakness of the INTERNIST-1 program as a model of scientific discovery. The data base of INTERNIST-1 is developed by first constructing a "disease tree." This is, in the words of the authors of the program, "a classification scheme for *all possible* diagnoses." We thus see that a *new* disease, akin to a novel or original hypothesis, is not generatable by INTERNIST-1. (This limitation was also part of the DENDRAL program, since in that program a hypothesis generator had to be programmed to generate a priori "every conceivable molecular structure"; I will return to this point about novelty again in a succeeding section.) The disease tree is constructed by selecting "successive general areas of internal medicine." Subcategories based on similar pathogenetic mechanisms are then specified within each general area. Further subdivision continues, terminating at the level of individual diagnoses or diseases of which there are about 600 in the most recent versions of INTERNIST-1 and its descendants. Each disease is characterized by a disease profile, which is a list of manifestations (signs, symptoms, and laboratory abnormalities) associated with that disease. Each manifestation in a disease profile has two clinical variables associated with it: an "evoking strength" and a "frequency." The evoking strength is a rough measure, on a scale of 0 to 5, of how strongly the manifestation suggests this disease as its cause and is employed in the generative phase of clinical diagnosis (though it is also used to suggest "clincher" questions in the pursuing phase). The crudeness of the scale is demanded because of the imprecision of data in internal medicine. Table 2.2 (from Miller, Pople, and Myers 1982) presents an interpretation of these numbers.

TABLE 2.2   INTERPRETATION OF EVOKING STRENGTHS

Evoking Strength	Interpretation
0	Nonspecific—manifestation occurs too commonly to be used to construct a differential diagnosis
1	Diagnosis is a rare or unusual cause of listed manifestation
2	Diagnosis causes a substantial minority of instances of listed manifestation
3	Diagnosis is the most common but not the overwhelming cause of listed manifestation
4	Diagnosis is the overwhelming cause of listed manifestation
5	Listed manifestation is pathognomonic for the diagnosis

TABLE 2.3   INTERPRETATION OF FREQUENCY VALUES

Frequency	Interpretation
1	Listed manifestation occurs rarely in the disease
2	Listed manifestation occurs in a substantial minority of cases of the disease
3	Listed manifestation occurs in roughly half the cases
4	Listed manifestation occurs in the substantial majority of the cases
5	Listed manifestation occurs in essentially all cases—i.e., it is a prerequisite for the diagnosis

The frequency used in both the preliminary and strong evaluative phases, on the other hand, is a rough measure of how often patients with the disease have that manifestation. This is measured on a 1 through 5 scale, an interpretation of which is given in table 2.3. The medical literature is the source for frequency numbers, though again, because of the quality of the data, a judgemental element figures in as well.

TABLE 2.4   INTERPRETATION OF IMPORT VALUES

Import	Interpretation
1	Manifestation is usually unimportant, occurs commonly in normal persons, and is easily disregarded
2	Manifestation may be of importance, but can often be ignored; context is important
3	Manifestation is of medium importance, but may be an unreliable indicator of any specific disease
4	Manifestation is of high importance and can only rarely be disregarded as, for example, a false-positive result
5	Manifestation absolutely must be explained by one of the final diagnoses

Source of Tables 2.2 − 2.4: Adapted from information appearing in *The New England Journal of Medicine*, 307: 468-476. Miller, R. A., Pople, H. E., Jr., and Myers, J. D. (1982) "INTERNIST-1: An ExperimentalComputer-Based Diagnostic Consultant for General Internal Medicine."

In addition to these two numbers, each manifestation is assigned an "import" on a scale of 1 through 5, as displayed in table 2.4. The import is a disease-independent measure of the global importance of explaining that manifestation. In addition to the disease profiles with their manifestations, INTERNIST-1 also contains "links" between diseases, which are meant to capture the degree to which one disease may cause or predispose to another. There are also relations among manifestations; for example, "sex: female" is a precondition of "oligomenorrhea." Finally, INTERNIST-1 contains a number of problem-solving algorithms that operate on the individual patient data entered, using the information contained in the data base.

As a specific case with the patient's manifestations is entered into the computer, the INTERNIST-1 program generates disease hypotheses that may account for each manifestation. As an example representing an actual clinical case, we can consider the following data entry.[9] Under *symptoms*, items of history (including age, sex, and so on), symptoms, signs, and laboratory tests are entered, with the computer requesting additional data through its "please continue" phrase until the doctor indicates by a "no" that the preliminary data is complete (items prefixed by a * are entered by the doctor presenting the case to INTERNIST-1; all other text is generated by INTERNIST-1).

Symptoms [recall these include "history" items (age, etc.) and laboratory results]:

```
*(DOCTOR)-SYMPTOMS?
*AGE-25-TO-50
*SEX-FEMALE
*FEVER
*JAUNDICE
*NAUSEA-VOMITING
*ANOREXIA
*URINE-DARK-HX
*LIVER-ENLARGED
*EOSINOPHILIA
*BILIRUBIN-CONJUGATED-BLOOD-INCREASED
*SGOT-GTR-THAN-400-UNITS
*SGPT-GTR-THAN-600-UNITS
*PROTHROMBIN-TIME-INCREASED
*SKIN-RASH-MACULOPAPULAR-ALLERGY-HX
*NO [ADDITIONAL ENTRY AT THIS TIME]
```

(The meaning of some of these manifestations will be obvious to any reader, but some are technical medical terms. I present this case as is without any attempt to define the medical terminology since I believe that the *logic* of the process is generally evident even without special medical knowledge. The terms employed are standard ones, however, and the interested reader can consult any standard medical dictionary for definitions.)

The generation or "evoking" of specific disease hypotheses by these "symptoms" is a simple and direct triggering process that employs the evoking strengths of the lists contained in the data base linking manifestations to diseases. This set of disease hypotheses, which is usually huge, is termed the master list. In addition, for each disease hypothesis four associated lists are maintained that represent the match and lack of match between the specific patient under consideration and the disease profile. Each disease hypothesis on the master list is assigned a score on the basis of the match between the patient's set of manifestations and the data base disease profiles. Counting *in favor* of a specific disease hypothesis are the manifestations explained by that hypothesis; credit is awarded based on the manifestations' evoking strengths. Counting *against* a specific disease are (1) manifestations expected but found absent in the specific patient, which are debited in terms of the frequency values, and (2) manifestations not accounted for by the disease hypothesis, which are debited in accord with the import of each manifestation. In addition, a bonus is awarded to any disease that is related to a previously diagnosed disease via the links mentioned above. This bonus is equal to 20 times the frequency number associated with the disease in the diagnosed disease's profile.

A disease's total score is based on a nonlinear weighting scheme that takes into account scores based on evoking strengths, frequencies, and imports. Such nonlinearity has often been found in descriptive studies of human judgment in a variety of disciplines, and thus it should not be a surprising feature of INTERNIST-1. The weighting scheme assigns "points" in the following fashion:

(i) for evoking strengths: $0 = 1, 1 = 4, 2 = 10, 3 = 20, 4 = 40, 5 = 80$

(ii) for frequencies: $1 = -1, 2 = -4, 3 = -7, 4 = -15, 5 = -30$

(iii) for imports: $1 = -2, 2 = -6, 3 = -10, 4 = -20, 5 = -40$

in accord with the crediting-debiting procedure mentioned in the previous paragraph. These nonlinear point assignments represent Myers's clinical judgement as honed by continuing experience with the INTERNIST-1 program applied to patient cases.

All the disease hypotheses on the master list are scored in accordance with the procedure outlined in the two previous paragraphs. Then the topmost set of hypotheses above a threshold is further processed by a simple but powerful sorting heuristic that partitions these hypotheses into several naturally competing subsets of disease hypotheses. This allows INTERNIST-1, as Myers has noted, to compare "apples with apples and oranges with oranges." The sorting heuristic can be stated in various ways. One recent formulation is: "Two diseases are competitors if the items not explained by one disease are a subset of the items not explained by the other, otherwise they are alternatives (and may possibly coexist in the patient)" (Miller, Pople, and Myers 1982, 471). This idea can be put another way by realizing that two different diseases, A and B, which meet this criterion, will not explain any more of the manifestations if taken together than either one does taken alone. This sorting heuristic thus creates a "current problem area" consisting of the highest-ranked disease hypothesis and its competitors. Miller, Pople, and Myers (1982) refer to this procedure for defining a problem area as "ad hoc" and note that, because of the procedure, INTERNIST-1's "differential diagnoses will not always resemble those constructed by clinicians" (1982, 471).

At this point INTERNIST-1 will either conclude with a diagnosis or will commence with one of its interactive searching subphases, such as *ruleout*, as described earlier. A diagnosis is concluded if the leading disease hypothesis is 90 points higher than its nearest competitor. This value was selected because it is just a bit more than the "absolute" weight assigned to a pathognomonic manifestation, that is, $5 = 80$, as presented on page 29. (It should perhaps be added here as an aside that pathognomonic manifestations which are only found in *one* disease are extremely rare in medicine.) It should be stressed here that this method of concluding a diagnosis is comparative with respect to its competitors, as defined by the sorting heuristic, and is not based on any absolute probabilistic threshold, such as 0.9.

If a diagnosis is not attainable, INTERNIST-1 enters one of its searching subphases. In the searching subphase additional information is requested from the user. The specific subphase that is entered, and thus the type of question posed, is determined by the number of competitors within 45 points of the leading diagnosis. If there is none, attention is focused on one strong contender and INTERNIST-1 enters the pursuing phase, posing specific questions to the user that have a high evoking strength for the topmost hypothesis. If the answer to these questions is "yes," the program will rapidly reach a conclusion. If, however, there are a number of competing hypotheses running neck-in-neck, specifically 5 or more within 45 points of the leading diagnosis, the program enters its ruleout subphase. Here, questions that have high frequency values for the competitors are asked of the user, the rationale being that negative answers will result in the rapid elimination of some of the contending hypotheses. Finally, if 2 to 4 hypotheses cluster within 45 points of the leading diagnosis, the program enters its discriminating subphase. Here, questions are posed to the user which are likely to yield answers which would increase the separation in scores between or among the competing hypotheses.

2.7 An Example of the Logics of Generation and Evaluation in Clinical Diagnosis

Let us continue with the example that had its "symptoms" entered in the previous section. In the example we are considering, it is the ruleout subphase that is entered in the first series of moves after the initial data entry (history, signs, symptoms and laboratory results) described above on page 28. Specifically, those moves are represented in our example by the following sequence of questions and answers (as before, items prefixed by * are entered by the doctor presenting the case to INTERNIST-1; all other text is generated by INTERNIST-1):

(RULEOUT: DRUG-HYPERSENSITIVITY-HEPATOCELLULAR-REACTION
HEPATITIS-B HEPATITIS-A INFECTIOUS-MONONUCLEOSIS CHRONIC-AC-
TIVE-HEPATITIS LEPTOSPIROSIS)
WEIGHT-LOSS-GTR-THAN-TEN-PERCENT ?
*NO
RIGOR ?
*NO
(RULEOUT: DRUG-HYPERSENSITIVITY-HEPATOCELLULAR-REACTION
HEPATITIS-B HEPATITIS-A TOXIC-HEPATOCELLULAR-DISEASEINFEC-
TIOUS-MONONUCLEOSIS DRUG-HYPERSENSITIVITY-CHOLESTATIC-RE-
ACTION)
PLEASE ENTER FINDINGS OF PAIN-ABDOMINAL
*NO
ABDOMEN-PAIN-GENERALIZED ?
*NO
ABDOMEN-PAIN-RIGHT-UPPER-QUADRANT ?
*NO
(RULEOUT: DRUG-HYPERSENSITIVITY-HEPATOCELLULAR-REACTION
HEPATITIS-B HEPATITIS-A INFECTIOUS-MONONUCLEOSIS DRUG-HY-
PERSENSITIVITY-CHOLESTATIC REACTION TOXIC-HEPATOCELLULAR-
DISEASE)
ARTHRITIS ?
*NO
SKIN-URTICARIA ?

*NO

PLEASE ENTER FINDINGS OF ABDOMEN-PALPATION

*NO

ABDOMEN-TENDERNESS-GENERALIZED ?

*NO

ABDOMEN-TENDERNESS-RIGHT-UPPER-QUADRANT ?

*YES

LYMPHADENOPATHY ?

*NO

(RULEOUT: DRUG-HYPERSENSITIVITY-HEPATOCELLULAR-REACTION
HEPATITIS-A TOXIC-HEPATOCELLULAR-DISEASE HEPATITIS-B-DRUG-
HYPERSENSITIVITY-CHOLESTATIC- REACTION)

EXPANDING

SKIN-SPIDER-ANGIOMATA ?

*NO

(RULEOUT: DRUG-HYPERSENSITIVITY-HEPATOCELLULAR-REACTION
ACUTE-TOXIC-HEPATOCELLULAR-INJURY HEPATITIS-A HEPATITIS-B
DRUG-HYPERSENSITIVITY-CHOLESTATIC-REACTION ACUTE-ALCO-
HOLIC-HEPATITIS)

PLEASE ENTER FINDINGS OF URINALYSIS-ROUTINE

*BILIRUBIN-URINE-INCREASED

*NO

UROBILINOGEN-URINE-INCREASED ?

*NO

PROTEINURIA ?

*NO

PLEASE ENTER FINDINGS OF LIVER-FUNCTION-TESTS

*NO

ALKALINE-PHOSPHATASE-80-TO-160-IU ?

*NO

ALKALINE-PHOSPHATASE-GTR-THAN-160-IU ?

*NO

PLEASE ENTER FINDINGS OF WBC-AND-DIFFERENTIAL

*NO

WBC-LESS-THAN-4000 ?

*NO

WBC-14000-TO-30000 ?

*NO[10]

The program continues in the ruleout subphase until either
the discriminate subphase is entered or the type of data requested has reached the level of laboratory specificity (the *type*

order is history, symptoms, signs, laboratory data). At this point, because of the cost or danger of obtaining new laboratory data, the program artificially shifts to the discriminate subphase, which usually is used only when the considered list is reduced to two to four disease models. In the discriminate subphase, evaluation is comparative between the two top models, with questions asked that are very likely to count heavily for one model while counting heavily against the other. In our example, the printout of the program for the discriminate subphase reads as follows:

```
(DISREGARDING: EOSINOPHILIA)
(NARROW: TOXIC-HEPATOCELLULAR-DISEASE DRUG-HYPERSENSITIV-
ITY-HEPATOCELLULAR-REACTION)
ANEMIA-HEMOLYTIC ?
*YES
PLEASE ENTER FINDINGS OF DRUG-ADMINISTRATION-HX
*HALOTHANE-ADMINISTRATION-HX
PLEASE CONTINUE
*NO
DRUG-ADMINISTRATION-RECENT-HX ?
*YES
PLEASE ENTER FINDINGS OF LIPIDS-BLOOD
*NO
CHOLESTEROL-BLOOD-DECREASED ?
*YES
(DISCRIMINATE: DRUG-HYPERSENSITIVITY-HEPATOCELLULAR-REAC-
TION HEPATITIS-B)
DRUG-ADDICTION-HX ?
*NO
LDH-BLOOD-INCREASED ?
*YES
PLEASE ENTER FINDINGS OF HEPATITIS-CONTACT-HX
*NO
HEPATITIS-CONTACT-ABOUT-180-DAYS-BEFORE-ILLNESS ?
*NO
```

When the considered list is reduced to only one highly plausible disease model, the program enters what I would term its strongest evaluative phase, termed "confirm," or *pursuing* by Pople, Myers, and Miller. The program asks additional questions that are "clinchers" — questions about manifestations which have a strong evoking strength for the specific model under consideration. The program continues in the pursuing phase until (1) either the spread between the two top models is sufficiently *increased* that it meets a specified *criterion*,[11] at which point the program *concludes*, or (2) until the spread is *reduced* sufficiently so that the program reenters the discriminate subphase. In our example, the pursuing phase is very rapid, one step:

(PURSUING: DRUG-HYPERSENSITIVITY-HEPATOCELLULAR-REACTION)
(CONCLUDE: DRUG-HYPERSENSITIVITY-HEPATOCELLULAR-REACTION)
(DIAGNOSIS: DRUG-HYPERSENSITIVITY-HEPATOCELLULAR-REACTION)
(CPU TIME UTILIZED: 61.569000 SECONDS)

In more complex examples, the pursuing phase is quite long.

An examination of this case, or any of the other patient cases in the literature (see for example either Miller, Pople, and Myers 1982 or Schaffner 1981), will disclose that several questions are asked at a time, that the program then recalculates its scores, and that it may well also repartition its diagnostic hypotheses. Questioning proceeds from the more easily obtained data to the more expensive and invasive information. Once a diagnosis is concluded, the manifestations that are accounted for by that diagnosis are removed from further consideration. This is an important point that should be noted, and I will comment on it again in connection with some of its deleterious consequences. If there are manifestations that are not accounted for, the program recycles and by this process can diagnose multiple coexisting diseases. There are two circumstances in which INTERNIST-1 will terminate without reaching a diagnosis. First, if all questions have been exhausted and a conclusion has not been reached, the program will "defer" and terminate with a differential diagnosis in which the competitors are displayed and ranked in descending order. Second, if all the unexplained manifestations have an import of 2 or less, the program stops.

INTERNIST-1 is a powerful program, surprisingly so in the light of its prima facie "brute force" methods of analyzing clinical data. A formal evaluation of its diagnostic prowess by Miller, Pople, and Myers (1982) indicates that its performance is "qualitatively similar to that of the hospital clinicians but inferior to that of the [expert] case discussants." The program does, however, possess a number of problems, on which work continues; these problems are pointed out in Miller, Pople, and Myers 1982, as well as in Pople 1982 and 1984.

The point of this rather detailed example from the logic of diagnosis was to underscore the difference between the logic of generation and the logic of preliminary evaluation, as well as to indicate that the latter phase may have considerable additional fine structure. Another feature of the example is that it indicates the necessity, in a fully developed logic of discovery, for a set of generators that will articulate the hypothesis that is to explain the data such that it can be evaluated in a preliminary way as part of the discovery process and in a stronger way as part of the logic of conclusive evaluation.

I argued above that Hanson, in his extensive writings, never made these distinctions clear. He also never provided "a way up," to use his terminology, a means of generating a hypothesis in the first place. As such, without a logic of generation, *the retroductive mode of inference is little more than the H-D model itself.*

What little more it is seems to lie in Hanson's and others conceptualization of a distinction akin to the distinction urged here between preliminary evaluation and fully developed justification. Hanson did press for a distinction between "(1) reasons for accepting a hypothesis H" and "(2) reasons for suggesting H in the first place" (1961, 22). In my view, however, Hanson equivocated on the word "suggesting," sometimes using it in the *generative* sense and sometimes in the preliminary *evaluative* sense. Hanson also wished to make a sharp distinction between reasons for (1), which he identified with reasons we might have for thinking H *true*, and reasons for (2), which he identified with those reasons which would make H *plausible*. Hanson distinguished his position from one he attributed to Herbert Feigl as follows:

> One might urge, as does Professor Feigl, that the difference [between (1) and (2)] is just one of refinement, degree, and intensity. Feigl argues that considerations which settle whether H constitutes a plausible conjecture are of the *same type* as those which settle whether H is true. But since the initial proposal of a hypothesis is a groping affair, involving guesswork amongst sparse data, there is a distinction to be drawn; but his, Feigl urges, concerns two ends of a spectrum ranging all the way from inadequate and badly selected data to that which is abundant, well diversified, and buttressed by a battery of established theories. (1961, 22)

On this issue I tend to agree with Feigl against Hanson. The *criteria* of acceptance which are the backdrop in the generative phase and which function weakly in the preliminary evaluation phase of the preliminary act of discovery stage are identical with those that will be proffered in the polished published research article — the context of justification. (See my 1974a for an example involving the discovery of the operon theory.) In the context of justification, however, the substantive evidence will be systematically organized, often further developed, and in general much more powerful. Let me hasten to add here that though in this chapter I have disagreed with the way the classical distinction between the context of discovery and the context of justification is drawn, I do not intend to label the difference between contexts as meaningless or completely mistaken. The difference in presentation that I believe we encounter between these contexts is frequently pragmatic and strategic. Scientists can, in the published paper announcing their discovery narrow down their reasoning to only several competing models and marshal arguments that discriminate the strengths of the new, favored hypothesis against alternatives. The criteria, it should be noted, do not differ, but now the scientist has caught her hypothesis and from that vantage point she is offering some still weak evaluational criteria in its support. Strong evaluational criteria may not be available for some time after a hypothesis is initially proposed.

These criteria of evaluation are familiar ones: empirical adequacy, coherence, and the like. Hanson argued that simplicity considerations were involved in the logic of discovery, but in my view he did not go far enough. Harman also has proposed similar criteria, as where he noted in his discussion of inference to the best explanation:

> There is, of course, a problem about how one is to judge that one hypothesis is sufficiently better than another hypothesis. Presumably such a judgment will be based on considerations such as which hypothesis is simpler, which is more plausible, which explains more, which is less *ad hoc*, and so forth. (1965, 89)

Harman, however, did not elaborate on these criteria.

The logic of discovery, then, comprises two phases: a logic of generation and a logic of preliminary evaluation. Actual discoveries in the biomedical sciences involve both these phases. Unfortunately, recollections of the generative phase are often couched in "illuminationist" terminology, in which irrational aspects are heavily stressed. These give support to Popper's and others' theses of the illogicality of discovery — a support that is likely unwarranted for reasons to be discussed in section 2.9. Application of the account of a logic of discovery sketched above can, I believe, accommodate *some* "intuitive" or irrational elements for two reasons. First, it is not essential for the thesis sketched above that *all* aspects of the generative phase of the discovery process be fully articulated; I believe we can make some progress in understanding the discovery process even if parts of the scenario are murky and contain gaps. Second, even in those cases in which a solution comes in a "eureka" experience without—it is often contended—conscious preparation, there is still the preliminary evaluative phase of a logic of discovery into which we should inquire.

It may be useful at this point to examine a specific case in which an irrational "eureka" element is contained and also in which a truly novel hypothesis was advanced. The case study is Burnet's discovery of the clonal selection theory of acquired immunity; it is a natural development from our earlier example of Jerne's natural selection theory of antibody formation. This case will then be analyzed with the assistance of Simon's "blackboard" theory of "selective forgetting" to provide a general interpretation within a logic of scientific discovery.

2.8 The Clonal Selection Theory

Burnet's theory was initially proposed in his 1957b and further elaborated at Vanderbilt in 1958 in the Abraham Flexner lectures on "Clonal Selection as Exemplified in Some Medically Significant Topics," published as *The Clonal Selection Theory of Acquired Immunity* (Burnet 1959). The theory initially encountered resistance and was even "falsified" several times in its early life, as I shall recount in detail in chapter 5. Such falsifications subsequently turned out to be experimental artifacts, and the power of the theory was gradually appreciated, with the theory becoming generally accepted by 1967.[12] Currently, the clonal selection theory serves as *the general theory* of the immune response, and all finer-structured theories involving detailed cellular and molecular components are required to be consistent with it.[13] We will examine some of the complexities of the logic of justification and the processes of acceptance with respect to this theory in chapters 3, 4, and 5, but here the logic of its discovery will be our focus.

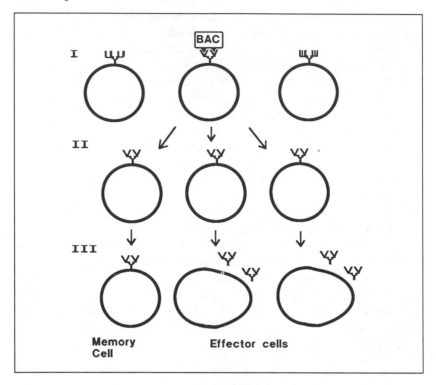

Figure 2.1   Diagram of a contemporary version of the clonal selection theory. Stage I shows representatives of three resting lymphocytes bearing receptors for antigens complementary to antibodies with U, V, and W types of specificity. A bacterium (BAC) with antigenic determinants which bind with V specific antibody activates the middle lymphocyte. In Stage II, the activated lymphocyte proliferates to form an expanded cloned population. In Stage III, some of these cells become long-term memory cells, but most differentiate into effector cells and release soluble antibody of the V type. (Also see figure 3.3, page 86.)

The discovery of the clonal selection theory was a major breakthrough in immunology and illustrates some important logical and epistemic features of scientific discovery in general.[14] In this immunological theory, Burnet proposed the existence of a set of cellular entities (lymphocytes) that bore specific receptors on their surfaces. These receptors or "reactive sites" were specific for particular antigens as a lock is specific for a particular key, and the cells were triggered (or "unlocked") only by very specific antigens (keys). A cell so triggered was genetically programmed to produce only that specific antibody which it bore as a receptor.

Binding of the antigen to the receptor thus stimulated the cell to reproduce its kind in a large clone of identical cells, which would then differentiate into plasma cells releasing soluble antibody (though a small subpopulation of triggered cells might remain undifferentiated, serving as "memory cells" should the stimulating antigen be reencountered at a later time). (For readers unfamiliar with immunology, a diagram indicating, in a simplified manner, how clonal selection works may well clarify these essential assumptions of the theory; see figure 2.1.)

First let me present Burnet's own account of the discovery;[15] I shall then comment on the philosophically interesting aspects of the example. Burnet recalls the episode in the following terms:

> In 1957, I had been deeply interested in immunity for many years and had published a good deal about the possible interpretations of antibody. They had necessarily been in terms of the concepts that had been current at the time in biochemistry and general biology. The development, first of ideas, and then of an experimental approach in the field of immunological tolerance, had already impressed me with the crucial nature of those phenomena for immunological theory.
>
> Then, in 1955, I had seen Niels Jerne's paper on a natural selection theory of antibody production.
>
> Niels Jerne is a Dane, a few years younger than I am, whom I met for the first time at Geneva in 1956. Since then I have come to know him well and I am sure that he is the most intelligent immunologist alive. I did not always think so because, in 1954 [actually in 1956], I had published what I now know was a rather bad, over-ambitious book with an interpretation of antibody production which was already beginning to look unconvincing by the time I finalized the proofs. Jerne did not like the interpretation and told me that I was merely creating metaphysical entities which explained nothing. This, of course, did not predispose me to adopt his quite different theory. (1968, 203–204)

At this point Burnet describes Jerne's natural selection theory, which I have presented above. Burnet critically focused on the uptake mechanism introducing the antigen—natural antibody complex into the macrophage, which would then process the antibody and initiate massive production of identical antibodies:

> The crux of the theory was that this complex of antigen and natural antibody was taken up by a phagocytic cell, inside which the antigen was destroyed and the natural antibody used as a pattern to make more antibody of the same type. This had many virtues in explaining tolerance and some other phenomena, but even in 1955 it did not fit at all with the way proteins were known to be synthesized, and there was still the awkward failure to account in any satisfactory fashion for the diversity of natural antibodies. So we were mutually unimpressed by the other's ideas.
>
> I came back to Australia pondering heavily on why Jerne's theory was so attractive, though obviously wrong. I said earlier that at that time I was then working with two phenomena which suggested (a) that auto-antibodies might be produced by *proliferating* semi-malignant cells, and (b) that the Simonsen spots on the membrane CAM of the chick embryo[16] resulted in part from the *proliferation* of lymphocytes reacting immunologically. Rather suddenly "the penny dropped." If one replaced Jerne's natural antibodies by the cells which produced them and applied a selective process in a Darwinian sense to the antibody-producing cells, the whole picture fell into shape. I wrote it out in a short paper of two pages which I published in *The Australian Journal of Science*. It still, I believe, gives a brief and clear account of the clonal selection theory basically acceptable in 1967. (1968, 204–205)

I shall return to Burnet's comments concerning his intercurrent work on autoantibodies and the Simonsen spots to provide some additional background. Let me, however, first quote Burnet's concise formulation of the basic postulates of his clonal selection theory. This formulation represents to Burnet the "*essence*" of his theory. It articulates in a somewhat more explicit, modern, and concise manner what was asserted in 1957.[17]

(1) Antibody is produced by cells, to a pattern which is laid down by the genetic mechanism in the nucleus of the cell.

(2) Antigen has only one function, to stimulate cells capable of producing the kind of antibody which will react

with it, to proliferate and liberate their characteristic antibody.

(3) Except under quite abnormal conditions one cell produces only one type of antibody.

(4) All descendants of an antibody-producing cell produce the same type of antibody.

(5) There is a genetic mechanism [Burnet preferred somatic mutation] capable of generating in random fashion a wide but not infinite range of patterns, so that there will be at least some cells that can react with any foreign material which enters the body. (1968, 213)

It will be useful to dwell for a moment on the background theories, generalizations, and experiments that were involved in the generation and preliminary evaluations of the clonal selection theory.

Note that Burnet identifies as relevant background his own earlier 1954 (or 1956) *theory*, Jerne's *theory*, and Jerne's *methodological* criticism imputing "metaphysical entities which explained nothing" to his earlier theory (this is probably the Burnet [and Fenner] "self-marker hypothesis"),[18] as well as his criticism of Jerne's theory that "even in 1955 it [Jerne's theory] did not fit at all with the way proteins were known to be synthesized." Apparently Burnet is referring here to what he noted in his 1957b essay announcing the clonal selection theory, namely, that "its major objection is the absence of any precedent for, and the intrinsic unlikelihood of the suggestion, that a molecule of partially denatured antibody could stimulate a cell, into which it had been taken, to produce a series of replicas of the [undenatured] molecule" (Burnet 1957b, 67). These considerations serve to provide the puzzles or problems with which inquiry leading to a new hypothesis or theory begins. However, it must be noted that in this case several key elements came from outside the specific area of focus—namely from the work with the Simonsen spots on the CAM, and from Burnet's speculations concerning cancer and autoantibodies.

"CAM" is an abbreviation for chorioallantoic membrane— that delicate sheath which surrounds the developing embryos of birds and which normally lies against the inside of the protective eggshell. Early in his career—in the early 1930s—Burnet had developed a means of exposing the CAM without destroying it, and he was able to use it as a fertile medium upon which to grow disease viruses. This was in itself an important contribution to research on the causes and cures of viral diseases.[19] Over twenty years later — in early 1957 — M. Simonsen discovered the graft-versus-host (GVH) reaction, in which transplanted cells immunologically attack the host into which they have been transferred.[20] The GVH reaction, often termed the Simonsen phenomenon, was investigated by Burnet through smearing blood cells from adult fowls on the CAM of chick eggs. Burnet found that *single* white blood cells were stimulated to divide and attack the host CAM, producing white spots on the membrane. The "recognition that single cells could produce immune responses on the CAM" was for Burnet an extremely important experimental background discovery leading to the clonal selection theory (Burnet 1968, 199), as we shall see in a moment.

Burnet also noted that he had considered that "auto-antibodies might be produced by *proliferating* semi-malignant cells" (1968, 204), and that this speculation had also played an important role in the discovery of the clonal selection theory. This may well be the case, though his articles on cancer, which were completed in 1956 and published in April 1957 in the *British Medical Journal*, do not explicitly discuss autoantibodies.[21] What we *do* find in Burnet's speculations on cancer, however, is the thesis that cancer is probably a consequence of a *series* of somatic mutations in cells, mutations which successively free the altered cells from those levels of biological controls — Burnet speculated these were about six in number — which maintain the cells in their appropriate locus and form and reproducing at their usual rate of replication. Burnet explicitly noted that "there is every reason to believe that mutation is at least as frequent in somatic cells as in the germ cells. The essential difference between a mutation occurring in a germ cell and . . . a somatic cell depends simply on . . . the cell's descendents. . . . A somatic mutation can influence only those body cells which directly descend from the mutant cell" (1957a, 843). We see here the essence of clonal branching (see figure 2.1) based on random somatic mutation, which later that year was incorporated into the clonal selection theory of acquired immunity. Clonal branching — that a somatic mutation in one cell will be replicated in all of that cell's descendants — and the Simonsen phenomenon — the ability of one white blood cell to be stimulated to replicate and mount an immune response — thus appear to have functioned as relevant analogies in the generation of the clonal selection theory.

Burnet's clonal selection theory serves as an illustration of the manner in which earlier and contemporaneous research markedly affects scientific discovery. It demonstrates the role of earlier theories and the function of criticism of those theories. Criticism on various levels, ranging from the experimental through the theoretical to the methodological, provides puzzles or problems that initiate the discovery process. We also appreciate, perhaps, with this background, what occurred in that creative moment described by Burnet when he noted that "Rather suddenly 'the penny dropped.'"

It would clearly be utopian to expect, at this point in the development of a logic of generation, that Burnet's discovery of the clonal selection theory could be fully rationally reconstructed, and its anticipation by such an applied logic would have been even less likely. (I would not rule out, however, that similar but future novel discoveries might be so reconstructible if the right data are gathered.) It may be useful, nonetheless, to speculate on the manner in which such a rational reconstruction, using the terminology developed thus far in this essay, might be employed to understand what was involved in the discovery of this theory.

The analogies of the Simonsen phenomenon and the clonal branching aspect of cells rendered malignant by somatic mutations were mechanisms in Burnet's repertoire of possible models.[22] They constitute what Simon might term "subsolutions to analogous problems" in neighboring fields in the biological domain. These are conjecturally evoked by the puzzles of natural antibodies and of self-tolerance that were highlighted by Jerne's theory. The linkages between the puzzles, p_1, p_2, p_3 — accepted facts or generalizations which are not adequately accounted for by extant hypotheses — and new hypotheses evoked to account for them are, however, extremely weak. If we were to attempt speculatively to develop this approach further, we might imagine a computer programmed with all known basic biochemical and genetic mechanisms and a combining operator that would associate combinations of these mechanisms to constitute "new" models. We might also envisage a subprogram that could operate on known mechanisms and construct analogical forms of them. The actual process of the combination or analogizing that occurred in Burnet's mind is not available for inspection and reconstructive imitation, though he may have given future investigations enough clues to at least partially mimic the private generative process involved in this case.

2.9 Simon's Theory of Selective Forgetting in Discovery

Herbert Simon has outlined a procedure for explicating an illu-
minationistic moment, such as Burnet refers to when he states
"the penny dropped." Simon's account is both consistent with
what we know of Burnet's research program and with the position I am developing in this chapter. According to Simon, an explanation of a scientist's illumination following on an often
prolonged period of incubation is provided by the process of "selective forgetting." This process is somewhat complex but is important, and I will develop it in some detail. Simon notes that:

> In the typical organization of a problem-solving program,
> the solution efforts are guided and controlled by a hierar-
> chy or "tree" of goals and subgoals. Thus, the subject starts
> out with the goal of solving the original problem. In trying
> to reach this goal, he generates a subgoal that will take him
> part of the way (if it is achieved) and addresses himself to
> that subgoal. If the subgoal is achieved, he may then return
> to the now-modified original goal. If difficulties arise in
> achieving the subgoal, sub-subgoals may be erected to deal
> with them. (1977, 296)

This goal hierarchy can be held in short-term memory and set
aside after a subgoal is achieved. It is a conceptual device, a tool,
designed to facilitate problem solution. The tree of *unattained*
goals, however, must be retained, though its precise structure
may be imperfectly recalled.

Simon adds that "during the course of problem solving, a
second memory structure is being built up" (my emphasis). This
second memory structure involves permanent or relatively long-
term memory and is termed by Simon *"the blackboard."*[23] The
blackboard contains new complexes that the problem-solver is
learning to handle as *units*. The blackboard also contains *newly
noticed* information that is accumulated while the problem-solver
is engaged in particular subgoal solutions. This newly noticed
information may be used at that point in the subgoal task and
may perhaps also influence new subgoal formulation, but the
new information may also be placed more permanently on the
blackboard. Simon summarizes this interaction between short
term (goal tree) and long-term (blackboard) memory as follows:

> The course of problem solving, then, involves continuous
> interaction between goal tree and blackboard. In the course

of pursuing goals, information is added to the blackboard. This information, in turn, helps to determine what new goals and subgoals will be set up. During periods of persistent activity, the problem solver will always be working in local goal contexts, and information added to the blackboard will be used, in the short run, only if it is relevant in those contexts. (1977, 297)

"Selective forgetting" enters when the problem-solver sets aside his or her problem. The information in short-term memory will fade more rapidly than the information on the blackboard, thus the finer structures of his goal tree will have disappeared. Returning to the problem will, on this account, necessitate a *reconstruction* of the goal tree beginning with one of the higher level goals, but *now* with the aid of new information available from the blackboard. Simon argues:

In general, we would expect the problem solver, in his renewed examination of the problem, to follow a quite different path than he did originally. Since his blackboard now has better information about the problem environment than it did the first time, he has better cues to find the correct path. Under these circumstances (and remembering the tremendous differences a few hints can produce in problem solution), solutions may appear quickly that had previously eluded him in protracted search. (1977, 297)

Though not a complete explanation of the incubation and illumination phenomenon, Simon believes that his "goal tree blackboard" paradigm does

account for the suddenness of solution without calling on the subconscious to perform elaborate processes, or processes different from those it and the conscious perform in the normal course of problem-solving activity. Nor does it postulate that the unconscious is capable of random searches through immense problem spaces for the solution. (1977, 298)

In connection with Burnet's account of the discovery of the clonal selection hypothesis, we can envisage the clonal branching mechanism for cell amplification being placed on his "blackboard" along with the Simonsen one-cell GVH immune response. The goal tree is complex but begins from the problems of antibody production by antigen and of self-tolerance and seems to have as a search strategy formulation of a Jerne-like theory — some type of a (Darwinian) selective theory, but one that does not employ unprecedented mechanisms of protein synthesis.[24] It would be rather speculative to pursue a tree-blackboard reconstruction of Burnet's discovery, but it should be reiterated that Simon's schema does appear to offer a naturalistic and plausible account of the outlines of the origin of the clonal selection theory.

I can now illustrate in the context of this example the possibly more public process of *preliminary evaluation*. Part of this involves speculation as to what occurred for Burnet immediately after "the penny dropped," namely a review of the problems with Jerne's and his own earlier theory in mind. Burnet has noted that he "wrote [the theory] out in a short paper."[25] It is *likely* that that paper closely reflects the state of mind of Burnet in the early stages of evaluation of the clonal selection theory. Inspection of the paper, which appeared in the 27 October 1957 issue of *The Australian Journal of Science*, shows striking parallels with Burnet's consideration of the relevant factors preceding and concomitant with the generation of the hypothesis, with the crucially important exception that in the paper *the hypothesis is now present* to give a focus to the related constraints and to solve in a preliminary and tentative way the problems that initiated the inquiry. Let us now examine that paper.

In the 1957 paper Burnet begins with a brief review of the extant theories of antibody production — the direct template theory, his and Fenner's own indirect template theory with self-markers, and Jerne's 1955 theory. He points out early in the paper that Jerne's theory offers a better explanation of self-tolerance than the self-marker theory, but that one of its basic flaws is that there is no "precedent for . . . a molecule of partially denatured antibody stimulat[ing] a cell, into which it had been taken, to produce a series of replicas of the molecule" (1957b, 67). Burnet then adds that he believes the "advantages of Jerne's theory can be retained and its difficulties overcome if the recognition of the foreign pattern is ascribed to clones of lymphocytic cells and not to circulating natural antibodies." A statement of the clonal selection theory follows (see note 17). Burnet closes his paper by repeating the advantages the clonal selection theory has (1) over his own earlier theory — namely its explanation of existing natural antibodies [recall this was the major empirical finding impelling Jerne to his theory] and a simpler interpretation of self-tolerance—and (2) over Jerne's theory, namely the unlikelihood of the partially denatured antibody stimulating replicas of itself (see p. 41). At this point Burnet also added a *new* advantage of the clonal selection theory over Jerne's theory: the clonal selection theory could account for the fact that some aspects of the immune response—namely certain types of sensitization and homograft immunity—seem to be mediated directly by cells, and do not involve liberation of classic antibody. The clonal selection theory could permit cells to be sensitized directly, whereas Jerne's theory seemed to demand the production of antibody for such a process.

Burnet's paper is very much a preliminary communication. Detailed deduction of consequences from the elaborated theory did not occur until later, though even in the preliminary communication we see the marshalling of *additional* evidence beyond what was used in the very early stages of hypothesis evaluation. The theory was not fully developed until the following year when Burnet gave the Flexner lectures, and was not extensively tested and criticized until several years later. As already mentioned, it was not generally accepted until about 1967.

It seems to me that Burnet's thinking in his original paper, when analyzed in the light of his autobiographical remarks quoted earlier (p. 40), constitutes an exercise in the logic of preliminary evaluation with respect to the clonal selection theory. His approach, however, seems to be more akin to the "discriminate" subphase of hypothesis evaluation discussed in connection with the logic of diagnosis, and is thus somewhat removed from the surmised earlier stage of evaluation commented on in the autobiographical note. I think the difference in presentation that this reference to the "discriminate" subphase reflects, suggests to an extent the classical distinction between the "context of discovery" and the "context of justification." Though in this chapter I have disagreed with the way the classical distinction is drawn, I have not characterized the difference between contexts as meaningless or completely mistaken.

The difference in presentation that I believe we encounter here between Burnet's analysis in his autobiographical notes and in his "finished research paper" (1957b) is pragmatic and strategic. What Burnet has done is to narrow down his reasoning to only several competing models (recall that the discriminate subphase of evaluation is entered when there are two to four competitors) and to marshal arguments that discriminate the strengths of his new clonal selection hypothesis against alternatives (principally Jerne's 1955 hypothesis). The criteria, it should be noted, do not differ, but now Burnet has caught his hypothesis and from that vantage point he is offering some yet weak evaluational criteria in its support. Strong evaluational criteria will not be forthcoming for several years post-1957, and then, as will be described in detail in chapter 5, in the years 1958–66 or so, the experimental data were not self-consistent.

2.10   Hempel's Objections to a Logic of Scientific Discovery

The distinguished philosopher of science, C. G. Hempel, has offered in his (1965) and (1985) a series of clear and powerful arguments against a logic of scientific discovery of a strong or Baconian form. Some of his arguments may apply to the two-aspect account of a logic of scientific discovery as a logic of generation and a logic of preliminary evaluation urged earlier. Let us turn to Hempel's precisely articulated views on this subject.

In his 1965 work, *Aspects of Scientific Explanation*, Hempel presented three arguments against the possibility of a logic of scientific discovery. First, a logic of discovery would presumably begin from *facts*, but there are an *infinite* number of facts and some sorting into relevant and irrelevant facts must be presumed. However, second, such a sorting cannot be based purely on a *problem* with which scientific inquiry might be said to begin, for a "problem" is too vague and general to provide criteria for the selection of relevant facts. The only candidate, Hempel argued, that qualifies as a sorting device for relevant facts is a *hypothesis*, and on his view relevance is a relation between a hypothesis and its consequences: a fact is relevant if and only if it or its negation is a deductive consequence of a hypothesis (1965, 12). Thus, Hempel argued, we must begin our inquiry with hypotheses that are "happy guesses," freely invented to account for facts.

Hempel offered a third argument against a logic of scientific discovery. "Scientific hypotheses and theories," he writes, "are usually couched in terms that do not occur at all in the description of the empirical findings on which they rest, and which they serve to explain."

> Induction Rules [a strong logic of discovery] . . . would therefore have to provide a mechanical routine for con-

structing, on the basis of given data, a hypothesis or theory stated in terms of some quite novel concepts which are nowhere used in the description of the data themselves. Surely, no general mechanical rule of procedure can be expected to achieve this. (1965, 12)

This (third) argument was further embellished by Hempel in his comments at a later conference on discovery and medical diagnosis by computers. Hempel noted that:

The discoveries achievable by programs of the kind just considered (such as DENDRAL and INTERNIST-1) are subject to various limitations, in particular (i) the limitation of all discoverable hypotheses to sentences expressible with the logical means of a given computer language; (ii) limitation of the available vocabulary to one that is antecedently given and fixed; (iii) limitations of the available principles of manifestation (more generally: limitations of the given empirical background assumptions). (Hempel 1985, 118)

Commenting further on such programs as meta-DENDRAL, Hempel added:

The rules, or general principles, however, that lend themselves to discovery in this manner are clearly limited to hypotheses that are expressible entirely in the given vocabulary of the program, and with the logical means embodied in its language. But the formulation of powerful explanatory principles and especially theories normally involves the introduction of a novel conceptual and terminological apparatus. The explanation of combustion by the conflicting theories of dephlogistication and of oxidation illustrates the point.

The new concepts introduced by a theory of this kind cannot, as a rule, be defined by those previously available; they are characterized, rather, by means of a set of theoretical principles linking the new concepts to each other and to previously available concepts that serve to describe the phenomena to be explained. Thus, the discovery of an explanatory theory for a given class of occurrences required the introduction both of new theoretical terms and of new theoretical principles. It does not seem clear at all how a

computer might be programmed to discover such powerful
theories. (Hempel 1985, 119-120)

At the conclusion of the remarks quoted above Hempel proposed a new, fourth argument against mechanizing discovery.
Noting that many (an infinite number of) hypotheses can be formulated to account for an aggregate of data, in the sense that
through two points an infinite number of different curves can be
constructed, Hempel concluded that some criteria of preference,
e.g., simplicity, must be involved. Hempel then cited Kuhn's
analysis of scientific revolutions in support of an argument
against a logic of discovery:

> There are, indeed, several such criteria of preference that
> are frequently invoked — among them simplicity and large
> range of potential applicability; but these notions have not,
> so far, received a precise characterization. Moreover, as
> Kuhn's account of scientific revolutions has emphasized,
> there are further considerations that affect the choice
> among competing theories in science; but these are to some
> extent idiosyncratic, and no exact and generally acknow-
> ledged formulation of corresponding criteria is presently
> available or likely to be forthcoming. (Hempel 1985, 121)

My response to these trenchant objections will be threefold.
First, I want to argue that scientific *problems* are such that they
can evoke a sufficient set of constraints to enable them to serve as
the source of regulated scientific inquiry.[26] This argument will
require me to anticipate somewhat an analysis of science that
will be explored in more detail in chapters 3, 4, and 5. Second, I
want to suggest that recently developed discovery programs that
implement Simon's approach, discussed earlier, indicate how
new theoretical terms can be introduced, and also how "analogy" may be formally introduced into scientific discovery.

2.11 Problems, Disciplinary Matrices, BACON, and Analogy

It should be obvious from the historical examples cited earlier
that scientific inquiry, as performed by trained, competent researchers, always begins in medias res. An individual working
on the forefront of biomedical science has been schooled for
many years in previously formulated theories, experimental results, and techniques of analysis and also usually has a rough

and ready set of standards by which he or she judges the work of scientific contributions. Kuhn has stressed this feature of science in his influential *Structure of Scientific Revolutions*. Kuhn saw the need to introduce a more general term to characterize the entity with which a scientist works, which he called a "paradigm" in the original text. As I shall show in chapter 5, that term occasioned much criticism, and in his later postscript Kuhn suggested the term "disciplinary matrix" to designate this more general entity. Such a disciplinary matrix is comprised of (1) symbolic generalizations, (2) models, and (3) standards or values, as well as (4) *exemplars*. Exemplars are "concrete problem-solutions that students encounter from the start of their scientific education." These exemplars are most important, and Kuhn sees them as involving the essence of scientific problem solving:

> The student discovers, with or without the assistance of his instructor, a way to see his problem as *like* a problem he has already encountered. Having seen the resemblance, grasped the analogy between two or more distinct problems, he can interrelate symbols and attach them to nature in the ways that have proved effective before. The law-sketch, say f = ma, has functioned as a tool, informing the student what similarities to look for, signaling the gestalt in which the situation is to be seen. (Kuhn 1970, 189)

Kuhn adds:

> The role of acquired similarity relations also shows clearly in the history of science. Scientists solve puzzles by modeling them on previous puzzle-solutions, often with only minimal recourse to symbolic generalizations. Galileo found that a ball rolling down an incline acquires just enough velocity to return it to the same vertical height on a second incline of any slope, and he learned to see that experimental situation as like the pendulum with a point-mass for a bob. (Kuhn 1970, 189–190)

A given scientific problem accordingly makes its appearance in concert with a rich set of other players. To Kuhn's constituents of a disciplinary matrix ought explicitly be added the *heuristics* which a scientist has learned to use in his problem-solving career. The notion of a disciplinary matrix also needs to be conceived to be appropriately narrowed in many contexts. Thus, in an account of Burnet's discovery, the area of focus of the problem is a subregion of immunology. This subregion is, I believe, closely analogous to what Shapere has termed a "domain" in science. For Shapere a "domain" is a set of "items of information" having an "association" displaying the following features:

(1) The association is based on some relationship between the items.

(2) There is something problematic about the body so related.

(3) That problem is an important one.

(4) Science is "ready" to deal with the problem. (Shapere 1977, 525)

Though suggestive, the concept of a domain is difficult to make precise, and Nickles (1977), for example, believes that domains are better characterized as determined by a theory (or previously successful theories) that explain the "items of information," thus providing a unifying principle. To me, however, this misses Shapere's important point, that a "domain" exercises an important *extrinsic* control over what is an acceptable and/or complete theory of that domain.

Fluid though the concepts of "disciplinary matrix" and "domain" may be, they suggest, contra Hempel, that actual scientific problems may be sufficiently associated with accessory informational structures as to provide a set of antecedent constraints that function as part of a logic of scientific discovery in both generating and evaluating new hypotheses or theories.[27] I would furthermore contend that Hempel's view, which analyzes the relevance of a "fact" on the basis of its (or its contrary's) deducibility from a hypothesis, is too strong to serve as an account of how facts govern hypotheses or theories in the preliminary evaluative stage. In the early stages of formulation of a new hypothesis, scientists offer weak guesses as to how a hypothesis might be extended to account for important phenomena in a domain. I believe that at this preliminary evaluation stage they will often speculate on hypothetical mechanisms that are *roughly analogous* to known mechanisms and offer at best "gappy" "explanation sketches" that will constitute elements of the "positive heuristic" of a new research program.[28] It would be difficult to reconstruct such arguments in a tight deductive form.

Accordingly, I would maintain that we have replies to Hempel's first two objections to a logic of discovery cited above. (1) There are *not* an infinite number of relevant facts; there are a limited number, selected in advance by a problem that is sufficiently precise to evoke a domain and a disciplinary matrix in a subarea of science. (2) Hempel's view of experimental relevance as essentially a deductive relation is probably too strong; I have tried to show that relevance can be extrinsically introduced by the domain and disciplinary matrix, together with exploratory plausibility considerations involving analogical reasoning and gappy explanation sketches. Hempel's third and fourth objections to a logic of discovery are more difficult to answer, but some recent developments in artificial intelligence research appear to point the way to a reply to the third criticism.

I shall begin by briefly describing a scientific discovery program developed by Pat Langley working with Herbert Simon and his colleagues. After a number of articles describing this work were published, a monograph summarizing much of this project appeared (Langley et al. 1987). This program, termed BACON, has evolved through some half-dozen stages, denominated BACON.1 through BACON.6. In addition, BACON has generated several spinoff programs known as GLAUBER, STAHL, and DALTON (Langley et al. 1987).[29] I will outline the structure and some of the accomplishments of the BACON.4 version, which will permit specific answers to Hempel's third objection, and then go on to comment on several additional features of the BACON spinoff programs.

BACON.4 represents an implementation of Simon's theory of scientific discovery as problem solving within an information-processing framework. It utilizes what is known as a production-system approach, in which discovery heuristics are represented as cue-action pairs or rules.[30] BACON in its first five versions is what is termed a data-driven program, in contrast to a theory-driven program such as Lenat's AM (see Lenat 1977); a variant of BACON.5 termed BLACK is, however, explicitly theory-driven. (The difference refers to the basic information source of the program. In accordance with what was argued above using suggestions by Kuhn and Shapere, the ultimate scientific discovery program will have to be *both* data and theory driven.) According to Simon, Langley, and Bradshaw (1981):

> BACON.4 employs a small set of data-driven heuristics to detect regularities in numeric and nominal data. These heuristics, by noting constancies and trends, cause BACON.4 to formulate hypotheses, define theoretical terms, postulate

intrinsic properties, and propose integral relations (common divisors) among quantities. The BACON.4 heuristics do not depend on the specific properties of the particular problem domains to which they have been applied but appear to be general techniques applicable to discovery in diverse domains. (1981, 12)

These heuristics fall into four classes: (1) detecting covariance, (2) conducting recursion and generalization, (3) postulating intrinsic properties, and (4) finding common divisors. It would take us beyond the scope of this book to describe BACON.4 in any detail, since it is primarily concerned with discovery in the physical sciences, but several examples of its employment, drawn from physics, will be cited to illustrate the strengths and limitations of BACON.4. (A similar, though more complex, program has been developed by Blum [1982] in the rheumatological disease area. This program, known as Rx, detects time-lagged covariance in patient data and produces generalizations.)

The "detecting covariance" heuristic can be applied to data of the type that might have been available to Kepler when he generated his third law of planetary motion — period^2 = constant (distance from sun)^3. Such laws can be utilized as input for further generalizations. Using its recursion and generalization, BACON.4 began with "level 0" data and produced Boyle's law for gases (pressure x volume = constant). It then induced the more complex Boyle-Charles law (Pressure x volume/temperature = constant) from Boyle's law and additional data, and finally the ideal gas law from the Boyle-Charles law and further data.

As noted above, Hempel expressed doubt that new theoretical properties could be generated by any algorithmical (logical) procedure. An attempt to reply to this type of objection can be made by pointing to the "postulating intrinsic properties" heuristic of BACON.4. One example of its use is in postulating the concept of "inertial mass," following a Mach-like approach. Mach, in his *Science of Mechanics* (1960 [1883]), disagreed with Newton's original attempts to define mass either in terms of density and volume or according to a particulate theory of matter, proposing an "operational" definition instead. The essence of Mach's approach was to use the law of conservation of momentum and to allow several blocks of matter to interact pairwise (by imagining them to be connected by an idealized stretched spring, for example) such that the blocks produce mutual, oppositely directed acceleration in each other. At any given instant the velocities produced in the system are such that the total momentum equals zero.

BACON.4 "performs" a series of Machian experiments (actually it does not perform the experiments but requires the data from such experiments).

TECHNICAL DISCUSSION 1

BACON.4's "experiment" works with a pair of blocks O_x and O_y (with acceleration of $O_x = a_x$, and acceleration of $O_y = a_y$). In the "experiment":

> BACON.4 treats pairs of objects O_x and O_y as the independent variables and their accelerations, a_x and a_y as the dependent variables. In addition, the program is told that the objects of a pair are interchangeable (i.e., that the same objects can be used for O_x or O_y). Thus, when an intrinsic property is discovered for O_y, BACON.4 knows it can associate that property with the same object when it appears as O_x (Simon, Langley, and Bradshaw 1981, 16).[31]

Then, according to Simon, Langley, and Bradshaw:

> Let BACON.4 experiment with five blocks, A, B, C, D, and E. At level 0 of the experiment, where O_x is the block A, BACON.4 will discover that each pair of objects, A, O_y, has a constant ratio of accelerations, K_{Ay}. Suppose that the ratios are $K_{ab} = 1.20$, $K_{ac} = 0.80$, $K_{ad} = 1.60$, and $K_{ae} = 1.80$. BACON.4 now defines a new variable, M_y, an intrinsic property associated with the second object in each pair, O_y, and sets its value equal to the corresponding K. At this point, BACON.4 cannot specify an M value for block A, which has not appeared in the experiment as O_y, and so it includes only blocks B, C, D, and E in the remaining experiments it carries out. At this point, BACON.4 also defines the term K_{xy}/M_y, which, by the definition of M_y as equal to K_{ay}, must always equal 1.0 whenever O_x is A.
>
> BACON.4 now collects data for new values of O_x. When O_x is the block B, it again discovers a constant ratio of accelerations for each value of O_y: 0.667, 1.33, and 1.50 for the pairs (BC), (BD), and (BE), respectively. Since these ratios, K_{By}, vary directly with the stored values of M_y, BACON.4 now varies the first block, and looks at the values K_{xy}/M_y obtained on the previous level. When the program retrieves the M_x values of each of the blocks and compares them with the previously mentioned ratios, it finds that their product, $K_{xy}M_x/M_y$, is a constant. Thus, for any pair of

blocks, O_x, O_y, $M_y/M_x = K_{xy}$, which is the desired law of conservation of momentum. (1981, 16–17)

In his original formulation Mach (1960 [1883], 303) suggested that two additional "experimental propositions" were needed in order to characterize the concept of inertial mass, namely *independence* from the physical state of the bodies and *independence* of the accelerations (which, e.g., blocks B, C, D, . . . induce in A). Let us assume that this information can be detected by BACON.4 in appropriate data. Would we, in that case, have a procedure which permitted a "theoretical term" to be generated by a heuristic program operating on experimental data? There are several objections that I believe a heuristic program can outflank, but there remains at least one difficulty for which there is only a speculative rejoinder.

Hempel has criticized the operationalistic approach due to Bridgman (with its roots in Mach) on several grounds. Operational definitions are dispositional and thus go beyond operationalist standards. Furthermore, the use of concepts such as mass that take on real number values is impossible because there is a nondenumerable infinity of reals whereas operationalistic analysis can only introduce a denumerable infinity of operations. (See Hempel 1965, 128-129.)

It seems to me, however, that both of these objections can be met by a heuristic program such as BACON.4, because it is *not* constrained by the operationalist philosophy. Surplus theoretical, nonoperational meaning is not barred from the problem-solving, information-processing approach of Simon and his colleagues, whether it be dispositional or involve higher order infinities. What is required is a set of heuristics that will *generate* the theoretical terms, not *reduce* those theoretical terms to experimental operations. On this score, then, the illustration involving the concept of inertial mass seems adequate. Other concepts such as electrical resistance (or its inverse, conductance) have also been generated by BACON.4.

What is less certain is whether such a program can generate the concepts of theoretical *entities* such as atoms, electrons, and genes. On this topic BACON.4 appears to be less successful. Though there is a fourth class of heuristics in BACON.4 termed "finding common divisors," which can obtain certain atomic terms such as atomic weights, these do not appear capable of working to an atomic theory. Simon et al. address this point as follows:

> The chemical formula $2H_2 + O_2 = 2H_2O$, provides a reductionist explanation of the formation of water vapor from hydrogen and oxygen, in terms of the atomic theory and hypotheses about the atomic compositions of the respective substances. BACON.4 using its GCD [greatest common divisor] heuristic discovers that water contains two "quanta" of hydrogen and one of oxygen, and that each "quantum" of the latter weighs sixteen times as much as a "quantum" of the former. Does this result support the claim the BACON.4 has discovered the atomic theory of the formation of water vapor? We would say that it does not, although it is not easy to specify what is missing.
>
> Perhaps we should only assert that a system has an atomic theory if it has some internal representation for atoms, each having associated with it its atomic weight and such other properties as theory attributes to it. Sets of such atoms would represent molecules. In addition to this representational capability, we might require that the system also have operators (representations of reactions) for rearranging sets of atoms. (1981, 20–21)

In their later work, Simon, Langley, and their associates developed spinoffs of BACON in several different directions, of which I shall comment on two. In a program known as STAHL — after the renowned chemist Georg Ernst Stahl who developed the phlogiston theory toward the end of the seventeenth century — "explanations" of various chemical reactions are generated. However, the inputs to STAHL contain the term "phlogiston" (see Langley et al. 1987, 229), thus the STAHL program is not likely to serve as an adequate counter to Hempel's critique with respect to such theoretical concepts as phlogiston. In their DALTON program, the situation appears to be similar; the concepts of atoms and molecules appear in the *inputs* rather than being generated by the program (see Langley et al. 1987, 260). DALTON is characterized as "theory-driven" (1987, 259), thus this limitation does not affect the operation of the program; it does not, however, allow DALTON to provide an answer to Hempel's concerns. Of interest to readers of this book, DALTON has also been used to explore the generation of simple Mendelian genetics (see Langley et al. 1987, 274–276), though this research is quite preliminary.

What I suspect is missing, and what gives rise to the difficulties of BACON, STAHL, and DALTON with respect to generating novel theoretical concepts, is the inability to *generate a model* (in DALTON an atomic model) that contains surplus antecedent theoretical meaning which is only obtainable by *analogical* information processing. In chapter 4 I shall discuss the source of this type of theoretical meaning in some detail, but the key idea is that antecedently understood notions are drawn upon and put together in a way different from, though analogical to, the way they are related in their source(s). In Burnet's discovery of clonal selection, this "antecedent theoretical meaning" is illustrated by his concept of a lymphocyte with specialized recognition receptors that allow it to be selected by antigen for clonal expansion.

The question then arises whether analogical information processing is possible: can an appropriate program be formulated which will permit a computer to reason analogically?[32] Work by Winston (1982) indicates that such analogical reasoning is programmable on a computer, and in recent years the investigation of analogical reasoning in AI has proliferated.[33] Winston proposed a theory that uses *precedents* to obtain solutions to problems based on analogical computations. The program has been tested on several simple stories drawn from diverse subject areas, called the "Macbeth world," the "politics world," and the "diabetes world," and has been extended to match semantic nets—standard tools of knowledge representation that present sentences diagramatically (Winston 1984, 1986). For Winston, "analogy is based on the assumption that if two situations are similar in some respect, then they must be similar in other respects as well" (1982, 326). Similarity is estimated by a *matching* program which has a "similarity function" that "uses properties, classes, acts, and other relations depending on what is important . . . and searches the space of all possible matches heuristically beginning by linking up the most similar parts from the two situations and then moving on to those that are less similar. The parts that are linked supply helpful evidence for those that are not" (1982, 326; also see Winston 1980).

The constraint relations in the precedent(s), especially causal relations, "suggest the right relations to check and the right questions to ask" (1980, 327). In addition, the program can generate rules which summarize the exercise solutions. Though the rules are valuable and can be used in later, different exercises, rules lack some of the detail contained in the precedent(s) from which the rules arise. Retaining both rules and precedents permits more powerful problem-solving behavior. (In this regard, it is interesting to recall Kuhn's 1970 comments, as quoted on page 51, concerning the role of exemplars and analogical reasoning in scientific education contexts.) Winston notes that, in doubtful conclusions where, for example, there are imperfect matches, use of the precedent can result in the program hypothetically creating a missing actor in order to solve the exercise. In such situations the program prints a "Beware . . ." statement, followed by the required creation. For example, in the "diabetes world" John and Tom are analogous diabetics. The program is told that John, in C1, is a diabetic with an unhealthy pancreas. Tom in, C2, shares several features with John but information regarding Tom's pancreas is absent. In an exercise designed to show that Tom takes the medicine insulin, the trace reveals the following:

> I am trying to show (TOM TAKE MEDICINE-INSULIN-2)
> Supply t = true, ? = don't know, l = look, or a precedent:
> c1
> Should I use the last match between C2 and C1?
> y
> Beware! Use of match require creating PANCREAS-2 for PANCREAS-1
> I note that (BLOOD-SUGAR-2 HAS-QUALITY HIGH) for use with C1
> I note that (TOM AKO DIABETIC) for use with C1
> All consequences of (PANCREAS-2-HAS QUALITY UN-HEALTHY) are confirmed.
> The evidence from C1 indicates (TOM TAKE MEDICINE-INSU-LIN-2).
> (Winston 1982, 344)

I conclude that Winston's results show that computer-based analogical reasoning is possible in scientific contexts. This or a similar approach, coupled with a program like BACON, should be able to generate theoretical terms, including entity concepts.

Several promising developments in recent years have advanced the prospect of powerful computational tools becoming available for analyzing and assisting scientific discovery; they cannot be treated further here but should be noted for their significant future potential. Kulkarni and Simon's KEKADA extension of a BACON-like approach (see note 29) has already been commented on. Also noted (in note 27) has been the approach of Holland et al. (1986). The latter group has developed a program known as PI (for "processes of induction") on the basis of initial work by Thagard and Holyoak (1985). Among PI's strengths is its ability to work with a "mental model" characterization of a scientific theory (see more below in chapter 3, section 7), as well as its ability to employ analogies as part of theory discovery (Holland et al. 1986, 336-342). These investigators note that PI is in its early stages of development and has primarily been tested on comparatively simple examples (1986, 127). In contrast to the more extensive research on BACON and the high-fidelity and complex example in KEKADA, PI awaits further elaboration and application. Nevertheless given its promise of a rich informational structure system (see above, note) as well as its ability to incorporate analogical reasoning, PI is an exciting system that bears watching.

Finally, I want to cite the very recent work of Peter Karp on scientific discovery in molecular biology. Karp's research developed in the context of Peter Friedland's Stanford-based MOLGEN project, and is concerned with the issues of knowledge representation and hypothesis discovery in the *trp* operon theory. Karp's research is in its comparatively early stages but employs some approaches rather distinct from what has been described thus far — approaches which seem to me to be both plausible for biomedical science and potentially very powerful. In the next few paragraphs a very brief overview of this research will be summarized; additional details can be found in Karp (1989a) and (1989b).

Karp's investigation has resulted in two computer programs: one known as GENSIM, which provides a framework for representing theories of molecular biology, and another termed HYPGENE, which formulates hypotheses that improve the predictive power of GENSIM theories (1989a, 1). Karp proposes that it will be useful to think of hypothesis formation as a *design* problem. He views "a hypothesis as an *artifact* to be synthesized," subject to design constraints such as matches to experimental evidence. His HYPGENE program is then a "designer" of hypotheses which uses *design operators* to "modify a theory to satisfy design constraints" (1989a, 1).

The GENSIM program is heavily theory-oriented and uses a general biological theory to describe specific experiments. It "contains a taxonomic hierarchy of over 300 classes of biological objects including strains of bacteria, genes, enzymes, and amino acids" (1989a, 3). This is the "class knowledge base" or CKB. Also included in GENSIM is a "process knowledge base" (known both as PKB and T) that constitutes a theory of chemical reactions.[34] In addition, the program creates another, separate knowledge base for the simulation of a specific experiment known as the SKB. The entire program is implemented in the Intellicorp™ Knowledge Engineering Environment™ (KEE). KEE is a very powerful system which enables the use of frame structures (to be discussed in some detail in chapter 3) as well as other information handling and processing tools. The general flavor of Karp's programs is what computer programmers call "object-oriented," though predicate calculus forms of knowledge representation are also used as needed.[35]

Karp's hypothesis-generating program, HYPGENE, employs a series of processing strategies similar to those discussed earlier in this chapter, though with modification to reflect the *design* orientation as well as the resources of KEE. HYPGENE's input includes GENSIM's knowledge bases CKB and T, as well as the initial conditions of an anomalous experiment, GENSIM's original prediction for this experiment (as well as dependency information as to how the prediction was computed), and an error term P_A describing the difference between what was predicted in the experiment and what was found.

HYPGENE's output is a set of alternative descriptions of new initial conditions, new theories, or both. The process of new hypothesis generation is complex but involves the *design operators* producing modifications of various assertions in CKB and T; this results in the creation of new "objects." One example is the creation of a new mutation (see Karp 1989a, 10–11). Additional details can be found in Karp (1989a, 1989b).

These modifications result in a potentially very large search space of alternative hypotheses (in some cases an infinite search space). HYPGENE then conducts a "best-first" search of the design space as defined by the application of the various design operators. A simple preliminary evaluation function is employed to order the search, a function which Karp describes as "based on the syntactic complexity of its unsatisfied goals [i.e., simplicity is preferred], and based on the number of objects modified in the hypothesis . . . (a measure of the cost of computing . . .) [i.e., the program is "conservative"]." Other information is also used to prune and rank the hypotheses, though not all plausible constraints, such as background knowledge principles (e.g., conservation of mass) are yet implemented. The search is facilitated by a KEE resource known as an assumption-based truth maintenance system (ATMS).

Karp's results are preliminary but very encouraging. Moreover, for reasons which will become clearer in the succeeding chapters, the means which Karp has chosen to represent biomedical knowledge resonate strongly with conclusions of this author reached through different routes. The existence of an implemented discovery system in molecular biology thus is significant support for many of the theses argued for above as well as themes to be developed below.

There is one additional feature of Karp's approach which may play an important role in our getting a purchase on both knowledge representation and discovery in the biomedical sciences. Though there is very strong evidence that human beings (and scientists involved in the scientific discovery process) reason analogically, the advances that have been made on this subject (and cited above) are still fairly rudimentary. It may be the case that the more traditional modes of knowledge representation using symbols cannot capture analogical thinking very well, and that a more "connectionist" approach might be needed. The difficulty with that tack is that the study of knowledge representation in connectionist systems and of their correlates with traditional modes of knowledge representation is in its infancy (see McMillan and Smolensky 1988 and Touretzky and Hinton 1988).

As I shall argue in more detail in chapter 3, object-oriented programming (OOP) techniques may provide a means of representing the abstraction and similarity needed to capture biomedical systems more appropriately. Since Karp's programs utilize such OOP techniques and seem to avoid analogical reasoning, they may point the way to a different and more tractable means of capturing what is described by analogy and analogical reasoning.[36]

At this point in my discussion of a logic of scientific discovery, I believe I have addressed in outline responses to Hempel's first three objections. A reply to his fourth objection, based partially on Kuhn's theory of scientific revolutions, that there is no likelihood of developing criteria of preference among competing theories, requires a rather extensive reply. I defer that reply until chapter 5, where Kuhn's theory is considered and a Bayesian logic of theory competition is developed.

Much of what is proposed in this chapter is tentative and somewhat speculative, but I believe that the evidence is in its favor. Appropriate attention to the nature of science and its complex constraints, coupled with heuristic problem-solving programs with a capacity for analogical reasoning and appropriate criteria for choosing among competing theories, should constitute the basis for a logic of scientific discovery, both in the biomedical sciences and in science in general.[37]

CHAPTER THREE

Theories and "Laws" in Biology and Medicine

3.1 Introduction

IN THE PREVIOUS CHAPTER I discussed the way in which the discovery of generalizations in biology and medicine occurs. Our focus there in terms of the illustrative examples, was on the discovery of theories, though the methodology does not distinguish in significant ways between more narrowly conceived generalizations and more general theories. The structure of theories has not been analyzed in general terms, nor has the question of whether the received view of theories, based on physics, been examined closely to see if it applies in the biological sciences.

A number of questions have been raised in the literature about the logical nature of laws and theories with respect to biology and medicine. Some authors, such as J. J. C. Smart (1963), have argued that there are *no* laws in biology, and, correlatively, that the structure of theories in biology is quite different from the structure of those theories found in physics and chemistry. Wimsatt (1976b) has suggested that we should focus our attention on *mechanisms* rather than on laws (or theories) in our approach to explanation (and reduction) in biology. More recently Philip Kitcher (1984) has questioned whether "laws" play a very important part in our analysis of biological theories. Finally, Rosenberg (1985, 219) has argued that there are at most two bodies of information that "meet reasonable criteria for being scientific theories" in biology, namely the theory of natural selection and some universal parts of molecular biology; all the rest of biology is constituted by *case study*–oriented research programs. In this chapter I will begin to analyze these issues, primarily concentrating on Smart's critique and the response of certain philosophers of biology to it as well as to Rosenberg's claims. In later chapters, closely associated but distinguishable notions such as causality, explanation, and what I shall term a *temporally extended* conception of theory will be introduced, explicated, and related to the themes of this chapter. I shall consider Wimsatt's and Kitcher's proposals both in chapter 6 (on explanation) and in chapter 9 (on reduction), where their views have the most relevance.

Because the subject matter of this chapter is quite complex, it will be helpful to the reader if I state my theses at this point in the discussion. I shall argue that many of the theories we encounter in the biomedical sciences are different from the standard type of theory we see in physics. In the medically related biological sciences such as molecular genetics, immunology, physiology, embryology, and the neurosciences, we find "theories of the middle range," midway, in a sense, between the universal theories of biochemistry and the universal mechanisms of neo-Darwinian evolution.[1] The problem of "generalizations" in biology and medicine is a complex one, and it has been addressed in several different contexts over the past nearly thirty years; I shall review that literature in the course of my arguments. I will maintain that further analysis of the senses of "universal," distinguishing *scope of application* from *causal generalizations which can support counterfactuals* within the framework of theories of the middle range, provides an important part of the solution to this issue. I also will suggest that the semantic approach to scientific theories, which has attracted considerable interest on the part of philosophers of biology in the 1980s, is a natural context in which to give added structure to these theories of the middle range. In my examination of the semantic approach, I generalize the set-theoretic characterization from previous accounts, such as Lloyd's (1988) and Thompson's (1989), and I also respond to some criticisms posed by Suppe in his recent (1989) book.

3.2 General Approaches to Analyzing Theory Structure in Biology and Medicine

Over the past fifteen years questions about the nature of theory structure in biology have received considerable attention. Early work in philosophy of biology on this issue, such as Woodger's (1937, 1939, 1959), assumed that axiomatization and formalization in the predicate calculus would capture the essential aspects of theory structure in the biological sciences.[2] Criticisms by philosophers of biology of the standard model for the analysis of scientific theories (also known as the "received view"), initially tended to focus on the explanatory dimension of theoretical reasoning, as in the work of Scriven (1959) and Goudge (1961). In his penetrating work, Beckner (1959) proposed analyses for "model" and "theory" in biology, in the latter case primarily directing his attention to the theory of evolution. Subsequently Ruse (1973) and Hull (1974), stimulated in part by Smart's (1963, 1968) critiques of theory in biology, propounded differing accounts of theory structure in biology, Ruse also reacting specifically to Beckner's account. (Simon [1971] also comments on Smart [1963, 1968], but his discussion of theory concentrates primarily on the theoretical entity problem rather than on theoretical structure.) More recently Beatty (1979, 1981, 1987), Lloyd (1984, 1989), Rosenberg (1985), Thompson (1983, 1987, 1989) and Waters (1990) have written on the nature of theory in biology, though primarily from the point of view of the theory of evolution.

Curiously, much of the earlier debate in the philosophy of biology concerning theory structure took place in isolation from major changes in the philosophy of science, and even the more recent work in this area has tended to be concentrated in the area of evolutionary biology to the exclusion of significant advances in molecular biology, genetics, and microbiology. This recent work has, in addition, tended to ignore advances on such generally relevant topics as scientific explanation and scientific realism. I will discuss this first claim in the next few paragraphs and also in section 3.4 below, though some further development on this point will be deferred until chapter 5.

The view that a scientific theory is most appropriately analyzed as a set of sentences, some small subset of which are the axioms, with the remaining theorems related deductively to the axioms, is to be found in Duhem (1914). This notion was developed by Campbell (1920) and ultimately accepted as the "received view" (so termed by F. Suppe, 1977) which dominated Anglo-American philosophy of science until the mid-1960s. A particularly clear and comprehensive account of this view can be found in Nagel (1961, chapters 5 and 6), and an excellent historical analysis of the rise and fall of the "received view," and of new developments in theory structure, is to be found in Suppe (1977). I shall return to some of these developments in section 3.4.

It would take us beyond the scope of this chapter to rehearse the details of the "received view" and the problems with it that led to its demise. It should be pointed out here, however, that philosophy of science has been significantly affected by the criticisms by Hanson (1958), Popper (1959), Feyerabend (1962), Kuhn (1962), Putnam (1962), Polanyi (1962), and Achinstein (1968) of a number of traditional distinctions, such as that between theoretical statements and observation statements, which undergirded the "received view." It also became clear from the work of Feyerabend (1962) and Kuhn (1962), and then Lakatos (1970), Toulmin (1972), Shapere (1974), and Laudan (1977), that the "unit" with which scientists worked was larger and more complex than what the "received view" understood by a theory. In fact, focus on this older sense of "theory" obscured a number of problems concerning scientific change, the dynamic character of scientific explanation, and the complex nature of inductive support of scientific theories. A fuller account of theory structure in biology necessitates discussing and taking into account these challenges to the "received view" and elaborating a concept of theory in biology and medicine which shows its interrelation with discovery, testing, explanation, and justification procedures. In addition, a fuller account requires the development of a diachronic or temporally-extended conception of "theory." Discovery was treated in the previous chapter and these other issues will be reserved for later chapters. Before we can tackle these subjects, however, it is necessary to get clearer about the less sweeping but crucially important issue for the logical structure of "static" or, better, synchronic theories and laws in biology and medicine.

3.3 Some Recent Debates Concerning Theory Structure in Biology

The "received view" of scientific theories as formalized axiom systems that (with the aid of boundary conditions and initial conditions) deductively organize specific subject areas in science, exhibiting empirical laws and individual occurrences as logical consequences, spawned an influential criticism of the applicability of such a notion in biology. J. J. C. Smart (1963) argued that there were no "laws" in biology, and in addition:

> Writers who have tried to axiomatize biological and psychological theories seem to me to be barking up the same gum tree as would a man who tried to produce the first, second, and third laws of electronics, or of bridge building. We are not puzzled that there no laws of

electronics or of bridge building, though we recognize that the electronic engineer or bridge designer must use laws, namely laws of physics. The writers who have tried to axiomatize biology or psychology have wrongly thought of biology or psychology as a science of much the same logical character as physics, just as chemistry is. (1963, 52)

On the basis of his argument against there being biological laws, Smart concluded that "biology is not a theory of the same logical sort as physics though with a different subject matter" (Smart 1963, 52). It will, accordingly be instructive to examine Smart's arguments concerning biological laws as well as his views concerning theory structure in biology.

Smart's thesis that there are no laws in biology is based on three arguments: (1) a condition that a sentence (or proposition) be a scientific "law" is that it be universally true, that is, hold for all places and all time; (2) a law also ought not contain individual constants or place names such as "the Earth"; and (3) a law ought not have exceptions. Smart claims that any attempts to outflank (2) above by generalizing will lead to a violation of (1), since we do not believe that full universalization of such generalizations as "all albinotic mice breed true" will hold on planets in the great nebula in Andromeda, for example.

Michael Ruse (1970, 1973) responded to Smart's arguments, which he saw as "extremely serious," with implications for a "second-rate" assessment of biology (Ruse 1973, 26). As regards "unrestricted universality," Ruse counters that that notion was too broad: We do not test our laws in physics and chemistry in the Devonian period or in Andromeda, but within a broad range of our roughly current experience. As long as there are new tests not "built into" the laws, the laws are susceptible of test in accordance with the more limited "unrestricted-universality" condition. But Mendel's laws of genetics, Ruse's favorite example contra Smart, are testable and confirmable in a way quite similar to procedures in physics and chemistry. As regards the place-name problem, Ruse replies with a *tu quoque*, citing Kepler's laws (which named the "sun").[3] Finally, Mendel's laws do have exceptions (involving linkage and crossing over, for example) but so does Snell's law (in Iceland spar) and Boyle's law (at high temperatures and pressures). Ruse's replies are, in my view, much to the point, though, as I shall argue in section 3.6, in general they go too far, while occasionally they do not go far enough.[4]

In regard to biological theories, since Ruse's general strategy is to provide counterexamples to Smart's views, he uses the theory of population genetics contra Smart's position.

Population genetics for Ruse is centrally important as an example of both biological theorizing and theorizing in evolutionary theory. He maintains:

> The obvious question which arises is in just what respects evolutionary theory . . . is a theory like physics and chemistry? The answer to this is that, by virtue of the fact that the theory of evolution has population genetics as its core, it shares many of the features of physical sciences. The most vital part of the theory is axiomatized; through this part (if through nothing else) the theory contains reference to theoretical (non-observable, etc.) entities as well as to non-theoretical (observable, etc.) entities; there are bridge principles; and so on (Ruse 1973, 49).

Thus, for Ruse, biological theories are typified by population genetics and are not different in structure from theories in physics and chemistry.

Ruse did not present the theory of population genetics in its full complex form (as it is presented, for example, in Crow and Kimura 1970 and in Jacquard 1974) but was satisfied to derive mathematically the Hardy-Weinberg law for genetic populations in equilibrium, to draw attention to its similarities with Newton's first law of motion, and also to show that population genetics employs "bridge principles," citing as an example the standard work of Race and Sanger (1954) on the distribution of the M-N blood groups in England. (In my view a stronger argument against Smart can now be made by laying out the assumptions of population genetics as elegantly presented in Jacquard 1974 [see section 3.4.5], though this will not introduce a qualitatively different argument.)

Ruse's view is worth contrasting with an earlier position taken by Beckner (1959). Beckner argued a different thesis as regards evolutionary theory in biology. To Beckner,

> if we look in evolution theory for the pattern of theoretical explanation exemplified in that paradigm of theory formation, Newton's explanation of Galileo's and Kepler's laws, we shall be disappointed. Evolution theory does not attain its ends by exhibiting, e.g., Williston's and Bergmann's

principles as consequences of one or more hypotheses of greater generality. There are a number of small hierarchies of this character scattered about evolution theory, but the theory as a whole does not approach this type of organization. It is impossible to be dogmatic on the point, but it does seem to be true that this fact is not due to the undeveloped state of biology, but to the nature of biological subject matter. Some biologists seem to think that greater order could be brought into their science by a single genius of the caliber of a Newton. And though one cannot say that in the nature of the case a Newton for biology will not in time appear, one can venture to say that, insofar as the theory of evolution is concerned, further advances in theory will not effect a revolution, but will result in filling out a sketch whose outlines are already apparent. My own view is that evolution theory consists of a family of related models; most evolutionary explanations are based on assumptions that, in the individual case, are not highly confirmed; but that the various models in the theory provide evidential support for their neighbors. The subsidiary hypotheses and assumptions that are made for the sake of particular explanations in one model recur again and again in other related models, with or without modification and local adaptation. To use the metaphor of Agnes Arber, biological theory is less "linear" than, e.g., physical theory, and is more "reticulate." (Beckner 1959, 159–60)[5]

I will not be able to review Beckner's views in more detail at this point (though I will return to them again in sections 3.4 and 3.5 below). Ruse's arguments against Beckner's construal of evolutionary theory and his defense of the thesis that population genetics constitutes the core of the theory (see Ruse 1973, 52–62) are still unsettled questions in the philosophy of biology and will be reconsidered later.[6] The main theme I wish to extract from this dispute is that differences that exist, even within the restricted context of evolutionary biology, among alternative views of the nature of theory structure.

In his book *Philosophy of Biological Science* (1974), David Hull does not address this specific debate between Ruse and Beckner but does articulate his own views about the structure of evolutionary theory. In a lucid summary of the spectrum of positions that have been taken on theory structure, Hull writes:

The currently popular paradigm of a scientific theory is that of a deductively related set of laws. Laws in turn must be universal statements relating classes of empirical entities and processes, statements of the form "all swans are white" and "albinic mice always breed true." Just as scientific laws must be universal in form, the class names which occur in these laws must be defined in terms of sets of traits which are severally necessary and jointly sufficient for membership. . . .

However, certain authorities are willing to accept something less than the deductive ideal in the organization of scientific theories. The laws in such theories might also be less than universal in form. Perhaps statistical laws, possibly even approximations, trend, and tendency statements might count as genuine scientific laws. Certain authorities are also willing to countenance definitions which depart from the traditional ideal of sets of conditions which are severally necessary and jointly sufficient. Perhaps definitions in terms of properties which occur together quite frequently but without the universality required by the traditional notion of definition might be good enough. . . .

Thus, at one end of the spectrum are deductively organized theories that contain nothing but laws that are universal in form and terms that are defined in the traditional manner; at the other end are inductively organized theories that contain less than universal statements and terms that can be defined by properties which vary only statistically. (Hull 1974, 46–47)

On Hull's view there is a sense in which evolutionary theory is statistical, since meiosis and fertilization involve a random component (Hull 1974, 60). This sense of statistical is articulatable and formalizable in population genetics. However, when environmental effects on species are taken into account, the randomness becomes unmanageable (Hull 1974, 60–61). Such systems are not sufficiently "closed" to permit useful predictions. Furthermore, stochastic elements such as "genetic drift" become crucially important in small populations, as has been stressed by Mayr (1963) in formulating his "founder principle" (Hull 1974, 62).

On Hull's view, however, there is also a sense in which evolutionary theory may be construed as "deductive." This sense of deductive is based on Williams's (1970) axiomatization of evolutionary theory that introduces new units, which she terms "clans and subclans." A "clan" is "defined as a set containing all of the descendants of some collection of 'founder' organisms; the clan contains not only all contemporary descendants but also all descendants in all generations between the founder organisms and contemporary organisms" (1970, 350). A "subclan" is a subset of a clan "held together by cohesive forces so it acts as a unit with respect to selection." Williams is using these units to exhibit a deductive structure in evolutionary theory.

I will return to a consideration of Williams's (1970) theory in chapter 7, I but should point out here that her axiomatization has elicited strongly opposed assessments from philosophers of biology. Ruse, for example, has criticized her axiomatization since it "succeeds only by avoiding all mention of genetics" (Ruse 1973, 50). On the other hand, Rosenberg writes that Williams's axiomatization "provides the best account available of the axiomatic structure of evolutionary theory" (1983, 464). Moreover, Rosenberg finds Ruse's focus on population genetics as the essential core of evolutionary theory indefensible, as we shall see in chapter 7. Sober (1984b), however, views Williams's axiomatization as severely limited.

Suffice it to note here that on Hull's view of theory structure in biology, some parts of evolutionary theory are inductively systematizable, and an evolutionary theory reinterpreted in Williams's (1970) terms may be deductively systematizable in certain subareas.[7] Hull, as mentioned, does not directly address the Ruse-Beckner disagreement. In section 3.4 I will argue that the intense focus on evolutionary theory as the main paradigm of theory in biology by philosophers of biology has led to an overly parochial notion of theory structure in biology and medicine. In section 3.5 I shall maintain that, in one sense, Beckner is "more correct" than Ruse, especially if his notion of a theory as a family of models is generalized to apply to other theories in addition to evolutionary theory. In another sense, however, I will maintain that Ruse is more correct than Beckner, in that, in the area of evolutionary theory, population genetics is "more equal" (in the Orwellian sense) than alternative models and serves as an important core in evolutionary theory. This has been disputed in recent years, especially by Rosenberg (1985) and to an extent Thompson (1989), and I shall comment on their views further below and also again in chapter 7.

I have discussed the main points of Smart's criticism and also looked at Ruse's reply. Rosenberg (1985, 219–225) proposes a view that is similar to Smart's in that it denies that most domains of biology and medicine contain universal theories. Rather, most of biology for Rosenberg is a series of *case study*–oriented research programs. Arguing largely from evolutionary considerations, Rosenberg maintains:

> The upshot of our long discussion [3 chapters in his 1985] of the theory of evolution, of fitness, and of the nature of species is a very radical one. For in the end it suggests that, strictly speaking, there are in biology at most two bodies of statements that meet reasonable criteria for being scientific theories. These will be the theory of natural selection and such general principles of molecular biology as are free from any implicit or explicit limitation to any particular species or indeed any higher taxon of organisms restricted to this planet. (1985, 219)

Rosenberg's view is similar (though reached by an independent route) to a view I proposed in my 1980a essay:

> It is a thesis of the present essay that most theories propounded in biology and medicine are not now and will not in the foreseeable future be "universal" theories. . . . There are some important exceptions. . . . The theory of protein synthesis and the genetic code appear to be (at least at present) universal on earth, . . . and at the level of abstraction and simplification of the simplest theories of population genetics we are also likely to find universality (even extraterrestrially, since it is difficult to imagine a natural process which is not based on Darwinian evolution). (Schaffner 1980a, 82–83)

Rosenberg and I draw somewhat different conclusions about the nature of the generalizations and theories found in biology, however, and these will be considered further after I have had a chance to introduce some examples that will make my points clearer.

3.4 Examples of Representative Theories in Biology and Medicine

One of the main sources of the difficulties I see in contemporary accounts of the structure of biological theories lies in the overly restrictive areas from which the examples are taken. Theories in science serve both as generators of philosophical concepts about such theories and as tests of our philosophical intuitions about sciences. One can imagine the skewed nature of a philosophy of science which has as its source of examples only, say, classical mechanics and Maxwell's electromagnetic theory, neglecting statistical mechanics, quantum mechanics, and relativity theory. I will maintain that preoccupation by a number of philosophers of biology with evolution theory and Mendelian (and population) genetics has a similar narrowing effect.[8] In the present section I will draw what I take to be representative examples of theories in the biomedical area, from molecular biology, regulatory genetics, and cellular and systemic immunology, and briefly compare and contrast them with genetic and evolutionary theories to provide a broader basis for speculations concerning theory structure in biology and medicine.

3.4.1 *The Theory of the Genetic Code*

My first example is from molecular biology, or molecular genetics. In a sense, the theory of the genetic code is actually only a component of a more comprehensive and powerful "theory of protein synthesis," which in the space of several pages would be too complex to elaborate (see Watson et al. 1987, chapters 13–15, for a detailed discussion). Almost all the philosophical points which the more powerful theory supports can, however, be articulated on the basis of its less elaborate component. The function of this example is to describe a set of generalizations that are (almost) universal in the current biological world. Subsequent examples (with the exception of "simplified" population genetics) contrast with this aspect of the genetic code exemplar.

The first glimmerings of the theory of the genetic code occurred independently to Dounce (1952) and Gamow (1954).[9] The basic idea was that the linear sequence of nucleic acids in DNA could constitute the information necessary to determine the sequence of amino acids in polypeptide chains (proteins). This notion was coherent with the confirmed "one-gene–one-enzyme" hypothesis of Beadle and Tatum (1941) and received increased emphasis by Watson and Crick's (1953a) discovery of the three-dimensional double-helix structure for DNA with its two complementary intertwined linear nucleotide chains. It occurred to Dounce and Gamow that, since there are four different nucleotides in DNA, namely, adenine (A), thymine (T), guanine (G), and cytosine (C), a code made up of combinations of two nucleotide bases would have sixteen (4^2) possibilities, where a code made up of combinations of three nucleotides would entail sixty-four possibly (4^3) available codons. Both Dounce and Gamow suggested that the code was composed of three nucleotides, since twenty different amino acids were known to be involved in proteins. They also proposed, incorrectly as it turned out, that the code was overlapping.

The breakthrough on the code determination came in 1961 after the discovery of messenger RNA (mRNA), which is an in-

TABLE 3.1   THE GENETIC CODE

Codon	Amino Acid	Codon	Amino Acid	Codon	Amino Acid	Codon	Amino Acid
UUU	Phenylalanine	UCU	Serine	UAU	Tyrosine	UGU	Cysteine
UUC	Phenylalanine	UCC	Serine	UAC	Tyrosine	UGC	Cysteine
UUA	Leucine	UCA	Serine	UAA	stop	UGA	stop
UUG	Leucine	UCG	Serine	UAG	stop	UGG	Tryptophan
CUU	Leucine	CCU	Proline	CAU	Histidine	CGU	Arginine
CUC	Leucine	CCC	Proline	CAC	Histidine	CGC	Arginine
CUA	Leucine	CCA	Proline	CAA	Glutamine	CGA	Arginine
CUG	Leucine	CCG	Proline	CAG	Glutamine	CGG	Arginine
AUU	Isoleucine	ACU	Threonine	AAU	Asparagine	AGU	Serine
AUC	Isoleucine	ACC	Threonine	AAC	Asparagine	AGC	Serine
AUA	Isoleucine	ACA	Threonine	AAA	Lysine	AGA	Arginine
AUG	Methionine (start)	ACG	Threonine	AAG	Lysine	AGG	Arginine
GUU	Valine	GCU	Valine	GAU	Aspartic acid	GGU	Glycine
GUC	Valine	GCC	Alanine	GAC	Aspartic acid	GGC	Glycine
GUA	Valine	GCA	Alanine	GAA	Glutamic acid	GGA	Glycine
GUG	Valine	GCG	Alanine	GAG	Glutamic acid	GGG	Glycine

Each codon, or triplet of nucleotides in RNA, codes for an amino acid. Twenty different amino acids are produced from a total of 64 different RNA codons, but some amino acids are specified by more than one codon (e.g., phenylalanine is specified by UUU and UUC). In addition, one codon (AUG) specifies the start of a protein, and three codons (UAA, UAG, and UGA) specify the termination of a protein. Mutations in the nucleotide sequence can change the resulting protein structure if the mutation alters the amino acid specified by a codon or if it alters the reading frame by deleting or adding a nucleotide.

U = uracil (thymine) A = adenine C = cytosine G = guanine

(Sources: Office of Technology Assessment and National Institute of General Medical Sciences, 1988.) Table and legend from Office of Technology Assessment (1988, 23).

termediary between DNA and the synthesized protein: RNA differs from DNA in that uracil (U) substitutes for thymine. (Interestingly enough, the discovery of mRNA was predicted by the operon theory, my next example.) Nirenberg and Matthaei (1961), using a synthetic messenger composed of uracil bases (...UUU...) in an in vitro system, demonstrated that protein chains composed only of the amino acid phenylalanine were synthesized. This indicated that the RNA complementary to a DNA sequence of an adenine triple (...AAA...) would code for a specific amino acid (phenylalanine, or *phe* in abbreviated form). Extensive work by a number of researchers, including Crick et al. (1961), resulted in the complete deciphering of the genetic code, which is presented in terms of the RNA-amino acid relation in table 3.1.

It should be noted, on the basis of a large number of experiments using cell-free extracts from a number of animals, that it is currently believed that the genetic code is almost universal, the exceptions being a few changes occurring in the mitochondria of certain species (Watson, et al. 1987, 453–456). Watson et al. (1987, 453) have pointed out that it is expected the code would be strongly conserved on evolutionary grounds since a mutation in the code would almost certainly be lethal.

3.4.2. *The Operon Theory*

Our next example of a biological theory is drawn from regulatory genetics, which is primarily a subbranch of molecular biology. The theory, which is principally due to the work of Jacob and Monod (1961), developed over a number of years.[10] The initial form of the theory dates from 1960–61 and has had a most important impact on both experiment and theory construction in molecular biology (and in embryology). It has been extraordinarily well corroborated by a variety of experiments. It was further developed in the sixties, seventies, and eighties. Let me first briefly outline the operon theory as it is illustrated by the *lac* operon or the lactose metabolism controlling region of the genome of the bacterium *Escherichia coli (E. coli)*. I will then quote the manner in which the theory was introduced in a standard genetics textbook (Strickberger's 2d edition of his excellent *Genetics*), for reasons which will become clearer in the subsequent section.

The theory proposed the existence of a new class of genes, termed regulator genes, that were responsible for the synthesis of a substance (later determined for the *E. coli lac* operon to be a protein of about 160,000 molecular weight) termed a *repressor*. The repressor, in inducible systems such as the lactose metabolizing system of *E. coli*, binds specifically with a DNA region termed the *operator locus* or *operator gene*. (The normal or "wild type" form of this gene is designated as o^+.) This operator has adjacent to it several structural genes, which are under the operator's control. When the repressor is bound to the operator, the associated structural genes are not transcribed into messenger RNA, and accordingly no proteins or enzymes associated with those structural genes are synthesized. An *inducer* can specifically interact with the repressor, altering its three-dimensional structure and thus rendering it incapable of binding to the operator. The enzyme RNA polymerase, which attaches to a promoter gene in the presence of a protein called CRP,[11] and which can transcribe the structural genes, is then no longer prevented from initiating transcription of the structural genes adjacent to the operator, and mRNA synthesis and then protein synthesis commence. Repressible systems employ a similar regulatory logic, only in that case the initially ineffective repressor is aided in its operator-binding capacity by an exogenously added corepressor. It has been often noted by biologists that such a regulatory system is most useful to the organism since it allows unnecessary genes to be turned off when the proteinaceous enzyme products of those genes are not required for a metabolic process (see, e.g., Lewin, 1985, 221). This results in energy saving and is conceived of as evolutionarily useful to the organism.

The description of the *lac* system just sketched is oversimplified in a number of respects. In research articles and advanced textbooks such theories are introduced by describing not only the "wild type" form but also various mutations. I know of no more concise and clear account than that provided by Strickberger, who, in addition to his text discussion, also outlines the theme by diagrams (see figure 3.1 A and B) and summary comments as given in Technical Discussion 2.

TECHNICAL DISCUSSION 2

Scheme for the regulation of *lac* enzyme synthesis through transcription control . . . is explained . . . in figure [3.1A and B]. (a) In the absence of repressor, transcription of the *lac* operon is accomplished by the RNA polymerase enzyme which attaches at the promoter site (p)

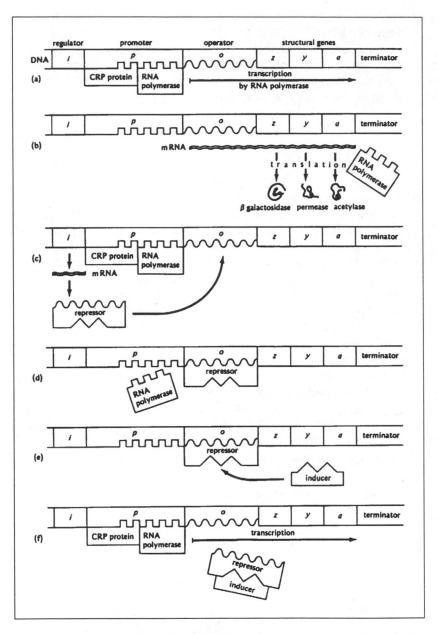

Figure 3.1 A. *lac* enzyme regulation and mutations (a–f). For details see Technical Discussion 2. Reprinted with the permission of the Macmillan Publishing Company from GENETICS, Second Edition, by Monroe W. Strickberger. Copyright © 1976 by Monroe W. Strickberger.

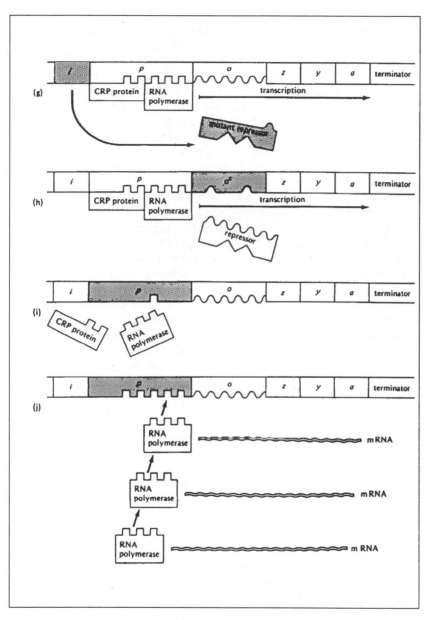

Figure 3.1 B *lac* enzyme regulation and mutations (g–j). For details see Technical Discussion 2. Reprinted with the permission of the Macmillan Publishing Company from GENETICS, Second Edition, by Monroe W. Strickberger. Copyright © 1976 by Monroe W. Strickberger.

Scheme for the regulation of *lac* enzyme synthesis through transcription control . . . is explained . . . in figure [3.1A and B]. (a) In the absence of repressor, transcription of the *lac* operon is accomplished by the RNA polymerase enzyme which attaches at the promoter site (p) in the presence of CRP [or CAP] protein, and then proceeds to transcribe the operator until it reaches the terminator sequence. (b) Subsequent translation of the *lac* mRNA leads to the formation of *lac* enzymes. (c) Synthesis of the *lac* repressor protein occurs via translation of an mRNA which is separately transcribed at the i regulator gene locus. (d) Attachment of the repressor protein to the operator prevents the polymerase enzyme from transcribing the operon. Some studies suggest that the repressor will also prevent the RNA polymerase from binding to the promoter. (e) An appropriate inducer attaches to a specific site on the allosteric repressor . . . causing it to change its shape and detach from the operator, thereby permitting transcription (f). In g–j the effects of various regulatory mutations (shaded sections) are shown: (g) A mutation of the regulator gene produces a repressor which is unable to bind to the operator thereby causing constitutive *lac* enzyme synthesis. (h) A mutation in the operator prevents binding of the repressor, and therefore also leads to constitutive enzyme synthesis. (i) A mutation or deletion in the promoter interferes with the attachment of RNA polymerase thus preventing transcription of the *lac* operon. (j) A mutation in the promoter ("up-promoter" mutation) . . . enables more rapid attachment of the RNA polymerase, thereby increasing the number of mRNA molecules and subsequent role of *lac* enzyme synthesis. "Down-promoter" mutations also exist which diminish the attachment rate of RNA polymerase, and some promoter mutations may reduce the requirement for cyclic AMP. (Strickberger 1976, 680–681)

One particularly important mutation encountered in the *lac* operon system is the o^c or constitutive operator mutation. This change in the DNA prevents binding of the repressor and results in continuous enzyme synthesis since the control system cannot be turned "off." In addition to these basic mutations described by Stickberger, it is important to note the even broader range of "mutant" types of *lac* operon systems that have been selected for by various investigators. For example, Gilbert and Müller-Hill (1970) recapitulate their superb work leading to the isolation of the repressor (this work is reviewed in chapter 4) and discuss *i* gene mutants of a variety of types: thermolabile (i^{TL}), temperature-sensitive synthesis (i^{TSS}), high quantity repressor (i^Q), very

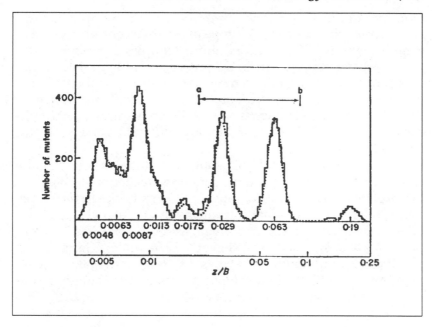

Figure 3.2 Variations of o^c mutations (from Smith and Sadler, 1971, p. 284.) Reprinted with permission.

high quantity repressor (i^{superQ}), and constitutive dominants (i^{-d}), in addition to the so-called normal or wild type i^+ and those mutations known to Jacob and Monod, including constitutive (i^-) (represented in figure 3.1 B [g]) and superrepressor (i^s). Jacob and Monod were also aware of a broad range of gene mutations, and in addition used several o gene mutations in their earlier investigation (such as the o^c mutation mentioned above and also by Strickberger in figure 3.1 B [h]).

The philosophical point to be made here is that there is a very wide range of subtle variations that occur in biological control systems even in the same type of organism. The extent of this variation is so broad that it even occurs *within* characteristically well-defined mutations. An excellent illustration of these superfine mutations appears in the work of Smith and Sadler (1971) on 590 o^c mutations. In figure 3.2, I represent the variety (almost continuity) of mutations of the o^c type. Such variation can be further underscored by noting that even the type of control found in the *lac* system, namely, negative control, varies in other operons in *E. coli*. In the *ara* (or arabinose) operon, for example, the operon control circuit involves a type of positive control in which a gene known as "*C*" produces, not a (simple) repressor, but a product that acts positively in the presence of arabinose to switch on production of three enzymes that catalyze the biosynthetic pathway leading from arabinose to more metabolizable breakdown substances.[12] This extensive variation has important implications for theory structure in biology and will be interpreted in that light in section 3.5.

There is an additional philosophical point occasioned by the operon theory. In contrast to the genetic code theory discussed in the previous subsection, the operon theory is clearly *interlevel*. This is a term that was first introduced by Beckner (1959, 37–38) in his analysis of models in biology, and the point has been appropriately restressed by Wimsatt (1974, 1976), Darden and Maull (1977), and Maull (1977); it is, I think, worth making again in connection with the issue of theory structure.[13] Though the entities such as operator, repressor-making gene (i^+), and the like are biochemical and have been completely sequenced,[14] the theory as originally presented involved entities specified on both genetic (e.g., *i* and *o* genes) and biochemical (e.g., messenger RNA) levels. (I will give a fuller explanation of the sense in which I use the term "interlevel" below after two additional interlevel examples have been introduced.)

3.4.3 *The Clonal Selection Theory*

The clonal selection theory was introduced in some detail earlier in chapter 2 above and is a useful example to employ in a discussion of theory structure. It will not be necessary to represent the theory in any detail again, but the reader may wish to review the discussion in the previous chapter to refresh his or her memory of the basic elements of that theory.

From the point of view of theory structure, the clonal selection theory has several very interesting features. First, like the operon theory, it is interlevel: It borrows from molecular characterizations (antibody), from genetics, and from cell theory. Second, the theory can be roughly axiomatized, as in Burnet's concise formulation given on page 41 of chapter 2. Its having this feature indicates that in certain circumstances there will be a "sharpening" of the subtle variation mentioned above in connection with the range of mutations in the operon theory. Such variation often makes it difficult to provide clear models or theories which hold in a variety of organisms within a species and across species, but at certain levels of abstraction the variation may sufficiently sharpen. I would speculate that such sharpenings (akin to those situations in the statistical theory of quantum mechanics which produce sharp results, such as the energy levels in the hydrogen atom) are a consequence of universal molecular mechanisms and strong evolutionary pressures tending to eliminate variation at the level under consideration. Such "sharpening" is not very mysterious; causally it may be understood here as the (natural) selection at some specified level of a very narrow range of variation from a set of more diffuse possibilities.

Another, more epistemic way to conceive of this sharpening might be to imagine the effect of superimposing a variety of specific models (based on a range of strains of the same organisms) at various levels of aggregation and looking for features common to (almost) all the models. Those features which are (almost) universal represent the "sharp" aspects. These sharp aspects may exist at one level of aggregation (or a level of abstraction) but not at others in the same system. Thus, though there is apparently a large amount of variation in the individual antibody types among individuals in a species (and among species), the general mechanism by which antigen stimulates antibody production is not variable. This is no doubt due in part to the (probably) universal character of the genetic code and protein synthesis which imposes considerable restrictions on mechanisms for the synthesis of antibody (a protein), and also to the strong evolutionary advantage enjoyed by those organisms which were the first to generate an antibody synthesizing (and immune response) capacity. Such an evolutionary argument would also have to show that mutations at the level under discussion would be lethal. From a speculative point of view, however, this is likely because of the damage that modifications to the immune system can wreak on their hosts—infection, autoimmune diseases, and the phenomenon of anaphylactic shock being primary examples.

A third important feature of the clonal selection theory lies in its clear "ontogenetic" dimension. An explicit part of the theory (postulate 5 on p. 41) introduces a mechanism for generating antibody diversity ontogenetically.[15] This feature can be generalized to bring out an aspect that is also implicit in the two theories previously considered (though more so in the overall theory of protein synthesis than in that specific part of it dealing with the genetic code), namely, that biological theories are usually given in the form of a series of temporal (and frequently *causal*) models. In physics, time is usually eliminated by making it implicit in differential equations, whereas in biology a temporal process, such as the sequence of events representing transcription and translation of the genetic code in protein synthesis, or the prising off of the repressor from the operator, is the rule. Such a temporal model appears not only in the course of theorizing about the development of antibody diversity but also in the fuller version of the clonal selection theory when the course of lymphocyte differentiation into plasma cells and the liberation of soluble antibody are considered.

3.4.4 *The Two-Component Theory of the Immune Response*

Our next example of a biological theory is also from the discipline of immunology.[16] This theory, however, is perhaps more closely associated with the clinical side of the biomedical sciences than the three previous examples, and it also exhibits more clearly a multi-level structure, involving biochemical, cellular, tissue, organ, and systemic (most specifically the blood and lymphatic system) features. The rudiments of the theory had two (or three) independent origins, which were first clearly articulated in the 1960s. For our purposes, the theory culminates in the important cellular distinction between T (thymus-derived) cells and B (bursa or bursa-equivalent) cells and the synergistic interaction between them in the immune response. The theory continues to be further elaborated at all levels, and there is sound evidence that a full understanding of its various components will lead to more rational therapies in the areas of organ transplantation rejection, cancer, and autoimmune diseases, such as lupus and rheumatoid arthritis. Already the theory has allowed the clearer interpretation of a wide range of immune deficiency diseases and has served as the intellectual source for successful life-saving treatments, including thymus and bone-marrow transplants. I will not have the opportunity in this brief summary of the theory to discuss these implications, tests, and applications of the theory, and I also can do no more than cite sources discussing the historical origins and elaboration of the theory (see Good and Gabrielsen 1964; Miller 1971).

The theory had what might be called its protosource in a chance finding of Glick, Chang, and Japp (1956) that a hindgut organ in birds known as the bursa of Fabricius had an important immunological function (see Glick 1964). This had been overlooked by numerous previous investigators because bursectomy only affects the immune system if it is done very early in life. Glick's work was further developed in Wolfe's laboratory at Wisconsin (see Mueller, Wolfe, and Meyer 1960), and the same principle — early or neonatal organ ablation — was then applied to the thymus, another organ with a then-unknown function, in the early 1960s by Archer and Pierce (1961) and Good, Martinez, and Gabrielsen (1964). This research, carried out in Good's laboratory at the University of Minnesota, had its groundwork prepared by an observation by Good in 1956 that an instance of a broadly based immunodeficiency disease was associated with a tumor of that patient's thymus gland (see MacLean, Zac, Varco, and Good 1956). Initial attempts by Good and his colleagues to associate thymectomy with immunodeficiency were not successful for the same reason that bursectomy beyond an early stage of development had failed to reveal the immunological function of the bursa.

The immunological function of the thymus was also discovered independently by J. F. A. P. Miller, who was working along an initially different line of research, attempting to determine the effects of thymectomy on virus-induced leukemia in mice. Miller (1961) noticed a wasting effect of neonatal thymectomy in his mice, and quickly determined by additional research that the thymus played an important immunological role in both graft rejection and lymphocyte production. Miller's work was particularly clear and is discussed in more detail in chapter 4, where we consider hypothesis and theory testing. A third possibly independent line of research culminating in a determination of the immune function of the thymus was pursued by Waksman and his colleagues at Harvard.[17] In late 1962, Warner and Szenberg (1962, 1964) proposed the "hypothesis" of "dissociation of immunological responsiveness," suggesting that the thymus was responsible for homograft immunity and the bursa for the production of antibody-producing cells. This notion was further clarified by other investigators and was termed the "two-component concept of the immune system" by Peterson, Cooper, and Good (1965). The importance of the synergistic interaction of the two systems and their cellular components was discovered by Claman, Chaperon, and Triplett (1966). The theory as presently conceived is outlined in simplified form in figure 3.3. (It should

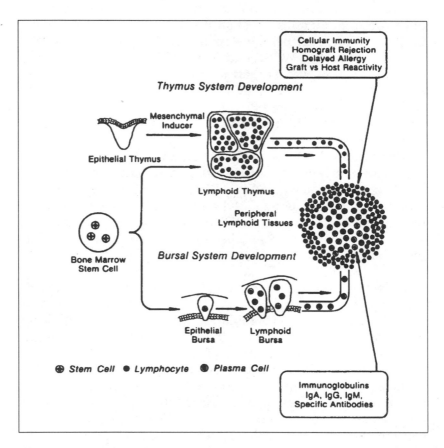

Figure 3.3 The two-component theory. "The two branches of the immune mechanism are believed to develop from the same lymphoid precursor. The central thymus system starts as an epithelial structure arising from the third and fourth embryonic pharyngeal pouches and becomes a lymphoid organ under stimulation by a mesenchymal inducer. The bursal system develops by budding from the intestinal epithelium. After release from the central organs into the bloodstream, the lymphoid cells reassemble in peripheral lymphoid tissues. Here the lymphocytes—thymus-dependent in origin—control cellular immunity, while bursa-dependent plasma cells synthesize serum antibodies." Reprinted with modifications, by permission, from R. A. Good, "Disorders of the Immune System" in *Immunobiology*, ed. R. A. Good and D. W. Fisher (Stamford, CT, 1971), 9. (Readers should be aware that immunology has become considerably more complex in the years since 1971. See Barrett [1988] or the very accessible articles on immunology in many recent issues of the *Scientific American*.)

be stressed that cellular [and molecular] interactions in immunology have become extraordinarily complex in the past thirty years, and this diagram is *very* much simplified in comparison with current knowledge.) To date no bursa equivalent in mammals has been discovered, and most investigators believe that bone marrow–derived cells can become B cells without a bursa equivalent.

The two-component theory is confirmed both by a wide range of experiments in the laboratory and by clinical findings. Immunology straddles the disciplines of biology and clinical medicine, and in its latter aspect had, by 1970, effected a reconceptualization of immune deficiency diseases in humans on the part of the World Health Organization (Fudenberg 1970) (see table 3.2).

The theory illustrates some of the previously asserted philosophical points concerning theory structure in biology and medicine in a different manner from the earlier examples. First, it should be noted that this theory is vigorously interlevel and contains entities which are biochemical and molecular (antibody molecules for which a full sequence of amino acids has been worked out), cellular (lymphocytes and plasma cells), tissue level (peripheral lymphoid tissue), organ level (thymus), and systemic (lymphatic system, circulatory system). Second, the *evolutionary* variation associated with the theory should be noted: The thymus is present in all organisms evolutionarily distal to the lamprey eel, but the lack of a bursa in mammals also underscores variation at the organ level. The range of diseases cited in table 3.2 illustrates the more extreme types of variation that can occur in humans. In addition to these features, it should be briefly noted that there is both an ontogenetic and a phylogenetic aspect to the theory. The ontogeny is illustrated in figure 3.3, and the continuing process of stem-cell differentiation has been confirmed in adult life in irradiated mice (see Miller, Doaks, and Cross 1963). The ontogenetic and phylogenetic roles of the thymus and the cellular immune system as a defense against neoplasms have figured extensively in the literature (see, e.g., Burnet 1968, Smith and Landy 1975) but cannot be examined here. Finally, it should be pointed out that this theory is closely integrated into immunology as a whole and also into general biology. It is difficult to separate out this theory from an analysis of antibody structure, from the clonal selection theory, from the

TABLE 3.2   CLASSIFICATION OF PRIMARY
IMMUNODEFICIENCY DISORDERS

Type	Suggested Cellular Defect		
	B Cells	T Cells	Stem Cells
Infantile X-linked agammaglobulinemia	+	...	...
Selective immunoglobulin deficiency (IgA)	+*	...	...
Transient hypogammaglobulinemia of infancy	+	...	...
X-linked immunodeficiency with hyper-IgM	+*	...	...
Thymic hypoplasia (pharyngeal pouch syndrome, DiGeorge)	...	+	...
Episodic lymphopenia with lymphocytoxin	...	+	...
Immunodeficiency with normal or hyperimmunoglobulinemia	+	+**	...
Immunodeficiency with ataxia telangiectasia	+ .	+	...
Immunodeficiency with thrombocytopenia and eczema (Wiskott-Alderich)	+	+	...
Immunodeficiency with thymoma	+	+	...
Immunodeficiency with short-limbed dwarfism	+	+	...
Immunodeficiency with generalized hematopoietic hypoplasia	+	+	+
Severe combined immunodeficiency: Autosomal recessive	+	+	+
X-linked	+	+	+
Sporadic	+	+	+
Variable immunodeficiency (largely unclassified)	+	+**	...

* Involve some but not all B cells.
** Encountered in some but not all patients.
Source: Fudenberg et al. (1970). Adapted from information appearing in *The New England Journal of Medicine*, Fudenberg et. al., 1970, "Classification of the Primary Immune Deficiencies: WHO Recommendation," 283, p. 656.

role of the HLA system in immunogenetics, from the role of other cells such as macrophages, and so on, not to mention its *connection* to genetics, to a theory of protein synthesis, and to a theory of evolution. This point cannot be appropriately developed even in a book of this size, but a review of Good (1971) and Watson et al. (1987) will support the thesis. The theory in its multiple interconnections thus illustrates, in a rather different biomedical discipline, Beckner's (and Arber's) point made earlier that theory in biology is "less linear" and "more reticulate" than is physical theory. In fact, the two-component theory displays "reticularity" in two different dimensions: horizontal in its interconnections with other biological theories and fields at the same level, for example, cell biology within and without immunology, and *vertical* in its interconnection with systems at different levels of aggregation as depicted in figure 3.3.

3.4.5 *The Theory of Evolution and Population Genetics*

As discussed in the earlier sections, it is one of the theses of this chapter that overconcentration on evolutionary theory and on population genetics has introduced a bias (in the statistical sampling sense) into analysis of theory structure in biology and medicine. This bias is also accentuated by a concentration of philosophers of biology on the simpler representations of population genetics; if a richer, more detailed perspective on population genetics were presented I believe we would find that even population genetics would be shown to have a number of features in common with the "middle-range" theories discussed above.

Evolutionary theory will have three functions in this section. First, I shall argue that evolutionary theory plays an important *metatheoretical* role in that it justifies central features of theories at *all* levels of biology and medicine. Second, the theory can be argued to have a universality at the most general level that is probably only mimicked at the "lowest" molecular level, typified by my earlier example of the genetic code. Because of this universality, the theory in its most general terms has unrepresentative features such as prima facie universality, lack of polytypy, and in its simplified textbook population-genetics aspects, overly neat mathematical axiomatizability. Third, I shall argue, following some of the work of Levins (1968), that close attention to the workings of evolutionary biologists on population genetics, not in the introductory textbook versions but on the forefront of research, would disclose that even population genetics lacks the neat mathematical axiomatizability and broad universality that matches the generality found in the axiomatic theoretical structures of the physical sciences. I do not intend to present a comprehensive introduction to evolutionary theory either in this chapter or in this book; see chapter 1 for the scope of this book and pointers to the vast literature on evolutionary theory. I do think, however, that the sections immediately below, as well as the discussions of evolutionary theory in chapters 7 and 8, will suffice to clarify my various points about the roles of evolutionary theory.

The Metatheoretical Function of Evolutionary Theory

We have seen in several of the examples mentioned above that evolutionary theory often functions as background, providing a degree of intelligibility for components of a theory. Recall, for example, that the (near) universality of the genetic code was explained evolutionarily, that the *lac* operon was conceived to have evolutionary advantages, that the "sharpness" of the clonal selection theory was justified evolutionarily, and that cell-mediated immunity was seen to confer important survival benefits as a defense against neoplasms in multicellular organisms. Evolutionary theory also allows us to understand why there is subtle variation in the organisms: Variation due to meiosis, mutation, and genetic drift, for example, should occur most frequently in evolving populations where strong selection pressures toward sharpness (involving lethal variations) are not present. Thus evolutionary theory at a very general level explains some of the specific and general features of other theories in biology and medicine.

The Unrepresentativeness of Evolutionary Theory

In part because of the generality of the theory of evolution — it does apply to all known organisms — the theory possesses certain atypical features when compared with theories such as the operon theory and the two-component theory of the immune response cited above. The factors underlying subtle variation that is responsible for blurring the universal applicability and clarity of those theories are made explicit in and explained by evolutionary theory in terms of mutations, genetic reshuffling (meiosis), genetic drift, migration, and other processes causing genetic change. In addition to (and perhaps because of?) the universality and the explicit incorporation of variation, the theory in certain of its aspects possesses a precision that permits mathematical axiomatizability and allows one to bring the powerful apparatus of deductive mathematical proof to bear on its elaboration and systematization. This is especially true if one confines one's attention to the "simpler" models in population genetics. Though population genetics is not, as Lewontin remarks, "the entire soup of evolutionary theory," it is, as he notes, "*an* essential ingredient" (Lewontin 1974, 12). (The extent to which population genetics constitutes a "core" in evolutionary theory has become quite controversial in recent work in philosophy of biology. These arguments and counterarguments are somewhat complex and do not affect the main theses of the present chapter, however, and thus further discussion of them can most fruitfully be postponed until chapter 7.)

Regardless of what position one takes on this recent controversy, however, because of the central importance of population genetics in evolutionary theory, it would be useful to discuss the theory briefly. In chapter 7 I will elaborate on the theory in considerably more detail.

The axioms of population genetics. There is a variety of ways in which one can represent population genetics. One of the most elegant presentations has been given by Jacquard (1974), and it is his representation which I will use in this subsection. One of the more interesting and elegant features of Jacquard's account is the presentation of six axioms that together entail Hardy-Weinberg equilibrium, followed by the demonstration that systematic progressive weakening of each of the axioms is sufficient to introduce the causes of evolutionary change. The approach also permits one in a very natural way to introduce one of the simplest but most powerful models of conjoint evolutionary change, due to Wright (1931, 1949).[18] Jacquard's axioms are as follows:

(1) Migration [into and out of the population] does not occur.

(2) Individuals from different generations do not breed together.

(3) Mutations do not occur.

(4) There is no selection [i.e.,] . . . the number of offspring an individual has is independent of his genotype at the locus in question.

(5) For the locus in question, mates are genetically independent of one another. [This condition can be strengthened to require that "mating is at random."]

(6) The population size is so large it can be treated as infinite. (Jacquard 1974, 42–48)

These assumptions, plus the background theory of Mendelian genetics, including its law of segregation applied to a single genetic locus, suffice for the demonstration of the Hardy-Weinberg principle that both gene frequencies and genotype frequencies will remain constant in successive generations. This formulation of population genetics is not only able to express the important Hardy-Weinberg condition of equilibrium in quantitative terms; it is also able to represent more realistic departures from axioms (1)–(6) in a quantitative manner. Some relatively simple complications which allow for easily computable variations from the Hardy-Weinberg situation are to be found when one considers sex-linked genes and multiple genetic loci. (In the latter case, for example, it can be shown that multifactorial genotypes gradually approach genetic equilibrium over many generations, rather than one, as in the case of a single locus.)[19]

Evolution and the Wright model. More interesting deviations from Hardy-Weinberg equilibrium occur in cases of evolution, which population genetics treats largely as the genetic change of a population. Population genetics specifies several causes of evolution, which can be associated with relaxations of some of axioms (1)–(6) presented above. For example:

(1) Migration is a relaxation of condition (1).
(2) Mutation is a relaxation of condition (3).
(3) Selection is a relaxation of condition (4).
(4) Mating influences by kinship represent a relaxation of condition (5).
(5) Genetic drift appears as a relaxation of condition (6) to allow consideration of finite populations.

These various agents of evolution can be characterized quantitatively; for example, the action of selection is normally introduced quantitatively with the help of the concept of "fitness" or survival into the next generation of a genotype. The effects of the various agents, quantitatively construed, can be brought together and represented as a general equation of motion, analogous to Newton's second law. Wright developed such a theory in the 1920s, which he later published (1931). It would take us beyond the scope of this chapter to present the mathematical axioms of Wright's theory, which will be developed in one form in chapter 7, but it will be instructive to refer to his general equation of motion for the reproductive unit at this point, as well as to indicate the strong analogies which this approach has with the physical sciences. Technical Discussion 3 below provides enough of the details of this analysis to indicate these parallels.

TECHNICAL DISCUSSION 3

Wright's equation of motion may be written, following Jacquard (1974), as:

$$\Delta p + \delta p = -\mu p + \lambda (1-p) + p(1-p)(t+wp) + \delta p \tag{1}$$

In this equation, Δ represents a small one-generational change, and p is the frequency of an allele at a specific genetic locus, whose other allele is $q = 1 - p$; δ_p represents the effect of chance fluctuations in gene frequency as a result of finite population size and mathematically captures the notion of "genetic drift"; p can be set equal to dp/dt "to obtain the approximate amount of change in a given number of generations (t) by integration" (Wright 1949, 369); μ and λ are simple functions of the mutation and migration rates, and t and w are relatively simple approximate functions of the selection coefficients (representing "fitness") but modified by a factor which takes nonrandom mating into account. The elements represented by p are, Jacquard notes, "fully deterministic when *p* is known, but the last term, δ_p, is a random variable" (Jacquard 1974, 391).

The solution of equation (1) above introduces some interesting additional features of population genetics which have not been commented on in the philosophical literature.[20] The variable p is assumed to be approximately continuous, on the hypothesis that the population size, N, though finite, is sufficiently large; $\Phi(p,g)dp$ is introduced as the probability that the frequency of a gene, say A_p, is between p and p + dp in generation *g*. Thus $\Phi(p,g)dp$ is a solution of equation (1). It can be shown that this equation indicates that the frequency $p_g + 1$ (in the next generation) is a binomial distribution with a specific expectation and variance. The terms p_g in successive generations are elements of a series of random variables and related by the transition law expressed by equation (1), which is equivalent to a Markov process. If p_g is not given, but a prior distribution represented by $\Phi(p, g)$ is specified, then the frequency of the distribution in the next generation g + 1 is given by:

$$\Phi(p, g+1) = \int_0^1 \Phi(x, g) f(x, p) \, dx \tag{2}$$

where f(x, p) is the probability that a gene frequency of x will shift to the frequency p in one generation. It can also be shown that f(x,p) is a binomial distribution with a known mean ($x_g + x_p$) and known variance $[x_g(1 - x_g)]/2N_e$, where N_e is the "effective" population number.

Now if the change in gene frequency in one generation is very small, the discrete time process can be approximated by a continuous process, and if in addition higher-order terms involving $f(x, p)$ are ignored, a fundamental equation known as the "diffusion equation" can be obtained for Φ (x, g) (for the derivation see Crow and Kimura 1970):

$$\frac{\partial}{\partial g} [\int_0^1 \Phi (x,g) \, dx] = \frac{1}{2} \{ \frac{\partial}{\partial p} [V (p,q) \Phi (p,q)] \} - \Delta \, p \, \Phi (p,q). \qquad (3)$$

This diffusion equation is analogous to equations in physics representing Brownian movement and other random processes. It can also be solved in a number of important special simple cases yielding accounts of specific genetic changes in equilibrium involving various population structures, such as the probability of a gene's survival, and the mean time that it takes for a neutral gene to become fixed or become extinct in a population (see Crow and Kimura 1970 and Kimura and Ohta 1971 for details).

The development of Wright's theory as elaborated in Technical Discussion 3 demonstrates the strong analogies which this type of evolutionary theory has to physical theories such as Newtonian mechanical theory and suggests, perhaps, why philosophers of biology who focus on such exemplars can be misled about the more typical structure of biological theories.

The Complexity of More Realistic Evolutionary Theories of Population Genetics

The presentation of the theory of population genetics outlined above, including the Wright model and an outline of some approximate solutions of general equation (1) via diffusion equation (3), might lead the reader to the conclusion that population genetics is clearly a theory like theories in the physical and chemical sciences. One has clear axioms, and one can use powerful mathematical techniques to develop consequences. In addition, the theory is unilevel, making use of genetic entities. I have, however, outlined only an introductory core of classical and neoclassical population genetics, and further exploration of the field would disclose that in reality there is a variety of models constructed to analyze genes in evolution. An excellent summary of the approach to theory construction in population genetics can be found in Levins 1968, and it is worth quoting him *in extenso* on these matters. Levins writes:

3. The basic unit of theoretical investigation is the model, which is a reconstruction of nature for the purpose of study. The legitimacy or illegitimacy of a particular reconstruction depends on the purpose of the study, and the detailed analysis of a model for purposes other than those for which it was constructed may be as meaningless as studying a map with a microscope.

4. . . . . A model is built by a process of abstraction which defines a set of sufficient parameters on the level of study, a process of simplification which is intended to leave intact the essential aspects of reality while removing distracting elements, and by the addition of patently unreal assumptions which are needed to facilitate study.

6. . . . . There is no single, best all-purpose model. In particular, it is not possible to maximize simultaneously generality, realism, and precision. The models which are in current use among applied ecologists usually sacrifice generality for realism and precision; models proposed by those who enter biology by way of physics often sacrifice realism to generality and precision. . . . A theory is a cluster of models and their robust consequences. [A robust consequence is a consequence "which can be proved by means of different models having in common the aspects of reality under study but differing in other details."] The constituent models fit together in several ways:

   (a) as alternative schemes for testing robustness;

   (b) as partially overlapping models which test the robustness of their common conclusions but also can give independent results;

   (c) in a nested hierarchy, in which lower-level models account for the sufficient parameter taken as given on a higher level;

   (d) as models differing in generality, realism, and precision (unlike the situation in formal mathematics, in science the general does not fully contain the particular as a special case. The loss of information in the process of ascending levels requires that auxiliary models be developed to return to the particular. Therefore, the "application" of a general model is not intellectually trivial, and the terms "higher" and "lower" refer not to the ranking of difficulties or of the scientists working at these levels but only levels of generality);

(e) as samples spanning the universe of possible models. (Levins 1968, 6–8)

In addition, Levins (1968) presents a summary picture of some of the relations among various components of evolutionary population biology theory. This picture is reproduced as figure 3.4, and discloses, together with the long quotation above, that population genetics in its rich reality is closer to the philosophical picture of theories in biology and medicine sketched in exam-

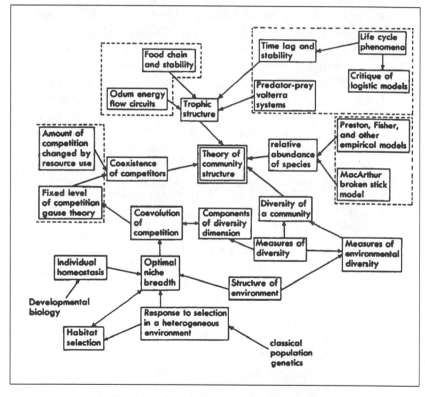

Figure 3.4 Relations among some of the components in evolutionary population biology theory. From Levins (1968, 430), © *American Scientist*, with permission.

ples in sections 3.4.2–3.4.4, in terms of its complexity and reticularity, than a more elementary or even advanced but narrowly focused perspective would indicate. This point is also a thesis developed in Beatty (1992).

3.5 "Middle-Range" Theories as Overlapping Interlevel Temporal Models

In this section I will attempt to extract some distinctions and generalizations from the examples discussed in the previous section. The first distinction which I think would be useful to make is a three-fold one between (1) biochemically universal theories, (2) theories of the "middle range" (with indebtedness for the term to R. K. Merton),[21] and (3) evolutionary theories.

The development of the notion of middle-range theories in biology and medicine is an attempt to specify and characterize a class of theories that I believe is prevalent in biology and medicine and that is typically represented by our examples in sections 3.4.2 through 3.4.4. The philosophically interesting features of this class of theories can be articulated both negatively (by distinguishing the characteristics from those in classes 1 and 3 in the previous paragraph) and positively (by enumerating the common characteristics found in the middle-range theories). In the following paragraphs, both positive and negative approaches will be taken.

It is a thesis of the present chapter that most theories propounded in biology and medicine are not now and will not in the foreseeable future be "universal" theories.[22] By universal I am here confining the scope of the theories to organisms available on earth. There are some important exceptions, and we have examined two in the previous section: the theory of protein synthesis and the genetic code appear to be essentially universal on earth—with a few exceptions in mitochondria—(and may even be so extraterrestrially). In addition, at the level of abstraction and simplification of the simplest theories of population genetics we are also likely to find universality (even extraterrestrially, since it is difficult to imagine a natural process producing organisms which is not based on Darwinian evolution).[23] However, I view these at least terrestrially universal theories, which have been taken as typical of theories in biology and medicine, as unrepresentative. I would suggest instead that most theories that are currently proposed and will be proposed in the areas of genetics, embryology, immunology, the neurosciences, and the like will be middle-range theories that are nonuniversal in the sense to be described. First, however, I need to discuss the general feature of middle-range theories.

The bulk of biomedical theories can be, I would maintain, best characterized as a series of overlapping interlevel temporal models. These theories also fall into what I term the "middle range." Each of the phrases in this characterization needs unpacking.

Theories in the middle range fall between biochemistry at one extreme and evolutionary theory at the other extreme on the continuum of levels of aggregation, from molecules to populations (albeit of the genic structure of the populations).[24] Components of such theories are usually presented as temporal models, namely, as collections of entities that undergo a process. The entities that appear in the model are idealized representations in the sense that they are partially abstracted from the full richness of biological details (at each entity's own level). The models as a whole are usually interlevel. In the characterization of such a middle-range theory, not all possible (or even existing) model variants are usually described explicitly. Rather, a subset of variants of the models are selected to constitute *prototypes* that represent the most *typical* of the wild-type and mutant models. It is these prototypes that "overlap" with respect to their assumptions.[25]

In established usage employed in the biomedical sciences, the term "model" usually refers to rather specific systems found in particular strains of organisms. Thus the *lac* operon in inducible (z^+) K 12 *E. coli* with "wild-type" β-galactosidase (z^+) and galactoside permease (y^+) is a model. As mentioned above, however, such models vary by mutation in closely related strains, such as the constitutive (i^-) and (o^c) strains of *E. coli*. This fact of variation, especially the extraordinary range and subtlety of the variation as indicated in the (o^c) mutations depicted in figure 3.2, suggests that we might usefully begin to represent the variation by first identifying the most *typical* variants as *pure-type models* or prototypes. These pure- or ideal-type models are the kind represented pictorially in figure 3.1. A linguistic representation could also be constructed and could even be presented in rough axiomatic form. These possibilities raise the question of theory representation in a rather general way, a topic to which I will now turn.[26]

3.6 The Semantic Approach to Scientific Theories

As an abstraction, the linguistic (or pictorial) representation can be said to *define*, in an implicit sense, the kind of systems to which it applies. Particularizing the pure-type abstraction by adding initial conditions of time, space, temperature, pH, and the like, one can construct a set of *abstract replicas* of empirically given or "phenomenal systems" (see Suppe 1974, 48).[27] Those abstract replica systems that satisfy the general linguistic representation can also be characterized as a class of what Suppe terms "theoretically induced models." It will then be an *empirical* question whether the *empirically given* systems or phenomenal systems are adequately modeled by those abstract replicas.

This rough characterization represents what has been termed by philosophers of science a *semantic conception of a scientific theory*. This approach to analyzing scientific theories was initially proposed by Beth (1949) and developed independently by Suppes (1957, 1964), Suppe (1974, 1977), and van Fraassen (1970, 1980) and has more recently been applied to biological theories by Giere (1979), Beatty (1981), Lloyd (1984, 1988), and Thompson (1984, 1989). At the moment I am only applying it to *pure* types, in the sense of prototypical biological models (and even this application will require a more developed formulation than I gave immediately above), but later in the discussion this restriction to pure types will be relaxed to accommodate variation. Even in this restricted application, however, there are certain advantages of the semantic conception over the traditional view which may be briefly mentioned. Let me review some of those advantages and then define the general notions more precisely.

First, the traditional "received view" of theories mentioned on page 66 characterized scientific theories primarily as *linguistic* structures in terms of a small set of sentences—the axioms—which would then be formalized. This required investigators to capture *the* form of a scientific theory; it is generally felt, however, that there are several *different* linguistic means of representing a theory, which is in point of fact an *extra*linguistic entity (Suppe 1974; 1977, 45). Second, emphasis on the linguistic form of a theory required some basic logic—usually the first order predicate calculus with identity—in which to express the theory.

This not only was clumsy but resulted in an impoverishment of theoretical language, since set theoretic language is richer than, say, first-order logic. In the semantic conception, though a clear characterization of the systems at an abstract level is essential, standard mathematical and biological English—as well as pictorial representations and computer languages—can be utilized. This is a most important point and I shall rely on it further subsequently, using some computer languages to give us a better purchase on biomedical theories.[28] Various equivalence arguments for syntactic and semantic approaches can be adduced, such as the fact that "an axiomatic theory may be characterized by its class of interpretations and an interpretation may be characterized by the set of sentences which it satisfies" (van Fraassen 1970). And, as van Fraassen notes,

> These interrelations, and the interesting borderline techniques provided by Carnap's method of state-descriptions and Hintikka's method of model sets, would make implausible any claim of philosophical superiority for either approach. But the questions asked and methods used are different, and with respect to fruitfulness and insight they may not be on a par with specific contexts or for special purposes. (1970, 326) [29]

Paul Thompson, in his recent monograph, differs with this view. Admitting that even in his 1985 essay on the subject he viewed the difference between the syntactic and semantic approaches to a scientific theory as primarily "heuristic and methodological," he writes in his 1989 monograph that his previous position "underestimates the difference between the two views. The fundamental logical difference is the way in which the semantics is provided" (1989, 73). I am not persuaded by Thompson's arguments, which develop this stronger position. Basically, Thompson maintains that the syntactic conception of a scientific theory employs a rather weak notion of "correspondence rule" to provide its semantics, whereas the semantic conception provides the semantics "directly by defining a mathematical model" (1989, 73). This is, however, only part of the semantics, and as we shall see in chapter 4, after additional requirements for theory testability are specified, the strong contrast is not supportable. Nevertheless, I do agree with Thompson and others on the flexibility and fertility arguments in favor of the semantic conception; it is easier to work with a theory that is not formulated in first order logic, and the naturalness of "model" language permits more facile elaboration and analysis.

Let me now further elaborate on the semantic approach to theory structure I want to employ. There are two general subapproaches to developing the semantic conception that have been advanced by its proponents, known as the "set-theoretic" and the "state space" analyses. Each is most suitable for a somewhat different area of implementation. Both have been discussed in the philosophy of biology literature, Beatty developing the set-theoretic approach in his 1981 and Lloyd favoring the state space account in her 1983 and 1988. Both are easily applied to versions of evolutionary theory. I shall begin with a general version of the state space account favored by van Fraassen (1970) and Suppe (1974b, 1989)[30] which is perhaps more intuitive, and then outline the somewhat more abstract set-theoretic approach developed by Suppes (1957), Sneed (1971), and Giere (1979, 1984).

3.6.1 *The State Space Approach*

We may define a *state space* in order to represent, in an abstract fashion, the states of a class of possible abstract models. This notion of state space needs to be taken in a very general sense to include not only standard metrical spaces such as Euclidean phase spaces and Hilbert spaces but also nominal and semiquantitative ordinal spaces, which are important in biology and medicine. The properties used to construct the state space have been termed by Suppe *the defining parameters of the theory*. Once the state space is constructed, one can then interpret those connected laws or generalizations, which constitute a theory, as representing restrictions on that state space. As an example, confining our attention to prototype (or pure–type) forms in the operon theory such as (o^+) and (i^+) wild types, we would need a state space defined by i^+ genes, o^+ genes, two repressor states, and inducer concentrations, which allows one to represent *at least* the states of repression and induction of the operon. These restricted regions of state space for induced and repressed operons would give us a representation of what have been termed "laws of coexistence" for biological models. We can say similarly that what "laws of succession" have as their biological model analogue here is a selection of the physically possible trajectories in the state space, as systems evolve in the state space over time. The constituent restrictions of the model tell us what happens, for example, when an inducer is added and inducer concentration exceeds that threshold value above which the repressor is prised off the operator.

The above representation of laws of coexistence and laws of succession obtains not only in deterministic systems but also in statistical systems. There, however, laws of coexistence are represented by sets of prior probabilities of the state variables and laws of succession by a transition–probability matrix relating successive states of the system.

In addition to a state space we also require a set of determinable biological properties — possibly magnitudes — in order to characterize the empirical components of the systems in this state space. These properties (whether they be continuous, discrete or dichotomous) are used to construct what has been termed variously "the set of *elementary statements* (E) about the systems (of the theory)" (van Fraassen 1970, 328) or elementary propositions (Suppe 1974, 50). These elementary statements or propositions roughly represent the "observation language" of the theory, though that interpretation can be misleading. The elementary statements assert in this context that a biological parameter has a biological quantity or quality q as its value at time t. Whether the elementary statements are *true* depends on the state of the system. One can define a mapping h(E), termed the *satisfaction function* by van Fraassen, which connects the state space with the elementary statements and "hence the mathematical model provided by the theory with empirical measurement results" (van Fraassen 1970, 329). The exact relation between elementary statements and actual experiments is complex, and though I shall return to this issue in chapter 4 where experiments are discussed, the reader must be referred to Suppe 1974 for a full discussion.

I have now introduced some simple pure type examples. It remains to be seen, however, if these notions can be applied to the interlevel and overlapping features of biomedical theories. These terms need further explication. The term "interlevel" here is being used to refer to entities grouped within a theory (or model) which are at different levels of aggregation. Roughly, an entity e_2 is at a higher level of aggregation than entity e_1 if e_2 has e_1 among its parts and the defining properties of e_2 are not simple sums of e_1's but require additional organizing relations. The notion of different levels of aggregation is a working intuitive one among biomedical scientists and has occupied the attention of a number of philosophers of biology, especially those with organismic tendencies. A clear exposition and useful examples can be found in Grobstein 1965 and in Wimsatt's 1976a and 1985. This rough characterization of levels of aggregation may not order entities in an unambiguous manner. There are also complexities associated with defining "parts." For searching analyses on this matter, see Simon (1962), Kauffman (1971), and Wimsatt (1974, 1976a). A definition of levels based on disciplinary lines (e.g., genetics, biochemistry) will not suffice, as N. L. Maull-Roth has pointed out (personal communication), since disciplines are usually interlevel (also see Maull-Roth writing as Maull 1977).

It will also be useful at this point to examine a more detailed characterization of the notion of "level." Wimsatt has suggested a kind of pragmatic notion of a level of organization in his 1976a:

> If the entities at a given level are clustered relatively closely together (in terms of size, or some other generalized distance measure in a phase space of their properties) it seems plausible to characterize a level as a *local maximum of predictability and regularity*. . . . [S]upposing that . . . regularity and predictability of interactions is graphed as a function of size of the interacting entity [for example,] . . . [t]he levels appear as periodic peaks, though of course they might differ in height or "sharpness." (Wimsatt 1976a, 238)

Wimsatt provides a graphical representation of this interpretation (1976a, 240) and also speculates on other, less "sharp" and less regular possibilities, where the utility of level individuation or separation would be much less valuable.

This pragmatic suggestion seems correct to me, and also suggests the reason why it is difficult to give any general and abstract definition of a level of aggregation, namely that a level of aggregation is heavily dependent on the generalizations and theories available to the working biomedical scientist.[31] Thus if we were to have no knowledge about the properties and functions of ribosomes, a ribosomal level of aggregation would not be one worth characterizing.

I do not see any difficulties with extending the semantic conception of theories, as outlined, to encompass interlevel theories. All that is required is that the appropriate interlevel parameters be utilized in defining the state space. The situation is not so straightforward, however, when it comes to dealing with the "overlapping" character of biomedical models. By the expression "a series of overlapping models," I intend that the subtle variation encountered in organisms, even in a specific strain, is presented as part of the theory, or at least part of the textual elaboration of the theory. Recall that we encountered this variation in the operon theory, in the different types of mutations and in the two types of control (negative and positive) to be found in operon systems, and in the two-component theory of the immune response, in that, for example, there is no mammalian "bursa." It is this variation which "smears out" the models and makes them more a family of overlapping models, each of which may be biochemically and genetically precise, but which collectively are prima facie related by similarity.[32] Some features of these models are more central, contained in (almost) all models — they can be termed "robust," following Levins (1966, 1968) — and are often introduced as part of the theory via a pure–type model such as the *lac* operon in (*i*+) *E. coli* organisms. These theories thus have a polytypic character, where "polytypic" can be defined following Beckner (1959), who notes:

> A class is ordinarily defined by reference to a set or properties which are both necessary and sufficient (by stipulation) for membership in the class. It is possible, however to define a group K in terms of a set G of properties $f_1, f_2, \ldots, f_n$ in a different [i.e., polytypic] manner. Suppose we have an aggregation of individuals (we shall not as yet call them a class) such that:
>
> (1) Each one possesses a large (but unspecified) number of the properties in G;
> (2) Each f in G is possessed by large numbers of these individuals; and
> (3) No f in G is possessed by every individual in the aggregate.
>
> By the terms of (3), no f is necessary for membership in this aggregate; and nothing has been said to either warrant or rule out the possibility that some f in G is sufficient for membership in the aggregate. Nevertheless, under some conditions the members would and should be regarded as a class K constituting the extension of a concept [C] defined in terms of the properties in G. (Beckner 1959, 22)

Now a concept C can be defined as polytypic with respect to the set G if it is definable in terms of the properties in G and its extension K meets conditions 1 and 2. Beckner introduces the notion of "*fully* polytypic with respect to G" if condition 3 is also met; however, we shall in general not need full polytypy in this inquiry since I think that full polytypy would usually take us outside of the realm of intelligible theory construction.[33]

Because of this polytypic character of biological theories, it is not very useful to attempt to axiomatize most middle-range theories precisely. In contrast to typical theories in the physical sciences that represent the "Euclidean ideal" — a simple and concise axiomatization which can be utilized to provide extensive deductive systematization of a domain — typical biomedical theories of the middle range would require a very complex repetitious axiomatization to capture the polytypic variation found in them. Though it is possible to speculate about extensions of the state space approach to scientific theories that might permit a felicitous representation of such middle-range theories (and I do so in the appendix to this chapter), it seems more natural to explore a generalization of the set-theoretic approach to the semantic analysis of scientific theories for possible alternatives.

3.6.2 *The Set-Theoretic Approach (in Generalized Form)*

Though the state space approach to scientific theorizing is the most useful in certain contexts, there is, as has been noted, an alternative to it that will be more useful to us in connection with representing the variation found in middle-range theories in biology and medicine. In point of fact, I will argue it is actually a generalization of the alternative, "set-theoretic" approach which will be of maximal utility in this connection. The "set-theoretic" approach takes its name from Suppes's preference for employing the vocabulary of set theory for articulating the axioms of any theory to be represented and for conjoining those axioms to constitute a "set-theoretic predicate" that is satisfied by those and only those systems in which the axioms are (jointly) true. The set-theoretic predicate thus defines a class of models that satisfy the set-theoretic predicate.

Now, set-theoretic vocabulary seems more appropriate in the physical (and mathematical) sciences than in the biomedical arena, even though the language of biomedicine could be translated into set-theoretic vocabulary (and in fact has been for some theories).[34] It seems more natural to me, and useful as well given the "frame system" approach to be developed in the next section, to employ a generalization of Suppes's set-theoretic approach and simply, following Giere (1984), to introduce the notion of a "theoretical model" as "a kind of system whose characteristics are specified by an explicit definition" (1984, 80). This way of characterizing the systems in which we are interested is looser than Suppes's, which uses set-theoretic language, but it is in the same spirit. It does not obviate the need to specify precisely the principles that characterize (define) the theoretical model, but it does not commit us to set theory as a preferred mode of specification. The degree of formalization we will require is suggested by the following general description (in later chapters specific examples of the entities $\eta_1 \ldots \eta_n$ and the scientific generalizations $\Sigma_1 \ldots \Sigma_n$ will be provided as I introduce extended exemplars containing such entities and generalizations):

We let $\eta_1 \ldots \eta_n$ be a set of physical, chemical, or biological entities that can appear in a scientific generalization Σ. Typically Σ will be one of a series of such generalizations $\Sigma_1 \ldots \Sigma_n$ that make up a set of related sentences. Let Φ be a set of relations among $\eta_1 \ldots \eta_n$ that will represent causal influences, such as bind-to, be-extruded-from, prise-off, and the like. Then $\Sigma_i(\Phi(\eta_1 \ldots \eta_n))$ will represent the ith generalization and

$$\prod_{i=1}^{n} [\sum (\Phi(\eta_1 \ldots \eta_n))]$$

will be the conjunction of the assumptions (which we will call Π) constituting the "biomedical system" or BMS. Any given system that is being investigated or appealed to as explanatory of some explanandum is such a BMS if and only if it satisfies Π. We understand Π, then, as implicitly defining a kind of abstract system. There may not be any actual system which is a realization of the complex expression Π. The claim that some particular system satisfies Π is a theoretical hypothesis which may or may not be true. This characterization of a BMS follows fairly closely Giere's (1979, 1984) semantic approach to the philosophical analysis of scientific theories.

In introducing this terminology, I have deliberately left unspecified the nature of the language in terms of which Π is expressed. We need, however, to say a bit more about how the variation mentioned above can be effectively represented and how such a representation interacts with the tasks that theories perform, such as their being discovered, tested, and used for explanatory purposes. In the following section I propose one such specification that I believe offers considerable promise for capturing such variation as we found difficult to characterize in the state space model.

3.7 The Frame System Approach to Scientific Theories

In this section I am going to examine in a yet largely exploratory way the extent to which several tools of knowledge representation developed in the area of artificial intelligence (AI) may offer a purchase on the problem of variation in regard to biological theories. It seems to me that these AI tools constitute a plausible approach to relating concept meanings to one another and also fit well with the structure of models that need to capture much diversity in their instances.

Ultimately, I am going to suggest that an "object-oriented," frame-based systems approach currently constitutes the most viable method for knowledge representation of the middle-range theories discussed earlier. In the past two years, "object-oriented" approaches to programming have received increasing attention, with "frames" being replaced by "objects" in some of the standard textbooks.[35] Further below I will discuss some of the advantages of the object-oriented approach, as well as one of its implementations in biology and medicine. However, because the "frame" is still likely to be more familiar to most readers, and because frames and objects are ultimately very similar, I shall begin by discussing the frame concept.[36] I would like to examine the motivatation underlying the frame approach by referring to one psychological and one philosophical position, each of which appear to offer background support for this thesis. The psychological source to which I will refer is Rosch's work on concepts; the philosophical is Putnam's view of stereotypes in meaning analyses.

3.7.1 *Rosch and Putnam on Prototypes and Stereotypes*

Rosch's work was initially grounded in psychological anthropology. In her investigation, Rosch found, to both her and others' surprise, that primitive peoples as well as advanced societies do not represent concepts or categories as collections of necessary and sufficient properties. Rather, a category is built around a central member or a *prototype*, which is a representative member that shares the most attributes with other members of that category and which shares the fewest with members of the contrasting category (Rosch and Mervis 1975). Thus a robin would be a more prototypical bird than either a penguin or a chicken. Rosch wrote:

> Categories are coded in cognition in terms of prototypes of the most characteristic members of the category. That is, .many experiments have shown that categories are coded in the mind neither by means of lists of each individual member of the category nor by means of a list of formal criteria necessary and sufficient for category membership, but, rather, in terms of a prototypical category member. The most cognitively economic code for a category is, in fact, a concrete image of an average category member. (Rosch 1976, 212)

Rosch went on to extend her views to learning in children, questioning the sharpness of boundaries between concepts. Her contributions are viewed as major advances in our understanding of memory and knowledge representation, and, though her account has been construed as needing supplementation for complex category representation by some (Osherson and Smith 1981), it has been defended by others (Cohen 1982, Cohen and Murphy 1984, Fuhrmann 1991).

The Roschean view of concepts as being built around prototypes shares certain similarities with Putnam's urging that we consider meanings as "stereotypes." Putnam's more a priori methods antedate Rosch's empirical studies but appear to comport with them. A stereotype of a tiger will ascribe stripes to that animal, but not analytically so: "Three legged tigers and albino tigers are not logically contradictory entities" (1975, 170). Though I do not agree with Putnam's general, complex Kripkean theory of designation and meaning, Putnam's suggestion that "there is great deal of scientific work to be done in (1) finding out what sorts of items can appear in stereotypes; (2) working out a convenient system for representing stereotypes; etc." (1975, 188) seems quite correct.

The (Roschean) prototype perspective on concept characterization has in the past dozen years received increased atten-

FRAME 1: <u>GENE</u>
    SLOT 1: MATERIAL; VALUE = DNA
    SLOT 2: FUNCTION; VALUE = HEREDITY- DETERMINER

FRAME 2: <u>REGULATOR-GENE</u>
    SLOT 1: IS-A; VALUE = GENE
    SLOT 2: FUNCTION; VALUE = CONTROL

FRAME 3: <u>I+-GENE</u>
    SLOT 1: IS-A; VALUE = REGULATOR GENE
    SLOT 2: ORGANISM; VALUE = E.-COLI
    SLOT 3: REGION; VALUE = LAC

Figure 3.5   These frames can easily be written in a programming language like LISP and run with a simple inheritance program. The "question" (GET-VALUE 'MATERIAL 'I+-GENE) entered after the above frames are read into the system will return the value (DNA).

tion by researchers working in artificial intelligence. I will, within the limitations of this chapter, be able to discuss the work of only a few of the many proponents and critics of frame-based reasoning and "default logic," though this literature is vast and continues to grow rapidly.

3.7.2 *The Frame Concept*

Minsky's 1975 article on frames is the locus classicus of a discussion of these entities, but in this discussion I will tend to stay closer to later implementations of the frame concept. From a structural point of view, frames are names of generalized property lists. The property list has general features, usually termed slots, which in turn may have facet names and values. For example, a *lac* regulator gene frame may have as slots "material" and "function," with those two slots' values being "DNA" and "control" respectively. A facet name (not shown here, but see Winston and Horn 1984, 312, for a discussion) allows any one of several procedures to be triggered, depending on specific conditions, such as a search of the knowledge base in some prearranged fashion. (Figure 3.5 depicts simple frames for the concepts of "gene," "regulator gene," and "I gene.")[37]

From a functional point of view, it may be simplest to think of a "frame-based" approach to knowledge representation as representing one of three, somewhat divergent strategies for capturing knowledge. The most structured approach is to use the predicate calculus of traditional philosophical logic in almost Woodgerean fashion (Woodger 1937), but this is seen by a number of investigators as requiring more consistency and completeness in the domains they seek to represent than is likely to be found. Predicate logic is also perceived as being too fine-grained a tool for useful general work (Friedland and Kedes 1985, Fikes and Kehler 1985). "Rule-based" approaches are a second means of knowledge representation, and where the knowledge is heavily procedural, the use of this strategy of encoding such information in a large number of "if-then" rules is quite appropriate. The third, or "frame-based," type of knowledge representation is widely perceived to have certain advantages over both the predicate calculus and rule-based methods. Fikes and Kehler in a recent article write:

> The advantages of frame languages are considerable: They capture the way experts typically think about much of their knowledge, provide a concise structural representation of useful relations, and support a concise definition-by- specialization technique that is easy for most domain experts to use. In addition, special deduction algorithms have been developed to exploit the structural characteristics of frames to rapidly perform a set of inferences commonly needed in knowledge-system applications.
>
> In addition to encoding and storing beliefs about a problem domain, a representation facility typically performs a set of inferences that extends the explicitly held set of beliefs to a larger, virtual set of beliefs. . . . Frame languages are particularly powerful in this regard because the taxonomic relationships among frames enable descriptive information to be shared among multiple frames (via *inheritance*) and because the internal structure of frames enables semantic integrity constraints to be automatically maintained. (1985, 904–905)

Fikes and Kehler also note, apropos our earlier discussion, that in a frame-based approach "the description of an object type can contain a *prototype description of individual objects of that type;*

these prototypes can be used to create a default description of an object when its type becomes known in the model" (1985, 904; my emphasis).

As an example of a simple frame system with a hierarchical structure, consider a system with the entity "gene" at its highest level and with "regulator gene" and "structural gene" at the next lower level. (See figure 3.5.) We may postulate under "regulator gene" such entities as "inducibility gene" (in the original form of the operon model) and "operator locus." We can provide a property list for each of these entities, such as a "material" slot for the high-level "gene" entity. We can then link more specific entities under the gene frame by what are termed "is-a" links (originally termed "virtual copy" or VC links by Fahlman 1979), such that all the lower–level entities automatically *inherit* those linked properties. Thus if the above is implemented in a simple frame system, and a query is put to the knowledge base of the form "get-value 'material' operator," the answer "DNA" will immediately be generated. I should also point out that, in addition to inheritance via the "is-a" links mentioned, we can easily introduce into a set of frames *causal* information by placing properties describing what the entities cause and what they are affected by on their property list. For example, in frame 1 in figure 3.5 we could add a new slot: causes; value = m-RNA-synthesis. We can then allow entities of a lower order of generality to inherit causal properties from higher level entities; for example, a regulator gene can inherit the capacity to cause m-RNA synthesis from the more general gene frame.

A frame-based system is generally acknowledged to be equivalent to what is termed a "semantic net" or network representation, with only several subtle differences. Both can also be seen as alternative representations of the predicate calculus (Charniak and McDermott 1985, 28), though, as mentioned previously, many researchers find a frame-based approach significantly more flexible than one based on the predicate calculus. Though when I examine inheritance relations and inferences written in a programming language such as LISP I tend to use a frame-based (and more recently an object-oriented) approach, for the purposes of visual communication it is simpler to use the semantic net representation. Accordingly, the next figure employs that mode of knowledge representation. The figure is designed to show how inheritance can function so that higher level generalizations—in the sense of those with broader scope, not

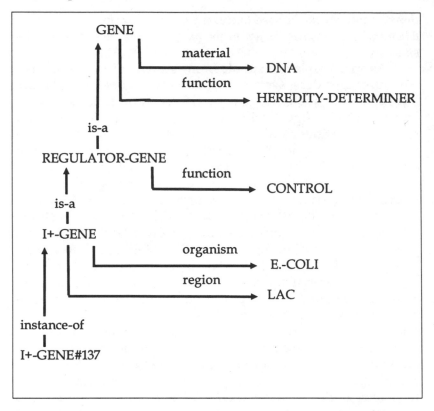

Figure 3.6 A semantic network form of the previous set of frames depicted in figure 3.5. A specific instance of an I+ gene, a prototype bearing number 137, is added here.

necessarily higher order of aggregation—can pass their values, including relevant causal properties, down to the more specific entities. Thus, since the I+ gene is linked through is-a links to the gene object, it can be allowed to inherit the capability of making m-RNA and any other properties we associate with such broader scoped entities. This affords a means of systematizing the knowledge in a complex domain.

3.7.3 Frames and Nonmonotonicity

This systematizing strength provided by inheritance, however, can lead to difficulties. In complex systems, we will occasionally want to block certain values from being inherited, so as to represent exceptions. Thus, though genes are usually or typically DNA sequences, if we are representing an AIDS viral genome we would have to cancel the link to DNA and instead link it with RNA. A more relevant example in our system is that the typical *lac o* locus will bind repressor in the absence of inducer, but typical o^c mutants will not, though we would like o^c mutants to inherit various noncancelled properties in our representation, such as their being DNA sequences. Cancellation in such systems provides increased flexibility, but at a price. The price is default logic's *nonmonotonicity*.

Traditional deductive logic is monotonic, by which we mean that if some theorem T can be proven on the basis of an axiom system A, then adding *another* axiom or piece of information to A will not result in the negation or withdrawal of that theorem T. In common sense thinking and in biological reasoning the matter is otherwise. To introduce the recurrent "Tweety" exemplar from the literature, we normally reason from the premise that "Tweety is a bird" to the conclusion that "Tweety can fly." If we find out that Tweety is a penguin, however, a new piece of information, the original conclusion is negated. (See McDermott and Doyle 1980.)

It has been shown clearly that the type of default logic used widely in frame-based systems described above has this nonmonotonic character (see, for example, Etherington and Reiter 1983). It has also been argued, by Brachman (1985) for instance, that permitting exceptions turns an inheritance hierarchy into one that holds only for *typical* entities but not for universally characterizable entities. It also follows from Brachman's arguments that natural kinds of the type that require necessary and sufficient conditions for their characterization cannot be defined in such a system. This is an interesting point, but one that may actually be a strength of such logics. The notion of a *typical* entity may allow for a different notion of "natural kind," one more suitable in biology, bearing a close relationship to Marjorie Grene's 1978 Aristotelian natural kinds, but this is not an issue I can pursue further in this chapter. There have been a number of papers in the AI and the logic literature attempting to provide a sound theoretical structure for nonmonotonic logics, but there is as yet no consensus. A very useful recent anthology edited by Ginsberg (1987) reprints and discusses many of these approaches.

My current view is that nonmonotonic logics are much weaker than generally thought. (See Hanks and McDermott

[1986] for a detailed argument to this effect. These authors indicate that, for those nonmonotonic solutions that seem to work, a fairly complex, problem-specific axiom will have to be articulated and justified in order to license the reasoning. This suggests that the nonmonotonic will lack generality and have a cumbersome, ad hoc structure.) Research on nonmonotonic logics continues to flourish, however, particularly on the subvariant of such logics known as "circumscription," and it may be that the problems of weakness and lack of adequate control may be resolved. At present I tend to be more conservative and recommend that more traditional monotonic reasoning processes be utilized in AI implementations.

It should be noted that the frame-system approach described above does not represent only structural (static) information. Frames can be constructed to describe processes and can be utilized in AI programs as components of dynamic simulations. Though "rule-based" or "production" systems have traditionally tended to be the form of knowledge representation employed for dynamic representations (see, for example, Holland et al. 1986), I believe that the sea change toward object-oriented programming in AI will produce more frame-based or object-oriented research programs in such areas.

3.7.4 Object-Oriented Programming Approaches

Object-oriented approaches appear to offer some important advantages for knowledge representation in the domains of increasingly complex sciences such as molecular biology. More specifically, large amounts of information pertaining to molecular biology, including information about DNA, RNA, and protein sequences, together with representations of the mechanisms of transcription and translation, will be required in any adequate system. Moreover, as I have noted several times earlier, this information will contain large variation in the types of mechanisms represented.

Object-oriented programming begins with the concept of "objects," which are "entities that combine the properties of procedures and data since they perform computations and save local state" (Stefik and Bobrow 1986, 41). Program activity works through "message sending" to objects, which respond using their own procedures called "methods." The same message can be sent to different objects, which, because they each have their own methods, can respond differently yet yield a common type of result. Thus the message "Area?" could be sent to some individual square object S_{37} and to a distinct circular object C_{78} and suitable answers in square meters returned for each object. Hidden from the inquirer (the message sender) would be the methods: "square the side" in the first case, and "multiply the square of radius by π" in the second. The concept is easily extended to messages such as "Protein?" which might be sent to the *lac* i+ gene in *E. coli*, to an HIV gene (which might be constituted of RNA or DNA depending whether it was in a virion or integrated in a human cell), or to the gene causing cystic fibrosis in humans. Messages can be designed in sets to constitute protocols. The capability of different classes of objects to respond in different ways to exactly the same protocols is termed "polymorphism," a feature that is seen as implementing modularity, whereby we can construct reusable and easily modifiable component pieces of code (see Stefik and Bobrow 1986).

In addition to modularity, another means of achieving useful and important abstractions without losing significant information, reflecting underlying biomedical diversity, in the process is by some combined technique involving both "multiple inheritance" and "information hiding." Multiple inheritance allows for different "parent" concepts to be used in building up a "child," an approach which permits the type of flexibility needed in the biomedical domain. This permits, for example, more efficient representation of the similarities and differences reflected in transcription, splicing, and translation mechanisms for viral, prokaryotic, and eucaryotic organisms. "Information hiding" allows for abstraction while at the same time permitting underlying diversity to be accessed as needed; we saw an instance of this in the use of "hidden" methods tied to objects above.

The features of modularity, multiple inheritance, abstraction, information hiding, and polymorphism form the essence of the relatively new style of writing code termed object-oriented programming (OOP).[38] The GENSIM program developed recently by Karp (1989a, 1989b) and discussed in chapter 2 is an example of a program written using the OOP approach, and the way it handles biomedical variation is worth some discussion. Recall that Karp's research resulted in two programs, GENSIM for knowledge representation of the *trp* operon (a close cousin of the *lac* operon discussed above), and HYPGENE, a hypothesis discovery and modification program which was intercalated with GEN-SIM. GENSIM implements its "objects," such as genes and enzymes, as frames (in KEE™) within the "class knowledge base" (CKB). In addition to CKB, however, GENSIM also has a "process knowledge base" known as both PKB and T, which encompasses a theory of chemical reactions (Karp 1989a, 3). Karp writes that:

> Each process is represented by a frame that lists:
>
> • the classes of reactant objects for its reaction (termed its *parameter objects*)
> • conditions that must be true of the objects for the reaction to occur (the process *preconditions*)
> • the *effects* of the reaction, which usually involve the creation of new chemical objects (1989a, 3)

In addition to CKB and PKB, a separate knowledge base for experiment simulation, SKB, is created from CKB and PKB.

I suggested earlier that the prototype concept seemed especially important in the selection of a (comparatively) small number of models from a potentially much vaster group of models which could be found empirically, given the large number of potential (and actual) mutations. Karp's knowledge bases utilize just such a strategy for knowledge representation. However, in addition, the various operators and control strategies permit the creation of new objects, for example new mutations in SKB, and (ultimately) additions or changes to the basic CKB and PKB.[39] Thus variation is represented in a complex manner, part explicitly in terms of prototype frames for both structures and processes, and part procedurally in terms of potential modifications in the system. Significantly, there are two ways in which GENSIM and HYPGENE do not take new approaches to reasoning and representation. The experimental simulations which HYPGENE creates are monotonic, and the control logic does not employ any analogical reasoning. Both of these choices seem appropriate at this point, based on what was said above about nonmonotonic logics and what was suggested in chapter 2 (p. 62) about analogical reasoning.

3.8 Additional Problems with Simple Axiomatizations in Biology and Medicine

The above discussion on frame-based and object-oriented systems suggests a means of representing knowledge about complex biomedical systems. It may be worth pointing out some additional features of biological knowledge that make the more traditional approach of capturing a scientific domain by a small number of axioms implausible.

In addition to the extensive variation, which defeats simple axiomatization of biomedical theories, the axiomatizations that are formulated are usually in qualitative biological (e.g., cell) and chemical (e.g., DNA) terms and thus do not facilitate deductive mathematical elaboration. Rather, what often seems to occur is an elaboration by more detailed specification, usually at a "lower" level, of aspects of one of the models, so that increased testing and explanation of particular phenomena can be explored.[40] Such elaboration is not deductive since it is ampliative and often rests on other biological theories and disciplines.[41]

The polytypic character of theories in the middle range does not prohibit occasional robust overlapping, with consequent sharpening or peaking of pure types at higher levels of aggregation, and where this occurs the results are usually striking and very useful. I examined such a case in connection with the clonal selection theory in chapter 2 and above, and I will return to that example in chapters 4 and 5. Even here, however, it is important to remember that polytypy will occur at lower levels of aggregation, so that the testing of the clonal selection theory will have to be individually tailored to specific systems.[42] (For example, an organism may be tolerant to certain antigens that are strongly cross-reacting to its self-antigens, and a knowledge of this would be important in testing the clonal selection theory in that organism, to control against misleading artifactual results.)

This notion of a theory as a series of overlapping temporal models can be analogized to overlapping populations in an n space, where n is the number of properties cited in the definition of polytypic above (p. 104). A core of necessary, distinctive features define the theory, but the theory is incomplete without some of the peripheral assumptions, which are variable and perhaps fully polytypic. A diagram that very crudely represents this by analogy with the *lac* operon theory is given as figure 3.7. The

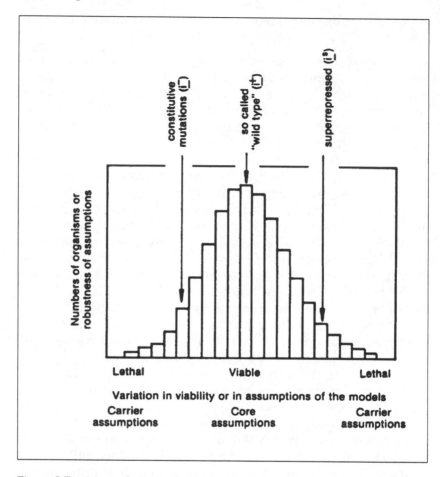

Figure 3.7   A speculative and crude analogical depiction of the variation in a biological theory such as the operon model. The X-axis depicts either various types of control in the *lac* region of varying numbers of *E. coli* in an average population or a continuum of varying assumptions holding in the overlapping models. A number of mutations may not differ significantly from their neighbors so as to be detectably different, whence the noncontinuous look to the "histogram." The peaked region would represent "robust" assumptions in Levin's (1966, 1968) terminology on the second interpretation of the X-axis, since these would hold in most (if not all) models.

similarity of this figure to figure 3.2 (from Smith and Sadler) (p. 81) should be noted.

Because of the interlevel character of middle-range theories, and because of the manner in which the theories become elaborated by development in the downward direction, there are strong interconnections among theories in a variety of prima facie separate biomedical disciplines. Thus a knowledge of genetics is usually indispensable in immunology, and immunological characterization of specificity is also of importance in genetics. Neurology requires biochemistry and cell biology, whereas embryology draws on transmission genetics, regulatory genetics, biochemistry, and cell biology in articulating and testing its theories. Again, it may be useful to point out that those interested in formally representing these complex interconnections are likely to find the features of modularity and multiple inheritance available in OOP techniques most valuable.

I have separated evolutionary theory from theories of the middle range. This was done in part because of the idiosyncratic character of the simpler forms of population genetics and in part because of evolutionary theory's universality at the most general level. Even in evolutionary theory, however, some of the significant features of middle-range theories, such as polytypy and interlevel elaboration, can be found, as I noted in the previous section (p. 97). These features are more characteristic of evolutionary theories that attempt to develop along Levins's lines of precision and realism rather than in the direction of generality. Such features are worth keeping in mind, however, since they indicate that the difference between middle-range theories and evolutionary theories is more like the separation of parts of a continuum rather than a sharp qualitative distinction.

3.9 A Proposal Regarding Current Debates on Theory Structure, Universality, and Biological Generalizations

I began this chapter with an examination of a series of current debates concerning theory structure in biology and medicine, and in this section I return to those views in the light of the examples and conception of theory developed in sections 4–8.

Smart's criticisms of law and theory in biology and medicine were noted to have served as a stimulus for several analyses of biological theory. The prevailing tendency (until quite recently) has been to defend universality of law and theory in biology.[43] From the perspective presented in this chapter, such defenses are somewhat limited and often beside the point. Universality, it has been argued, is most typically a feature at very low and very high levels of aggregation. Biomedical theories in the middle range are better conceived of as not possessing universality even within a given species. This feature, however, does not strike me, as it does Ruse (1973), as "extremely serious" for the status of biology. Nor do the types of theories we have encountered seem to fit Rosenberg's (1985) rubric of "*case-study*-oriented" research programs. Theories of the type I have characterized in the previous sections admit of *all the important features of theories in physics and chemistry*: biomedical theories of the middle range are testable and have excess empirical content, they organize knowledge in inductive and sometimes even deductive ways, they change and are accepted and replaced in accordance with rational canons, they have a generality that applies outside their original domains (though this generality is frequently partial and complex), and they are applicable for prediction and control in crucially important areas such as agriculture and health-care delivery.

It should now be obvious that I am steering a middle course between Smart and his critics, and also between Rosenberg and the defenders of a universal biology. There is a possible interpretation of Smart's thesis, however, that should be countered insofar as it concerns the predictability and control aspects of biomedical theories. Smart implies that such "generalizations" as are encountered in biology are the result of natural history and are thus "accidental" as opposed to lawlike generalizations, at best more like principles we might encounter in electronics or engineering. There are, he suggests, no "first, second, and third . . . laws of electronics" (Smart 1963, 52).[44] Smart illustrates his view by an interesting example based on an analogy with radios. Smart asks us to

> consider a certain make of radio set. Can we expect to find universal truths about its behavior? Surely we cannot. In general, it may be true that if you turn the left-hand knob you get a squeak from the loudspeaker and that if you turn the righthand knob you get a howl. But of course in some sets this will not be so: a blocking condenser may have broken down or a connection may have become loose. It may even be that the wires to our two knobs may have been interchanged by mistake in the factory, so that with some sets it is the left-hand knob that produces a howl and the right-hand knob that produces a squeak. (Smart 1963, 56)

Smart concludes his analogy by suggesting that "while roughly speaking radio engineering is physics plus wiring diagrams, biology is physics and chemistry plus natural history" (Smart 1963, 57). This reasoning seems to imply that the natural history component of biology introduces "accidentality" into the subject, eliminating any lawlike status.

In response to this possible interpretation of Smart, I believe a distinction which has, to the best of my knowledge, not previously been made in the philosophy of biology may be of some assistance in replying to Smart.[45] I want to distinguish two types of accidentality: "essential" and "historical."[46] Essential accidentality is what one encounters in universal generalizations of the type: "All of the screws in Smith's car are rusty." There are strong *background reasons* for believing that this generalization represents a *chance* event, such that the generalization would not support a counterfactual "if a screw [not at present in Smith's car] were in Smith's car, then it would be rusty."[47] Historical accidentality, on the other hand, though initiating from a chance event, is augmented by additional nomic circumstances, such as strong natural selection. Thus, though the origin of specific coding relations in the genetic code may have (likely) been due to a chance mutation, the occurrence of which could have been otherwise, at present the code is sufficiently entrenched by natural selection that it is only historically accidental. Assertions involving the genetic code can support counterfactual conditionals, at least as restricted to this planet. Historical accidentality thus represents accidentality "frozen into" nomic universality.

I also believe that the same situation holds with respect to theories of the middle range, appropriately restricted in scope to specific organisms, and within the context of the "overlapping" interpretation of such models as characterized above. It will, however, be useful to make a further set of distinctions that will clarify the nature of those generalizations, of both the universal and statistical type, that appear in middle-range theories.

First, I wish to distinguish *generalizations* into (1) universal or exceptionless and (2) statistical. Second, I want to maintain that we can distinguish "universal" generalizations into two subsenses: universal generalizations$_1$, referring to *organism scope*, to the extent to which a physiological mechanism will be found in *all* organisms, and universal generalizations$_2$, referring to the property illustrated by the phrase "same cause (or same initial conditions and mechanisms), same effect." This second sense of "universal" is roughly equivalent to a thesis of causal determinism. Biomedical theories employ many generalizations which, though they are not universal generalizations$_1$, are universal generalizations$_2$. As such, they possess counterfactual force.

This distinction between the two types of universality in generalizations has been characterized as difficult to understand (by one anonymous reviewer of an earlier version of this book). In addition, van der Steen has urged (in personal communication) that this distinction should be further clarified (also see van der Steen and Kamminga 1990 for similar distinctions regarding senses of "universal"). Furthermore, though the distinction introduced above (or reintroduced, since its basic form appears in my 1980a essay) is also made, if I follow them correctly, in Beatty (1992), these authors do not draw the important conclusion stated above that the second, *causal* sense of generalization will support counterfactuals. Thus the distinction in the two senses of "universal" mentioned above *is* a critically important one, and perhaps needs to be restated yet again. The claim is that, *biological and medical theories* employ many generalizations that though they do not have broad *scope* of application nonetheless are *causal* generalizations. By virtue of their causal character they support counterfactuals.

A still further comment should be made about the sense of "contingency" recently emphasized in Gould 1989 and elaborated on in Beatty 1992. I will call this sense of contingency *trajectory contingency* since it refers to different ways in which the evolutionary story on this earth could have developed; many different trajectories may be envisaged, each dependent on "accidents" of history. This type of contingency does seem to resemble the "essential accidentality" found in the rusty screws in Smith's car (or the universal claim that all the coins in my pocket are silver, to use Chisholm's example from the days of silver coins). This trajectory contingency, however, does *not* undermine the "causal laws of working" in systems that are the results of those trajectories. If they did, biologists, physicians, and drug companies would *really* be concerned about their laboratories and their liability! The diversity of evolutionary trajectories may even provide an explanation of the *narrowness of scope* of causal generalizations, as are found in biological organisms, but again, this does not undermine support for the counterfactual character of the narrow generalizations, since that is supported by their causal character.

I should add that, in addition, largely because of biological variation, system complexity, and the inability fully to specify and control for all relevant initial conditions, even when various pure types and intermediate types have been well defined, biological theories often have to employ statistical generalizations. These also have a type of counterfactual force, but it is probabilistic; that is, one can assert with confidence that, if X has not occurred, Y *probably* (at some level of probability < an error range) would not have occurred.

With these distinctions, then, it should appear that theories of the type I have mentioned are not troubled by Smart's critique of laws and theories in biology. I also believe that what this analysis yields are generalizations of varying scope and not "case studies," to use Rosenberg's (1985) term.[48] It seems to me that Ruse (1970, 1973), Munson (1975), Rosenberg (1985), and others are really concerned more about the *honorific* character possessed by laws and theory analyses, which is more suitable for less complex sciences, than they are about the role laws and theories rightfully play in biology and medicine. I would tend to agree with Simpson's (1964) position on the role of biology vis-à-vis physics (though not with all of his arguments elaborating his position) that:

> Einstein and others have sought unification of scientific concepts in the form of principles of increasing generality. The goal is a connected body of theory that might ultimately be completely general in the sense of applying to all material phenomena.
>
> The goal is certainly a worthy one, and the search for it has been fruitful. Nevertheless, the tendency to think of it as the goal of science or the basis for unification of the sciences has been unfortunate. It is essentially a search for a least common denominator in science. It necessarily and purposely omits much the greatest part of science, hence can only falsify the nature of science and can hardly be the best basis for unifying the sciences. I suggest that both the characterization of science as a whole and the unification of the various sciences can be most meaningfully sought *in quite the opposite direction*, not through principles that apply to all phenomena but through phenomena to which all principles apply. Even in this necessarily summary discussion, I have, I believe, sufficiently indicated what those

latter phenomena are: they are the phenomena of life.

Biology, then, is the science that stands at the center of all science. It is the science most directly aimed at science's major goal and most definitive of that goal. And it is here, in the field where all the principles of all the sciences are embodied, that science can truly become unified. (Simpson 1964, 107; my emphasis)[49]

In his recent book, Ernst Mayr also quotes some of the material cited from Simpson's (1964) book, and adds his own similar view:

Simpson has clearly indicated the direction in which we have to move. I believe that a unification of science is indeed possible if we are willing to expand the concept of science to include the basic principles and concepts of not only the physical but also the biological sciences. Such a new philosophy of science will need to adopt a greatly enlarged vocabulary—one that includes such words as biopopulation, teleonomy, and program. It will have to abandon its loyalty to a rigid essentialism and determinism in favor of a broader recognition of stochastic processes, a pluralism of causes and effects, the hierarchical organization of much of nature, the emergence of unanticipated properties at higher hierarchical levels, the internal coherence of complex systems, and many other concepts absent from—or at least neglected by—the classical philosophy of science. (Mayr 1988, 21)

There is much that I agree with in Mayr's view as expressed above, but I will also disagree in several of the chapters below with a number of Mayr's interpretations of the new concepts and implications of those concepts.

We have seen in the discussion in the previous sections that Beckner's view (following Arber) of the "reticulate" character of biological theory is more appropriate than Ruse's "physics" model or Rosenberg's "case-study" model, but with two important qualifications. First, Beckner's view was articulated in the area of evolutionary biology; it seems even applicable in the middle range (and also at the frontiers of evolutionary theory, oriented toward increasingly realistic models). Second, to the first approximation Ruse's claim for the prominence and centrality of population genetics in evolutionary theory seems more correct than Beckner's characterization. (In chapter 7, after I have elaborated more details of population genetics than are feasible to introduce in this chapter, I will consider Beatty's [1981] and Rosenberg's [1985] contentions that this view of Ruse's is misguided.)

Hull's view of biological theory as spanning a continuum from deductive, with concepts defined via necessary and sufficient conditions, to inductive, with polytypic concepts, is coherent with the view defended in the present chapter, with perhaps one exception and some elaboration. The exception is that Hull does not seem to have entertained the possibility of a *deductive* statistical form of systematization, in addition to deductive nomological and inductive statistical systematizations. Probability theory and the concepts of expectation values and standard deviations, however, are most important deductive statistical tools in population genetics. The elaboration is to stress the overlapping temporal models, the interlevel character of biological (and biomedical) theories, and the nondeductive (though deductively recastable) amplification of those theories in connection with testing and the development of their consequences, and to embed this analysis in the context of the semantic conception of theories extended to semiquantitative theories using a frame-based or OOP approach.

3.10 Summary

In this chapter I have argued that an overly narrow focus on examples drawn from biochemistry, elementary genetics, and simplified population genetics has skewed philosophers' analyses of theory structure in biology and medicine. Attention to other areas of these sciences indicates there are theories of the middle range which are best characterized as overlapping series of interlevel temporal models. Such theories lack universality but are important since they do organize their subject areas, are testable (often by elaboration in an ampliative, interlevel way through their lower–level elements), and are technologically significant with respect to their use in health care. I have also suggested how these theories can be construed in the light of the semantic conception of scientific theories and given a more structured, formal representation via some tools from artificial intelligence work on knowledge representation. Characterizing as "legitimate" biomedical theories only those theories that fit the analyses more

appropriate for physics and chemistry would impoverish existing biomedical sciences and would methodologically misdirect
ongoing research. In subsequent chapters I will examine both the
manner in which these biomedical theories, laws, and generalization are tested and elaborated over time and how they are used
to explain.

APPENDIX

One way in which we might, in the context of a *state space* semantic
approach, represent the polytypic aspects of biomedical theories is
by introducing some fuzzy set theory.[50] Here I shall only sketch these
notions and suggest in outline fashion how they can be developed in
the context of the semantic conception of scientific theories.

We might begin to represent variation by first constructing a
general state space as defined earlier, with various regions identified
as pure-type regions. These can be as narrowly defined as one wishes
for the degree of resolution provided by the currently available state
of experimentation. Then one introduces the concept of a *membership
function*, which specifies the degree to which an element is a member
of a particular *fuzzy set*. More generally, we could specify an intergrade vector, which would assign membership in several mutually
exclusive sets. Let me illustrate these notions of membership function, fuzzy set, grade of membership and intergrade vector with
some elementary examples, define the concepts more precisely, and
finally show how they might be employed in the area of our concern.

Suppose we consider the set of real numbers *much* greater than
1. This is an example of a *fuzzy set*, contrasted for example with the
set of numbers greater than 1. The set of men who are bald is another
instance of a fuzzy set. Zadeh developed the conception of a *grade of
membership* to quantify membership in such a fuzzy set by specifying
appropriate membership functions, μ ( ), defined on the interval [0,1]
(where 0 denotes *no* membership and 1 full membership, respectively). Zadeh (1965) illustrates the set of real numbers much greater
than 1, say A, by suggesting as representative values $\mu_A(1) = 0$,
$\mu_A(10) = 0.2, \mu_A (100) = 0.95, \mu_A (500) = 1$, etc. He notes that the value
of $\mu_A (x)$ provides a "precise, albeit subjective, characterization of A,"
but there may be clustering techniques available for obtaining a high
degree of *inter*-subjective agreement. Many classification schemes
utilize fuzzy set techniques implicitly. Woodbury (1978) and his colleagues at the Duke Medical Center have suggested, for example,
that Sheldon's tripartite classification of human physiques into three
ideal types of endomorph, mesomorph, and ectomorph constitutes

such an example. Most individuals are, of course, partial instances or combinations of these ideal or pure types.

One important point which should be stressed is that a membership function is *not a probability*. To check one's intuitions on this, consider a complex membership function termed an "intergrade vector," which assigned to a hermaphrodite 0.25 male and 0.25 female, construing male and female as pure types. It would be nonsensical to say of that hermaphrodite that this individual's probability of being male was 0.25. I stress this distinction because the *form* of statements where fuzzy sets are needed will look very much like probability statements. I hasten to add, however, that the use of fuzzy set analysis does not *exclude* or *replace* probabilistic analysis. In point of fact, probability and statistics are often widely employed in definitions of both pure and intermediate types. The distinction is important, and complex, and the reader is urged to consult Woodbury's 1978 article.

In an extension of the state space approach to the semantic conception of theories, these notions of fuzzy sets might be used to represent the kind of polytypic theories we find at the middle range of biomedical theorizing by proceeding as follows. Subsequent to defining regions of pure types in our state space, we characterize the state space *between and among* pure types in terms of the values of intergrade vectors. If the parameter space is sufficiently rich, there will be a number of regions where intermediate types will be located. Thus the state space will be characterized by a complex state function composed of quantitative parameters and more qualitative classificatory intergrade vectors. Using the o^c example from figure 3.2, the amount of β-galactosidase synthesized in the absence of inducers would be such a quantitative parameter, and an intergrade vector defining various mutants in terms of pure-type μ_o^c ( ) membership would be a semiquantitative classificatory function. Both parameters would be needed in order to characterize both the subtypes of o^c and the phenotypic expression of constitutive β-galactosidase synthesis. Here variation would be subtle, but other regions may be demarcated by sharp shifts in *some* of the parameters, as when transition is made to positive control from negative control. Even here, however, some of *the other* parameters may vary continuously, such as those that characterize the connected and coordinated structural genes. We can, accordingly, describe in terms of this state space a set of widely varying models and a set of permissible trajectories of those models over time.

I want to close this appendix by briefly remarking on the resurgence of interest in the AI, computer science, and engineering areas since I first proposed the use of Zadeh's fuzzy representation for biological theories (following Woodbury and his colleagues [1978]), leading to Suppe's criticisms at a symposium in which we participated in 1980 (Suppe 1989, chapter 8). Fuzzy set theory encountered an almost–visceral rejection in the AI community in the United States but was accepted and further developed in Japan, where it was progressively applied to a wide variety of control devices from air conditioning thermostats to television focus mechanisms. Apparently driven by these practical successes, fuzzy set theory has experienced a renaissance in the United States, where it has begun to be integrated synergistically with both research on algorithms and investigations into neural networks (see Karr 1991). Whether it becomes sufficiently powerfully developed to assist us with general biological knowledge representation as explored in this appendix is less clear, but the prospect is more encouraging now than it was a dozen years ago. Also of interest is a recent in-depth analysis by Fuhrmann (1991) relating fuzzy set theory and the prototype approach discussed in the main body of the chapter above.

CHAPTER FOUR

The Logic and Methodology of Empirical Testing in Biology and Medicine

IN THE PREVIOUS CHAPTERS I discussed the conditions and logical aspects of the discovery process in biology and medicine, and also the logical nature of the theories, models, and hypotheses which are discovered. In this and the succeeding chapters I would like to turn to a consideration of the factors affecting the activities of scientists *after* a hypothesis or theory has been generated and articulated. This aspect of scientific inquiry has been characterized as the "context of justification," as opposed to the "context of discovery," which was analyzed earlier. As we shall see in the examples to follow, however, the distinction is not a very clear one, and imaginative and creative thought often is found in the process of deducing the consequences of new hypotheses and theories.

This chapter covers a number of issues and it will be helpful to the reader if I provide a brief overview of its structure. The first two sections develop the general philosophical position that underlies the discussion of experimental testing, to be found in this chapter, and that of evaluation, to be found in the next. This position I call "generalized empiricism"; it places a premium on empirical foundations, but I believe it does so in a way that is more flexible than, say, Shapere's (1982), and more in accord with Hacking's (1983) and Galison's (1987) views about experiments. (In the next chapter, after Feyerabend's and Kuhn's positions have been discussed, "generalized empiricism" will be used to critique the sociological "constructivist" account of scientific knowledge.) Generalized empiricism departs from positivism and logical positivism to accept theoretical discourse as "meaningful" per se; how this works in detail is part of section 4.2. Section 4.3 reviews some preliminary points about experimental testing and then elaborates on them using as an example

the Nossal-Lederberg experiment, the first experiment designed
to test the clonal selection theory introduced in chapters 2 and 3.
Section 4.4 discusses how theories assist in defining observations
as relevant. Special considerations about "initial conditions" in
biology and medicine are described in section 4.6, and the problem of distinguishing an experimental effect from an artifact, an
issue which has received increased attention in the past five
years, is scrutinized. These preliminaries pave the way for an in-
depth analysis of the "methods of experimental inquiry" from
the perspectives of John Stuart Mill, Claude Bernard, and more
contemporary commentators. Finally, the issue of "direct evidence" discussed in physics by Shapere (1982) and Galison
(1987) is examined in molecular biology, employing an extended
example of Gilbert and Müller-Hill's isolation of the repressor of
the operon theory (introduced in chapter 3). This chapter closes
with some comments on Glymour's (1975, 1980) "bootstrapping"
approach to theory testing.

4.1 Epistemological Considerations: Generalized Empiricism

It will be useful to provide a brief conspectus of the philosophical
position to be taken in this and the following chapters. The position, which was implicit in the previous chapters, may not inac-
curately be termed "generalized empiricism." The sense which I
wish to give this term is that there are several levels of control
over the adequacy of scientific hypotheses and theories: (1) the
scope of direct experimental or observational evidence, which
shades into (2) the scope of indirect experimental or observational evidence, (3) theoretical support (or possibly intertheoretical discord), and (4) conformity to certain methodological
desiderata such as simplicity and unity of science. (Readers will
note that these factors are primarily "internalist"; the role of "ex-
ternalist" or social factors will be touched on in chapter 5, but
also see my 1982 for a discussion of the relations of these types of
factors. For a recent inquiry into the interplay among these factors see Hull 1988.) Each of these levels will be defined and examined in detail in the remainder of the chapter (and the
succeeding chapters). Suffice it to say for now that it is the con-
viction of this author—to be defended later—that level 1 is ultimately of decisive importance, that level 2 is next in importance,
and that the other levels of control (3 and 4) have as their ulti-

mate warrant the *empirical* success (in the sense of levels 1 and 2 and *scope* of experimental support) of their application. Thus the warrant for the desideratum of simplicity is not thought of as a priori, but is seen rather as resting on the historical (and empirical) thesis that simpler theories[1] have generally been ultimately supported experimentally over other, more complex competitors. (This focus on empiricism, however, does not entail that we cannot or should not investigate and employ what have traditionally been considered "metaphysical" aspects in analyses of science. The extent to which a metaphysical component is needed in an account of causation will be explored in chapter 6.)

4.2 Interpretative Sentences and Antecedent Theoretical Meaning

To those readers who are familiar with empiricist tenets in the philosophy of science, it might appear paradoxical that, prior to embarking on a discussion of the empirical testing of scientific theories and hypotheses, I need to introduce the concept of "antecedent theoretical meaning." Some comments on this notion are, however, required, for reasons which I believe will become evident. Traditional philosophy of science of the type represented by Nagel, Carnap, Reichenbach, and the early Hempel construed scientific theories as a collection of sentences employing theoretical terms connected by logical and mathematical relations, such as conjunction or differentiation. The theoretical terms, such as gene, electron, or 1 function, did not per se have meaning but could obtain empirical meaning by being connected to observational terms, which were per se meaningful. The principles of connection between theoretical terms and observational terms were called variously correspondence rules, dictionaries, or interpretative sentences (Schaffner 1969a). In contrast to this view, I want to argue that theoretical terms *are* meaningful per se, though this does not, of course, guarantee that what is designated by such terms actually exists. "Phlogiston" and "natural endogenous inducers" are good cases in point of theoretical terms which lack referents. I believe I can make my point of view clear on the need for "antecedent theoretical meaning" by means of an example from earlier chapters.

In the previous chapters, we considered the genesis (and logical structure) of the clonal selection theory of acquired immunity. Recall that Burnet proposed a set of cellular entities (lymphocytes) bearing specific receptors on their surfaces. These receptors or "reactive sites" were specific for particular antigens as a lock is specific for a particular key, and the cell was genetically programmed to produce only that specific antibody which it bore as a receptor. Binding of the antigen to the receptor stimulated the cell to reproduce its kind in a large clone, which would then differentiate into plasma cells releasing soluble antibody.

It should be clear that Burnet was not introducing a "meaningless" term when he proposed a lymphocyte with these properties. Though the philosophers of science of the logical empiricist persuasion referred to above might likely say that the clonal selection theory could be analyzed into a set of abstract terms plus a *model* or *analogy*, I believe this construal does not do justice to the fact that the theoretical properties are crucial for *reasoning to* empirical consequences of a theory. (In the empiricist tradition referred to, a model or analogy is heuristic at best, and not part of the empirical content of a theory, which is exhausted by the theoretical sentences and the correspondence rules.) It would seem much more direct and natural if we were to say that Burnet was not simply providing an analogy or model but rather was *creating the theoretical meaning* of the term "lymphocyte" by drawing on antecedently understood notions and putting them together in a radically new way.[2]

Thus scientific theories on this account are meaningful per se, but what makes them "scientific" rather than science fiction or fantasy is that, even in their initial stages of formulation, they have some connection with sense or laboratory experience. But this latter experiential content does not exhaust the "meaning" of the theory, nor do the interconnections of the theory's postulates plus their connections with experience fully exhaust the antecedent theoretical meaning. A theory is like a historical novel with a cast of characters, some of whom are known to have existed, some of whom are quite different from any known historical personage, but who, if they had existed, would explain history. The scientist proposes such a historical novel in the hope that it will turn out to be accurate history. But if it turns out to be false or nonconfirmable or nonfalsifiable, it may be read as fiction; it is not a "meaningless" story.

Only *after* theoretical terms have been given a relatively precise meaning, by providing a list of some of the important properties of the hypothetically proposed theoretical entities, does it even *become* possible to consider relevant experiments or observations which might test the theory. Otherwise there is no control over the admissibility of those interpretive sentences or correspondence rules that connect the presence of a theoretical entity or the occurrence of a (sensually) remote theoretical process with more immediate laboratory phenomena.

4.3 An Introduction to the Logic of Experimental Testing

Empirical control over the adequacy of a new theory or hypothesis in biology and medicine is achieved by *deducing consequences* from the proposed theory or hypothesis in the context of specific assumed test conditions, and then checking these consequences against empirically given evidence. Let us examine the nature of the deduction, the test conditions, and the consequences. In what follows, for the sake of convenience of expression, I shall use the term "hypothesis" for "hypothesis or theory," unless conditions require specific clarification or further distinction.

4.3.1 *Deduction: A Syntactic Approach to Testing*

Deduction is a form of inference which can be succinctly characterized as requiring the truth of the conclusion, assuming the truth of the premises. From our point of view the premises consist of (1) the hypothesis (or hypotheses) under scrutiny, (2) the initial conditions of the particular envisioned test (or type of test), and (3) the auxiliary hypotheses which are obtained from background theories. For the moment we shall ignore the complication of the auxiliary hypotheses in order to look at a more simplified or idealized logic of empirical testing. Hypotheses, whether they be in the physical or biomedical sciences, possess a *logically* universal form in the sense discussed in the previous chapter.[3] From these premises specific conclusions can be derived which can be compared with laboratory observations.[4] The necessary role of test or initial conditions can be seen more clearly in terms of a biomedical example. Let us return once again to the clonal selection theory.

4.3.2 *The Nossal-Lederberg Experiment*

Very shortly after the initial publication by Burnet of the clonal selection theory, Joshua Lederberg began a visit to Burnet's laboratory.[5] Though initially Lederberg's reason for visiting was to collaborate with Burnet and his colleagues on research on the genetics of influenza virus, Lederberg became very interested in the clonal selection theory, in part because of its potential unification of immunology and genetics. In point of fact, in an influential article published in *Science* in 1959, Lederberg outlined a rational molecular basis for the clonal selection theory. In the early 1960s the theory was often referred to as the "Burnet-Lederberg Theory."[6]

Lederberg seized on one of the hypotheses of the clonal selection theory that sharply distinguished it from the up-to-then dominant instructive theories. As mentioned in chapter 2, the clonal selection theory postulated in part that "except under quite abnormal conditions, one [immunocompetent] cell produces only one type of antibody." We will call this assumption the "one cell–one antibody" hypothesis.

This assumption differed from the instructive hypothesis, which held that any potential antibody-producing cell can respond to a wide range of antigenic specificities and synthesize antibodies complementary to a very great variety of antigens. What was needed, Lederberg saw, was to isolate individual cells and stimulate them with two quite different (i.e., noncross-reacting) antigens. Working with G. J. V. Nossal, Lederberg found that lymph cells obtained from an adult Wistar rat that would respond to one antigen, *Salmonella a*, and produce antibody to that antigen, would *not* respond to a different antigen, *Salmonella b*, to produce a different type of antibody. A similarly exclusive relation was found in the case of cells that would respond to *Salmonella b* but not to the *a* type.[7] See Technical Discussion 4 for the details of such an experiment. The reasoning entails that immobilization of the normally free-swimming bacteria in the cells examined under the microscope is taken as evidence of the production of antibody by the cells. In this experiment, no single cell was found to immobilize both strains of bacteria.

Technical Discussion 4

It will be worthwhile to examine the fine structure of the Nossal-Lederberg experiment, since specific details of their work will disclose important logical and epistemological features of hypothesis testing by experiment. Nossal and Lederberg began with two types of *Salmonella* bacteria (*S. adelaide* and *S. typhi*) associated with two specific antigens. The hind footpads of adult Wistar rats were injected with 0.25

ml of solution containing the two specific *Salmonella* antigens, grown in a broth culture. These injections were repeated at weekly intervals for three weeks. Three days after the last injection the rats were killed and their lymph nodes removed, pooled, sliced, and then allowed to disperse into a saline solution buffered to pH 7.0 to yield a solution of suspended lymphoid cells. These cells were sedimented in a centrifuge and then washed three times to remove any soluble antibody. Single cells were subsequently isolated into very small drops termed microdroplets (volume = 10^{-7}–10^{-6} ml) on a coverslip, which was then inserted into an oil chamber. The oil chamber was incubated at 37°C for 4 hours, following which the chamber was placed before a microscope of 100×. Using a micropipette and a micromanipulator, about ten bacteria were introduced into each droplet, with half of the droplets being given one type and the other half the other type of bacteria. After twenty minutes at room temperature, the droplets were examined to determine if the *Salmonella*, which in their normal state are free to swim in their host cells, had become immobilized. Immobilization is accomplished by a factor, thought to be made up of the specific antibodies, which coats the flagella or hair-like swimming organs of the bacteria. Total loss of mobility was recorded as "inhibition." If a cell immobilized the bacteria, then a second injection with 10 bacteria of the other *Salmonella* strain was performed. No single cell was discovered to immobilize both strains of bacteria.

This fairly detailed account of the Nossal-Lederberg experiment discloses a number of aspects of hypothesis testing. First, it is important to note the specific conditions under which the general hypothesis is tested. The cells are specified as individual rat lymphoid cells. They are treated by a very precise process with the temperature, time, pH, number of washings and type of centrifugation carefully controlled and recorded. Eventually the process terminates in several "observations." In this experiment, the observations were what are usually termed qualitative: the swimming behavior of the bacteria was looked for under a low-powered microscope, and if the bacteria were immobilized, the observers recorded a verdict of "inhibition." It is an important and explicit hypothesis that immobilization signified antibody specific for the strain of bacteria immobilized.

To a first and rather crude approximation,[8] the reasoning involved in the Nossal-Lederberg experiment can be schematized as follows:

Premise 1: If a cell is an antibody producer, it can synthesize antibody against only one type of antigen.

Premise 2: Each of these particular adult Wistar rat lymph cells are antibody producers.

Conclusion 1: Each of these particular adult Wistar rat lymph cells can synthesize antibody against only one type of antigen.

Premise 3: The adult Wistar rats were immunized against two different types of antigens, *a* and *b*.

Conclusion 2: These particular rat cells can synthesize antibody against either *a* or *b* type antigen but not both.

Premise 4: If antibody specific to *Salmonella a* is present, it will immobilize those salmonella within twenty minutes of the injection of *Salmonella* into the droplet containing the lymph cell. An identical situation holds for *Salmonella* of the *b* type. Both *a* and *b* are injected.

Conclusion 3: The cells will immobilize *Salmonella* of either the *a* or *b* type but not both.

Observation: The cells immobilized *Salmonella* of either the *a* or *b* type but not both.

Since Conclusion 3 is observable and is confirmed in the laboratory, the premise under scrutiny, namely Premise 1, is tested and confirmed.

There are, however, several logical and epistemological features inherent in this example, at which it is important to look closely. I will first comment on the *relevance* of the observations made, then on the significance and role of the initial conditions, and finally on the role of the other premises, such as Premise 4, which function as auxiliary hypotheses.[9]

In both the syntactic and semantic approaches to testing, one ultimately resorts to *observations*. This notion has been explored extensively in the philosophy of science and, because of its centrality in experimental testing and the generalized empiricism urged above, requires some detailed discussion.

4.4 Observation in Biology and Medicine — The Issue of Relevant Observations

The relation of theory to observation illustrated in the Nossal-Lederberg experiment described above is, I believe, quite representative of the manner in which theories are connected with observations — both in science in general and biology and medicine in particular. Earlier I spoke of interpretive sentences or correspondence rules, which in the approach of Carnap, Nagel, and the early Hempel, provided the empirical content for the theory. Just as I argued for an alternative construal of the source of theoretical meaning, however, I shall now urge a different view of these interpretive sentences and also of the observations in which they terminate.

Interpretive sentences or correspondence rules are best conceived of, in my view, as collapsed causal sequences. A "theoretical" process has many consequences (or effects), some of which can be argued, often in the light of *other* theories, to be observable. Expressed in the formal mode we can say that a theoretical sentence will, with the addition of premises borrowed from other theories and a sentence describing initial conditions (see below), entail a sentence (or sentences) describing an observation. Recourse to antecedent theoretical meaning is crucial for this account, for it is by virtue of that antecedent theoretical meaning that other theories are seen as appropriate auxiliary theories. For example, when Burnet postulated that an "antibody" equivalent to the antibody the cell could produce was present on the cell's surface, all of the antecedent theoretical meaning associated with the term "antibody" becomes available to draw upon for other knowledge to use in testing that postulate.

Observation sentences are those sentences that describe intersubjectively testable experiences such as meter readings patterns, colors, tastes, odors, and sounds.[10] Some degree of variation is expected among observers, but this is usually slight and is almost never, *contra* such philosophers of science as Hanson (1958), Kuhn (1962), and Feyerabend (1962), determined by the theory the observer holds. In those rare cases where proponents of different theories claim they "see different things," a negotiated withdrawal to a common description is, I would contend, always possible. This type of "negotiated" resolution is, however, not so readily available with respect to a determination of the *relevance* of an observation. Since an observation is, on the view urged here, connected with a theoretical process by virtue of a (usually) complex reasoning chain, a proponent of a different theory may construe the same observation as being *ir*relevant to his or her own theory, and the observationally verifiable occurrence may be dismissed as falling into the province of another discipline or subdiscipline.

It is here that the concept of a Shaperean domain, introduced in chapter 2 (p. 52), can be reinvoked as an additional control over observations.[11] The domain concept is frankly historical — it represents a cluster of items of information which cohere together, partially as a result of earlier generalizations' and theories' successes in binding them together. For example, the phenomenon of tissue transplantation rejection was not clearly seen as immunological in the early days of immunology. Ehrlich believed that transplanted cells died due to exhaustion brought about by malnutrition whereas others suspected the cell death might be caused by an immune response.[12] Thus, for Ehrlich, the death of transplanted cells would *not* be seen as falling into the *immunological* domain.

In the domain, however, are items of information, often observations, sometimes low-level experimental generalizations, which call out for explanation by any new theory proposed as a candidate to succeed the then current theory, particularly insofar as these are explained by the currently accepted theory. Observations that are closely related in kind or by virtue of accepted theories are also relevant to the test of a theory proposed in that subdiscipline. A new theory can diminish the previous scope of a domain by successfully explaining much (if not all) of the pre-existent domain and (usually) by extending the new domain in a heretofore unanticipated direction. (This occurred, for example, in physics in the nineteenth century when optics was removed from the domain of mechanics and situated in the domain of electricity and magnetism by Maxwell.) Factors that legitimate such theories in their competition cannot be pursued here but must be deferred until chapter 5, after I have developed a logic of comparative theory evaluation. Suffice it to say at this point that the relevance of an observation is Janus-faced: one face looks to the domain and the other looks to the theory which entails it. Disputes in this type of situation can and do arise, and settling them often takes time, during which protracted argument plus increased experimental scope and degree of resolution usually generate consensus. We shall examine such a case in depth in chapter 5.

4.5 The Special Nature of Initial Conditions in Biology and Medicine; Auxiliary Hypotheses

Both Premise 2 and Premise 3 in the deduction of section 4.3 specify the test conditions or the initial conditions of the experiment. Though initial conditions, because of the logic of testing, must appear in all empirical scientific inquiry whether it be in the physical or biological sciences, in biology and medicine the specification of the initial conditions takes on an added complexity and importance, a point I return to in section 5. It has often been remarked, especially by biologists of an antireductionistic or organismic persuasion, that biological systems display holistic traits which are closely associated with or caused by the extensive degree of interdependence of the parts (or of subsystems) of biological organisms. This holism and interdependence is thought to be qualitatively different from any correlates in naturally occurring *physical* systems. This claim will be analyzed in chapter 9, but there is an aspect of this interdependence that affects our discussion of the initial conditions involved in the experimental testing of biomedical hypotheses. The point may be put by asserting that often there is a greater need in biological experimentation to specify both *more* initial conditions and at least *one additional type* of initial condition than there is in the physical sciences.

There appear to be two types of initial conditions worth distinguishing in biology and medicine which I will term (1) strain type and (2) laboratory type. The "strain type" of initial conditions refers to the type of organism used in the experiment, though it might also be interpreted to refer to a specific chemical, say an enzyme, obtained from a particular strain. The "laboratory type" of initial conditions refers to those specific factors manipulable in the laboratory as part of the experiment, such as times, temperatures, pH, speed of centrifugation, solution composition, and the like. The "laboratory type" of initial conditions appears to be the same as one encounters in the physical and chemical sciences. The specification of both types of initial conditions is important to insure repeatability and checkability of experimental tests. Specifying the strain type is a guard (but not a guarantee) against varying physiologies in different organisms, or against the appearance of mutants in a strain which might have a significant interfering influence on a test of a hypothesis. Careful specification of the laboratory type of initial conditions is critical for excluding a fairly pervasive problem affecting testing in biology and medicine, the problem of the experimental artifact.

Briefly, an artifact is something produced by the experimental situation itself that, if not recognized and minimized through appropriate control of initial conditions, can be misinterpreted erroneously as a significant finding. In recent years, the importance of distinguishing an artifact from an experimental result has been commented on in the history and philosophy of physics. For example, Franklin writes:

> Although all scientists and philosophers of science are agreed that science is based on observation and experiment, very little attention has been paid to the question of how we come to believe rationally in an experimental result, or in other words, to the problem of the epistemology of experiment. How do we distinguish between a result obtained when an apparatus measures or observes a quantity and a result that is an artifact created by the apparatus? (1986, 165)

An illustration from biology, again based on the Nossal-Lederberg experiment, will make the problem and the epistemological point clearer. Though the Nossal-Lederberg experiment seemed to corroborate the one cell–one antibody hypothesis, subsequent experiments by Nossal and Mäkelä (1962) using a bacterial adherence test and by Attardi, Cohn, and Lennox (1959) using a sophisticated plaque technique for T_2 and T_5 bacteriophage indicated that there were circumstances in which statistically significant numbers of single cells could respond to at least two different antigens. Attardi et al.'s experiments of 1959 and 1964 were subsequently subjected to a very careful repetition by Mäkelä in 1967. Significantly, Mäkelä used strains of T_2 and T_5 bacteriophage (some of which he obtained from Lennox), which he found sufficiently typical and similar to the earlier organisms used by Attardi, so that his experiment would retest the earlier work. Mäkelä introduced several refinements into the procedure, all designed to avoid any contamination of the experiment. In particular, a new method of washing cells was employed to eliminate any undetected cell debris from being carried along.

His results, in contradiction to those of Attardi et al., strongly *supported the one cell–one antibody hypothesis*. In a brief commentary on Mäkelä's 1967 paper, Nossal, who was present at the paper, noted:

> I would like to comment on the very rare so-called double producers in the *Salmonella* system. Frequently these formed good amounts of one antibody, and gave a weak cyto-adherence reaction against the second. These, as pointed out in our original publications, may have represented an artifact. Perhaps there were weak cross reactions between *Salmonella* not detectable by classical serology; perhaps single cells occasionally contained adherent fragments from other cells that had been close to them in the body. (1967, 430)

It should have been evident in the discussion of the Nossal-Lederberg experimental test of the clonal selection theory that the connection of the one cell–one antibody hypothesis with an observational report required several stages of reasoning. At the time of the experiment, and even now, individual cell receptors and individual serum antibody molecules are not visible with the detail required for a straightforward empirical test of the hypothesis. At least one explicitly noted additional assumption, as well as several implicit assumptions, were employed in obtaining the conclusion (3) that could be compared with a laboratory observation. Let us now examine these in some detail.

In the Nossal-Lederberg experiment it was explicitly assumed (in Premise 4, p. 136) that the immobilization of the initially free-swimming *Salmonellae* was a sign of antibody production directed against the antigen borne by that type of *Salmonella*. This is known as an auxiliary hypothesis. There were additional but silent auxiliary hypotheses employed. For example, a microscope of 100x was used to observe the immobilization of the *Salmonellae*. The laws of geometrical optics that undergird the construction of the microscope thus help warrant the assertion that the *Salmonellae* have become immobilized, serving as silent assumptions in the reasoning leading to the empirical test of the hypothesis.

The fact that auxiliary hypotheses (or even initial conditions) are often of importance in empirical test situations weakens the asymmetry between confirmation and falsification. If there is an auxiliary hypothesis A (*in addition to* a hypothesis H being tested) that is required in order to deduce an experimentally checkable conclusion C, then the *falsification* of H by observing not-C is blunted. For it is a logical truth that, from the argument "H & A ⊃ C" and "C is not the case," it deductively follows only that "either H is not the case *or* A is not the case." (*Both* H and A, of course, may be false.) Though the auxiliary hypothesis A may be either a specific initial condition or a universal hypothesis, the logical problem involved in falsification is the same. This is the logical basis of the well-known Duhemian thesis (see Duhem 1914), which adds to this logical point the claim that it is always possible to introduce a *new* auxiliary hypothesis A' different from A that permits the *retention* of H, since now H & A ⊃ not-C.[13] This situation is not simply an abstract possibility, for we noted a case above in which Attardi et al. (1959) apparently obtained evidence falsifying the clonal selection theory. The one cell–one antibody hypothesis was saved by Mäkelä's introduction of an altered auxiliary condition, a new washing technique, yielding observations that confirmed the clonal selection theory.

4.6 The Methods of Experimental Inquiry

The case we have examined thus far employs a method of testing wherein an observable consequence of a hypothesis (or a theory) is observationally verified in the laboratory. The example we considered is, however, only *one* means of obtaining experimental control over hypotheses. There are other means than looking for (but not necessarily finding) consequences of positive instances of hypothetical processes. In biology and medicine, perhaps more so than in the physical sciences, those additional methods are of at least equally great importance. Especially significant are control experiments that are essentially equivalent to following John Stuart Mill's *method of difference*, appropriately interpreted with the aid of some (partially unjustified) criticism of Mill by Claude Bernard, and retitled *the method of comparative experimentation*. Also important is the *method of concomitant variation*. Let us discuss each of these methods and their applicability.[14]

The traditional methods of empirical verification (often also interpreted as methods of discovery)[15] were usually articulated as methods of establishing causal claims. These methods, following the great methodologists of the nineteenth century (who in turn followed Francis Bacon), have been known as the methods of agreement, difference, residues, and concomitant variation. These methods are largely methods of eliminative induction, and may thus not be thought sufficiently general to encompass the full scope of scientific methodology. (I will, however, later discuss what Mill termed the "deductive method" and also the "method of hypothesis," which will give us an opportunity both to consider more general methods and also to relate the foregoing discussion to Mill's concerns.) In this section I shall begin from Mill's characterization of the experimental methods, since Mill's analysis is *provisionally* adequate for our purposes and is also well known.

4.6.1 Mill's Methods

I begin with the "method of agreement." This was stated by Mill as follows:

> If two or more instances of the phenomenon under investigation have only one circumstance in common, the circumstance in which alone all the instances agree, is the cause (or effect) of the given phenomenon. (Mill 1973 [1843], 390)

It should immediately be pointed out that this method is most difficult to satisfy in biomedical inquiry because of the complexity of organisms. To vary every relevant character, save one, is largely unrealizable, though it may occasionally be done in very narrowly circumscribed investigations in molecular biology, for example in genetic codon analysis.

The applicability of the method of agreement is also suspect in complex biological organisms for two other general reasons, originally pointed out by Mill in his *System of Logic*. These general reasons were referred to by Mill as the *plurality of causes* and the *intermixture of effects*. With respect to the former, Mill noted that in those complex cases where the same consequence could be the result of different, jointly sufficient antecedents, the method of agreement yielded uncertain conclusions. In complex and adaptable biological organisms, such a situation is often likely. Even greater difficulties for the method of agreement arose in cases where effects were "intermixed," where either the effects were not separable into clearly defined components or else the result was emergent and incalculable on the basis of the causal components. As an example of the "intermixture of effects," Mill cited the production of water from oxygen and hydrogen, in which "not a trace of the properties of hydrogen or of oxygen is observable in those of their compound, water" (1973 [1843], 371).[16] Mill also believed that biological properties were emergent with respect to the physicochemical, with attendant difficulties. Mill does not offer a biological analogue of the hydrogen-oxygen case, but one could easily be imagined, for example the temperature of the organism resulting as the complex "sum" of several connected thermal regulating systems. Suffice it for now to note that the method of agreement possesses serious imperfections in its application to such complex circumstances as are found in biological organisms.

The "method of difference" was stated by Mill in the following manner:

> *If an instance in which the phenomenon under investigation occurs, and an instance in which it does not occur, have every circumstance in common save one, that one occurring only in the former; the circumstance in which alone the two instances differ is the effect or the cause, or an indispensable part of the cause of the phenomenon.* (1973 [1843], 391)

The application of the method of difference, like the other methods, is not automatic in any experimental situation and, as has been observed by a number of thinkers, *presumes* an analysis of the situation into all relevant factors, that can be examined one at a time.

Mill's methods also include, beside the better known method of agreement and the method of difference, the "method of residues," and the "method of concomitant variations." The latter, according to Mill, may be stated in canonical form as

> *Whatever phenomenon varies in any manner whenever another phenomenon varies in some particular manner, is either a cause or an effect of that phenomenon, or is connected with it through some fact of causation.* (401)

This method has important uses in biology and medicine, and an illustration of the method will be considered in the following section on direct and indirect evidence. Again, as in the case of the method of agreement, the complexity of biological organisms makes a simple and straightforward application of the method of concomitant variations uncertain. When we are attempting to determine the major causal role that, say, an entity plays in a system, a simple recording of concomitant variations is almost always insufficient. For example, if we compared a series of correlations in the level of a toxic substance in the blood with the titer of the substance in the urine excreted by the kidneys, we would not be able to ascribe an unambiguous causal role, such as clearing the blood of that substance, to the kidney. In such a case one would have to control for other possibilities, such as excretion via sweat glands, or be satisfied with a weak, indirectly supported causal claim. In point of fact, a direct causal judgment of the type indicated is possible only by picking cases in which the kidney is malfunctioning and using these as instances of the method of difference, a point to which I shall return again below.

The method of residues is likewise suspect in its simple application to biological causation. This method, in which one "*subduct[s] from any phenomenon such part as is known by previous inductions to be the effect of certain antecedents*," and considers "*the residue of the phenomenon . . . [to be] the effect of the remaining antecedents*" (398), is similarly difficult to apply in complex systems in which the residues are likely to be very large both in number and in their interactions.

I will argue shortly that the method of difference supplemented with a statistical interpretation, a combination which bears certain analogies to Mill's method of concomitant variation, is often the most appropriate method of experimental inquiry to establish empirically and directly scientific claims.[17]

4.6.2 Bernard's Method of Comparative Experimentation and Its Relation to Mill's Views

In his influential monograph *An Introduction to the Study of Experimental Medicine*, Claude Bernard noted that Mill's presumptions of an antecedent analysis of the experimental situation and of the ability to examine factors one at a time did not necessarily hold in experimental medicine, and he urged that the method of difference be further distinguished into (1) the "method of counterproof" and (2) the "method of comparative experimentation" (Bernard 1957 [1865], 55-57). According to Bernard, in the method of counterproof one assumes that a complete analysis of an experimental situation has been made, that all complicating and interfering factors have been identified and controlled. Subsequently, one eliminates the suspected cause and determines if the effect in which one is interested persists. Bernard believed that experimental medical investigators avoided counterproof as a method since they feared attempts to disprove their own favored hypotheses. Bernard defended a strong contrary position, and maintained that counterproof was essential to avoid elevating coincidences into confirmed hypotheses (Bernard, 55). He argued, however, that those entities that fell into the province of biology and medicine were so complex that any attempt to specify *all* of the causal antecedents of an effect was completely unrealistic. As a remedy for this problem he urged the consideration of the method of comparative experimentation. It is worth quoting him on this notion *in extenso:*

> Comparative experimentation bears . . . solely on notation of fact and on the art of disengaging it from circumstances or from other phenomena with which it may be entangled. Comparative experimentation, however, is not exactly what philosophers call the method of differences. When an experimenter is confronted with complex phenomena due to the combined properties of various bodies, he proceeds by differentiation, that is to say, he separates each of these bodies, one by one in succession, and sees by the difference what part of the total phenomenon belongs to each of them. But this method of exploration implies two things: it implies, first of all, that we know how many bodies are concerned in expressing the whole phenomenon, and then it admits that these bodies do not combine in any such way as to confuse their action in a final harmonious result. In physiology the method of differences is rarely applicable, because we can never flatter ourselves that we know all the bodies and all the conditions combining to express a collection of phenomena, and in numberless cases because various organs of the body may take each other's place in phenomena, that are partly common to them all, and may more or less obscure the results of ablation of a limited part. . . .
>
> Physiological phenomena are so complex that we could never experiment at all rigorously on living animals if we necessarily had to define all the other changes we might cause in the organism on which we were operating. But fortunately it is enough for us completely to isolate the one phenomenon on which our studies are brought to bear,

separating it by means of comparative experimentation from all surrounding complications. Comparative experimentation reaches this goal by adding to a similar organism, used for comparison, all our experimental changes save one, the very one which we intend to disengage.

If for instance, we wish to know the result of section or ablation of a deep-seated organ which cannot be reached without injuring many neighboring organs, we necessarily risk confusion in the total result between the effects of lesions caused by our operative procedure and the particular effects of section or ablation of the organ whose physiological role we wish to decide. The only way to avoid this mistake is to perform the same operation on a similar animal, but without making the section or ablation of the organ on which we are experimenting. We thus have two animals in which all the experimental conditions are the same, save one, — ablation of an organ whose action is thus disengaged and expressed in the difference observed between the two animals. Comparative experimentation in experimental medicine is an absolute and general rule applicable to all kinds of investigation, whether we wish to learn the effects of various agents influencing the bodily economy or to verify the physiological role of various parts of the body by experiments in vivisection. (127-128)

This recommendation of Bernard's is a characteristic feature of most inquiries in biology and medicine into the functions of organisms' parts and was, for example, utilized in the experimental investigations into the function of the thymus in the 1960s. Comparative experimentation, termed "sham operation" in the current literature on ablation, is thus one of the basic methods to insure a rational determination of causes or functions in biology and medicine. Bernard referred to comparative experimentation as "the true foundation of experimental medicine" (129).[18]

Bernard's account of comparative experimentation is useful but askew in important respects. It misrepresents the logic of causal inquiry in essentially two ways: (1) it overstates the distinction between the "method of difference" as classically conceived and the "method of comparative experimentation," and (2) it ignores the crucial necessity for a statistical approach in biomedical inquiry.

Let me first argue for essential identity of the methods of difference and the method of comparative experimentation. To see clearly what the relations between the methods are I shall first reformulate the method in terms of an abstract case. Let us suppose that an investigator wishes to apply the method of comparative experimentation to determine if an organ O plays a role in bringing about some physiological process I.[19] Let us also suppose that ablation of O involves at this point of time in medical science the need to injure severely or perhaps ablate an additional organ X that is adjacent to or surrounds O. (This introduces one aspect of the complexity with which Bernard was concerned in articulating his method of comparative experimentation.) The operative procedure also subjects the animal to general stress, S, which may also have an effect on process I. Implementation of Bernard's suggestions, then, will involve the investigator choosing (at least) two animals as similar as possible and creating the following comparative experimental situation:

$$\overline{X} \;\&\; S \;\&\; \overline{O} \;\&\; \overline{I} \quad (1)$$

in the first animal, and:

$$\overline{X} \;\&\; S \;\&\; O \;\&\; I \quad (2)$$

in the second. Here the bar over the capital letter asserts ablation of that organ, or cessation or severe attenuation of the process, in the case of I. This notion of attenuation raises a point to which I shall have to return below. Such ablation is normally surgical, but in some cases could be done by genetic means (i.e., by selecting mutants not possessing the organ) or by hormonal methods applied in the development of the organism (with appropriate modification of the stress term). Accordingly, (1) reads: animal 1 has organs X and O ablated, has been subject to operational stress S, and does not manifest (the usual level of) I.

Now it is important to note that the *minutely specific* details of X (the ablation of X) such as detailed reports of the trauma to surrounding blood vessels, and the details of stress S, do *not* need to be known as long as there are reasonable grounds for assuming that X and S in the two animals are equivalent. This is emphasized by Bernard in his comments quoted above. It must be added, however, as a criticism of Bernard's overly strong distinction between the methods of comparative experimentation and of difference, that when one examines the logic of the method represented by (1) and (2) above, it appears equivalent to the method of difference, and that he was not entirely fair to Mill.

Bernard was not fair to Mill since Mill himself made the following comment concerning the application of the methods of experimental inquiry, including the method of difference:

> The extent and minuteness of observation which may be requisite, and the degree of decomposition to which it may be necessary to carry the mental analysis, depend on the particular purpose in view. . . . As to the degree of minuteness of the mental subdivision, if we were obliged to break down what we observe into its very simplest elements, that is, literally into single facts, it would be difficult to say where we should find them: We can hardly ever affirm that our divisions of any kind have reached the ultimate unit. But this, too, is fortunately unnecessary. The only object of the mental separation is to suggest the requisite physical separation, so that we may either accomplish it ourselves, or seek for it in nature; and we have done enough when we have carried the subdivision as far as the point at which we are able to see what observations or experiments we require. It is only essential, at whatever point our mental decomposition of facts may for the present have stopped, that we should hold ourselves ready and able to carry it farther as occasion requires, and should not allow the freedom of our discriminating faculty to be imprisoned by the swathes and bands of ordinary classification. . . . (Mill 1973 [1843], 380–381)

Our contention that, logically and epistemologically, the method of comparative experimentation is equivalent to the method of difference, can be substantiated by noting what the experimenter is attempting to do in (1) and (2) above is to fulfill Mill's conditions for application of the method of difference; in other words, the experimenter is searching for *one* difference (O versus) associated with the presence (I) or absence (Ī) of the process I.

Let me now turn to my second general point, namely that Bernard ignores the crucial need for a statistical approach in inquiry in biology and medicine. Bernard's dislike of statistical analyses in scientific inquiry and his general scorn for statistics, as illustrated by several colorful examples, are generally well known, almost to the point of notoriety. For example, I. Bernard Cohen, in his foreword to Bernard's *Introduction to the Study of Experimental Medicine,* wrote:

> Anyone would agree with the absurdity of making a "balance sheet" of every substance taken in and excreted by a cat during eight days of nourishment and nineteen days of fasting, if on the seventeenth day kittens were born and counted as excreta. . . . Another example given by Bernard is the physiologist who "took urine from a railroad station urinal where people of all nations passed, and who believed he could thus present an analysis of *average* European urine!"[20]

Unfortunately for Bernard's position, statistical analysis has become a cynosure in the methodological armamentarium of biology and medicine. For reasons discussed in the previous chapters, such as the complexity and variability of organisms, statistical assessments of the empirical evidence corroborating hypotheses have become mandatory even in those areas where it is believed the processes are generally nonstochastic. This is the case for inquiry into the functions of organs and other biological entities.

Let us review some of the research which led to the two-component theory of the immune response discussed in the last chapter. In his classical article on "Immunological Function of the Thymus," J. F. A. P. Miller (1961) reported that there were significant differences between thymectomized and sham-thymectomized mice.[21] Miller analyzed both groups of mice with respect to two aspects of cellular immunity. He provided evidence showing that skin grafts on genetically dissimilar mice survived significantly longer on thymectomized mice compared with their sham-thymectomized counterparts. No formal statistics were used here even though the "comparative experiment" was clearly statistical, presumably because the comparison was not (at this point in time) distinctly quantifiable. The second aspect of Miller's experiment involved counts of the average lymphocyte : polymorph (or polymorphonuclear leukocyte) ratio of his two groups of mice. Here Miller reported *specific statistical differences* in the standard notation. His graph is reproduced as figure 4.1. It would take us beyond the scope of this chapter to dwell extensively on the interpretation of the statistics in Miller's experiment, but these issues will be considered in chapter 5. Suffice

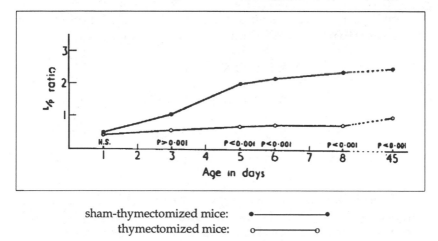

sham-thymectomized mice: •————————•
thymectomized mice: o————————o

Figure 4.1 Average lymphocyte : polymorph ratio of mice thymectomized in the neonatal period compared to sham-thymectomized controls. Statistical differences indicated. From Miller (1961), with permission.

it to say that in complex biological organisms, even of highly in-bred strains, variability (whether the source be genetic, environmental, or due to the measuring instruments) almost always requires a statistical analysis of the results of ablations in operated and sham-operated biota.

Let me now consider the question of complexity (and complex redundancy) from several other perspectives, from which it might be alleged one could call into question the methodology thus far developed. First, let us imagine the existence in our above schema of some alternative organ P which assumes O's role only when O is ablated or damaged. P then will mask O's function, since I will still occur following ablation of O. This biological phenomenon whereby there exist alternative pathways to the same end has been variously termed "multiple causation" or "parastasis."[22] I would argue in this case that the only way to determine experimentally that O's function is being masked by P is by applying a *reiterated method of comparative experimentation* (or difference) to an augmented experimental situation. Accordingly, the way to determine causes experimentally is not to es-chew the method of comparative experimentation in such circumstances but rather to apply it more vigorously. Schemati-cally we can represent this reiterated application as follows: If P (or any other organ) is suspected of masking O's function, then one creates experimentally the following situation:

$$\overline{X} \,\&\, S \,\&\, O \,\&\, P \,\&\, I \quad (1)$$

$$\overline{X} \,\&\, S \,\&\, \overline{O} \,\&\, P \,\&\, I \quad (2)$$

$$\overline{X} \,\&\, S \,\&\, O \,\&\, \overline{P} \,\&\, I \quad (3)$$

$$\overline{X} \,\&\, S \,\&\, \overline{O} \,\&\, \overline{P} \,\&\, \overline{I} \quad (4)$$

This shows that in O's absence P promotes I and also that O can promote I without P, but that with joint ablation of O and P process I does not occur. Therefore, O *or* P, in the weak sense of "or," is necessary for I.[23]

This qualitative account might have to be further developed into the more sensitive statistical, *quantitative* account hinted at above in certain circumstances involving interdependence. For example, one might suppose that, though P promotes I, it does so significantly less efficiently than does O. It might also be the case, however, that O requires P in order for O to function at peak efficiency. In such a circumstance, (2) above would have as a schematic analogue

$$\overline{X} \,\&\, S \,\&\, \overline{O} \,\&\, P \,\&\, \hat{I} \quad (2')$$

with (3) becoming:

$$\overline{X} \,\&\, S \,\&\, O \,\&\, \overline{P} \,\&\, \hat{I} \quad (3')$$

where $\hat{I}$ reflects a significant attenuation of I. Such a situation would warrant asserting that O promotes or causes I but would depend on a quantitative analysis and almost certainly involve statistical calculations.

Having defended the suitability of a generalized method of comparative experimentation in the case of parastasis, let us now turn to another type of criticism which might be directed against our thesis of the pre-eminence of a generalized method of comparative experimentation.

4.6.3 *The Deductive Method*

We have looked at the four classical methods of experimental inquiry above, namely the methods of agreement, difference,
residues, and concomitant variation. Our major source, John
Stuart Mill, however, believed that in certain complex sciences
involving, for example, the *intermixture of effects,* that none of
these four methods was sufficient. For such inquiries he recommended the *deductive* method. This method he characterized as
follows, "in its most general expression the Deductive
Method . . . consists of three operations—the first one of direct
induction; the second, of ratiocination; the third, of verification"
(Mill 1973 [1843], 454).

Mill believed that one had to ascertain the simple laws and
tendencies by direct induction and then, from a conjunction of
these simple tendencies, deduce consequences which could in
turn be verified. He noted, however, that there were considerable difficulties involved in applying this prescription to the
biomedical sciences of physiology and pathology. He wrote:

> Accordingly, in the cases, unfortunately very numer-
> ous and important, in which the causes do not suffer
> themselves to be separated and observed apart, there is
> much difficulty in laying down with due certainty the
> inductive foundation necessary to support the deductive
> method. This difficulty is most of all conspicuous in the case
> of physiological phenomena: it being seldom possible to
> separate the different agencies which collectively compose
> an organized body, without destroying the very phenom-
> ena which it is our object to investigate:

> "Following life, in creatures we dissect,
> We lose it in the moment we detect."

> And for this reason I am inclined to the opinion that
> physiology (greatly and rapidly progressive as it now is) is
> embarrassed by greater natural difficulties, and is probably
> susceptible of a less degree of ultimate perfection than even
> the social sciences, inasmuch as it is possible to study the
> laws and operations of one human mind apart from other
> minds much less imperfectly than we can study the laws of
> one organ or tissue of the human body apart from the other
> organs or tissues. (456)

Mill added that "pathological facts, or, to speak in common language, diseases in their different forms and degrees, afford in the case of physiological investigation the most valuable equivalent to experimentation properly so called, inasmuch as they often exhibit to us a definite disturbance in some one organ or organic function, the remaining organs and functions being, in the first instance at least, unaffected" (1973 [1843], 456). Even these observations, however, were contingent on *early* observations, inasmuch as diseases quickly had complicating systemic effects.

Mill further noted that "Besides natural pathological facts, we can produce pathological facts artificially; we can try experiments . . . by subjecting [for example] the living being to . . . the section of a nerve to ascertain the functions of different parts of the nervous system" (457). Such experiments, Mill suggested "are best tried . . . in the condition of health, comparatively a fixed state . . . [in which] the course of the accustomed physiological phenomena would, it may generally be presumed, remain undisturbed, were it not for the disturbing cause of which we introduce" (457). Mill summed up the utility of these approaches, which all appear to be the application of the method of difference or comparative experimentation as we have characterized it above, as follows:

> Such, with the occasional aid of the Method of Concomitant Variations, (the latter not less encumbered than the more elementary methods by the peculiar difficulties of the subject), are our inductive resources for ascertaining the laws of the causes considered separately, when we have it not in our power to make trial of them in a state of actual separation. (457)

4.6.4 *The Hypothetical Method*

In Mill's writing, the deductive method was sharply distinguished from the method of hypothesis or "Hypothetical Method." This latter method was denigrated by Mill since it "suppresses the first of the three steps, the induction to ascertain the law, and contents itself with the other two operations, ratiocination and verification, the law which is reasoned from being assumed instead of proved" (492). For Mill, the inductions which provided the laws necessary for the first step in the deductive method could be replaced by "a prior deduction," which would, of course, be dependent for its inductive force on *previously established* inductive truths.

Mill defended his view by arguing that certain classical examples that had been interpreted as examples of the hypothetical method were in fact subject to special constraints that relied on more acceptable methods. His most famous example is perhaps his interpretation of Newton's reasoning about universal gravitation:

> Newton began by an assumption that the force which at each instant deflects a planet from its rectilineal course, and makes it describe a curve round the sun, is a force tending directly towards the sun. He then proved that if this be so the planet will describe, as we know by Kepler's first law that it does describe, equal areas in equal times; and, lastly, he proved that if the force acted in any other direction whatever, the planet would not describe equal areas in equal times. It being thus shown that no other hypothesis would accord with the facts, the assumption was proved; the hypothesis became an inductive truth. . . .
>
> I have said that in this case the verification fulfills the conditions of an induction; but an induction of what sort? On examination we find that it conforms to the canon of the Method of Difference. It affords the two instances, A B C, *a b c* and B C, *b c*. A represents central force; A B C, the planets plus a central force; B C, the planets apart from a central force. The planets with a central force give *a*, areas proportional to the times; the planets without a central force give *b c* (a set of motions) without *a*, or with something else instead of *a*. This is the Method of Difference in all its strictness. (Mill (1973) [1843], 492-493)

In my view there is an important kernel of truth in Mill's position here. The hypothetical method in Mill's sense is essentially identical to what philosophers of science, for example, Hanson, Hempel, and Popper, have termed the hypothetico-deductive method. This method, without additional constraints, yields only *indirect* evidence. When the hypothetical method is supplemented by an additional constraint similar to that found in Mill's Newtonian example, however, the evidence, though *laced with hypotheses*, amounts to *direct* evidence and is broadly accepted as strong support for a scientific claim.[24] Let me elaborate on this.

4.7 Direct versus Indirect Evidence: Arguments for a Continuum

Experiments providing confirmation or falsification of a hypothesis are often discussed in terms of yielding "direct" or "indirect" evidence for a hypothesis or process. Whether an experiment can be classified as yielding direct or indirect evidence would seem to depend on such factors as (1) the degree of scientists' confidence in the auxiliary hypotheses (including control of the initial conditions) used in obtaining the observable implication and (2) the existence (or nonexistence) of proposed plausible competing hypotheses accounting for the same observations. The issue of the "directness" of evidence has been the subject of several inquiries into experiments and sophisticated examples of "observation" in the past ten years, and though most of this discussion has focused on examples from the physical sciences, the analyses have relevance for biology and medicine.

The most sophisticated philosophical analysis of "observation" to appear recently is Shapere's discussion of the topic in solar astronomy. Shapere argues that astrophysicists' usage of the term "observation" licenses the claim that we can have a "*direct view* of the solar core" (Shapere 1982, 488 quoting Ruderman 1969). This direct "seeing" involves the use of a prototypical "theoretical entity," a neutrino, which transmits the information. For Shapere, more generally:

> *x is directly observed (observable) if:*
>
> *(1) information is received (can be received) by an appropriate receptor; and*
> *(2) that information is (can be) transmitted directly, i.e., without interference, to the receptor from the entity x (which is the source of the information).*
> (Shapere 1982, 492)

What Shapere demonstrates is that "direct observation" can be, and is in astrophysics, heavily theory-laden. Shapere's analysis has been criticized by Hacking (1983, 185) who, though he generally favors it, finds that it is committed to the "old foundationalist" view of knowledge that attempts to base knowledge on observation. In my view, in conformity with the position of "generalized empiricism" discussed at the beginning of this chapter, this is a virtue and not a vice of Shapere's account. I must add, however, that Shapere does not seem to be sufficiently sensitive to the *provisional* character of the "directness" of such observation, along the lines of the two factors stated above (confidence in the auxiliary assumptions and the nonexistence of alternative, competing explanations of the observations).

This view seems to be in agreement with Galison's (1987) discussion of the *directness* of measurements and what he terms the *stability* of experimental results. Galison's account of directness seems to owe something to Shapere's account discussed above, and seems to be a comparative concept. "By directness," he writes, "I mean all those laboratory moves that bring experimental reasoning another rung up the causal ladder: measurement of a background previously calculated . . . or the separate measurement of an effect only previously measured together. . . . Or directness may refer to the signal itself" (1987, 259-260). Though this is somewhat obscure, Galison couples his notion of "directness" closely to his concept of "stability," which roughly captures "an underlying stubbornness of the phenomenon." Galison writes:

> By "stability" I have in mind all those procedures that vary some feature of the experimental conditions: changes in the test substance, in the apparatus, in the arrangement, or in the data analysis that leave the results basically unchanged. . . . Each variation makes it harder to postulate an alternative causal story that will satisfy all the observations. (1987, 260)

Galison adds that this resistance to alternative causal stories has implications for views about scientific realism, and in point of fact cites Hacking's (1983) position about the epistemological force of "intervening" as being closely related to this resistance. The issue of scientific realism is best deferred to chapter 5, where it can be pursued in more depth than at present; suffice it to note that the factors I mentioned above concerning the continuum from indirect to direct evidence appear born out in inquiries focused on (generally) very different subject matters than biology and medicine, suggesting the issues are both robust and significant ones.

A fairly extended historical case will help to bring out more clearly these points about the force of "direct" evidence and its role in experimental inquiry in biology and medicine. The operon theory of Jacob and Monod as it is understood today was briefly discussed in the previous chapter. Here it would be appropriate to reintroduce the theory. I wish to use this illustration to indicate how the experimental evidence for the theory's hypotheses became increasingly more direct in the years 1961 through 1967, though it remained dependent on both auxiliary hypotheses and the existence (and nonexistence) of plausible competing theories. The strong evidence for the theory provided by Gilbert and Müller-Hill, to be discussed below, also illustrates the important application of the methods of difference or comparative experimentation and concomitant variation.

The 1961 form of the Jacob-Monod operon theory was presented in chapter 3, and for readers interested in seeing exactly how those authors characterized their theory as a "model" a quotation from their 1961 paper is provided in Technical Discussion 5.

TECHNICAL DISCUSSION 5

A convenient method of summarizing the conclusions derived in the preceding sections of this paper will be to organize them into a model designed to embody the main elements which we were led to recognize as playing a specific role in the control of protein synthesis; namely the structural, regulator and operator genes, the operon, and the cytoplasmic repressor. Such a model could be as follows:

The molecular structure of proteins is determined by specific elements, the *structural genes*. These act by forming a cytoplasmic "transcript" of themselves, the structural messenger, which in turn synthesizes the protein. The synthesis of the messenger by the structural gene is a sequential replicative process, which can be initiated only at certain points on the DNA strand, and the cytoplasmic transcription of several, linked, structural genes may depend upon a single initiating point or *operator*. The genes whose activity is thus co-ordinated form an *operon*.

The operator tends to combine (by virtue of possessing a particular base sequence) specifically and reversibly with a certain (RNA) fraction [later understood to be a protein and not RNA] possessing the proper (complementary) sequence. This combination blocks the initiation of cytoplasmic transcription and there-

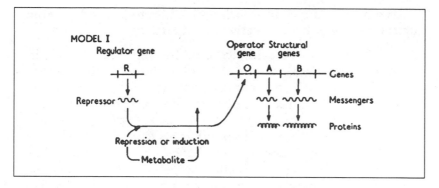

Figure 4.2   From Jacob and Monod (1961), with permission.

fore the formation of the messenger by the structural genes in the whole operon. The specific "repressor" (RNA?), acting with a given operator, is synthesized by a *regulator gene.*

The repressor in certain systems (inducible enzyme systems) tends to combine specifically with certain specific small molecules. The combined repressor has no affinity for the operator, and the combination therefore results in *activation of the operon.*

In other systems (repressible enzyme systems) the repressor by itself is inactive (i.e., it has no affinity for the operator) and is activated only by combining with certain specific small molecules. The combination therefore leads to *inhibition of the operon.*

The structural messenger is an unstable molecule, which is destroyed in the process of information transfer. The rate of messenger synthesis, therefore, in turn controls the rate of protein synthesis. This model was meant to summarize and express conveniently the properties of the different factors which play a specific role in the control of protein synthesis. (Jacob and Monod 1961, 352)

(A diagram of the mode of interaction of the postulated entities as understood in 1961 is given in figure 4.2.)

In spite of the breadth of evidence for the operon theory in 1961, it can be said that the evidence was primarily of an *indirect* genetic type. Monod in his Nobel lecture suggested, for example, that in the early 1960s the repressor — the crucial regulatory entity — seemed "as inaccessible as the matter of the stars." He characterized the indirect approach which had to be made to studying the repressor by a detective novel analogy:

What is to be said, then, of the repressor, which is known only by the results of its interactions? In this respect we are in a position somewhat similar to that of the police inspector who, finding a corpse with a dagger in its back, deduces that somewhere there is an assassin; but as for knowing who the assassin is, what his name is, whether he is tall or short, dark or fair, that is another matter. The police in this case, it seems, sometimes get results by sketching a composite portrait of the culprit from several clues. This is what I am going to try to do now with regard to the repressor.

First, it is necessary to assign to the assassin—I mean the repressor—two properties: the ability to recognize the inducer and the ability to recognize the operator. (Monod 1966, 480)

The difficulty of being able to provide more direct biochemical evidence for the existence of the repressor and its postulated properties stimulated at least one alternative theory of genetic regulation. Ames and Hartman in 1963, and subsequently Gunther Stent in 1964, proposed that regulation might take place, not at the genetic level of transcription, but rather in the cytoplasm at the level of translation.[25] Stent's (1964) account was quite complex, but basically what had been genetically mapped as the "operator gene" was reinterpreted in terms of a mechanism that acted in the cell's cytoplasm.[26] Stent's theory was complicated, but one not excluded by the genetic evidence. Importantly, it proposed different entities than did the Jacob-Monod theory, for example, an "operator-less operon."

In 1966 Walter Gilbert and Benno Müller-Hill reported that they had been able to isolate the elusive repressor, and in 1967 the same authors were able to demonstrate that the repressor bound directly to the operator DNA.[27] These experiments were most important for the field of regulatory genetics, and they were confirmed by Mark Ptashne's essentially simultaneous isolation of the repressor in the phage λ system and discovery that it also bound to DNA (Ptashne 1967). In the discussion below, I will focus on Gilbert and Müller-Hill's experiments. Some comments on their techniques and experimental methodology will help to elucidate the nature of "direct" evidence in the biomedical sciences. (For details see Technical Discussion 6.)

Gilbert and Müller-Hill noted in the paper reporting their results that, though they felt the Jacob and Monod theory to be the simplest, other models would also "fit the data" available. "Repressors," they continued, "could have almost any target that would serve as a block to any of the initiation processes required to make a protein. A molecular understanding of the control process has waited on the isolation of one or more repressors" (1966, 1891).

Isolating the repressor was particularly difficult because of the hypothesized very low concentration of repressor in the *E. coli* cells. Gilbert and Müller-Hill were aided in their task by looking for and finding mutant strains of the bacteria that allowed them to devise several different types of controls. In addition, they employed a radioactive form of the inducer to determine its presence in bacteria whose operons were alternately turned on and turned off.

Gilbert and Müller-Hill discovered that the enzymes that would attack DNA and RNA would not destroy the inducer binding ability of the presumed repressor but that an enzyme that attacked proteins would. Heating (above 50°C) also destroyed the ability to bind inducer. This was rather direct evidence that the repressor *was* a protein, though still conditional on hypotheses (1) that the enzymes possessed anti-DNA/anti-RNA capacity and (2) that heat denatures proteins. In addition, they determined, using standard methods, that the repressor had a molecular weight of about 150,000-200,000 daltons.

TECHNICAL DISCUSSION 6

Isolating the repressor was most difficult because of the hypothesized very low concentration of repressor in the *E. coli* cells. Gilbert and Müller-Hill solved this problem by looking for and finding a mutant form of the bacteria (i^t or tight-binding) that produced a repressor with about a 10-fold greater affinity for the inducer. As an inducer they used a radioactive form of the chemical IPTG (isopropylthiogalactosidose), which induces enzyme synthesis via the *lac* operon but which, in contrast to lactose, is not metabolized by the induced enzyme. (This type of inducer, discovered in Monod's laboratory in the early 1950s, is known as a "gratuitous inducer"). The repressor was detected by placing an extract of the i^t mutant in a dialysis sac in a solution of the radioactive IPTG and looking for an increased concentration of IPTG inside the sack after about thirty minutes (at 4°C).

Using the increased concentration as a sign of the presence of repressor, Gilbert and Müller-Hill purified the extract and analyzed the binding component. They discovered that the enzymes that would attack DNA and RNA would not destroy the inducer binding ability of the presumed repressor, but that an enzyme that attacked proteins would. Heating (above 50°C) also destroyed the ability to bind inducer. This was rather direct evidence, though still conditional on hypotheses (1) that the enzymes possessed anti-DNA/anti-RNA capacity and (2) that heat denatures proteins, that the repressor *was* a protein. The repressor (labeled with the radioactive inducer) was centrifuged and sedimented on a glycerol gradient. The "profile" of the sedemented repressor indicated that it had a molecular weight of about 150,000–200,000 daltons.

In their paper, Gilbert and Müller-Hill cited what they termed "negative and positive controls" on their supposition that they had isolated the repressor product of the *i* gene. The most important "negative controls" involved examining the extracts from *i*s (the superrepressed) and *i*- (constitutive) mutants. The former type (*i*s) presumably synthesizes a repressor which has lost the ability to bind inducer, and the latter *i*- had been hypothesized to produce an incomplete repressor. For both of these mutants no binding of IPTG was observed. (Gilbert and Müller-Hill noted that "the various mutant forms of the *i* gene were put into identical genetic backgrounds, so that unknown variations from strain to strain could not confuse the issue.") As "positive controls" Gilbert and Müller-Hill plotted graphs representing the binding constants of the wild type and *i*t mutant to demonstrate the essential identity of the repressors. An examination of the binding ability of the repressor for various other substances including galactose and glucose (yielding a decreasing *sequence* of affinities) "gave further support for the [thesis that the isolated] material . . . [was] the repressor."

In the following year (1967), Gilbert and Müller-Hill used this partially purified radioactive repressor to test for in vitro binding to the operator of *lac* DNA. In this experiment Gilbert and Müller-Hill used strains of bacteriophage which carried different forms of the *lac* operon in their DNA. By sedimenting mixtures of the various strains of the phage DNA with the radioactive repressor Gilbert and Müller-Hill found that:

(1) In the absence of inducer the radioactive chemical binds to the DNA.

(2) In the presence of IPTG, which releases the repressor from the DNA, no binding is observed.

(3) The effect of the IPTG is specific, for substitution by a chemical ONPF (a substance which binds to the DNA but does not induce) has no effect.

(4) Use of two mutant phage o^c strains, in which the affinity of the operator for the repressor is expected to be weaker by factors of 10 and 200 respectively, yielded sedimentation profiles in rough quantitative conformity with these binding expectations.

In their paper, Gilbert and Müller-Hill cited what they termed "negative and positive controls" in their experiments. The most important "negative controls" involved examining repressor molecules from mutants that on other evidence were known to produce defective repressors. These isolated defective repressors did *not* bind inducers, confirming Gilbert and Müller-Hill's expectations. As "positive controls" Gilbert and Müller-Hill plotted graphs representing the binding capabilities of their various mutant repressors. Their results here "gave further support for the [thesis that the isolated] material. . . [was] the repressor."

In the following year (1967), Gilbert and Müller-Hill used their isolated repressor, now made radioactive so it could be followed, to test for binding to the operator of *lac* DNA in the test tube (in vitro). In this experiment they found that:

(1) In the absence of inducer the radioactive repressor bound to the DNA.

(2) In the presence of an added inducer no binding was observed.

(3) Substitution of a close analogue of the inducer, which bound to the DNA but had a slightly different structure, did not induce; thus the inducer had a very *specific* action.

(4) Use of two additional mutants, known to have quantitatively different binding strengths for the repressor, yielded independent evidence, scaled according to these binding strengths, in conformity with the expectations.

These experiments, which appear to utilize the methods of comparative experimentation or difference (the "negative controls") and concomitant variation (the "positive controls"), have been characterized as offering "direct" evidence and "proving" the hypotheses of the Jacob-Monod theory. Clearly they do so, however, with the aid of auxiliary hypotheses involving, among other considerations, (1) the effects of growth in radioactive media so as specifically to label the "observed" entities and (2) the analysis of centrifugation and sedimentation techniques in density gradients (described in Technical Discussion 6). The experiments require a chain of reasoning and so, accordingly, also fit into Mill's characterization of the "deductive method." There is, in addition, (c) a general, negative auxiliary assumption (of a ceteris paribus type) that what is observed is not an artifact. It must be further emphasized that the "direct proof" of the Jacob-Monod operon theory is contingent on the assumption that other, and perhaps more important and overriding factors are not involved; that is, that some competing but as yet unarticulated hypothesis could not account for all these results. (As noted in chapter 3, in the years since 1967 it *has* in fact been discovered that there are several additional controls in the *lac* region. Though the discovery of additional control mechanisms certainly does not invalidate either the Jacob-Monod theory nor Gilbert and Müller-Hill's elegant experiments, it should provide an indication of the complexity of biological mechanisms.) The proposal of a novel mechanism of control that would account for the genetic data as well as Gilbert and Müller-Hill's findings (perhaps by showing some of them to be artifacts) but that would disagree with basic tenets of the operon theory cannot be logically excluded. The existence of Gilbert and Müller-Hill's experiments thus constitutes a *conditional* direct proof, the conditions depending on (1) the truth of auxiliary hypotheses and (2) the nonexistence of an inconsistent competing theory that would account for the same data as the operon theory.

Let us now generalize from this example and also relate these notions of direct evidence or "proof" to two current views concerning testing and evidence. The "directness" and force of the evidence is obtained by choosing one or more *central* (roughly equivalent to "essential") properties of the hypotheses in the theory to be tested. In the operon theory's case these properties were initially suggested in the quotation from Monod on p. 160, namely the repressor's "recognition" of the inducer and the operator. In addition, plausible competitor theories are scanned to determine if the test condition(s), if realized, would support the theory under test while falsifying the competitors. Recall that *genetic* evidence was insufficient to do this, whereas the Gilbert-

Müller-Hill experiments (as well as Ptashne's) were. The evidence was considerably strengthened by providing both positive and negative controls. Having these controls makes the methodology essentially equivalent to Mill's well-known methods of difference and of concomitant variation discussed earlier.

4.8 Glymour's Analysis of Relevant Evidence

In several articles and in his important book *Theory and Evidence*, Clark (1980), Glymour has proposed a new theory of hypothesis and theory testing. He claims that it is in important respects different from the hypothetico-deductive account of confirmation outlined in the earlier portions of this chapter. Glymour argues that his analysis provides a better idea of the *relevance* of evidence to a hypothesis, that it permits one to test specific hypotheses in a theory rather than testing the theory globally, and that it rationalizes and reinterprets scientists' preferences for evidential variety and for simplicity.

It would take us beyond the scope of this book to subject each of Glymour's claims to scrutiny, but there are interesting relations of his account to the views on direct and indirect evidence outlined above, so some exposition of his views is warranted at this point.[28] Glymour's theory is primarily directed at theories that are expressed in the form of equations relating various quantities. Glymour's approach in a sense stands the H-D approach on its head, by urging that we test theories by computing specific values of the quantities from observations (and from other theories) and substituting them in the to-be-tested theoretical statement. The theoretical statement under test can *itself* be used to compute a value of unknown quantity, as long as the statement is not an identity. Thus in the general gas equation relating pressure (P), volume (V), and temperature (T):

$$PV = kT$$

one specific set of values, say p_1, v_1, t_1, can be used to calculate the value of the constant k, and then another triple of values, p_2, v_2, t_2, used to test the hypothesis. It is the use of the theory which itself is being tested to generate the data used to test the theory that has led Glymour to label this procedure "bootstrapping." In general, Glymour maintains, such a determination or computation may be represented by a finite graph. The initial, or zero-level, nodes of the graph will be experimentally determined quantities; n-level nodes will be quantities or combinations of quantities such that, for each n-level node, some hypothesis of the theory determines a unique value of that node from suitable values of all the (n – 1)-level nodes with which it is connected. The graph will have a single maximal element, and that element will be a single quantity. We permit that two connected or unconnected nodes may correspond to the same quantity or combination of quantities. I will call such a graph a *computation*. (1975, 409)

Computations can be used to *test* hypotheses:

A plausible necessary condition for a set I of values of quantities to test hypothesis h with respect to theory T is that there exist computations (using hypotheses in T and h) from I of values from the quantities occurring in h, and there exist a set J of possible values for the same initial quantities such that the same computations from J result in a negative instance of h — that is, the values of the quantities occurring in h which are computed from J must contradict h. (1975, 411)

Glymour contends that this method of testing is in fact that used by Newton in arguing for the inverse square law of gravitation, and he discusses the Newtonian approach and the necessary approximation qualifications *in extenso*.

The similarity of this illustration to Mill's account of the deductive method and Glymour's method is suggestive. What it appears to indicate is that, though Glymour goes beyond Mill in his analysis, what Glymour is *explicating* is what I have termed above "direct evidence." If this interpretation is defensible, several corollaries follow. First, Glymour's account is likely to be incomplete as a theory of testing, since indirect tests are important at a variety of stages in a theory's evolution. Second, this interpretation suggests that there are *other* means of obtaining the type of tests which Glymour envisions as significant, which may be particularly suited to nonquantitative theories. In point of fact the methods of difference or comparative experimentation and roughly concomitant variation discussed above could be construed as providing the evidence that tests the operon theory with the strictness at which Glymour aims.

In addition to the H-D analysis, Glymour considers two other general views of theory testing, (1) analyses based on inductive logic accounts and (2) the conventionalist approach. The latter approach holds that the relevance of evidence is a matter of education — purely conventional — and this is, rightly I think, summarily dismissed by Glymour. The inductive logic accounts, such as Hempel's qualitative and Carnap's quantitative explications, are criticized as not providing linguistic connections between theoretical and observational subvocabularies that would permit an explication of support for the theory as a whole or for specific theoretical hypotheses. In addition, Glymour discusses the Bayesian approach to inductive support, of which he is quite critical for reasons which will be discussed in chapter 5.

There I shall argue (contra Glymour) that a Bayesian account is the best *general* analysis of hypothesis and theory testing and acceptance presently available. It seems to me that, given the fact that we need an analysis which rationalizes both indirect and direct testing, the flexible Bayesian account is potentially more general than Glymour's. That it can also do as well as his vis-à-vis other desiderata for an inductive logic, such as providing reasons why evidential variety and simplicity are valuable, will also be demonstrated in later chapters. I have argued above that the distinction between direct and indirect evidence actually falls on a continuum, and that support is a function of available competing hypotheses. These features are naturally incorporated in the Bayesian analysis, as will be shown in chapter 5.

4.9 Summary

This chapter has covered a number of issues. The first two sections developed the general philosophical position that underlies the discussion of experimental testing in this chapter and evaluation in the next. I termed this position "generalized empiricism"; it places a premium on empirical foundations, but I believe it does so in a way that is more flexible than, say, Shapere's 1982 (though it has affinities with it) and more in accord with Hacking's (1983) and Galison's (1987) views about experiments. Generalized empiricism departs from both positivism and logical positivism and accepts theoretical discourse as "meaningful" per se; how this works in detail was shown in section 5.2. Section 5.3 reviewed some preliminary points about experimental testing and then illustrated them using the Nossal-Lederberg experiment — the first experiment designed to test the clonal selection theory — introduced in chapters 2 and 3, and section 5.4 discussed how theories assist in defining observations as relevant. Special considerations about "initial conditions" in biology and medicine were described in section 5.6, and the problem of distinguishing an experimental effect from an artifact, an issue which has received increased attention in the past five years, was considered with reference to Franklin's (1986) comment on the importance of distinguishing these notions. These preliminaries pave the way for an in-depth analysis of the "methods of experimental inquiry" from the perspectives of John Stuart Mill, Claude Bernard, and more contemporary commentators. Finally, the issue of "direct evidence," discussed in physics by Shapere (1982) and Galison (1987), was examined with respect to molecular biology, employing an extended example of Gilbert and Müller-Hill's isolation of the repressor of the operon theory (introduced in chapter 3). This chapter closed with some comments on Glymour's (1975, 1980) "bootstrapping" approach to theory testing, and foreshadowed elements of the Bayesian analysis to be introduced in the next chapter.

Evaluation: Local and Global Approaches

Part I: Local Evaluation and Statistical Hypothesis Testing

5.1 Introduction

IN THE PREVIOUS CHAPTER I developed an account of how hypotheses and theories are tested; in the present chapter we shall turn to considering how hypotheses and theories are evaluated. Initially I will concentrate on the (comparatively) *local* evaluation of hypotheses. By this term I refer to those types of evaluation which have a high degree of specificity and in which very general and sweeping considerations of evaluation do not enter. The latter type of evaluation I term *global*. Global evaluation refers in part to evaluational problems of the type that Kuhn (1970) characterized as "revolutionary science" in his classic *The Structure of Scientific Revolutions*. Local evaluation, however, indicates somewhat more than just evaluation within Kuhnian "normal science," for I intend by the term to refer to evaluation using rather highly developed methodological techniques from statistics. Issues arising in global evaluation, such as "meaning variance" and "truth," will be considered in later sections of this chapter.

I shall begin by focusing on hypotheses that are largely of the statistical sort, in conformity with the thesis of the importance of statistical reasoning cited in chapter 4 and to appear again in chapter 6 with respect to explanation. These considerations apply, however, also to nonstatistical or deterministic universal hypotheses. In point of fact, if it is acknowledged that evaluation of deterministic hypotheses involves likelihoods of less than one because of observational error, then the discussion of this chapter applies fairly straightforwardly to deterministic hypotheses.[1]

In the previous chapter we considered the testing of several "deterministic" hypotheses. In chapter 2 I noted that under certain conditions we might have a sufficient "sharpening" of the "smeared out" character of biological processes. This sharpening can occur by natural selection at various levels or by artificial selection for pure types of mutants. Such sharpening will result generally in a more "deterministic" system.[2] In the case of the Nossal-Lederberg test of the clonal selection theory and in Gilbert and Müller-Hill's isolation of the repressor, we saw instances of such deterministic results. Where we can obtain direct evidence in the sense described in chapter 4, we obtain what amounts to a crucial experiment, and the evaluation of such well-confirmed hypotheses is, for the period of time until alternative, competing hypotheses appear, particularly compelling.

Many hypotheses in the biomedical sciences, however, are not testable in such a direct manner and, in addition, even hypotheses that initially appear deterministic often turn out to require statistical analysis. The experiments by Mäkelä on the "double producers" discovered subsequent to the Nossal-Lederberg experiment represent an example of experiments requiring such probabilistic or statistical analysis, and the work of J. F. A. P. Miller on the thymus outlined in chapter 4 is another illustration. As we shall see later in this chapter, even deterministic results of a theory are embedded in an evaluation of the temporally extended theory which is best treated probabilistically.[3]

The approach in this chapter will be essentially *normative*. Though what scientists actually do when they evaluate hypotheses is of crucial importance in assessing any account of local evaluation, I believe I provide sufficient evidence that the examples discussed in this chapter are representative of actual scientific activity, so that any question of adequately capturing actual scientific practices need not arise. The main objective in this chapter is to develop a consistent general account of both local and global evaluation that has normative or prescriptive force and generality.

5.2 Can Evaluations of Hypotheses and Theories Be Represented by Probabilities?

The discussion of local evaluation in the early parts of this chapter (and the generalization later in the chapter) will be in terms of *probability*. Whether hypotheses (and theories) can be evaluated in terms of probability, and whether varying intensities of scientific beliefs are captured by the probability calculus at all, is an issue that has occupied the attention of philosophers and scientists for literally hundreds of years.[4] The meaning of "probability" itself is no less controversial. Many lengthy books have been written on these topics and, accordingly, it will be necessary to treat these problems rather briefly and without explicit argumentation. It is hoped that reference to the literature will suffice for those who desire to pursue these topics in more depth.

I am going to take the position in this book following the work of Richard Jeffrey (1965, 1975, 1983), Abner Shimony (1970), and others (but with some differences and emendations), that rational commitments to a hypothesis or scientific theory can be interpreted as a tempered personal probability or a judgmental probability. The theses I will defend will be Bayesian, both in this chapter and in other chapters of the book.[5] Bayesians, following Ramsey (1931) and DeFinetti (1937), have tended to justify the axioms of probability by the use of an argument which is usually termed the "Dutch book argument."[6] Briefly, this argument begins by examining what it is to be a rational bettor. This notion is explicated as one who places one's bets so that he cannot be trapped into accepting a combination of bets which *guarantees a loss* (apparently a practice pursued by Dutch bookies?) regardless of the outcome of events. The reasoning about the sufficient conditions for such rational betting leads directly to the axioms for the probability calculus.

Considerable debate has developed as to whether this justification makes sense for scientific belief commitments.[7] Essentially, the problem arises because it is difficult to determine what conditions characterize "winning" if one has bet on a scientific hypothesis. Not all philosophers are sanguine about the application of the Dutch book justification, and Dorling (1979) in particular has urged reconsideration of the argument using a version developed by Teller (1976).

Regardless of the suitability of the Dutch book justification, alternative defenses of the appropriateness of personal probability as an explicandum of degree of rational commitment to scientific beliefs have appeared. One such is Shimony's proof that *tempered* personalism, in which any seriously proposed hypothesis is given a probability (ever so slightly) greater than zero, satisfies the axioms of the probability calculus. Following some earlier work by Cox (1947, 1961), Good (1950), and Aczel (1966), Shimony (1970, 104-110) proved a theorem and provided some additional argumentation to demonstrate the consistency of tempered personalism with the probability calculus.[8] Earman, in his recent book, reviews several versions of the Dutch book justification, as well as Shimony's (1970) defense and Rosenkrantz's (1981) and Carnap's (1950) justifications of the probability axioms as suitable for capturing degrees of belief. Earman concludes that, "although Dutch Book and other methods of justification investigated . . . are all subject to limitations and objections, collectively they provide powerful persuasion for conforming degrees of belief to the probability calculus" (1992, 2–46).

A Bayesian explication resolves to some extent the troublesome question of *acceptance*. I take the position, similar to Rosenkrantz's (1977) views, that scientists can pursue their research and their explanations from an essentially probabilistic perspective. The approach taken here will be *inferential*, but it can easily (and appropriately) be embedded in a decision-theoretic context. Probabilities can be multiplied by utilities and decisions made that maximize (or only "satisfice") expected utility.[9] I view the inferential approach permitted by the Bayesian position as more flexible and in better accord with scientists' activities than the inductive-behavior alternative favored by Neyman and more recently, if I understand him correctly, by Hacking (1980). I should add at this point that Earman (1992) disagrees with a unitary inferential Bayesian type of position, contrasting the notion of "acceptance" (actually two notions, one Kuhnian and one pragmatic) with the evaluation of hypotheses and theories in probabilistic terms that one encounters in the Bayesian approach. In the later sections of this chapter I shall discuss the Kuhnian notion, both disagreeing with it and arguing that we can capture the type of commitments we find in cases of theory competition within a Bayesian framework as comparatively high probabilities or "odds." As regards "pragmatic acceptance," this appears to me to amount to a conditional commitment based on the same sorts of considerations. I believe that one can work with a theory or hypothesis and explore its consequences without requiring a new notion of "acceptance" beyond what the Bayesian framework licenses. However, to develop this idea fully and to show how it can adequately model scientists' deliberations and decision-making processes from the planning of experiments to publication, as well as the process of community affirmation (e.g., the awarding of Nobel prizes), would take me far beyond the scope of this book, so it is appropriately left for a future research program.

5.3 Classical Approaches

I will begin this inquiry into local evaluation of statistical hypotheses by examining the two major classical approaches, the Fisherian approach and the Neyman-Pearson theory of testing.

5.3.1 *The Fisherian Approach*

That R. A. Fisher had a major influence on statistical inference through his analysis of experimental design and his advocacy of randomization is generally accepted. In the area of "hypothesis testing" or, in our terminology, in the area of local evaluation of hypotheses, the Fisherian approach has largely been superseded by that of Jerzy Neyman and Egon Pearson, though incompletely so since (perhaps under Fisher's influence) significance levels (or P values) are often given without the correlative power functions being calculated.[10] Giere, for example, concluded that:

> Fisher's account of significance tests yields at best an incomplete interpretation of the general testing paradigm applied to statistical hypotheses. A better interpretation would include explicit criteria for the choice of a rejection set and provisions for considering the probability of not rejecting a false hypothesis. These are just the elements introduced by . . . Neyman and . . . Pearson. (1977, 26–27)[11]

Fisher can of course be modified and extended, and both Hacking (1965) and Seidenfeld (1979) have specifically indicated how this might be done. For our purposes, however, since the predominant methodology for local evaluation *in the biomedical sciences* is due to Neyman and Pearson, and also because many of the positive, pro-Bayesian theses elaborated in this and the next chapter do not require reference to Fisher, an examination of the Neyman-Pearson account will suffice to characterize the details of the classical alternative.[12]

5.3.2 *The Neyman-Pearson Theory of Testing*

It is generally acknowledged that the most widely accepted and employed theory of the evaluation of a statistical hypothesis is due to Neyman and Pearson.[13] Termed a "theory of testing" in the statistical literature, the Neyman-Pearson theory provides a mathematical explication of the intuitive idea that a statistical hypothesis ought to be evaluated in terms of the numbers of events, relevant to the hypothesis, observed in some specified sample of trials.

In a book of this scope, it will not be possible in the text proper to elaborate in any detail the various concepts of the Neyman-Pearson classical model that at present dominates statistical testing in biology and medicine. I have included in appendix 1 to this chapter an example drawn from Mendelian genetics that will permit the interested reader to appreciate the seductive clarity and force of the concepts of significance level, or " P value," and power of the test. A perusal of any of the leading biological or medical journals will disclose the extent to which this approach has become the "received view" of statistical hypothesis evaluation. Here I am going to provide some bare outlines— essentially what I perceive are the "intuitions" behind the Neyman-Pearson approach—and relate it to a schematic characterization of the Mendelian example developed in detail in appendix 1. This should suffice to introduce the basic ideas, which will be necessary background for my arguments for the Bayesian alternative developed later in the chapter.

Suppose we are given a hypothesis from Mendelian genetics, for example, that for two contrasting traits or "unit characters" represented by pea color, namely yellow peas and green peas, Mendelian genetics predicts that yellow seed color (albumen color) will dominate the green color. On the basis of the simple dominance observed in Mendel's classical experiments, Mendel's theory predicts that random segregation of the factors or "genes" will yield four hybrid classes with the genotypes yy, yg, gy, and gg that display a phenotypic 3 : 1 ratio of yellow to green seeded progeny in the F_2 generation.

We represent a test of the hypothesis that the ratio of a pea selected at random will be yellow as a test of the hypothesis H_0: $p = .75$. Suppose that our walk in the garden and pea picking yields 70 yellow and 30 green peas. We wish to know if this empirical data supports the Mendelian hypothesis, H_0, since $70/100$ $= .70$; in other words, we want to know if this value is *sufficiently close* to .75 to support the theory. This notion of "sufficiently close" requires us to consider more specifically what type of a mistake or *error* we might make with respect to accepting the hypothesis on the basis of the empirical data we obtained. The Neyman-Pearson theory says that an evaluation or "test" is not made solely in terms of *one* hypothesis and the experimental data but is made *comparatively*: in addition to the primary hypothesis,[14] an *alternative hypothesis*, H_1 (or even a *class* of alternative hypotheses) must be proposed. As an alternative hypothesis in our Mendelian example, we will fancifully suppose that the *gy* genetic class (but not the *yg* class) has half yellow and half green progeny, yielding a prediction of $H_1 : p = 5/8$, as an example of a bizarre maternal dominance hypothesis.[15] The Neyman-Pearson theory is strong enough to enable us to test other types of alternatives, such as $H_1 : p\ 3/4$, but it would lead us into a complex discussion to indicate how that is done (but see appendix 1). With this comparative character of hypothesis testing in mind, we can define two different states of the world and two different decisions we might make about these two hypotheses and thus exhibit two different kinds of mistakes and their probabilities, as displayed in the following table:

	H_0 accepted	H_1 accepted
H_0 true	correct decision	type I error (α)
H_1 true	type II error (β)	correct decision

The key point for our purposes is to focus on the probability (a) of making the mistake of accepting the alternative hypothesis when the primary hypothesis is true. The Neyman-Pearson theory suggests that type I error is the most important kind to control. The control is exercised by making a decision, on *non-statistical grounds*, as to how serious an error might be committed by rejecting a "true" hypothesis. This decision fixes a *level of significance* which is expressed in terms of a number such as 0.05, 0.01, 0.001, and the like. A significance level, sometimes called the "P value," indicates what the chances are of rejecting a true hypothesis, H_0. The level of significance is usually denoted algebraically by the greek letter α, as shown above.

It turns out that we can calculate (the calculations appear in appendix 1) that what we observed in our garden (the 70 : 30 empirical ratio) *is* close enough that it supports a statement that "H_0 *is significant at the 0.05 level*." We could also calculate what the probability is of the second kind of error, which turns out to be about 0.13. This can be made smaller, but only if we let α become larger (see appendix 1). Both α and β could be made smaller if we *increased* the sample size (ours was 100 in the example). There are formal relations in many cases among the two types of error and the sample size, and statisticians are typically consulted as part of the design of experiments (and clinical trials) and asked to determine sample sizes for prechosen error probabilities.[16]

The above considerations offer the bare outlines of how the Neyman-Pearson approach is applied to a prototypical example of biological hypothesis testing. The approach is not without its limitations as well as its critics, with the strongest opposition to the Neyman-Pearson classical model coming from the Bayesian school of statistics, which I will defend. There are a number of reasons for pursuing a Bayesian approach. Though the school takes its name from Thomas Bayes, an eighteenth-century cleric who published an essay introducing "Bayes's theorem" into the literature for the first time, it was the contributions of Ramsey (1931) and DeFinetti (1937), and then Good (1950), Jeffreys (1961), and Savage (1954), that reinvigorated this approach to probability and statistics. Since the 1950s, the number of statisticians who describe themselves as "Bayesians" has grown significantly. Beginning in the mid-1960s many philosophers of science began to climb on the Bayesian bandwagon, and this shift has continued in spite of recognized foundational problems with Bayesianism and of some prominent holdouts and critics, such as Glymour (1980).

It is of interest to note that, in contrast to earlier work in inductive logic by such eminent philosophers as Reichenbach (1938, 1947) and Carnap (1950), recent inquiries in this discipline have moved much closer to the writings of statistical theorists. The preponderant move of inductive logicians has been toward the Bayesian position and is exemplified in Jeffrey's (1965, 1983), Salmon's (1967), Hesse's (1974), Rosenkrantz's (1977), Franklin's (1986, 1990) and Howson and Urbach's (1989) monographs. Kyburg's (1974) position and Levi's (1967, 1980) analyses have some affinities with a Bayesian view but are also importantly different. Hacking (1965), Seidenfeld (1979), and the early Giere (1975, 1976, 1977) dissent from a Bayesian orientation, the latter preferring the Neyman-Pearson approach, and the former two scholars a modified Fisherian account. More recently (in his 1988), Giere has been critical of Bayesianism and defended a "satisficing" account of hypothesis evaluation. Glymour (1980) as noted is anti-Bayesian, developing his own "bootstrapping" theory (also see Earman 1983), and more recently has begun to pursue a generalized learning theory as a strong alternative to Bayesianism. It is clear that philosophers are examining the foundations of statistical inference much more closely than previously, and that most have tended toward accepting the Bayesian approach.

Recently John Earman (1992) has surveyed and analyzed the strengths and weaknesses of Bayesianism and concluded that he is "schizophrenic" about the approach: there are many stunning successes but at the same time a number of significant flaws in Bayesianism. Among the successes, Earman lists a clarification of hypothetico-deductive qualitative confirmation, a resolution of Hempel's raven paradox, an explication of the force of variety of evidence as well as of the role of theories in scientific inference, and a solution to the Quine-Duhem problem. The flaws, such as Glymour's "old evidence" problem, will be pursued at appropriate points later in this discussion. In the present chapter, Bayesianism serves as a *general framework* in terms of which to introduce comparative and (in local as well as in some idealized global cases) quantitative features of hypothesis and theory evaluation. Because of the scope and complexity of the details of the Bayesian position, I am going to confine myself to introducing the basic essentials of Bayesianism as needed, to show how it can function as an evaluative framework in both local and global situations.

5.4 The Bayesian Approach to Probability and Statistics

In the sections immediately above I have been presenting the classical Neyman-Pearson view of evaluating tests of statistical hypotheses. In this and the following sections I want to introduce some rather different foundational ideas concerning the evaluation of statistical hypotheses in the light of evidence. As already noted earlier, the viewpoint outlined here is characterized as "Bayesian" after the work of Thomas Bayes, who published a theorem on inverse probability in 1763. There is considerably more to the Bayesian point of view than is to be found in Bayes's early exploration, however, and it has only been in this century, and primarily since the 1950s, that significant advances have

been made on the technical foundations of statistics. These, intercalated with the personal interpretations of probability,[17] have
resulted in a significant alternative to the more classical Neyman-Pearson and Fisherian approaches. I will first introduce
Bayes's theorem in two of its forms and then touch on some general but important issues involving varying interpretations and
uses of the theorem.

5.4.1 *Bayes's Theorem*

One of the features that distinguishes the Bayesian approach
from more traditional analyses of statistics is that Bayesians
have, on the basis of their views, many more chances to use
Bayes's theorem. This theorem can easily be proven on the basis
of uncontroversial axioms of probability theory; it states that the
probability of an event A conditional on another event B, $P(A \mid B)$,
is given by:

$$P(A \mid B) = \frac{P(A) \cdot P(B \mid A)}{P(B)} .$$

Here $P(A)$ is the "prior probability" of A, which for the typical
Bayesian refers to the degree of belief prior to any knowledge
about B. $P(BA)$ is the likelihood of B given A, and $P(B)$ is the non-
conditional probability of B, sometimes termed the "expected-
ness" of B on any theory whatsoever. $P(A \mid B)$ is known as the
"posterior probability" of A, given that we know B to be the case.
If we interpret A as a hypothesis, H, and B as some sample purportedly supporting A, say e (for evidence), the theorem can be
rewritten:

$$P(H \mid e) = \frac{P(H) \cdot P(e \mid H)}{P(e)} .$$

For a list of n different, mutually exclusive independent hypotheses H_i (where i ranges from 1 to n), the theorem can be written:

$$P(H_i \mid e) = \frac{P(H_i) \cdot P(e \mid H_i)}{\sum_{i=1}^{n} P(H_i \mid e) \cdot P(e \mid H_i)} .$$

A particularly useful form of the theorem is the so-called
odds form. If one writes Bayes's theorem for two hypotheses H_i

and H_j in the form given immediately above, and divides the former by the latter, one obtains:

$$(O) \qquad \frac{P(H_i \mid e)}{P(H_j \mid e)} = \frac{P(H_i) \cdot P(e \mid H_i)}{P(H_j) \cdot P(e \mid H_j)} \, ,$$

indicating that the ratio of the posterior probabilities, the posterior odds that one should offer for H_i against H_j, is a function of the prior odds multiplied by the likelihood ratio. The denominator for Bayes's theorem in both cases is identical and accordingly disappears.

Much of the opposition of classical theorists to the Bayesian approach has been grounded in the introduction of the prior probability P(H). It has been characterized as useless and unsatisfactory, and dispensable for statistical tests.[18] We will not be able to consider in detail all of the various arguments and counterarguments that have been directed at each school by the other, but it might be useful even at this juncture to make several points. The first is that the Bayesians consider *all* probabilities conditional, a consideration that could be formulated in an expansion of the above short form of Bayes's theorem to include conditionalization on an accepted background of theories and evidence, b. We would then rewrite the theorem as:

$$P(H \mid e\&b) = \frac{P(H \mid b) \cdot P(e \mid H\&b)}{P(e \mid b)} \, ,$$

a form that will be used extensively further below. My remaining three points concerning the Bayesian approach are more controversial and each requires a subsection for elaboration.

5.4.2 *Bayesian Conditionalization*

Bayesian conditionalization is generally recognized even by thinkers sympathetic to the Bayesian approach as insufficient to warrant a complete probability kinematics. By a probability kinematics I mean a "law of motion" which governs transitions to new belief states from a combination of prior belief states and new evidence. Several writers have explicitly recognized that the type of coherence required by the Dutch book argument mentioned earlier (p. 171) does not mandate the use of Bayes's theorem as such a law of motion.[19] A considerable amount of attention has been focused on probability kinematics by Jeffrey (1965, 1983), Levi (1967), Kyburg and Harper (1968), Teller (1973), Hesse (1974), Field (1978), Seidenfeld (1979), Garber (1980), van Fraassen (1980), Domotor (1980), Armendt (1980), Williams (1980), and most recently Howson and Urbach (1989, 284–288). It would take us far beyond the scope of this book to examine these arguments in depth, but a brief review of them and an indication of where they fit into the themes of the present book is presented in Technical Discussion 7. Suffice it to note that Bayesian conditionalization need not have all encompassing scope in order to capture rational belief changes. In comparatively simple situations such as the example developed in detail in appendix 2, Bayesian belief change is relatively uncontroversial. In cases reminiscent of Kuhnian paradigm competition, conditionalization can still play an appropriate role. To make the case for it in such contexts, however, I shall first have to discuss issues such as theory comparability and commensurability, and these are best deferred until later in the chapter, after more straightforward Bayesian issues have been covered.

TECHNICAL DISCUSSION 7

Jeffrey's and Field's Alternatives to Bayesian Conditionalization.

In his 1965 (chapter 11), Jeffrey proposed a generalized form of Bayesian conditionalization in which the simple Bayesian conditionalization:

$$P_1(A) = P_0(A \mid E)$$

is generalized to:

$$P_1(A) = qP_0(A \mid E) + (1 - q)P_0(A \mid E)$$

where $q = P_1(E)$, the degree of belief in E after observing the event which E describes.

This generalization was motivated in part by the observation that any evidence that is accepted subsequently must be assigned a probability $= 1$,[20] which seems both too strong epistemically and also contrary to the evidential revisability one finds in science.

Jeffrey has been criticized by Levi (1967) and Hesse (1974, 120–123) as not providing, among other things, a complete probability kinematics. Field (1978) proposed that Jeffrey's approach could be amplified, partly along lines initially suggested by Carnap. Field proposes that the q value is a combination of the prior probability of E *and* "the sensory stimulation that the agent was subjected to" (1978, 363). Field introduces an input parameter, roughly a measure of subjective certainty, which he terms α, and which allows for a reparametrization of Jeffrey's conditionalization expression.[21] On Field's proposed definition of α, Jeffrey's q is equal to:

$$pe^{\alpha}/(pe^{\alpha} + (1 - p)e^{-\alpha})$$

where e is the base of the natural logarithms.

Field's reparametrization has certain nice features, including simple and symmetric results for reiterative observations. Nonetheless it has been questioned as regards its correctness (see Garber 1980). Also, van Fraassen has argued that Field's parameter can be analyzed into two components, and that epistemic transitions can be shown on reanalysis to conform to Jeffrey's law. Domotor (1980) has argued that Jeffrey's and Field's conditionals cannot be reduced to Bayesian conditionals.[22] Finally, Howson and Urbach (1989) maintain that there is no *one* way of generalizing conditionalization but in point of fact an *infinity* of ways (1989, 287).

Whether observational uncertainty should be incorporated into conditionalization is accordingly both an important and an unsettled issue. Earlier, Hesse (1974) argued that an alternative means of representing uncertainty within Bayesian conditionalization was desirable and outlined a procedure for this. If it turns out that Jeffrey's conditionalization or some other form is more suitable than a simple Bayesian approach for representing probability kinematics, then hypothesis testing will in turn likely require additional complications.[23] Just as the Jeffrey and Field approaches are refinements and extensions of the basic Bayesian approach, however, it seems appropriate to elaborate the extant and extensive preexisting Bayesian apparatus in the directions of both local and global evaluation, and then to use these developments as (at least) limiting cases on the basis of which to develop a more sophisticated probability kinematics.[24]

5.4.3 *Bayes's Theorem and Novel Predictions*

It should be noted that a number of philosophers of science, including W. C. Salmon (1967), M. B. Hesse (1974), and Howson and Urbach (1989) (as well as Schaffner 1974) have suggested that Bayes's theorem *seems* to agree immediately with our intuitions for those cases in which a new hypothesis predicts a novel fact. Here, though P(H | b) is quite low, the likelihood is reasonably high (1 if e is a deductive consequence of H & b and the observational error is small). Most importantly, P(e | b) is usually construed to be very low since, by supposition, e is novel. Arthur Pap's version of the thesis is most direct.[25] Defining P(e | b) as "expectedness" (for Pap b only includes old evidence), Pap writes:

> If . . . [e] is a deductive consequence of [H] . . . we obtain
>
> $$\text{Posterior probability} = \frac{\text{antecedent probability}}{\text{expectedness}} \, .$$
>
> This theorem accords with the intuitive inductive logic of scientists, for it says that, assuming a finite antecedent probability of the tested hypothesis, the latter is confirmed by a favorable test all the more, the less such a confirming observation could have been expected *without* assuming the hypothesis. (1962, 160-161)

Unfortunately, this apparently elegant way of representing scientists' intuitions about novel predictions is spurious, and based on a misinterpretation of what Pap termed "expectedness."[26] The denominator expression p(e | b), as indicated in the expansion given on page 178, actually refers to the expectation on *any* theory whatever.[27] This issue is, interestingly, closely related to another problem with Bayes's theorem raised by Glymour (1980), and has, I believe, a common resolution. (I shall discuss Glymour's argument in the next section.)

It seems to me that in the area of local statistical hypothesis testing the problem can be at least preliminarily bypassed by using the "odds form" of Bayes's theorem given on page 179.[28,29] As I will show, this form is extensively used in Bayesian statistical hypothesis testing. In addition, the force of novel or unexpected experimental results can be captured by the odds form if the new hypothesis explains the new empirical result e, while the alternative hypotheses "poorly" explain that result (perhaps only by an ad hoc addition to the hypothesis). In such a case the support ratio in expression (O) on page 179 above is dramatically affected by novel predictions. Old evidence, however, can also be a severe test of a hypothesis, the relative support between or among competing hypotheses being a function of prior probability and ability of the hypothesis to account for the evidence (expressed in the likelihood term). Note, however, that if we are dealing with two deterministic hypotheses in which the likelihood expressions equal 1, the posterior probabilities' odds are equal to the odds of the prior probabilities so no new support accrues. I shall reconsider this type of situation in the next section.

5.4.4 *The Old Evidence Problem*

Glymour (1980, 85–93) questions whether Bayes's theorem in its simple form accurately captures scientific practice. He contends that Einstein's general theory of relativity was better tested by *old, expected* evidence than by new, unexpected evidence (such as the red shift). A similar point could be invoked in connection with many of the biological and medical theories we have examined, such as the well-recognized phenomenon of self-tolerance that would be used to test the adequacy of any new immunological theory. Old evidence is important, and any confirmation theory which disallows it is in serious trouble.

Glymour points out the following paradox: if previously accepted evidence is used to evaluate a new theory, the new theory *cannot* increase its (the theory's) probability. Glymour's argument is straightforward: we assume that e is known before the theory T is introduced, thus $p(e) = 1$. Glymour also assumes that T entails e with likelihood = 1. Then by Bayes's theorem:

$$P(T \mid e) = P(T) \cdot P(e \mid t)/P(e) = P(T).$$

Thus e *cannot* raise the probability of T, which is the paradox.

There have been several proposals made to outflank this disturbing conclusion.[30] A consensus seems to have emerged among the Bayesians that some form of *counterfactual* assessment of the likelihood that places restrictions on logical and/or empirical omniscience must be employed.[31] As Howson and Urbach note, "it is clear that the [Bayesian] theory has been incorrectly used and that the mistake lies in relativising all the probability to the *totality* of current knowledge: they should have been relativised to current knowledge minus e" (1989, 271).

TECHNICAL DISCUSSION 8

Bayesianism and Old Evidence

One of the best developed formal approaches to the old evidence problem is Garber's (1983). Analogous suggestions can be found in Jeffrey (1983b) as well as in Niiniluoto (1983). Even in a technical discussion I cannot examine Garber's approach in depth, and the reader is encouraged to consult Earman's full-chapter treatment of this difficult problem in his 1992. Suffice it to say that Garber defines a language in which a connective '$\Rightarrow$' is primitive but is intended to represent logico-mathematical implication. He then shows that, under reasonable constraints, there are probability functions defined in his language that permit $1 > P(T \Rightarrow e) > 0$ and $P(T \mid T \Rightarrow e) > P(T)$. Garber's suggestion has been criticized (Eells 1985, van Fraassen 1988) and defended to an extent (Earman 1992, chapter 5).

Glymour himself is actually willing to consider fairly complex counterfactual procedures that *might* allow the use of prior evidence, though he expresses considerable doubts about this tack, in part because he finds that in the case of historical (and deterministic) theories there is no clear, single counterfactual degree of belief in the evidence (1980, 88). This is not envisaged as a serious problem by Howson and Urbach (1989, 272–275), however. Howson and Urbach suggest that the acceptance of the *data* can for many purposes be treated outside of the Bayesian framework. In my view, this point, taken together with those situations in which Bayesian convergence of opinion is present, permits a sufficient degree of flexibility to allow reasonable variation in individuals' degrees of belief in the evidence (excepting the extreme values of 0 and 1 as argued by Shimony 1970), and yet supports appropriate Bayesian confirmation.

Glymour's additional point about the difficulties associated with computing likelihoods in those cases where it is the *discovery* that h entails e that is an important component of the computation can be similarly answered, namely that Bayesianism does not require that *all* the probabilities that appear in Bayes's theorem need be computed by Bayesian methods (see Howson and Urbach 1989, 272). Even if one were to want to follow Glymour (as well as Garber 1983 and Niiniluoto 1983[32] and weaken the probability calculus axiom to permit Glymour's emendation of replacing the likelihood expression by $P(h \mid e \ \& \ (h \Rightarrow e))$[33] in certain contexts, it is not clear that this would be a damaging modification for Bayesianism.

The problem of old evidence and the consequences of restricting logical omniscience can be viewed from either pessimistic or optimistic perspectives. Earman adopts the former writing:

There seem to me to be only two ways to deal with the residual problem of old evidence. The first is to ignore it in favor of some other problem. That, in effect, is the route pioneered in the G[arber]-J[effrey]-N[iiniluoto] approach. . . .

But if the problem is not to be ignored, the only way to come to grips with it is to go to the source of the problem: the failure of (LO2) [logical omniscience, which "involves the assumption that the agent is aware of every theory that belongs to the space of possibilities."] (1992, 134)

Earman argues that there are only two approaches that might be taken to deal with the failure of the strong form of logical omniscience (his LO2), and that both of them involve counterfactual degrees of belief, thus yielding the following pessimistic assessment:

I have no doubt that counterfactual enthusiasts can concoct ways to get numbers out of one or both of these scenarios. But what has to be demonstrated before the problem of old evidence is solved is that the numbers match our firm and shared judgments of the confirmational values of various pieces of old evidence. (1992, 135)

In my view, the old evidence problem, as well as the problem of when to conditionalize, has set a research agenda for those of a Bayesian persuasion. The development of a series of case studies — Earman, in his 1992 uses the example of Einstein's general theory of relativity and old evidence for it to good effect in such an inquiry — that will permit the finetuning of a more realistic Bayesianism is needed. The case study of the clonal selection theory as developed in this chapter, and also in its earlier stages discussed in chapter 2, is, I think, ripe for such use. Thus I believe that there is an "optimistic" perspective on the old evidence problem suggesting that a richer, more historically relevant variant of the Bayesian approach will emerge from such a research program.

Such case studies can often suggest perspectives that may offer hints toward piecemeal solutions of the old evidence problem. For example, there is another way in which we might extend the reply to Glymour developed in chapter 5, making use of the suggestion raised above that the likelihood expression is frequently less than 1. In the view developed in the present book, and supported by the case studies, almost all evaluation including global evaluation is comparative. Thus the most important form of Bayes's theorem is the odds form, which in Glymour's notation (letting T^1 be our alternative theory) is:

$$\frac{P(T^1 \mid e)}{P(T \mid e)} = \frac{P(T^1)}{P(T)} \cdot \frac{P(e \mid T^1)}{P(e \mid T)} .$$

This form would yield an analogous form of Glymour's paradox, since the ratios would be equal if e followed deductively from both T and T^1. (Note that in this form it is not the fact that $P(e) = 1$ that is the source of the problem.) However, as suggested above, we may often expect that $1 \neq P(e \mid T^1) \neq P(e \mid T) \neq 1$ in many cases in the biomedical sciences and in most other sciences too. But if this is the case then the paradox disappears (also compare Salmon 1990).

5.4.5 Bayes's Theorem and the Convergence of Personal Probabilities

A final, general point that would be appropriate to make about the Bayesian approach concerns the convergence of initially disparate personal probabilities. Savage and other Bayesian statisticians and philosophers (e.g., Shimony in his 1970) have argued that, even though personal probabilities may be subjective and widely divergent *initially*, the application of Bayes's theorem (or any appropriate kinematical law for probability transition — see Hesse 1974, 117) will lead ever closer to intersubjective agreement on the basis of the evidence.

A formal proof of this convergence was given by Savage (1954), but some of the assumptions on which the proof is based have been questioned by Hesse (1974, 115–119), who argues that the randomness and independence assumptions are "not always valid in scientific contexts" (1974, 118). There are, however, more powerful results entailing convergence than even those argued for by Savage (see Gaifman and Snir 1982), though they also depend on some rather restrictive assumptions.[34]

From a global point of view, Hesse's concerns are legitimate. However, in connection with more local types of statistical examples, convergence may be demonstrated. Savage and his colleagues outlined some such procedures in 1963 under the rubric of the "principle of stable estimation." This principle claims that if a prior density "changes gently in the region favored by the data and not itself too strongly favors some other region," convergence will occur. Savage and his coworkers developed some fairly complex mathematical explications of these terms and also provided an example (see Edwards, Lindman, and Savage 1963, 201–208). A lucid discussion of this principle and a clarification of the apparently vague terms such as "gently" and "strongly favors" can be found in Howson and Urbach's 1989, 243–245. At this stage I will not pursue this further, but in appendix 2 I provide an example to demonstrate how this convergence occurs in practice in the local examples involving Mendelian tests with different priors. Importantly, Hesse contends that, even though convergence cannot be demonstrated to hold a priori in a global sense for science, there are some conditions which can be adopted, such as the Bayesian transformation law (or Bayes's theorem), which collectively will be *sufficient* (but not necessary) to insure convergence. It would take us beyond the scope of this inquiry to develop these sufficient conditions, since they are quite complex and in general constitute Hesse's view of the scientific enterprise. Suffice it to say, however, that the appropriateness of the Bayesian approach is ultimately justified in a pragmatic manner by being able to make sense of actual scientific inductions.

In the next section, I shall argue that the Bayesian perspective captures all that is sound in the previous classical approach to hypothesis testing, and that on the balance it provides a more adequate account of both local and, as I will term it in the remainder of the chapter, global, evaluation.

5.5 Bayesian Hypothesis Testing

Let me begin my Bayesian argument by first indicating how a Bayesian approach to hypothesis testing (local evaluation) works and then providing a more general defense of the approach.[35] In this section I will assume a general knowledge of the Mendelian example discussed in the classical Neyman-Pearson section earlier (and in more detail in appendix 1). Let us begin by analyzing the manner in which a Bayesian might approach the Mendelian example. The first point to stress is that, from the Bayesian perspective, we are not seeking any special decision rules to govern inductive behavior. Therefore we will not generally choose α's, β's, and sample sizes in advance but rather will work with a more flexible set of procedures. As will be noted, we can *add* a decision rule to this approach, though it will have an odd, exogenous flavor.

One way we might formulate the Bayesian approach to hypothesis testing is to use the odds form of Bayes's theorem given for a hypothesis and an appropriate alternative and to compute the *posterior* odds from the prior odds and the likelihood ratios.[36] The Bayesian approach is accordingly *inferential*: it provides modified beliefs via conditionalization on the prior odds.[37] Bayesian statistics can also demonstrate the "sharpening" of belief which occurs as further data becomes available and the variance and standard deviation of the prior distribution of belief narrows. Earlier we encountered the objections of classical theorists to prior probabilities as being hopelessly vague and subjective. It was noted there that, as empirical data became available, diverse priors would converge as long as the prior probabilities were not too sharply concentrated outside a region favored by the data and also were reasonably gentle within that region. The Bayesian reformulation of the Mendelian illustration discussed earlier shows that this is the case (see appendix 2 for the argument).

One Bayesian approach to the Mendelian example is to proceed as suggested above. That is, we look at the two hypotheses we considered in the example, we compare them on the basis of their "prior" odds if there are prior probabilities that can be formulated, and then we examine what effect the empirical data have on the posterior odds.[38] In appendix 2, I discuss both the possibility that we have no prior probabilities and that we have some priors based on a theory. Calculations can be made for both cases, but the important feature of the example is that, regardless of the priors, the empirical data can "swamp" any posterior differences due to contrasting alternative priors. Evaluation is comparative here, as in the Neyman-Pearson analysis of the example, though alternative Bayesian approaches permit noncomparative posterior probability determinations.

It should be reemphasized (see endnotes 34 and 35) that at present there is no *general theory* of Bayesian *hypothesis testing*. Many of the problems of comparing the Neyman-Pearson approach with the Bayesian may well be found to be vestigial in nature, relics from classical considerations that will vanish in the light of a strong and consistent Bayesian orientation (see Kadane and Dickey 1980). In spite of the lack of consensus about a general theory of Bayesian hypothesis testing, the Bayesian approach, as a treatment of the examples in appendix 2 shows, seems general enough to encompass all the precise and powerful results of classical statistics, and to place it in a flexible inferential context that permits generalization to more global contexts, a topic to which I turn in the section after the next.

5.6 Some Additional Arguments Favoring Bayesianism

The Bayesian approach in statistics has in the past decade been the subject of a number of analyses scrutinizing its foundations and comparing them with the classical approach.[39] This book is not primarily a monograph in the foundations of statistics and accordingly I will not be able to give the debate the in-depth examination it deserves.[40] It will be useful, however, to summarize some additional salient strengths (and weaknesses) of the Bayesian approach to indicate why I am taking it as one of the thematic elements in this book.[41]

What is widely construed as the strongest single argument for a Bayesian approach *against the classical school* is known as the Lindley-Savage argument. The classical work of Neyman and Pearson was given a decision-theoretic interpretation by Wald in the 1940s. The addition of utilities (or equivalent loss functions) does not indicate, however, how to choose between two pairs of error probabilities of the type that I discussed earlier (α, β) (α', β') for a given sample size n in a test situation. Lindley and Savage have argued that a selection of such a pair is *equivalent* to holding prior probabilities.[42] The technical details supporting the claim are given in the note, but the argument can be summarized nontechnically (see Giere 1976, 47–48, for additional information). If we consider any test of a simple hypothesis against another simple alternative (our Mendelian example introduced above and developed in more detail in the appendixes is a good example), the test can be represented as a pair of error probabilities (α, β). From within classical statistical theory supplemented with Waldian decision theory, selecting a specific value of α and a sample size n that will then fix β is tantamount to accepting a value for the ratio of the prior probabilities of the hypothesis under test and its alternative.

Giere disagrees with the Lindley-Savage argument, objecting to the legitimacy of what are termed mixed tests such as (α', β'). For further discussion of Giere's arguments the reader must be referred to his article, and it should be noted that Allan Birnbaum (personal communication) was also persuaded that the Lindley-Savage argument could be blocked by such a move.[43] Birnbaum, who like Giere was disposed toward the classical approach, was also convinced, however, that the Lindley-Savage proof was a powerful *tu quoque* argument against the classical school that was having a profound effect on statisticians in making a Bayesian approach more attractive.

The reason why such a *tu quoque* argument, indicating the classical school is committed to prior probabilities, is so significant lies in the fact that the Neyman-Pearson proponents' (and Fisherians') main criticism of Bayesianism is the Bayesians' acceptance of prior probabilities. As already indicated, these priors are conceived of by the classical school as vague and as too subjective to capture the presumed objectivity of science, though we have seen above that the principle of stable estimation and convergence somewhat outflanks this problem. There exist, however, Bayesian proponents who believe that one can go even further than this and establish *objective* prior probabilities.[44]

My own position as defended in this book is similar to Richard Jeffrey's view that prior probabilities are too objective to be termed personal or subjective but not so objective as to be characterized in what Savage called "necessarian" terms. Jeffrey (1975) suggests the term "judgmental" be used to refer to the Bayesian probabilities:

> To my ear, the term "judgmental" strikes the right note, conveying my sense that probabilistic judgement need not be idiosyncratic, and may be founded on broadly shared critical standards. I take it that our standards of judgement undergo secular and occasionally revolutionary changes, and that there is no eternal, objective [i.e., "necessarian"] standard by which to control such evolution and revolution, over and above standards we may discern in our overall patterns of judgement and which we may revise if we can discern them. Inherited or inchoate, such standards inform our judgmental probabilities no less than do particular observations and experiments. They are our very standards of criticism. (1975, 155-156)

This view is consonant with the modeling of the expert approach taken in the chapter 2 discussion of INTERNIST-1 and in the discussion of the logic of discovery. In part 2 of this chapter the manner in which these (changeable) standards appear in the *b* or background term will be discussed explicitly.

There are a number of other arguments adduced in the continuing foundational debates between Bayesians and classical theorists. Savage and others have argued that the Bayesian approach, though self-referentially termed "subjective," is actually more *objective* than classical analysis. Part of this claim is based on the Lindley-Savage argument discussed above, but another aspect of this contention is based on the fact that, from a Bayesian perspective, classicists throw away data, since they refuse to incorporate the knowledge that Bayesians use in their prior probabilities. Rosenkrantz quoted C. A. B. Smith on this point, indicating that ignoring such a prior can lead classical significance tests to make serious errors. Smith wrote:

> A significance test . . . may reject a hypothesis at a significance level P, but P here is not the probability that the hypothesis is true, and indeed, the rejected hypothesis may still be probably true if the odds are sufficiently in its favor at the start. For example, in human genetics, there are odds of the order of 22 : 1 in favor of two genes chosen at random being on different chromosomes; so even if a test indicates departure from independent segregation at the 5 per cent level of significance, this is not very strong evidence in favor of linkage. (Smith 1959, 292)

Renwick, writing in the *Annual Review of Genetics,* also introduced a related point:

> Since the introduction of Bayesian methods into this field [the mapping of human chromosomes] by [C. A. B.] Smith, these [methods] have become the basis of most linkages in man because among other advantages, they are appropriate even when the sample is small. (1971, 84)

Bayesians have still further arguments in their favor. What is known as the likelihood principle in statistics indicates that the experimental import of two sets of data D and D' is equivalent if $P(D \mid H) = P(D' \mid H)$. This principle is robust and it arises naturally out of the Bayesian approach (Edwards, Lindman, and Savage 1963). It entails another feature of the Bayesian account: the irrelevance of stopping rules, rules which specify when a trial should end. Savage sees this as still another argument for the Bayesian position. He and his colleagues maintained:

> The irrelevance of stopping rules is one respect in which Bayesian procedures are more objective than classical ones. Classical procedures (with the possible exceptions implied above) insist that the intentions of the experimenter are crucial to the interpretation of data, that 20 successes in 100

observations means something quite different if the experimenter intended the 20 successes than if he intended the 100 observations. According to the likelihood principle, data analysis stands on its own feet. The intentions of the experimenter are irrelevant to the interpretation of the data once collected, though of course they are crucial to the design of experiments. (Edwards, Lindman, and Savage 1963, 239)

A good discussion of stopping rules and how they favor a Bayesian position can be found in Howson and Urbach (1989, 169–171). The importance of this position to clinical inquiry, where sometimes an experiment must be terminated or reevaluated in process, should be obvious and has been widely discussed.[45]

The Bayesian account of statistics and hypothesis testing is extensive and obviously cannot be pursued in all its richness in these pages. There is a good introductory article by Savage and his colleagues as well as several textbooks to which readers must be referred for more details.[46] I do not want to leave readers with the impression that there are not unresolved problems for Bayesians. Some of these, such as the old evidence conundrum, have already been mentioned and others will be touched on in the following chapter, but the problem of the "catchall hypothesis" should be mentioned before closing this chapter. Special problems for Bayesian approaches also arise in clinical situations, though they can generally be met by obtaining additional empirical data.

What I refer to as the problem of the "catchall hypothesis" arises because Bayes's theorem, in its usual (non-odds) form, explicitly contains in its denominator the set of all available hypotheses or theories. Since we do not *know* all theories yet, this can be represented by the conjunction of a last term, representing the *disjunction* of all known and explicitly cited theories to the sequence in Bayes's theorem. This last term will be:

$$P(H_n) \cdot P(e \mid H_n) = P[\neg (H_1 \vee ... \vee Hn-1)] \times P[e \mid (H_1 \vee ... \vee H_{n-1})] .$$

The problem is how to assign a prior probability and a likelihood in such an expression. There have been several suggestions. Savage and his colleagues have proposed that "the catchall hypothesis is usually handled in part by studying the situation conditionally on denial of the catchall and in part by informal appraisal of whether any of the explicit hypotheses fit the facts well enough to maintain this denial" (Edwards, Lindman, and Savage 1963, 200). Shimony proposes three means of dealing with the problem and in his 1970 favored treating the catchall hypothesis H_n differently from the explicit hypotheses $H_1...H_{n-1}$ and not attributing a numerical weight to it. Shimony was concerned that this might lead to a "departure from Bayesianism" but had "not worked it out in detail." A promising direction might, however, be to follow Jeffrey's suggestion that Robinson's analysis of infinitesimals can be introduced into the probability calculus and conceive of the catchall hypothesis as possessing an infinitesimal probability.[47]

Part II: Global Evaluation And Extended Theories

5.7 Transition to More Global Approaches

Thus far in this chapter the discussion has been rather narrowly focused, concentrating on the confirmation and falsification of specific hypotheses. Beginning with this section I will broaden these subjects to address a series of interrelated problems which I group under the term "global evaluation." This term was introduced earlier, where it was distinguished from the highly developed methodologies that have figured prominently in statistical hypothesis testing. As there, I associate the term with a cluster of themes that have arisen in relatively recent philosophy of science, predominately in the writings of Hanson (1958), Kuhn (1962, 1970), Feyerabend (1962, 1975), Shapere (1974, 1984), Toulmin (1960, 1972), Lakatos (1970), Laudan (1977), and Kitcher (1984, 1989). Among the themes I will need to touch on (full treatments are obviously beyond the scope of this book) in this part 2 are "truth," scientific realism, commensurability, and the need for a methodological unit more general than a scientific theory, such as a "paradigm," "discipline," "domain," "research program," "research tradition," or "practice." Lest the reader be overly concerned about the sweep and scope of these themes, let me hasten to add that I will be primarily focusing on the latter topic, the need for a methodological unit, and will introduce only as much discussion about truth, realism, and commensurability as is needed to make sense of my arguments concerning global evaluation.

One of the major debates over the past nearly thirty years in the philosophy of science has been the extent to which scientific change is rational and represents objective progress. "Global evaluation," in the sense I wish to give to it, is more centrally related to this problem as it is concerned with the conditions and methods of evaluating competing general theories in their evolving historical dimension. The approach to be taken to global evaluation will be a generalization of the Bayesian approach introduced in part 1. Prior to elaborating that generalization, however, it would be appropriate to outline some epistemological positions that function as presuppositions of this approach. Issues of truth, realism, and commensurability are, in an epistemological sense, prior to a logic of global evaluation and will significantly affect such a logic. It is, accordingly, first to those issues that I turn in the next two sections.

5.8 Scientific Fallibilism and Conditionalized Realism

5.8.1 *Lessons from the History of Science*

An examination of the history of science in general and of the biomedical sciences in particular would lead one to the conclusion that there have existed many "good" scientific theories that have not survived to the present day. These theories have gone through the stages of discovery, development, acceptance, rejection, and extinction. Further examination of these extinct theories, however, would show that they possessed a number of beneficial consequences for science. Incorrect and literally falsified theories have served several explanatory functions and have systematized data, stimulated further inquiry, and have led to a number of important practical consequences. For example, the false Ptolemaic theory of astronomy was extraordinarily useful in predicting celestial phenomena and served as the basis for oceanic navigation for hundreds of years. Newtonian mechanics and gravitational theory, which is incorrect from an Einsteinian and quantum mechanical perspective, similarly served both to make the world intelligible and to guide its industrialization. In the biological sciences, the false evolutionary theory of Lamarck systematized and explained significant amounts of species data, and in medicine Pasteur's false nutrient depletion theory of the immune response nonetheless served as the background for the development of the anthrax vaccine (Bibel 1988, 159–161). Such examples lead one toward what has been termed an *instrumentalist* analysis of scientific theories (or hypotheses). The basic idea behind such a position is to view theories and hypotheses as *tools* and not as purportedly true descriptions of the world. For a thoroughgoing instrumentalist, the primary functions of scientific generalizations are to systematize known data, to predict new observational phenomena, and to stimulate further experimental inquiry.

Though such a position is prima facie attractive, it is inconsistent with other facets of scientific inquiry. I noted in chapter 4 above that scientists view the distinction between direct and indirect evidence as important. Even though it was then argued that the distinction is relative, it is nonetheless significant to note that scientists *behave* as if the distinction is important, and that "direct evidence" would seem to support a more realistic analysis of scientific theories (or hypotheses). A realistic type of alternative to the instrumentalist position would characterize scientific theories as candidates for *true* descriptions of the world. Though not denying the importance of theories' more instrumentalistic functions, such as prediction and fertility, the realist views these features as partial indications of a theory's *truth*.

5.8.2 *Current Debates Concerning Realism in Science*

The history of recent philosophy of science has seen an oscillation between these realist and instrumentalist positions, as well as the development of some interesting variants of these positions. Subsequent to the demise of traditional logical positivism in the early 1960s, many philosophers of science shifted to a realistic position. The works of Quine (1969), Sellars (1970), and Hesse (1966, 1974) are cases in point. More recently the types of historical considerations alluded to above seem to have led a number of philosophers of science away from a realist position and back toward a more instrumentalist stance. Van Fraassen (1980) has distinguished the antirealists into two subtypes: "The first sort holds that science is or aims to be true, properly (but not literally) construed. The second [more instrumentalist view] holds that the language of science should be literally construed, but its theories need not be true to be good" (1980, 10).

Under the first type one could group those more sophisticated realists who hold that well-confirmed scientific theories are "approximately true" (such as Shimony) or are approaching the truth either in some Peircean sense or in the sense of Popper's (1962) notion of verisimilitude or Sellars' (1977) similar view. These attempts to find a more adequate explicandum than "literal truth" for the property possessed by highly confirmed scientific theories, such as Shimony's (1970) "rational degree of commitment to h given e," have met with a variety of problems.[48] These recalcitrant conundra have led several philosophers either toward neutral ground on this debate, for example, Laudan in his 1977 (but not in his 1981), or toward van Fraassen's specific form of the second species of antirealism (in his 1980). Van Fraassen (1980) supports his brand of empiricist antirealism with a variety of sophisticated arguments, and his analysis has generated a vigorous set of criticisms from the philosophy of science community, and a spirited reply from van Fraassen (see Churchland and Hooker, eds., 1985). Putnam has evolved through several forms of realism from his early preference for metaphysical realism (1975–76) to his increasingly complex "internal realist" views (in his 1978 and 1988). It would take us beyond the scope of this chapter (and book) to rehearse all of these views, arguments, and counterarguments, and the reader must be referred elsewhere for them.[49]

It will suffice for our purposes to review briefly Putnam's (1978) argument against metaphysical realism, which will both illustrate the nature of the reasoning involved about realism and illuminate the position to be taken in these pages. On Putnam's view, what he terms "metaphysical realism" is incoherent. This type of realism assumes that truth is "radically nonepistemic." (Putnam still accepts a kind of Peircean realism, which he terms "internal realism." See his 1978 and also his 1988 for his evolved views.)

Basically, Putnam argues as follows. Suppose we use model–theoretic considerations to construct a correspondence between some pragmatically "ideal" theory, T (which meets all "operational constraints" such as consistency, empirical adequacy, simplicity, and so on), and the world, W (equals external reality). The correspondence exists between a model, M, of the theory (with the same cardinality as W) and the world, via a one-to-one mapping between the individuals of M and the pieces of W, and any relations in M and in W. This correspondence, then, is a satisfaction relation, "SAT," and the theory, T, is true just in case "true" is interpreted as "TRUE(SAT)." (Here "TRUE(SAT)" is the truth property determined by the relation "SAT" exactly as "true" is defined in terms of "satisfied" by Tarski; see Putnam 1978, 123–126.) If it be claimed that SAT is not the *intended* correspondence, this claim becomes unintelligible, because there are *no other constraints* on reference which "could single out some other interpretations as (uniquely) intended, and SAT as an unintended interpretation."

The metaphysical realist, on the other hand, contends that truth is "radically nonepistemic," and that a theory satisfying all the above pragmatic characteristics *might be false*. But, on the basis of the above argument, Putnam contends this claim that the pragmatically ideal theory "might *really* be false appears to collapse into *unintelligibility*" (1978, 126), since by supposition everything that can be said about the theory and its relation to the world has been duly considered and found satisfactory.

5.8.3 *Conditionalized Realism*

If metaphysical realism is incoherent and a type of Peircean realism in which scientific theories that achieve consensus belief at the end of time is utopian, at best a regulative ideal,[50] is there any defensible position one can take in the present day? It seems to this author that these two "extreme" or "idealized" positions of realism and instrumentalism each contain important elements of the position to be argued in this book. According to this view, which has analogues with previous and current thinkers' suggestions,[51] the position that is most in accord with scientists' attitudes, as revealed in the history of science, and in contemporary science can be expressed by the phrase *conditionalized realism*.

If one analyzes the notion of scientific "truth" involved in the realistic position from the perspective of an empiricist position, the notion soon becomes suspect. The empiricist denies any direct intuitive experience of the certitude of scientific hypotheses or theories. Recall the discussion in chapter 4 (p. 130) on generalized empiricism. Hypotheses and theories are universal and thus cover (infinitely) many more cases than have been examined in tested situations. Furthermore, theories generally have observationally inaccessible aspects to them and these cannot usually be completely checked via "direct" observation. A believer in scientific intuitionism, perhaps of a Kantian type whereby a scientist could directly intuit the truth or falsity of a scientific hypothesis,[52] would not be in such a position of uncertainty, but it is difficult to find recent scientific or philosophical proponents of such an intuitionist view who have offered convincing arguments for their positions.

If one accepts the generalized empiricist position advocated in the previous chapter, then the most that one can assert regarding the adequacy of a hypothesis is that there is (relatively) direct evidence in its favor. But as we saw in connection with the analysis of direct evidence, such testimony or proof is *conditioned* by the acceptance of both (1) auxiliary assumptions, and (2) the nonavailability of plausible alternative, incompatible theories that account for the same "direct" evidence. An examination of the realistic position within the framework of the epistemological tenets advocated in this book leads, then, to a *conditionalized realism* at most.

A similar examination of the instrumentalist position will disclose a convergence of the two prima facie very different positions of realism and instrumentalism. An instrumentalist will not deny the importance of deductive consequences of a hypothesis or a theory, especially insofar as those consequences lead to further observable predictions. One subclass of those implications will be tests that scientists characterize as "direct evidence" for a hypothesis. Scientists, moreover, will view such direct evidence as crucial for an estimation of their confidence in further predictions of the hypothesis in new domains and its likely "elaborability" and fertility in scientific inquiry. Consider, for example, what the "falsification" of a hypothesis by a generally agreed upon "direct test" would mean even to a scientist who asserted (verbally) that he was an instrumentalist. It is exceedingly likely that such a negative outcome would engender serious qualms on his part about the future reliability and heuristic character of such a hypothesis. As far as the *behavior* of all scientists is concerned, then, the two positions converge, and it therefore seems permissible to attribute, at least behavioristically, a conditionalized realism to all scientists. (I should add that I believe that this conditionalized realism has an inferential or epistemological dimension that is quite coherent with the Bayesian view defended in this chapter.) It is this conditionalized realism, along with its correlative relativized notion of truth and falsity, that will be employed in this and later chapters.[53]

This explicit reference to the *conditionalization* of realism allows for an important aspect of the "acceptance" of hypotheses and theories. As noted earlier, there have been many theories that have had a most important impact on the historical development of science but have turned out to be false. The conditions cited concerning the limits of direct evidence would seem to rationalize the provisional and tentative "acceptance" in the sense of high probability of hypotheses.[54] When, however, the conditions regarding auxiliary assumptions and the availability of plausible alternative, incompatible hypotheses or theories change, one is likely to see a change in the acceptance status of a hypothesis or theory by the scientific community. An analysis of evaluation and acceptance from the perspective of conditionalized realism will accordingly importantly depend on the precise articulation of these conditions in specific cases. With the possibility of a conditionalized realism it becomes unnecessary to subscribe to the (naive) instrumentalist's conception of scientific theories because of the existence of many false but "accepted" theories in the history of science. It might be wise to point out, however, that the significance of "direct evidence" in connection with evaluation and "acceptance" should not be overemphasized. In accordance with the generalized empiricism outlined earlier, it will be argued in section 5.11 that there are other, less directly empirical factors that are important in both an individual's and a scientific community's decision to (conditionally) accept a hypothesis or theory.

5.8.4 *Social Constructivism*

In recent years a number of sociologists of science have emphasized the "conditionalized" aspect of what I have above termed conditionalized realism, suggesting in their more extreme moments that all scientific "facts" are in truth "socially constructed" rather than objective features of the scientific world. Latour and Woolgar's *Laboratory Life* (1979, 1986) is prototypical in this regard, arguing that scientists engaged in "discovering" neuroendocrinological "releasing factors" are not finding something that is "pregiven." Rather these "substances" are *constructed* socially as part of a complex give-and-take among laboratory machine readings and discourse among laboratory scientists.

There is a kernel of truth in the constructivist program, which has been further advanced by Knorr-Cetina (1981) and recently criticized by Giere (1988), but it is developed in the wrong direction as I interpret it. As noted in chapter 4 and reexamined in connection with the "incommensurability" thesis in the following section, the relation of scientific theory to "observations" in the laboratory is exceedingly complex. In spite of the weblike connections between theoretical postulation and laboratory experimentation, multiple empirical constraints on theoretical speculations generate a stability and "stubbornness" of both data and theory, to use Galison's terms, that I believe to be best described according to the "conditionalized realism" presented in this book. Thus, though scientific progress does not yield certainty and absolute objectivity, the situation is far less socially subjective than depicted by the constructivist program.

5.9 The Problem of Commensurability

In the past three decades the interest both of scientists and of philosophers of science in the problems of evaluation and "acceptance" (and rejection) of scientific theories has been stimulated by the contributions of P. K. Feyerabend and T. S. Kuhn. Feyerabend appears to have developed his ideas from his association with and initial commitment to Sir Karl Popper's philosophy of science and also from his acquaintance with the arguments pro and con Bohr's "Copenhagen" interpretation of quantum theory. Kuhn's prior work was in physics and the history of science, and while he was a junior fellow at Harvard he produced a clear and eminently readable account of the Copernican revolution. During the late 1950s and early 1960s, Kuhn and Feyerabend were both associated with the philosophy department at the University of California, Berkeley, and through extensive conversation developed their initially fairly similar views of the relation of scientific theories and of scientific revolutions.[55] Important aspects of their views had been anticipated by the monographs of N. R. Hanson (1958) and S. Toulmin (1961). Neither Hanson nor Toulmin, however, developed their positions in the direction of "incommensurability," which is the problem to be considered in this section, so it is thus appropriate to focus on the views of Feyerabend and of Kuhn.

The problem of incommensurability is of interest to us in connection with the evaluation and acceptance of scientific theories, since it implies that intertheoretical standards of evaluation and comparison are impossible. The impossibility of such standards has three sources: the theory-ladenness of criteria, that of scientific terms, and that of observation terms.[56]

5.9.1 *The Theory-ladenness of Criteria*

In his book, *The Structure of Scientific Revolutions*, Kuhn (1962) suggested that the standards by which groups of scientists judge theories are heavily conditioned by the theory itself, or, in Kuhn's term, by the *paradigm*. A paradigm is broader than a theory and contains within it not only the abstract theory per se but also metaphysical commitments, methodology and rules, specific examples of application, and standards of evaluation. Thus an æther theorist of the late 19th century viewed an æther, a commitment of his paradigm, as a condition of intelligibility of any field theory, and would have rejected Einstein's special theory of relativity because the latter denied that the existence of any æther was necessary. Similar instances in the history of science can be found in Einstein's opposition to the essentially statistical character of quantum mechanics, in the dispute between Metchnikoff and von Behring in the late nineteenth century on the role of macrophages and antibodies in immunology (see Bibel 1988, 12–15 and 119–124), and in the furor over Darwin's evolutionary theory in England and America in the 1860s and 1870s (Hull 1973).

5.9.2 *The Theory-ladenness of Scientific Terms*

Both Kuhn and Feyerabend have argued that prima facie cases of intertheoretic comparability are illusory because of the radically different meanings that scientific terms in different theories possess. Thus, though it appears that Newtonian mechanics is a limiting case of Einsteinian mechanics (for velocities much less than light), Kuhn asserts that what one obtains in such a limiting case is *not* Newtonian theory but at best an explanation as to why Newton's theory has worked at all. A term such as "mass" in Einsteinian theory has associated with it the ideas of variability with relative velocity and intercovertibility with energy (expressed by the famous equation $E = Mc^2$). These notions are foreign and inconsistent with the concept of Newtonian "mass," and, accordingly, any identity, even under restricted conditions such as v << c, is incorrect and misleading. In the area of the biomedical sciences a similar problem arises with different concepts of the classical and molecular characterization of the gene, a position which has been forcefully argued by Hull (1974), Rosenberg (1985), and others (see chapter 9).

5.9.3 *The Theory-ladenness of Observations*

Kuhn and Feyerabend also assert that observations or experimental results, which a scientist might be disposed to think would be independent of theory, are actually heavily conditioned by theory. (I considered this view earlier in chapter 4, but it is worth reexamining here in connection with incommensurability.) The position of Kuhn and Feyerabend in this regard can be set forth by noting that they do not subscribe to the thesis that there is a theory-neutral observation language. Thus basic meterstick and volume measures, pointer readings, solution colors, sedimentation coefficients, and the like are viewed as meaningless per se, and as noncommon to proponents of two inconsistent theories. Any evidential weight of observational results, on this view, is dependent on the assumption of the truth of the theory explaining those results.

There are several instances in current biomedical science which offer prima facie support for this view of the theory-ladenness of observational reports. For example, data regarding the sequence of amino acids in immunoglobulins were interpreted significantly differently by proponents of the germ-line and somatic mutation theories to explain the source of antibody diversity (see Burnet 1964 and Hood and Talmage 1970). As briefly mentioned in chapter 4 (and to be discussed again later in this chapter), the double antibody-producing plasma cells were interpreted in different ways by proponents and opponents of the clonal selection theory.

These three aspects of the incommensurability problem have led Kuhn and Feyerabend to assert that it is impossible to compare and evaluate paradigms and very general theories disinterestedly and objectively. Proponents of different general theories live in "different worlds," worlds which are noncomparable or "incommensurable" with one another. Such a position, though it does explain scientific inertia and the resistance of scientists to give up their preferred theories, raises the specter of subjectivism in science (Scheffler 1967).

5.9.4 *Responses to the Problem of Incommensurability*

There have been a number of responses to this problem of incommensurability. One suggestive direction which has been taken is to hold that, though the syntactical meaning of terms may vary diachronically, the *reference* of the term is stable. Thus we have whatever the term "electron" refers to named less adequately by prequantum theories than by quantum theories of the electron, but *objectively* it is the same entity. Scheffler (1967) has argued eloquently for this position.

In an article critical of this view, Field (1975) contended that no consistent interpretation for Newtonian and Einsteinian notions of mass could be provided, but he was subsequently criticized by Fine and Earman (1977). Putnam (1988) as well as Scheffler (1967) have championed a referential approach to meaning stability, but unanticipated difficulties have arisen. Problems similar to those cited in section 5.8.1 on realism are encountered with any referential approach, and I suspect that a referential solution is at best empty and is most likely self-contradictory. I suspect this for the following reason: Choose two theories, T_1 and T_2, which are thought to be incommensurable, for example, Newton's and Einstein's. Suppose Putnam's conditions, as elaborated in section 5.8.2, are to be met now for the two ideal theories. Then we have *both* theories TRUE(SAT), and this conclusion violates the assumption of referential stability because of logical inconsistency.

An alternative means of resolving the incommensurability problem is to accept it but to deny that it significantly affects global evaluation. This is exemplified in one of Laudan's suggestions, developed in the context of his problem-solving approach. He proposes:

> It was observed . . . that rationality consisted in accepting those research traditions which had the highest problem-solving effectiveness. Now, an approximate determination of the effectiveness of a research tradition can be made *within* the research tradition itself, without reference to any other research tradition. We simply ask whether a research tradition has solved the problems which it set for itself; we ask whether, in the process, it generated any empirical anomalies or conceptual problems. We ask whether, in the course of time, it has managed to expand its domain of explained problems and to minimize the number and

importance of its remaining conceptual problems and anomalies. In this way, we can come up with a characterization of the progressiveness (or regressiveness) of the research tradition.

If we did this for all the major research traditions in science, then we should be able to construct something like a progressive ranking of all research traditions at a given time. It is thus possible, at least in principle and perhaps eventually in practice, to be able to compare the progressiveness of different research traditions, *even if those research traditions are utterly incommensurable in terms of the substantive claims they make about the world!* (1977, 145–146)

This route, however, if accepted without qualification would lead one into the "two different worlds" problem introduced by Kuhn. It is unclear how *common* comparable weights could be involved which would allow even an intersubjective means of assessment.

Laudan proposes an alternative means of outflanking incommensurability, which assumes that problems can be *common* between competing research traditions (1977, 142–145). This, in my view, is more plausible and accords well with the thesis urged in chapter 4 that intertheoretic observational identity is more the rule than the exception.[57] Basically, the claim that will be defended in this book is that incommensurability is a *false* thesis, that it depends (1) on a perhaps initially plausible theory of meaning which is at root incoherent and (2) on unproven and historically falsified assumptions concerning value and observational lability.

That the theory of meaning is incoherent is shown by an argument sketched by Hempel (1970). Hempel pointed out that if the terms that appear in a scientific theory obtain their meaning from the sentences in which they appear, that is, if they are only implicitly defined, then the terms in two very different theories cannot conflict. But the historical arguments given by the proponents of incommensurability depend on just this conflict; for example, Newtonian mass is *not* interconvertible with energy, but Einsteinian mass is, since in Einstein's theory $m = E/c^2$ (see Kuhn 1970, 101–102).

Arguments that measurements and observations utilized in comparing competing extended theories possess a requisite stability for commensurable global evaluation have been discussed on page 137; further below a historical example indicating how general observation agreements function in practice will be presented. I believe that the problem of incommensurability is, accordingly, a pseudoproblem. What is not a pseudoproblem, however, is locating the actual source of scientific inertia and extended conflicts. It appears to me that the source of what has been interpreted by Kuhn and Feyerabend as incommensurability is in fact simply the Quinean (1960) *underdetermination of theories* by what I will term in the next section the theories' "constraints," such as empirical adequacy and theoretical context sufficiency. In later sections, especially in the example of the clonal selection theory, this thesis will be explored and illustrated in more detail.

5.10 Metascientific Units of Global Evaluation: Paradigms, Research Programs, and Research Traditions

In the discussion in chapter 3 on theory structure in the biomedical sciences, I indicated that a number of philosophers of science have argued for a larger and more complex "unit" than what had been earlier construed as a scientific theory. A close examination of these units is a prerequisite to an analysis of global evaluation, since these are in point of fact what are evaluated.

In the 1962 version of his classic *The Structure of Scientific Revolutions*, Kuhn introduced the notion of a "paradigm" that was both prior to and more general than a scientific theory. I shall have a number of specific comments to make later in this section about the "paradigm" notion, but suffice it to say at this point that the term as initially introduced was *too* general and contained a number of inherent ambiguities and obscurities. Shapere, in an influential review, argued that Kuhnian scientific relativism,

> while it may seem to be suggested by a half-century of deeper study of discarded theories, is a *logical* outgrowth of conceptual confusions, in Kuhn's case owing primarily to the use of a blanket term. For his view is made to appear convincing only by inflating the definition of "paradigm" until that term becomes so vague and ambiguous that it cannot easily be withheld, so general that it cannot easily be applied, so mysterious that it cannot help explain, and so misleading that it is a positive hindrance to the under-

standing of some central aspects of science; and then, finally, these excesses must be counterbalanced by qualifications that simply contradict them. (Shapere 1964, 384–385 and 393)

Masterman (1970) similarly discerned some 21 different senses of the term "paradigm." Kuhn (1970) himself admitted there were "key difficulties" with the concept of a paradigm and proposed replacing it with the term "disciplinary matrix." As already indicated in chapter 2 (p. 51), the disciplinary matrix, similar to the paradigm, contains four components: (1) symbolic generalizations, such as $f = ma$ in "Newtonian" mechanics, or presumably Mendel's Laws in genetics, (2) models, which refer to the ontological aspects of theories as well as to analogical models, such as billiard ball models of gases, (3) values, by which scientific claims are assessed, such as predictive accuracy and simplicity, and (4) exemplars. Exemplars are "concrete problem-solutions that students encounter from the start of their scientific education whether in laboratories, on examinations, or at the ends of chapters in scientific texts." (Kuhn 1970, 187).

In his earlier definition of a paradigm, which included all of the above components of a disciplinary matrix, Kuhn also characterized a paradigm as a "concrete scientific achievement" that functioned as a "locus of professional commitment" and which was "*prior* to the various laws, theories, and points of view that . . . [could] be abstracted from it" (my emphasis). Such a paradigm was usually embodied in a scientific textbook or, earlier, in books such as Ptolemy's *Almagest* or Newton's *Principia* but obviously could also be found in a (collection of) scientific article(s). This aspect of a paradigm has at least two significant but interacting components; one is sociological and the other is temporal.[58] In introducing the notions of professional commitment and scientific communities as defined by (and defining) a shared paradigm, Kuhn identified an important characteristic of scientific belief systems that has had a major impact on the sociology of science.[59] In stressing a temporal developmental aspect of a paradigm — normal science is the solving of a variety of puzzles not initially solved by the paradigm, as well as the paradigm's further elaboration and filling in of fine-structured details — Kuhn focused attention on the temporally extended and subtly varying features of a scientific theory. What a falsification-ist-minded philosopher might be inclined to see as a refuting instance of a theory Kuhn interpreted as a puzzle that a modified form of a theory, derived from the same paradigm, could turn into a confirming instance.

Lakatos, initially trained as a Popperean, discerned in Kuhn's monograph a most serious critique of Popperean falsificationist methodology — one that not only had significant methodological consequences but which also raised profound moral and political questions.[60] In attempting to come to a rapprochement between Popper and Kuhn while being sensitive to Duhemian problems with falsificationism, Lakatos developed his "methodology of scientific research programmes."

A research program (I will adhere to the American spelling convention) captures, among other elements, the temporal dimension of a paradigm but introduces a somewhat different internal dynamic structure. A research program is constituted by methodological rules — "some tell us what paths of research to avoid (*negative heuristic*), and others what paths to pursue (*positive heuristic*)" (Lakatos 1970, 132). A research program also contains a "hard core" — in general this contains the essential hypotheses of a theory — and a "protective belt," a set of auxiliary hypotheses "which has to bear the brunt of tests and get adjusted and readjusted, or even completely replaced, to defend the hard core." (The negative heuristic instructs us not to subject the hard core to falsification.)

An excellent example for Lakatos of a research program was Newton's gravitational theory. Lakatos noted:

> When it [Newton's gravitational theory] was first produced, it was submerged in an ocean of 'anomalies' (or, if you wish, 'counterexamples'), and opposed by the observational theories supporting these anomalies. But Newtonians turned, with brilliant tenacity and ingenuity, one counterinstance after another into corroborating instances, primarily by overthrowing the original observational theories in the light of which this 'contrary evidence' was established. In the process they themselves produced new counter-examples which they again resolved. They 'turned each new difficulty into a new victory of their programme.'
>
> In Newton's programme the negative heuristic bids us to divert the *modus tollens* from Newton's three laws of dynamics and his law of gravitation. This 'core' is 'irrefutable' by the methodological decision of its protagonists:

anomalies must lead to changes only in the 'protective' belt of auxiliary, 'observational' hypothesis (sic) and initial conditions. (Lakatos, 1970, 133)

The temporally extended and continual modifications of the (protective belt portions of the) theory thus characterize a notion which is more general than what philosophers had understood by the term "theory."

Other philosophers of science, as already mentioned in previous chapters, have similarly seen the need to work with a unit that is more general than the traditional time-slice snapshot of a scientific theory. Earlier I discussed briefly Shapere's concept of a "domain."[61] Toulmin (1972) has introduced a notion of *conceptual* evolution in a *discipline*, and Laudan subsequently proposed the term "research tradition." For Laudan:

1. Every research tradition has a number of specific theories which exemplify and partially constitute it; some of these theories will be contemporaneous, others will be temporal successors of earlier ones;
2. Every research tradition exhibits certain *metaphysical* and *methodological* commitments which, as an ensemble, individuate the research tradition and distinguish it from others;
3. Each research tradition (unlike a specific theory) goes through a number of different, detailed (and often mutually contradictory) formulations and generally has a long history extending through a significant period of time. (By contrast, theories are frequently short-lived.) (Laudan 1977, 78–79)

In general for Laudan:

a research tradition is a set of general assumptions about the entities and processes in a domain of study, and about the appropriate methods to be used for investigating the problems and constructing the theories in that domain. (Laudan 1977, 81)

More recently, Kitcher increased by one more the number of terms proposed for a metascientific unit by introducing the notion of a "practice." Kitcher first outlined his notion of a "practice" in his 1983, but I will confine most of my discussion to the manner in which he used the concept in connection with classical and molecular genetics. For our purposes we are interested in (1) the structure of a practice and (2) the manner to which it is put in scientific development and application. In connection with classical genetics, a practice is characterized as follows:

> There is a common language used to talk about hereditary phenomena, a set of accepted statements in that language (the corpus of beliefs about inheritance . . .), a set of questions taken to be appropriate questions to ask about hereditary phenomena, and a set of patterns of reasoning which are instantiated in answering some of the accepted questions; (also: sets of experimental procedures and methodological rules, both designed for use in evaluating proposed answers . . .). The practice of classical genetics at a time is completely specified by identifying each of the components just listed. (1984a, 352)

It is the "pattern of reasoning" which I take to be most important for Kitcher's notion of practice. This idea is further elaborated:

> A pattern of reasoning is a sequence of schematic sentences, that is sentences in which certain items of a nonlogical vocabulary have been replaced by dummy letters, together with a set of filling instructions which specify how substitutions are to be made in the schemata to produce reasoning which instantiates the pattern. This notion of pattern is intended to explicate the idea of a common structure that underlies a group of problem-solutions. (1984a, 353)

Kitcher relates this account to what beginning students learn:

> Neophytes are not taught (and never have been taught) a few fundamental theoretical laws from which genetic "theorems" are to be deduced. They are introduced to some technical terminology, which is used to advance a large amount of information about special organisms. Certain questions about heredity in these organisms are posed and answered. Those who understand the theory are those who know what questions are to be asked about hitherto unstudied examples, who know how to apply the technical language to the organisms involved in these examples, and who can apply the patterns of reasoning which are to be instantiated in constructing answers. More simply, success-

ful students grasp general patterns of reasoning which can
be used to resolve new cases. (1984a, 354)

Though moving in the correct direction, I believe that
Kitcher has understated the extent to which the nature of
biomedical theorizing requires an increased emphasis on what
might be called prototype organisms, an issue I discussed in
chapter 3. In addition, I do not find enough fine structure in
Kitcher's notion of "practice" to enable it to account for the complexity of interlevel interactions and progress. Kitcher has extended his notion of a practice and provided a rich set of
examples in his recent (1989) essay, but, in contrast to the temporally extended version of the account of theory structure I favor
(and develop below), I find it still lacks sufficient detail to account for "high fidelity" historical development, though I also
think that Kitcher could extend his analysis still further to accomplish this. Let me elaborate on this point, which I believe also
affects other proposed metascientific units.

One difficulty with each of these more general units, such as
"paradigm," "disciplinary matrix," "research program," "research tradition," or "practice," is that they are *too* general for
our purposes in the sense of lacking sufficient structure. They
may have their utility in explicating *extraordinarily* encompassing
scientific belief systems, but they lack both sufficient internal
structure and limits to be useful in illuminating issues of global
evaluation in contemporary biology and medicine. For example,
Laudan notes in connection with a "research tradition," that "*research traditions are neither explanatory, nor predictive, nor directly
testable*. Their very generality, as well as their normative elements, precludes them from leading to detailed accounts of specific natural processes" (1977, 81–82).

Later I shall argue that the lack of *direct* testability does not
entail lack of testability, and that some additional distinctions involving more specific levels of realization of a very general theory indicate how this testability can be and has been achieved.
Also, later in this chapter, I shall discuss an example of global
justification which exhibits certain similarities with the types of
historical conflicts discussed by the above cited authors. I shall
argue, however, that the appropriate metascientific unit, which I
will term an *extended theory*, has a more explicit structure than is
allowed by the theorists of scientific change discussed thus far
(though my proposal will be closest to that of Lakatos). The ex-

tended theory will be a temporal (and logical) generalization of the type of middle range theory introduced in chapter 3.

5.11 The Extended Theory as the Appropriate Metascientific Unit of Global Evaluation in the Biomedical Sciences

In this section I want to outline a concept of what I shall argue is the appropriate metascientific unit of global evaluation in the biomedical sciences. An extraordinarily complex set of issues are intertwined here, and it will be impossible to do more than sketch my suggested solution to those problems comprising, among others, (1) theory individuation, (2) diachronic theory structure, (3) the relation of various levels in biomedical theories, and (4) the relation of problems (1) through (3) to scientific rationality. I find it useful to begin from Lakatos's account as outlined above. I shall introduce various features of what I term an extended theory through criticisms of some of Lakatos's essential characteristics of research programs.

As briefly suggested above, I am using the notion of an *extended theory* to introduce a diachronic unit that (1) permits *temporal* theory change and (2) also allows for some *logical* changes — namely, some of the assumptions within the diachronic unit will change while the integrity of the whole is preserved. The latter is a necessary condition, since we must be able to individuate one extended theory from another (or others) with which it competes.

5.11.1 *Centrality*

Returning to Lakatos's notion of a research program, let us begin by suggesting that there is no absolute distinction between hard core and protective belt but rather a roughly continuous (and often shifting) set of commitments of varying strengths, ranging from hypotheses that are *central* to those that are *peripheral*. Peripheral hypotheses are not dispensable without replacement and often do serve to help individuate an extended theory from its competitor(s). "Intrinsic centrality" refers to those entities and processes conceived of as essential elements in a Shaperean domain, which are designated by the selected postulates or laws in a representation of an extended theory.[62] (Other essential elements in the domain that are explained by derivation from these postulates are of crucial importance but do not figure as central features in the extended theory.) It is difficult to give a more precise general characterization of intrinsic centrality than this, though I do not think that there would be problems with recognized scientific experts relatively easily reaching a consensus on the intrinsically central features of a scientific theory, even if they thought the theory false or unsupported. There may also be other postulates in the extended theory that will be central in the sense of individuating the theory from other competitors but that may not be sanctioned by preexisting consensus as constituting domain elements. These will be *extrinsically* central hypotheses, by which I mean hypotheses that cannot be given up easily without turning the extended theory of which they are a part into one of its competitors. Detailed illustrations of these notions will be provided later, but as a simple example an *intrinsically* central assumption of the operon theory is the sequence hypothesis, namely that the genes dictate the primary, secondary, and tertiary structure of proteins, such as the repressor protein and the structural genes' proteins.[63] An *extrinsically* central assumption is that the regulation takes place at the level of transcription via repressor-operator binding, since this assumption is just the one called into question in Stent's (1964) "operatorless operon" competitor to the standard operon model. The utility of this distinction will become more evident in the following section, in which we discuss a Bayesian kinematics and dynamics of belief change for competitions between extended theories.

5.11.2 *Generality*

The second distinction I make between Lakatos's account and the structure of an extended theory is that the hard core is not unilevel but is distinguishable into at least three different *levels* of *generality*. "Generality" here must be distinguished from vagueness. The essence of the notion of generality is that a hypothesis which is general can be instantiated at a lower level by a broad range of more detailed specific hypotheses, each of which may be logically inconsistent with the other specific hypotheses. This occurs naturally because of the *ampliative* character of theory elaboration at lower levels (see chapter 3, p. 119). Provisionally I will distinguish three levels of decreasing generality or increasing specificity, though these distinctions both are initially subjective[64] and also may simply represent points on a continuum. The most *general* hypothesis I will term the γ-level hypothesis. I will assume a set of more specific *subsidiary* hypotheses, termed the σ-level hypotheses, and finally a most specific, highly *detailed* level on which are found the δ-level hypotheses. In this terminology, there may be many, mutually inconsistent σ realizations of γ-level hypotheses, and similarly many mutually inconsistent δ realizations of σ level hypotheses (different hypotheses at a single level will be indicated here by different subscripts). The relation of being a realization may jump the level, and a γ-level hypothesis may be directly realized by a δ-level hypothesis.

Hypotheses at the γ, σ, or δ level may be central *or* peripheral. In general, δ level hypotheses will, de facto, turn out to be molecular-level hypotheses, but there is no reason in principal why a molecular level hypothesis cannot be γ-level. The reason for the de facto relation between levels of generality and levels of aggregation has to do with the number of plausible realizations one can envision, and when one gets to the molecular level there are such a considerable number of constraints and so much auxiliary knowledge available that this level of aggregation usually will utilize the δ level of generality for hypotheses (or for mechanisms).

5.11.3 *Change of Central Hypotheses*

My third point of difference with Lakatos involves the fact that investigators often *do* direct their experiments and theoretical modifications at the hard core of essential hypotheses. In the terminology of extended theories, this means that modifications of central hypotheses at the σ or δ level of generality will be considered, though Lakatos is correct as regards a ban against falsification at the γ level for central hypotheses, since this would be equivalent to giving up the theory. We reexamine such a situation in sections 5.13 and 5.14.5.

5.11.4 *Factoring the Extended Theory into Components*

In order to examine the effect of new experimental evidence (or new relevant intertheoretical results) on an extended theory, and also to represent change within the extended theory, it is necessary to provide some substructure using the above notions. In many test situations, a number of the assumptions of the theory are (conditionally) taken as true, and the brunt of the test is directed at one (or a few) of the theory's assumptions (though which of the assumptions are accepted as true for a test situation will change from one situation to another). Let us then factor the theory into two parts, κ and τ, where κ represents the conditionally accepted kernel of the theory in that situation and τ the hypothesis (or hypotheses) under test. The only restriction on the range of τ is, as noted above, that it cannot include central γ-level assumptions in its range. In a typical test situation involving a theory with seven postulates:

$$k = \gamma_1 \& \gamma_2 \& \sigma_3 \& \delta_4 \& \sigma_6 \& \delta_7,$$
and
$$t = \sigma_5.$$

In section 5.14.7 I shall show how some simple numbers for priors and likelihoods can be obtained which should make this strategy both clearer and more plausible.

5.11.5 *The Semantic Conception of an Extended Theory*

An extended theory also needs to be understood in the polytypic sense elaborated in chapter 3. Thus one must construct, using the semantic conception, an adequate definition of the theory (using whatever conjunction of axioms is warranted) in the appropriate language.[65] (In the notation of chapter 3, this means that we must specify appropriate generalizations, Σs, which can be conjoined to constitute Π, a definition of the theory.) Using the notion from model theory of a "reduced model," we extensionally represent increasing generality by increasing reductions of the detail in the model (or in the state space, if that approach should be feasible) by simply eliminating the more specific axioms from consideration at that level of generality (for example, deleting a δ_i which further specifies some σ_i). On the basis of these notions, we can then introduce the *temporal* property of theory change by specifying a new time dimension in terms of which to represent the evolution of semantically characterized theories *over* time. This we do by a series of numerically increasing superscript integers, applying either to specific hypotheses (e.g., $\delta_4^1 \to \delta_4^2$) or to an evolving theory $T^1 \to T^2$ (or, in our alternative notation, $\Pi^1 \to \Pi^2$).

The important feature of biomedical theories that involves *similarity* between models can be represented, as in chapter 3, by appealing to a frame or object-oriented programming language in which to embed any required variation. (Diachronic as opposed to synchronic variation, however, is represented as just suggested, using the numerically successive superscripts to denominate successive modifications of the theory. I shall present a detailed case later on to show how this works in practice.) Notions of inductive support are complicated by this potential variation in biomedical theories, but appropriate weighted averaging should in principle resolve this problem. The question as to how exactly to weigh different models vis-à-vis the theory as a whole does not at present have a general answer and must await further research. (In the comparatively simple historical example presented below, this variation does not appear since we can work with reasonably sharp hypotheses.)

The above constitutes the outlines of a diachronic extension of the structure of biomedical theories initially presented in chapter 3. Further details will be provided in part by a biomedical illustration in section 5.13 and in part through a discussion of the kinematics of belief change, to be investigated from a generalized Bayesian perspective in the following sections.

5.12 A Bayesian Logic of Global Evaluation

In part 1 it was argued that the personalist Bayesian approach to statistical hypothesis testing was preferable to classical alternatives such as the Neyman-Pearson accounts. It was also contended there that degree of confirmation or support can be construed as a judgmental probability. In this section I will argue that the Bayesian approach can be generalized to cover extended theories and the type of competition that arises between alternative theories, such as the instructive theory of the immune response and the clonal selection theory. I believe that the Bayesian approach provides a natural formalism for developing the criteria of comparative global theory evaluation which are often explicitly employed in such debates.

Though a Bayesian analysis *could* be articulated that would not depend either on a common set of general background assumptions or (more restrictively) on a language for reporting experiments that is sufficiently common for empirical (or "observational") comparison, I will argue that these conditions of commonality as a matter of fact *do hold*. The formalism can function without this commonality, since one could compare the difference between, say, (1) the time slice of an extended theory T_i with its own set of experiments {e} against its own background b to obtain a value $p(T_i \mid e \& b)$ and (2) an alternate T_j with *its own* {e}′ and b′. This comparison might yield a judgment, for instance, that $p(T_i \mid \{e\} \& b) > p(T_j \mid \{e\}′ \& \beta′)$. It would presumably hold for incommensurable theories treated as Laudan suggests.[66] This is not very satisfactory, however, since not only does it not accord with a considerable degree of commonality found in science but it also could lead to the nonsensical comparability of Mendelian genetics with Einsteinian relativity. To reflect the type of dispute over common ground discussed in the interesting, historical cases by philosophers such as Kuhn and Feyerabend, commonality must exist.[67]

Global evaluation in science is almost always comparative. The "almost" qualifier is introduced to cover those situations where a domain exists on the basis of a folk tradition and where (1) *any* proffered theory is *so* poor vis-à-vis accounting for well-supported experimental results that the existence of this aggregate of stable facts can result in the proffered theory's rejection, or (2) a proffered theory accounts for a reasonable number of the results in the domain and is thus accepted at least provisionally.

In examining the factors philosophers have employed in global theory evaluation and choice, I suggested in my 1970 that they can be grouped under three general headings: theoretical context sufficiency, empirical adequacy, and simplicity. Other proposed criteria can be seen as more specific forms or combinations of these criteria, for example, precision generally is a species of empirical adequacy, scope and consilience are also species of empirical adequacy, and ad hocness is a combination of the lack of empirical adequacy and simplicity.[68]

Theoretical context sufficiency is intended to cover both a theory's self-consistency and its consistency or entailment relations with other well-confirmed theories. Empirical adequacy refers to the ability of a theory to explain empirical results, whether these be singular reports of experimental data or empirical generalizations such as Snell's law in optics. Simplicity is the most difficulty notion to define explicitly; roughly, it is a comparative notion, with greater simplicity accorded those theories with fewer entities, fewer independent hypotheses, and fewer terms such as the number of constants required to characterize an equation. (I return to a discussion of several senses and explications of simplicity on page 232.)

Each of these factors can vary in strength and each can be weighted differently. As Kuhn (1970) has noted:

> Judgments of simplicity, consistency, plausibility, and so on often vary greatly from individual to individual. What was for Einstein insupportable inconsistency in the old quantum theory, one that rendered the pursuit of normal science impossible, was for Bohr and others a difficulty that could be expected to work itself out by normal means. . . . In short, . . . the application of values is sometimes considerably affected by the features of individual personality and biography that differentiate the members of the group. (1970, 185)

Such variation is important in permitting creativity to function, leading to the pursuit of new theories.[69] It is interesting to note, however, that though such variation does occur, there is not as much as Kuhn suggests, and as time passes this variation converges toward a mean among scientists. (We will see an example of this subsequently in a discussion of the clonal selection theory, as viewed in 1957 and in 1967.) This convergence, I believe, is an illustration of the swamping effect discussed in the Bayesian section of part 1, illustrated by the Bayesian approach to the Mendelian example in appendix 2 (p. 256). (Also see the comments by Einstein on "simplicity," page 232.)

It is difficult to provide much more in the way of a general set of factors affecting a logic of comparative global theory evaluation beyond what is cited above a priori; for more detail one must go to specific cases. (In this section and in section 5.14 these factors will, however, be further combined and elaborated on in the context of a Bayesian dynamics.) A more detailed specification of these factors will be given in section 5.13 in the context of one such specific case, but prior to doing so, it will be useful to see how these factors can be applied to *extended* theories and embedded in a generalized Bayesian kinematics. (A discussion of Bayesian dynamics will occur in section 5.14.)

Recall the formulation of Bayes's theorem given in part 1 above: $P(H \mid e\&b) = P(H \mid b) \cdot P(e \mid H\&b)/P(e \mid b)$. Using the factoring approach introduced in section 5D, we may replace H by T = κ & τ and rewrite Bayes's theorem in its simple form as:

$$P(κ\&τ \mid e\&b) = \frac{P(τ \mid κ\&b) \cdot P(κ \mid b) \cdot P(e \mid τ\&κ\&b)}{P(e \mid b)}.$$

Each of these terms need explication. In addition, the effect of dealing with an extended *diachronic* theory needs to be considered carefully, for as we shall see, the appropriate comparison vis-à-vis confirmation is somewhat complex.

The expression on the left side of the equation is the posterior probability of the theory conditionalized on the truth of a new experimental datum e. (For simplicity I will illustrate the kinematics using new experimental knowledge represented by e, though some new *intertheoretical* result, say t, could be accommodated with appropriate switch of e and t in the formula. Accordingly, what Laudan terms "conceptual problems" [in chapter 2 of his 1977] could easily be accommodated in this generalized Bayesian schema.)

The term $P(τ \mid κ\&b)$ represents the prior probability of test assumption τ, say a postulate of middle level generality, central or not, on the conditional truth of the *other* assumptions of theory T and the background assumptions. Similarly, $P(κ \mid b)$ is the prior probability of these other assumptions on the assumption of the background only. The expression $P(e \mid τ\&κ\&b)$ is the likelihood of obtaining the experimental result e on the (conditional) truth of the theory and the background. In general e will not be obtainable from τ and b above but will essentially involve (some other postulates in) κ. If, however, τ can be made sufficiently independent of T, as in those cases where each of the nonlogical parameter values of the expression τ can be simultaneously fixed on the basis of b,[70] then we can obtain a powerful and specific test of τ in a non-Duhemian manner (with respect to T but not, of course, to b). In such a special situation, the above expression has the κ terms stricken, $P(κ\&b)$ is also eliminated, and we have a test of $P(τ \mid e\&b)$.[71]

For the sake of simplicity we initially consider b constant in such tests, though this assumption will have to be relaxed, as it is unrealistic, and a changing b is actually needed to make sense of a number of cases of theory evolution and revolution.[72] I will also assume that b, for any specific situation, contains not only accepted experimental results and well-entrenched background theories but also methodological rules. This is controversial[73] but it allows the "prior" probability, $P(T \mid b)$, to express the joint assessment of theoretical context sufficiency, prior empirical adequacy, and simplicity. The importance of this will be seen further below.

Now let us examine the effect of a prima facie falsifying experiment on the extended theory, a situation that will require a modification of T. We will consider the following three situations in which extended theory T can find itself, as summarized in Table 5.2. This will require us to represent the extended theory in two states, T^1 and T^2. (In general, changes in an extended theory and in its constituted parts will be indicated by changing *super*scripts; *different*, competing extended theories will be indicated by different *sub*scripts, T_1 versus T_2, or, more realistically, T_1^3 versus T_2^5, for example.)

State	Situation	Internal Structure
T^1	Prior to experiment e	$(\kappa \ \& \ \tau^1) \rightarrow -e)$
T^1	Falsified by a new experiment	$(\kappa \ \& \ \tau^1) \rightarrow -e) \ \& \ e$
T^2	Explaining a new experiment	$(\kappa \ \& \ \tau^2) \rightarrow e) \ \& \ e$

(The $\rightarrow$ arrow can be read as logical entailment.)

In the table above we assume for simplicity that T^2 is the only plausible modification to make at this point to outflank the falsifying effect of e on T^1.[74] This type of transition (of T^1 to T^2) *can* be ad hoc under certain conditions, which will be explored in section 5.14 after we have had a chance to examine a detailed case illustration to provide appropriate material for analysis.

A question can be raised concerning the legitimacy of the comparison of T^1 with T^2 on the evidence e&b, since T^2 is not exactly equivalent to T^1.[75] This, however, is one of the main points at issue in attempting to characterize an *extended* theory. I would contend that, as long as central γ-level hypotheses are maintained in such transitions and "enough" of the σ- and δ-level hypotheses also retained, comparison of T^1 with T^2 is legitimate. What constitutes "enough" of the hypotheses is in part a function of the internal hypothesis structure of a theory's competitors and in part a matter of the centrality of those assumptions that are preserved. A general response to these issues must await general solutions of the problems of theory individuation,[76] but some specific answers to particular questions can, however, be offered, and it is now to a specific case that I turn. I will return to further general methodological elaborations of this Bayesian dynamics of extended theory development and evaluation in section 14.

5.13 The Clonal Selection Theory as an Extended Theory

In this book we have referred to the clonal selection theory as an example of a biomedical theory several times: in connection with discovery in chapter 2, in chapter 3 on theory structure, and in chapter 4 on empirical testing. The clonal selection theory, however, is really an *extended theory* in the sense characterized in sections 5 and 6. Recall that the theory was formulated in 1957, elaborated in 1959, and tested a number of times by a variety of experiments from 1957 on. It was "accepted," in the sense of being granted high probability by the immunological community, by 1967, as indicated by a review of the papers in the 1967 Cold Spring Harbor Symposia of Quantitative Biology volume *Antibodies*, consisting of the proceedings of a conference and attended by 300 of the most prominent immunologists of that time. Even in that book, however, Felix Haurowitz exhibited a kind of "Kuhnian" resistance when he wrote:

> It may be a heresy to talk in this group about direct template action. However, I would like to show in a diagram [fig. 5.1] that template action of the antigen could still be reconcilable with our present views on protein biosynthesis. As shown in the diagram, the antigenic determinant might force the nascent peptide chain to fold along its surface, and thus might prevent the incorporation of certain amino acids. Growth of the peptide chain would continue as soon as a suitable amino acid is incorporated. Such a process might also cause the elimination of one amino acid, or of a few amino acids from the peptide chain,

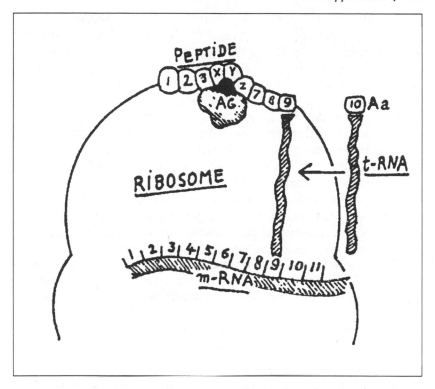

Figure 5.1 "The diagram shows the hypothetical template role of an antigen fragment (Ag) during the translation phase of antibody biosynthesis. The amino acid residues 1–3 and 7–9 have been assembled according to the triplet code provided by the messenger RNA molecule (mRNA). The antigenic fragment interferes with the incorporation of the amino acid residues 4, 5, and 6 since these cannot yield a conformation which would allow the growing peptide chain to fold over the surface of the antigenic determinant (black area in Ag). For this reason, the aminoacyl-tRNA complexes no. 4–6 are rejected and the sequence 4, 5, and 6 either replaced by three other amino acids x, y, and z, as shown in the diagram, or omitted. The latter process would result in a deletion." The figure and the caption quoted are reproduced from Haurowitz 1967, p. 564, © 1967 by Cold Spring Harbor Laboratory, with permission from the Cold Spring Harbor Laboratory.

but would otherwise not alter the amino acid sequence. (1967, 564)

In addition, Morton Simonson, in his (1967) article in those proceedings, indicated doubts about the simple form of the clonal selection theory.

What is most interesting about the clonal selection theory's route to "acceptance," however, is that it was, at least according to its opponents, significantly "refuted" in 1962. The peregrinations and modifications of the theory, and the factors affecting "rejection" and "acceptance" should serve as an excellent illustration and test of the notions of an extended theory and of a generalized global Bayesian logic of comparative theory evaluation.

It is also worth pointing out here that these "peregrinations and modifications of the theory" we will encounter in the following pages indicates that much of this story involves "the context of discovery," though of a less dramatic form than we saw in Burnet's original discovery discussed in chapter 2. The reader should recall that in chapter 2 I indicated that an important phase of the "logic of discovery" included those episodes in which preliminary evaluations of new hypotheses were being undertaken by working scientists. Thus some aspects of what is characterized as a "logic of global evaluation" overlap with periods in which a hypothesis is being fine-tuned or modified as part of an extended theory. This is consistent with the views developed in chapter 2, but it seems worth recalling as we embark on an account in which this preliminary evaluation is presented in detail.

5.13.1 *The Form of the Clonal Selection Theory, 1957–1959*

The simple form of the clonal selection theory has been discussed in chapters 2, 3, and 4. In this section of the book I will need to be somewhat more detailed concerning the main features of the theory as it was proposed in its earliest form. I shall then indicate the nature of some aspects of its temporally changing structure, thus exhibiting it as an illustration of an extended theory.

In its simple form the clonal selection theory (hereafter abbreviated as CST) is as explained in chapters 2 and 3. However, if we employ the 1957 (and 1959) articulations of the theory, it is useful to distinguish the following hypotheses employing the γ, σ, δ notation discussed above on p. 213:

γ_1 Antibody formation is the result of a selective process: no structural information is passed from the antigen to the antibody.

σ_2 Antibody specificity is encoded in the genome of the antibody-producing (plasma) cell.

δ_3 Antigenic determinants are recognized by (gamma-globulin) surface receptors on lymphocytes, and this receptor is identical in specific type with the soluble antibody produced by the cell's clonal descendants.

σ_4 Antigen reacting with the surface receptors stimulates the cell to proliferate as a clone.

δ_5 All antibodies produced by a cell or its descendants are of the same specific type(s) (in primary, secondary, and tertiary structure).[77]

γ_6 There is a mechanism for the generation of antibody diversity σ_6 (probably somatic mutation).

σ_7 One cell (most probably) produces only one type of antibody (however, since cells are diploid, it is possible that two different types of antibody might be produced by one cell).

These seven hypotheses can be considered the *central* hypotheses of the clonal selection theory. Some of these are more detailed realizations of higher level hypotheses, such as σ_6 is of γ_6. Several less central but important hypotheses of the theory are:

σ_8 Some descendants of proliferating cells differentiate into plasma cells and release soluble antibody, but others persist in the parental (lymphocyte) state and carry long-term immunological memory (for the secondary response).

σ_9 Self-tolerance is generated by elimination (in the embryo) of forbidden (anti-self) clones.

σ_{10} Some cells function directly (i.e., not via release of soluble antibody), as in the homograft response.[78]

The distinction I make between central and less central assumptions is based on my interpretation of remarks made by Burnet in his 1959 and his retrospective 1968. Each of the hypotheses should be conceived of as having "1" superscripted to it, as the formulation of some of these hypotheses will change over time. On the basis of my previous claim (p. 213), γ_1 and γ_6 cannot change; other hypotheses may or may not change depending on historical circumstances. The postulates probably do not constitute a minimal nonredundant set, and some may be consequences of others, especially if background theories are taken into account.[79] Nevertheless, this seems to be an accurate and useful reconstruction of the clonal selection theory in its earliest form. Finally, it should be noted that, though γ-level hypotheses are generally systemic, σ-level generally cellular, and δ-level usually molecular, there are exceptions. Hypothesis σ_2 is actually genetic and δ_3 is clearly interlevel. Recall that the provisional distinctions between γ, σ, and δ are intended to represent levels of *generality* and not necessarily levels of aggregation.

5.13.2 The Main Competitor of the CST: The Extended Instructive Theory

There were several competitors to the CST when it was proposed by Burnet in 1957. As noted in chapter 2, Jerne's natural selection (but noncell-based) theory, Talmage's selection theory, and Burnet's (and Fenner's) own earlier indirect template theory had been proposed and were still fairly plausible accounts.[80] The main competitor theory at this time, however, was the direct template theory or, to use Lederberg's term, the instructive theory (hereinafter abbreviated as IT). This theory had initially been proposed in the early 1930s, first by Breinl and Haurowitz (1930), then independently by Alexander (1931) and by Mudd (1932).[81] Initially Breinl and Haurowitz had believed that an antigen might interfere with the lining up of amino acids in the peptide chain, and that this might result in differences in the order and orientation of the amino acids (Haurowitz 1963, 28). Later an elegant chemical mechanism (at the atomic molecular and δ level of specificity) based on hydrogen bonding and other weak bonding effects was developed for this theory by Pauling (1940). According to this hypothesis, it was only the *tertiary* structure (or folding) of the antibody molecule that was interfered with by the antigen. The theory in its post-1940 form (which persisted largely unchanged until the later 1950s) can be characterized in terms of the following hypotheses:

γ_1 Antigen contributes structural information to the antibody.

δ_2 The function of antigen is to serve as a template on which the complementary structure of antibody molecules is formed.

δ_3 The order of amino acids in the active site of the antibody molecule is irrelevant.

δ_4 Template action is by stabilizing of the hydrogen bonds and other weak bonds in the antibody molecule. (This is actually a $\delta_4{}^2$ hypothesis, the Breinl and Haurowitz (1930) hypothesis being $\delta_4{}^1$ — see above.)

σ_5 Antigen penetrates into the antibody-producing cell.

It follows from γ_1 that antigen must be present whenever antibody is formed, whether it be initial formation or renaturation (refolding) of the antibody after chemical denaturation (unfolding).

There are several additional, less central hypotheses which have been abstracted from later versions of the direct template theory, principally from Haurowitz's writings:[82]

γ_6 Immunological memory (secondary response) is attributed to persisting antigen interacting with antibody. No σ or δ level mechanism is proposed. (Note that this is a *general* hypothesis but also a *molecular level* hypothesis.)

γ_7 Tolerance is attributed to a common mechanism of immunological paralysis which occurs without excess of antigen (see Haurowitz 1965).

This theory was again modified with respect to the mechanism of tertiary folding by Karush (1958), who proposed $\delta_4{}^3$: covalent disulphide (S-S) bonds are instrumental in stabilizing the tertiary structure of antibody molecules. Thus the $\delta_4{}^2$ of Pauling goes in the Karush version to $\delta_4{}^3$ (in our formalism).

5.13.3 *Arguments between Proponents of the CST and Proponents of the IT*

The main objection of the instructional school against any type of selection theory (initially directed against Ehrlich's early 1900 side-chain theory) arose in the late 1920s out of Landsteiner's classic work on eliciting antibody responses to a variety of artificially synthesized antigenic determinants.[83] It was thought extremely unlikely that the antibody-producing animal (or its ancestors) could have earlier experiences with these previously nonexistent, newly synthesized molecules, and also unlikely that as much information as would be required to *anticipate* such antigenic structures could be carried in the organisms' genomes. Instructional theories provided a simple explanation of the ability of animals to synthesize antibody against "various artifacts of the chemical laboratory" (to use Haurowitz's phrase), such as azophenyltrimethylammonium ions.

Burnet found this objection "intuitive" and not compelling, and he suggested that the information necessary to encode about 10^4 different antibody types should not overly tax a genome. In 1962 he proposed:

> A majority of immunologists find it difficult to accept the hypothesis that 10^4 or more different patterns of reactivity can be produced during embryonic life without reference to the foreign antigenic determinants with which they are 'designed' to react. This response is perhaps more intuitive than logical. After all[,] we know that in the course of embryonic development an extraordinary range of information—probably many million 'bits'—is interpreted into bodily structure and function. There is no intrinsic need to ask for another 10,000 specification[s] to be carried in the genetic information of the fertilized egg. (1962, 92)

Burnet suggested there were at least three ways the some 10,000 patterns could be obtained: by germline mutation, by somatic mutation, and (a then-recent suggestion of Szilard) by production and manipulation by the cell's own enzymes. No special stress on somatic mutation appears at this point in Burnet's account.

In the early 1960s, after the initial confirming experiment of Nossal and Lederberg discussed in detail in chapter 4, the clonal selection theory ran into considerable experimental difficulties. Burnet had begun with the simple form of the CST. In 1962 he characterized this form as follows:

> It is the simplest self-consistent theory, and because it is so inherently simple it is probably wrong. As yet however no decisive evidence against it has been produced and it is a

good rule not to complicate assumptions until absolutely necessary. Occam's razor is still a useful tool. (1962, 90)

Simplicity, however, as has been argued in connection with the thesis of generalized empiricism, is of lesser import than experimental results, and as Burnet noted in his 1967 address to the Cold Spring Harbor meeting, experiments did begin to raise difficulties for the CST:

There is one aspect of the ten years I am talking about that has interested me enormously. Most of the crucial experiments designed to disprove clonal selection once and for all, came off. Attardi et al. (1959) showed that the same cell could often produce two different antibodies if the rabbit providing it had been immunized with two unrelated bacteriophages. Nossal much more rarely found a double producer in his rats. Trentin and Fahlberg (1963) showed that, by using the Till-McCulloch method, a mouse effectively repopulated from the progeny of a single clone of lymphoid cells could produce three [or four] different antibodies. Szenberg et al. (1962) found too many foci on the chorioallantois to allow a reasonable number of clones amongst chicken leukocytes and so on. (1967, 3)

These experiments, such as the double producer, Trentin's triple or quadruple producer, and the work of Szenberg et al. on the Simonsen phenomenon, for a time moved Burnet toward a considerably modified selection view known as *subcellular selection*. Adoption of this temporary fall-back view by CST proponents was seen by instructionists such as Haurowitz as indication of a refutation of the CST,[84] though Burnet saw the modification as still consistent with a selection hypothesis of the γ_1 type.

In a 1962 paper, Burnet wrote "Further study of the [Simonsen or graft-versus-host] phenomenon in Melborne has . . . shown conclusively that the simple form of the clonal selection theory is inadmissible. The first difficulty is that competent cells have a proportion of descendants whose specificity is different from their own . . . the second difficulty is that too high a proportion of cells can initiate foci" (1963, 13). Earlier, writing with his colleagues Szenberg, Warner, and Lind, it was asserted that: "A selectionist approach (Lederberg 1959) is still necessary but for the CAM-focus system it must be a sub-cellular selection" (1962, 136).

The Simonsen phenomenon continued to trouble the CST.[85] The mystery of the double producers was resolved, however, partly by discovering the artifactual nature of those results by 1967 — recall the discussion of Mäkelä's analysis earlier — and partly by interpreting the double producers as Nossal did in the quote given in chapter 4 (p. 141), in terms of artifacts produced by weak cross-reactions and/or impure preparations. This was also Burnet's most recent view before his death (personal communication).

In the quotation given above from his 1967 Cold Spring Harbor address, Burnet noted that "crucial experiments designed to disprove clonal selection once and for all, came off." In a later paragraph in that address he drew a distinction between these experiments and new *heuristic advances*. He stated:

> But, on the other hand, every new heuristic advance in immunology in that decade — and it has been a veritable golden age of immunology — fitted as it appeared easily and conformably into the pattern of clonal selection. With each advance some minor ad hoc adjustment might be necessary, but no withdrawals or massive re-interpretations. Sometimes the new discovery was actually predicted. The statement (Burnet 1959, 119) that the lymphocyte "is the only possible candidate for the responsive cell of clonal selection theory" was validated by Gowans' work in vivo and by Nowell (1960) and many subsequent workers, especially Pearmain et al. (1963), in vitro. The thymus as a producer of lymphocytes must have immunological importance and Miller's work in 1961 was the *effective* initiation of the immunological approach to the thymus (Miller 1962). The origin of thymic cells from the bone marrow was the logical extension of this.
>
> In quite different directions, Jerne and Nordin's (1963) development of the antibody plaque technique provided a precise demonstration of two very important presumptions of the theory that in a mouse a few cells capable of producing anti-rabbit or anti-sheep hemolysin are present before immunization and that on stimulation with sheep cells a wholly different population of plaque forming cells develops from what appears if rabbit cells are used as

antigen.

The findings by several authors in 1964–65 that pure line strains of guinea-pigs responded to some synthetic antigens but not others; the analysis of the classic Felton paralysis by pneumococcal polysaccharide which showed that in the paralyzed mice there was a specific *absence* of reactive cells—these facts just don't fit any instructive theory.

Finally, there is the immensely productive field that opened when the work of Putnam and his collaborators led to a progressive realization of the monoclonal character of myelomatosis and the uniformity of the immunoglobulin produced. . . . [G]iven the established facts of human myelomatosis you have almost a categorical demonstration of (a) clonal proliferation, (b) phenotypic restriction and precise somatic inheritance, (c) the random quality of somatic mutation, and (d) the complete independence of specific pattern on the one hand and mutation to metabolic abnormality such as failure of maturation of the plasmablast, on the other. Almost all the essential features of clonal selection are explicitly displayed. (Burnet 1967, 3)

This distinction between heuristic and experimental results, though suggestive, will not, I think, stand up under closer scrutiny. To an extent, some of the work Burnet reports under heuristic results *are* experimental findings. More important are the experiments on renaturation of antibody molecules, which were considered in 1964 and 1965 by both Burnet and Haurowitz as most significant.

In an article entitled "The Unfolding and Renaturation of a Specific Univalent Antibody," which appeared in the November 1963 issue of the *Proceedings of the National Academy of Sciences USA*, Buckley, Whitney, and Tanford (1963) noted that "the chemical basis for antibody specificity has not, so far, been determined" (1963, 827). They suggested that there were three possibilities: (1) specificity was encoded in the primary structure of the amino acid sequence (the Burnet and Lederberg approach); (2) variability was dependent on disulphide (covalent) bonds (the Karush modification); and (3) variability was dependent on noncovalent bonds, with the specificity directed by a complementary antigenic structure (based on Pauling's work). Buckley and his colleagues worked on small fragments of antibodies, employing an important discovery made by Porter in 1959 that a digestive enzyme could cleave the antibody into fragments. They directed their attention to the fragment that was equivalent to the larger (parent) molecule as regards antibody specificity and affinity for antigen (later called the Fab part).

Buckley, Whitney, and Tanford caused the Fab part of the rabbit antibody specific to bovine serum albumin to unfold by adding a certain reagent to the antibody, testing their result by examining the optical rotation power of solutions of the antibody fragments. Reversal of the unfolding was brought about by slow removal of the reagent by dialysis. In analyzing their results they asserted that "these data provide very strong evidence that different antibody specificities cannot be generated by different arrangements of non-covalent bonds in molecules of identical covalent structure" (1963, 833), citing other investigators' related work on both covalent and noncovalent mechanisms. They summed up their position by noting that "one must conclude from these considerations that antibody specificity is generated primarily by differences in amino acid sequence in some portion of the antibody molecule." Also cited in support of this notion was a then recent important discovery by Koshland and Engleberger (1963) that two different antibodies for the same animal had different amino acid sequences. Previously this had been masked by insufficiently sensitive experimental techniques.

Burnet recognized these experiments in an article he wrote in 1964. In Burnet's view these experiments constituted "evidence from several sources [that] seems to render [the instructive theory] untenable." He noted:

> Koshland and Engleberger have shown differences in amino acid constitution of two antibodies from the same rabbit, Buckley, *et al.* have shown that completely denatured γ-globulin fractions can regain immunological specificity on renaturation. (1964, 452)

Haurowitz also took note of both of these results in a review article, writing that the Pauling version "has lost much of its appeal by the discovery of different amino acid composition of two antibodies formed simultaneously in a single animal . . . , and by the observation that unfolded and denatured anti-BSA from rabbit serum refolds and regains its antibody activity after removal of the denaturing guanidine salt [the reagent] by dialysis" (1965, 36).

It is important to realize that Haurowitz did not question these *observations*, though he did call into question some of the *auxiliary assumptions* made by these experimenters. For example, he expressed doubt whether in the work of Buckley et al. discussed above, "the unfolding of the antibody fragments . . . is indeed complete as concluded from the change in optical rotation" (1965, 16). Haurowitz also questioned whether the amino acid differences found by Koshland and Engleberger "involve the combining groups of these antibodies or whether they are *merely* a consequence of the heterogeneity of the two antibody populations" (Haurowitz 1965, 40; my emphasis). Acceptance of a relatively stable observation language and of many of the assumptions of these experiments did not result in Haurowitz's yielding of the instructive kernel, however, for he wrote in his review article that "the reviewer would attribute the small changes in amino acid composition [discussed by Koshland and Engleberger] to a disturbance of the coding mechanism by serologically determinant fragments of the antigen molecule, resulting in a change in the cellular phenotype but not its genotype" (1965, 36). What we have here, then, is a modification of one of the central δ-level assumptions, namely the Pauling hypothesis—stable since the early 1940s in this extended theory though questioned by Karush in 1958—and its replacement by a new δ-level assumption: the disturbance of the coding mechanisms of protein synthesis. (This approach is further developed in Haurowitz's 1967 in the quote on page 220 and in figure 5.1 and it will be reconsidered again in the next section as an instance of an ad hoc hypothesis.) The 1965 modification amounts to still another δ-level hypothesis, $\delta_4{}^4$ in the instructive theory, after Haurowitz and Breinl's (1930) $\delta_4{}^1$, Pauling's (1940) $\delta_4{}^2$, and Karush's (1958) $\delta_4{}^3$, and underscores the kind of diachronic variation that exists at levels of generalization lower than γ in an extended theory.

5.14 Types of Factors Involved in the CST-IT Debate

In section 5.12 I discussed three types of factors which influence theory "acceptance" and "rejection." We have now examined a fairly detailed illustration of extended theory competition and can return with profit to the Bayesian logic outlined above both to relate that logic to the example and to elaborate further on that logic.

Since we are dealing with both a normative logic and a logic which permits some variation in its application, one must anticipate deviations from the logic in individual cases.[86] I submit, though, that the individual assessments can in a sense be "averaged" so as to demonstrate a change in consensus among scientists over time. Individual variation, as has been noted implicitly, is in part a function of what that individual knows — not all scientists hear of an experimental or theoretical innovation at the same time, nor do all scientists react to such news in the same way: an individual's own background knowledge and "prior probabilities" will affect his or her interpretation of novel results. It is clear, however, at least in the example I have sketched, that in the 10 years from 1957 to 1967 the *consensus* of immunologists shifted from a commitment to the instructive theory to a commitment to the clonal selection theory.[87] In the present section I investigate the dynamics — in the sense of the factors which *forced* that shift — of this change in consensus.

I shall begin by discussing "simplicity." This, as has been noted several times, is generally the weakest of the types of dynamic factors involved in theory change, though in situations in which other, stronger factors are individually or jointly indeterminate it can become significant.[88] I then progress to a discussion of the role of intertheoretic considerations (what I termed theoretical context sufficiency), which also affect the prior probability. Finally, I turn to considering empirical adequacy. I will at that point also discuss how ad hoc modifications affect theory assessments. Some general comments on comparability of probability assessments will close this section and also this chapter.

5.14.1 *Simplicity*

There is no consensus definition of the important notion of simplicity. As Einstein has noted: "an exact formulation of [what] logical simplicity of the premises (of the basic concepts and of the relations between these which are taken as a basis) . . . [consists in] meets with great difficulties" (1949, 23). Logical simplicity has nonetheless "played an important role in the selection and evaluation of theories since time immemorial" (1949, 23). Einstein also suggested that agreement was usually found among scientists in assessing logical simplicity or determining which formulation of a theory contained "the most definite claims." Terming such factors as logical simplicity "inner perfection," he wrote that, in spite of the difficulty of defining various senses of simplicity, "it turns out that among the 'augurs' there usually is agreement in judging the inner perfection of the theories" (1949, 23–25). A review of Hesse's (1974, chapter 10) discussion of simplicity will disclose the variety of senses the term has had for philosophers and scientists.

Earlier I suggested that "simplicity" determinations affect the prior probability of hypotheses and theories. We saw an instance of this in section 5.13, in which Pauling's (1940) modification of the instructive theory's assumption resulted in increased simplicity and, according to assessments in review articles, increased commitment by immunologists to the extended instructive theory. Other inductive logicians of a Bayesian persuasion have also located the effect of simplicity assessments in the prior probability component of Bayes's theorem. Most notable are the suggestions of Sir Harold Jeffreys, who first (with Dorothy Wrinch) proposed that simple laws have greater prior probability than more complex laws. Jeffreys and Wrinch (1921) use a paucity-of-parameters criterion for simplicity, ordering laws from the simpler to the more complex as they move from $y = ax$ to $y = ax^2$, $y = ax^3 \ldots y = an^n$, for example. Jeffreys and Wrinch realized that one would have an infinity of hypotheses whose prior probability must sum to unity, and, they provided a scheme for assigning that probability. Jeffreys later modified this approach in his *Theory of Probability*; his explication has been criticized from several different points of view by Popper (1959, chapter 7 and appendixes vii and viii) and others.[89] It is unclear that a paucity-of-parameters criterion is a suitable one, in any event, to apply in semiquantitative sciences such as biology and medicine, though insofar as it can be generalized to an Occam type of simplicity (presupposing the minimum number of entities required), Jeffreys' approach may be a good approximation.

I have suggested, along with Jeffreys, that simplicity is best conceived of as affecting the prior probability. In his 1977, Roger Rosenkrantz proposed a quite different but still Bayesian explication of simplicity but located the notion in the *likelihood* term of Bayes's theorem. Distinguishing plausibility from simplicity, Rosenkrantz writes:

while simpler theories may or may not be plausible, they typically have higher likelihood than less simple theories which fit the data equally well. That is *they are more confirmable* by *conforming data*. (1977, 93)

While I would agree with Rosenkrantz's plausibility-simplicity separation, preferring to interpret plausibility in terms of a combination of theoretical context sufficiency and prior empirical adequacy, I am less in agreement with Rosenkrantz's analysis of simplicity. The central notion of Rosenkrantz's "Bayesian" explication of simplicity is "sample coverage." He defines it as follows:

By the *sample coverage* of a theory T for an experiment X, I mean the chance probability that the outcome of the experiment will fit the theory, a criterion of fit being presupposed. The smaller its sample coverage over the range of contemplated experiments, the simpler the theory. (1977, 94)

Rosenkrantz believes that simplicity as sample coverage captures the common intuition that simplicity decreases if we add to a theory's "stock of adjustable parameters" (1977, 93). As examples he suggests that "polynomials of higher degree are more complicated, as are various well-known refinements of Mendel's laws, among them polygenes, multiple alleles, pleiotropic effects, and the introduction of additional parameters for linkage, partial manifestation, differential viability of recessives, and so on" (1977, 94).

It is worth considering two points where simplicity enters into the above example of competition between the CST and the instructive theory. First, recall Burnet's "complication" of the original, simpler CST to account for double and triple or quadruple producers, and the later-detected strong Simonsen effect (in the strong version of the effect, 1 out of every 40 lymphocytes would produce the effect). Some type of *sub-cellular* selection was proposed to explain the ability of the cell to respond to several antigens. This does increase sample coverage by the introduction of a modification — sub-cellular selection — analogous to introducing new parameters. The correlation between complexity and sample coverage is intuitive here but reasonably clear, but it goes *against* Rosenkrantz's views.

Now consider Pauling's $\delta_4{}^2$ modification of the earlier, Breinl-Haurowitz instructive theory hypothesis $\delta_4{}^1$. Pauling proceeded by attempting to answer the following questions:

What is the simplest structure which can be suggested, on the basis of the extensive information now available about intramolecular and intermolecular forces, for a molecule with the properties observed for antibodies and what is the simplest reasonable process of formation of such a molecule? (Pauling 1940, 2643)

There are several ways in which Pauling was guided by simplicity, for example, in his assumption that antibodies had a common primary structure. Pauling also noted that antibody-antigen complexes precipitate, and that in forming such a precipitate lattice or framework, "an antibody molecule must have two or more distinct regions with surface configuration complementary to that of the antigens" (1940, 2643). Pauling added:

The role of parsimony (the use of minimum effort to achieve the result) suggests that there are only two such regions, that is that the antibody molecules are at most bivalent. The proposed theory is based on this reasonable assumption. It would, of course, be possible to *expand the theory* in such a way as to provide a mechanism for the formation of antibody molecules with *valence higher than two*, but this would make the theory *considerably more complex*, and it is likely that antibodies with valence higher than two occur rarely if at all. (1940, 2643; my emphasis)

Now in this case it is unclear that complication by increasing the valence would result in increased sample coverage. The sense of simplicity here appears closer to Occam's: presuppose the minimum number of entities required.

Because of his objective Bayesianism (discussed briefly in part 1), Rosenkrantz cannot easily locate simplicity in the prior probability (since other factors such as minimum entropy determine the prior). His intuition is a good one, but the Jeffreys-Occam *type* of alternative proposed above seems (1) to accommodate simplicity more naturally in the prior, and (2) to square with the cases as described reasonably well.

There are other arguments against Rosenkrantz's identification of simplicity with sample coverage. In his book Glymour suggests that "sample coverage does not correlate neatly with simplicity" because, with respect to the conjunction of an irrelevant hypotheses h' to h, h and h' will have the same sample coverage as h but be more complex (1980, 82). Also "deoccamized" hypotheses (for example, one obtained by replacing a simple force function, F, in Newton's laws of motion with one in which F is given by $F_1 + F_2 + \ldots + F_{99}$) will have the same sample coverage but obviously different simplicity (Glymour 1980, 82).

It would seem then that the desideratum of simplicity interpreted in accord with a generalized "Occam's razor" notion is best located as a factor affecting prior probability. The determination of what specific weight to attach to simplicity, and a detailed explication of simplicity, are at least partially empirical questions, and the answers may vary from historical case to historical case. Here we can only give rough comparative indications as in the above quotations. Further elaboration of a detailed, partially empirical theory of simplicity will require extensive additional research.

5.14.2 Theoretical Context Sufficiency

Issues involving conformity with well-confirmed theories of protein synthesis significantly affected the acceptability of the CST and the IT in the early to middle 1960s. Burnet's and Haurowitz's comments in the preceding sections clearly support this point; Haurowitz felt constrained to keep his views in approximate conformity with the increasingly detailed mechanism of protein synthesis emerging from the work of geneticists and molecular biologists. How this was done and the decreasing flexibility protein synthesis theory offered proponents of the IT were noted on page 220.

It is probably difficult for biologists today to realize that during the late 1950s and the early 1960s what has been termed the "sequence hypothesis" — that primary structure dictates tertiary structure — was not generally believed. As will be discussed later in chapter 9, though Cohn and Monod, in their early work that was background for the operon model, accepted the "one gene–one enzyme" hypothesis of Beadle and Tatum, they were at that time reluctant to accept the only much *later* established truth that genes completely determine the structure, especially the three-dimensional "tertiary structure," of the enzyme. The sequence hypothesis was advanced by Crick in his 1958 essay, but this was not in conformity with the then current IT and the still widely believed Pauling model (1940). For a detailed discussion of work done on enzyme synthesis during this period, see my 1974a.

In the Bayesian schema outlined earlier, I proposed to accommodate this intertheoretic effect on acceptability by locating it in the prior probability. For any hypothesis h at any level of specificity (γ, σ, or δ), a scientist assesses the $P(h \mid b)$, where b, the background knowledge, includes other well-confirmed theories. Each hypothesis can be assessed alone as well as jointly. If a theory is factored into the h in question and into the complement θ, then one assigns a value (usually informally or judgmentally) to

$$P(h \mid b) \cdot P(\theta \mid b)$$

for any h in determining the prior probability of a theory. For nonindependent hypotheses, this prior assessment is made on the basis of:

$$P(h \mid b \,\&\, \theta) \cdot P(\theta \mid b) \ .$$

For a theory consisting of n independently assessable hypotheses, the joint prior probability from theoretical context sufficiency can be given by:

$$\prod_{i=1}^{n} P(h_i \mid b) \ .$$

For the more realistic situation of n nonindependent hypotheses in a theory, we use:

$$\prod_{i=1}^{n} P(h_i \mid b \,\&\, \theta_i) \ .$$

Thus far we have assumed a stable background b. This, however, is only good to the first approximation in limited contexts, and in point of fact, in our historical example, the b changed with respect to the general theory of protein synthesis and also, more specifically, with the development of the sequence hypothesis concerning the primary structure determination of the tertiary structure of proteins.

In representing the dynamics of theory change, then, one must reconditionalize with a modified b in a number of cases. The exact procedure is not well understood,[90] but as long as the shift from b at time 1 to b at time 2 is applied consistently to any given case of theory competition—in other words, it would be inappropriate to compare $P(T_1{}^i | b_1)$[91] with $P(T_2{}^i | b_2)$—special problems regarding this background change should not arise.

Since both theoretical context sufficiency and simplicity judgments affect prior probability in the view being urged here, some consideration as to how these operate jointly is needed. In treating simplicity above, I alluded to the possibility that both the simplicity determination and the *weight* scientists might attribute to that determination might vary from individual to individual. This point can be accommodated together with a theoretical context sufficiency assessment in the prior probability expression by taking a weighted product:

$$P(T | b) = \alpha P_{Tcs} (T | b) \cdot \beta P_{Sim} (T | b)$$

where $\alpha + \beta = 1$, and in general $\alpha > \beta$, since theoretical context sufficiency judgments usually figure more prominently than simplicity assessments in global comparative theory evaluation.

As discussed in part 1 earlier, however, divergent prior probabilities are often "swamped" by increasing experimental evidence, and we saw such an instance in the case above. Determinations of the force of empirical adequacy have certain problems in a Bayesian dynamics of theory evaluation, to which I now turn.

5.14.3 *Empirical Adequacy*

The Bayesian approach suggests that we *revise* our probability by conditionalization as new evidence becomes available. This means, as noted earlier, that as new experimental evidence e^1 becomes available, we update our probability by Bayes's theorem:

$$P(T | b^1 \& e) \propto P(T | b^1) \cdot P(e^1 | b^1 \& T) .$$

We can construct a new $b^2 = b^1 \& e^1$ and assess the effect of a later new e^2 by rewriting

$$P(T \mid b^2 \& e_2) \quad \propto \quad P(T \mid b^2) \cdot P(e^2 \mid b^2 \& T)$$

where $\propto$ is the symbol for "is proportional to." In providing a global evaluation of two competing theories, say the CST and the IT, we compute

$$\frac{P(T_{IT} \mid b^i \& e^i)}{P(T_{CST} \mid b^i \& e^i)} = \frac{P(T_{IT} \mid b^i) \cdot P(e^i \mid b^i \& T_{IT})}{P(T_{CST} \mid b^i) \cdot P(e^i \mid b^i \& T_{CST})}$$

each time as $i = 1$, $i = 2$, and so on, reincorporating the "old" e^i into the new b^{i+1} and assessing the effect of the "new" e^{i+1}. Let us call this *the reiterative odds form* of Bayes's theorem. As shown by Savage and his colleagues, this reiterative process will result in a convergence, even if the priors are divergent, if the conditions of the principle of stable estimation are met.[92]

There is a difficulty arising in connection with deterministic hypotheses and theories that has received scant attention in the Bayesian literature and that must be commented on at this point. In the testing of statistical hypotheses of the type discussed extensively in part 1 and in appendixes 1 and 2, the likelihood expression $P(e \mid h)$ has been generally thought to be well defined. Savage, in fact, used to contrast the more subjective judgment involved in the prior probability $P(h)$ with the more "public" calculation of the likelihood term in Bayes's theorem.[93] This may be the case for hypotheses that suggest well-defined distributions, such as the binomial or beta distributions illustrated in the examples of appendix 2, though recently some Bayesian statisticians have questioned even this assumption.[94]

When the hypothesis under test is deterministic and entails the evidence, as is usually the assumption in such a context, philosophers have suggested setting $P(e \mid h) = 1$ (see Howson and Urbach 1989, 82). Some statisticians have suggested, though, that since any measurement involves uncertainty, one could use the uncertainty inherent in the measuring apparatus to obtain a likelihood of < 1 (see Box and Tiao 1973, 15).[95] If, however, there is a (conditional) probability < 1 for the likelihood, and the likelihood expression is viewed as a Bayesian probability measuring how well the hypothesis *accounts for or explains* the evidence e, the likelihood expression takes on characteristics more similar to a "prior" probability—it measures the "belief" of the individual scientist that h accounts for or explains e (see section 5.14.7 for some specific illustrations of this). This view would apparently not trouble some Bayesian statisticians, who have urged that the likelihood cannot legitimately be separated from the prior (see Bayarri, DeGroot, and Kadane 1988), but it does introduce an additional, explicit subjective element into the Bayesian approach. If, on the other hand, one views subjectivity masquerading as objectivity as worse than a frank acknowledgment of the subjective aspects of judgments, as Savage frequently suggested,[96] the Bayesian position may represent as much objectivity as can be obtained. In point of fact, the recognition of a subjective element in likelihood determinations does not eliminate the ability of the Bayesian approach to enforce a consistency of belief on an individual's judgments, but it may open the door to additional (though rationalized) disagreement among proponents of competing hypotheses.

Sometimes a mathematically equivalent but notationally different form of Bayes's theorem can clarify a methodological point or make a calculation somewhat easier. We considered the "odds form" of Bayes's theorem at several points above, and here I would like to indicate that there is still another way in which the odds form of Bayes's theorem is illuminating. As noted above in the reiterative odds form, one is comparing the explanatory abilities of T_{CST} with T_{IT} in comparing likelihood ratios. If T_{CST} gives a more precise explanation and e is more in accord with T_{CST} than with T_{IT}, then the likelihood ratio of CST to IT will be greater and favor the former over the latter. This is a sequential process, and the reiterative form of Bayes's theorem can represent this process of competition over time.

Suppose, however, a γ-level hypothesis of CST were falsified, for instance by a proponent of the CST being *un*able to provide a new unfalsified σ- or δ-level hypothesis consistent with CST. Then its (CST's) likelihood becomes arbitrarily close to zero, and the alternative triumphs.[97] Thus the theorem incorporates an analogue of Popperean falsification.[98]

Though "falsification" is important, the *saving* of a prima facie refuted theory was encountered many times in the course of the historical example developed in section 5.13. We saw two types of outflanking moves in such rescues. One type was to assign provisionally the force of the refutation to one or more *aux-*

iliary hypotheses (as in Haurowitz's initial assessment of the Buckley et al. experiment). The other type of move made to outflank falsification was to *change* one or more of the central hypotheses (exemplified for example by the sequence of δ_4 changes in the instructive theory above). Both of these moves are often associated with the name of Pierre Duhem (1914), who first clearly identified and described them. In more recent years, similar theses have been associated with the name of W. V. Quine, who argued persuasively in an influential article (Quine 1951) that there was no sharp separation between analytic and synthetic statements, and later developed this thesis into a view that all assertions and theories about the world are underdetermined by the evidence (Quine 1960). This later, more general thesis of Quine explains to an extent why the two outflanking strategies can work. This Quinean point of view also, I think, satisfactorily accounts for any "incommensurability" discernable in the historical case examined in section 5.13.

Quinean underdetermination, however, is not all that persuasive; in point of fact, as experimental evidence increases, the flexibility a proponent has in outflanking falsification decreases. It is in these circumstances, moreover, that extraempirical considerations such as simplicity and theoretical context sufficiency can exercise considerable constraint on hypothesis modification. These considerations also suggest a deeper Bayesian explanation for the force scientists attribute to the notion of "direct evidence" discussed in chapter 4 and again in this chapter. The power of "direct evidence" arises from the very low probability of any *competing* explanation of that evidence; the odds form of Bayes's theorem indicates quite clearly why this is the case.

I believe that the Bayesian perspective, as outlined thus far, can illuminate the way in which these increasing constraints on rescuing options arise. I also think that such a Bayesian analysis will be closely connected to an account of what are termed ad hoc hypotheses, in the pejorative sense of that term.

5.14.4 *Ad Hoc Hypotheses and Global Evaluation*

The Bayesian approach outlined in the previous subsections 5.14.1–5.14.3 can also be developed to provide an analysis of *ad hoc* hypotheses. This is important, since in a comparative debate between proponents of a theory charges of ad hoc moves are often made. The sense of *ad hoc* to be developed below is a pejorative one; there are other senses of the term which are *not* pejorative, but are used to describe hypotheses that, though they are not part of a theory to which they are conjoined, are *not* added solely to outflank an experimental (or theoretical) result which falsifies the theory but rather because (1) they are part of the *elaboration* of the theory and (2) they are expected to be further testable.

We can use either the simple form of Bayes's theorem or the odds form, as necessary, to analyze the notion of *ad hoc*.[99] As above, we let $T^1 = H^1 \ \& \ \theta$. Primarily for notational simplicity, I will assume independence between θ and H^1, and between θ and H^2, where H^2 is an ad hoc modification of H^1. (Non-independence can easily be assimilated by conditionalizing any $P(H^1)$ or $P(H^2)$ on b & θ rather than on b alone. Though θ should be superscripted in principle, since it is constant here I will not do so, again primarily for notational simplicity.)

A hypothesis H^2 is ad hoc from the perspective of this analysis if it is the consequence of the prima facie falsification of theory T^1, such that it is proposed as a modification of T^1, and there is virtually no additional support for H^2 in b, either of a theoretical or experimental nature. This characterization of ad hocness represents the historical aspect of an ad hoc hypothesis. It should be noted, however, that there is a *logical* aspect to ad hocness that is importantly *a*temporal, and that does not depend on whether H^2 was proposed after the falsification of T^1 or before e either became available or came under explicit consideration. This logical aspect of ad hocness is contained in the formalism of Bayes's theorem:

$$P(T^2 \mid e\&b) = \frac{P(\theta\&H^2 \mid b) \cdot P(e \mid T^2\&b)}{P(e \mid b)}$$

$$= \frac{P(\theta \mid b) \cdot P(H^2 \mid b) \cdot P(e \mid T^2\&b)}{P(e \mid b)} \ .$$

But $P(H^2 \mid b)$ is necessarily close to zero, since by assumption, e is the only empirical evidence for H^2 (and H^2 possesses virtually no theoretical support). Therefore, the expression on the right hand side of the equation becomes close to zero, and, a fortiori, e does not support T^2. Clearly it is desirable that this be the case, since e could only support T^2 by virtue of its incorporation of H^2, which is *ad hoc*. Note that, according to the logical formalism, H^2 need not have been elicited by a clash between e and T^1; H^2 *could have* appeared earlier in the scientific literature. If, however, $P(H^2 | b)$ is at any and all times close to zero, T^2 cannot be supported by e. The fact that H was historically elicited by e falsifying T^1 does make H^2 historically ad hoc, and this temporal property of H^2 probably does increase its lack of attraction for scientists. This would seem to be more psychological than logical, but still important from a historical point of view.

The notion of support or confirmation employed here, and *what* is supported, needs some further discussion. The appropriate theories to be compared vis-à-vis the conjunction of the ad hoc hypothesis are T^1 on the assumption of b but *prior* to e, and T^2 (which includes the ad hoc H^2) on the assumption of b but *posterior* to e. What one is interested in is the comparative support for the *extended theory* at times prior to and posterior to the acceptance of the T^1-falsifying e. This point of view is consistent with the views expressed thus far on extended theories.

The fact that e cannot strongly support T^2 (compared with T^1) does not preclude further experiments from increasing the support of T^2. To determine the effect of a new experiment e^1 on T^2, we form a new background knowledge b^1, now *including* e. Bayes's theorem then is written as:

$$P(T^2 | e^1 \& b^1) = \frac{P(\theta | b^1) \cdot P(H^2 | b^1) \cdot P(e^1 | T^2 \&)b}{P(e^1 | b^1)}$$

using the expanded form of T^1 introduced above, mutatis mutandis. Now the term $P(H^2 | b^1)$ is somewhat larger than $P(H^2 | b)$ (approximately by a factor $(P(e | b))^{-1}$) since $b^1 = b \& e$, the increase being given by Bayes's theorem. The value of $P(H^2 | b^1)$ is still low, however, and thus H^2 still continues to weaken T^2 in contrast to H^1's support of T^1. We can, however, consider T^2 via-à-vis its rivals in connection with the new experiment e^1 by examining the "odds form" or ratio of $P(T^2 | e^1 \& b^1)/P(T_i | e^1 \& b^1)$, where $T_i = T^1$ and is another extended theory. This ratio equals

$$P(H^2 | b^1) \cdot P(\theta | b^1) \cdot P(e^1 | b^1 \& T^2) / P(T^1 | b^1) \cdot P(e^1 | T_i \& b^1).$$

If T^2 is the only theory conveying a high likelihood on e^1, then the likelihood expression can "swamp" the weakening effect of H^2 on T^2 and result in a high probability of T^1 relative to its rivals. This abstract situation was actually realized in concreto in the physical sciences when Lorentz's theory with its ad hoc contraction hypothesis later received high support by being able to explain the Zeeman effect. (In this case e = the Michelson experiment, H^2 = the contraction hypothesis, and e^1 = the Zeeman effect.) A similar effect can be found in the expansion of the somatic mutation hypothesis of the CST to incorporate genetic recombination as *the* major generator of diversity, and in the ability of the thus modified CST to receive support from the phenomenon of "class switching" (see Watson et al. 1987, 852–853).

The hypothesis H^2, even though it allows T^2 to maintain some acceptability by screening off the falsifying effect of e on its earlier form T^1, is likely to be considered suspect and as weakening the theory T^2. It is of interest to note that the analysis so far provided permits an account of the quantitative seriousness of the ad hoc character of such a hypothesis. If H^2 is ad hoc, however, an assessment of its demerits cannot be based on empirical considerations, since by supposition, e was the only experimental result associated with H^2. It is at such a point that simplicity and theoretical context sufficiency considerations enter into the assessment of an ad hoc hypothesis, and allow, I believe, a determination of the seriousness of the ad hoc character of H^2.

Recall that there are two types of considerations different from direct empirical support, that significantly affect a theory or hypothesis. These are (1) the effect that other well-confirmed theories have on a particular theory in question and (2) the simplicity that a theory possesses relative to its competitors. Suffice it to say that the new hypothesis H^2 introduced above will be judged as more or less acceptable depending on (1) the theoretical accord or discord that it introduces and (2) the simplicity of its entities and logical form. If intertheoretic accord or discord and simplicity can be quantified, as I believe they can, then we possess a means of judging the seriousness of the ad hoc character of a hypothesis. This becomes particularly important if all competing theories that are attempting to explain a set of experiments are thought to be ad hoc in certain respects.

The above constitutes a Bayesian analysis of the pejorative sense of "ad hoc hypothesis" in the context of the global evaluation of extended theories. This analysis is a development of a somewhat oversimplified earlier analysis (Schaffner 1974), which was criticized by Grünbaum and Laudan.[100] Redhead (1978) also directed some sustained criticism against that account, which conceivably might be thought to hold against the current analysis. In my view Redhead's criticisms are incorrect, and his own Bayesian explication is seriously flawed. In point of fact I do not think he even explicates a sense of ad hoc but rather, instead, mistakenly analyzes the quite different notion of Bayesian irrelevance.[101]

Something like the analysis of ad hoc given above is necessary to understand the changes in scientific *consensus* regarding the merits of the instructive and clonal selection theories of the immune response. As presented in the historical account of section 5.13, several seriously ad hoc hypotheses were proposed that strongly and negatively affected belief commitments of scientists, such as Burnet's subcellular selection hypothesis (Haurowitz thought this tantamount to a refutation of the CST) and Haurowitz's attempt to save the instructive theory by his 1965 modification of the δ_4 hypothesis.

By 1967, as already mentioned, most immunologists had been convinced of the correctness of the CST and had abandoned the IT. Haurowitz, then (and even ten years post-1967)[102] still its ablest elaborator and defender, was not convinced an instructive approach *had* to be abandoned. Recall he proposed in his article in the 1967 Cold Spring Harbor volume that the presence of antigen in protein synthesis might lead to the rejection of some fragments of t-RNA-bearing amino acids and favor other t-RNA—amino acid complexes.[103] This would preserve a positive quasi instructive role for antigen and represent still another return, in a sense (now a $\delta_5{}^5$), to the original 1930 Breinl-Haurowitz analysis. The modification is ad hoc in the sense that it is meant to outflank the falsifying experiments that eliminated the instructive modification of Pauling while preserving the γ instructive hypothesis as well as one other, σ-level hypotheses, entrance of antigen into the cell. The analysis sketched above shows why this move is objectionable. The $P(H^2 | b) = P(\delta_{IT}{}^5 | b_{1967})$ is very low, since the hypothesis finds no support from the then-extant theory of protein synthesis and is antagonistic to selective processes found in all other areas of biology.

5.14.5 Hypothesis Centrality, ad Hoc Theory Modifications, and Theory Integrity

At several points in my discussion above I have employed the odds form of Bayes's theorem to explicate global evaluation of extended theories. I would like to argue now that this form of the theory can also be used in clarifying one of the senses of centrality discussed earlier on page 213, namely *extrinsic* centrality. This notion was defined as a property of a hypothesis that served to distinguish the extended theory of which it is a part from a competitive extended theory. A hypothesis obtains this property, which is relative to competitors, by being able to explain an item(s) in the theor*ies'* domain on the basis of itself and a common complement θ. The Bayesian factor in this case is the likelihood ratio, for recall that:

$$\frac{P(T_1 \mid e)}{P(T_2 \mid e)} \quad \frac{P(e \mid T_1)}{P(e \mid T_2)} = \frac{P(e \mid H_1 \,\&\, \theta_1)}{P(e \mid H_2 \,\&\, \theta_2)} .$$

Now it often happens, as a science progresses, that initially quite disparate extended theories begin to *converge*. This occurs because modifications of the non-γ central hypotheses in the light of increased experimental and intertheoretical constraints lead toward overlap of hypotheses. In the extreme case $\theta_1 = \theta_2$ and then H_1 and H_2 are the only distinguishing characteristics. H_1 and H_2 may or may not be *intrinsically* central (see p. 213), but by convergence of θ_1 and θ_2, the hypotheses H_1 and H_2 become the extrinsically central or essential *differentiating* characteristics.

Now if the likelihood ratio is much different from unity, which will be the case in the above situation if either H_1 or H_2 (but not both) explains e much better than its competitor, we have, in the situation which produces e, an (almost) crucial experiment. If we reinvoke the previous subsection's analysis of an ad hoc hypothesis, we see that, if H_1 or H_2 represents a γ-level hypothesis and if the only possible more detailed realizations of the γ-level hypothesis are ad hoc in the pejorative sense (because of very low prior probability), a massive shift of relative support between T_1 and T_2 will occur because of e. When this happens we encounter a major consensus shift, as happened in the years from 1964 to 1967 as regards the clonal selection theory — instructive theory competition. A theory which has evolved to the point of major overlap with its competitors *has major attention focused on the differentiating hypothesis*. This hypothesis cannot be yielded without the theory *becoming* identical with its competitor, and this type of change represents the limit of modifiability of the extended theory. Notice that it may only be a relative or comparative limit, but then, on the basis of the view expressed in this book, that is the nature of global theory evaluation in most situations.

5.14.6 *General Bayesian Comparative Considerations*

I will close this section by reviewing some general issues of comparative hypothesis and theory evaluation. The problem of the comparative increase in support of two hypotheses (or theories) on the basis of evidence that may be different has received some attention by Richard Jeffrey (1975). It is relevant to our concerns since, in comparing two extended theories, not all the evidence, whether it be in the background b or in the empirical e, may be the same for two different extended theories. Jeffrey considers several different ways one might on Bayesian grounds compare such theories. Jeffrey confines his attention to hypotheses H and H^1 and evidence E and E^1. I shall follow his formalism, but the arguments hold mutatis mutandis if we change H and H^1 to T_1 and T_2, and E and E^1 to $e_1\&b_1$ and $e_2\&b_2$ respectively. Should E = E^1, we obtain the limiting case of identical evidential support.

$$P(E|H) > P(E^1|H^1) \qquad \text{(likelihood)}$$

$$\frac{P(E|H)}{P(E)} > \frac{P(E^1|H^1)}{P(E^1)} \qquad \text{(explanatory power)}$$

$$\frac{P(E|H)\,P(H)}{P(E)} > \frac{P(E^1|H^1)\,P(H^1)}{P(E^1)} \qquad \text{(posterior probability)}$$

$$P(E|H) - P(E) > P(E^1|H^1) - P(E^1) \qquad \text{(likelihood difference or } \Delta L)$$

$$P(H|E) - P(H) > P(H^1|E^1) - P(H^1) \qquad \text{(posterior probability difference or } \Delta P)$$

Jeffrey (1975) proposed the five measures and terminology for comparative confirmation given in the text box at the bottom of the previous page. He rejects the first (likelihood), since it is not sensitive to differences in the prior probabilities of the different evidence, which seems correct; we want to take into account the effect of bold hypothesis and novel predictions. Explanatory power is dismissed since it does not distinguish the effect of evidence on two conjoined and completely independent theories compared with a relevant theory (i.e., if E = Kepler's laws and their data, M = Mendel's theory, and N = Newtonian theory, $P(E|MN) = P(E|N)$, which seems counterintuitive, since E is *not* as good evidence for MN as for N). The third explication of the comparative effect of evidence meets this last desideratum, according to Jeffrey, but is defective since, even when E is unfavorable and E^1 is favorable, the difference in the prior probabilities may swamp the effect of experiments. Jeffrey finds the fourth explication wanting since it fails on the Newtonian-Mendel example and also "seems to give the wrong sort of weight to the prior probability" (1974, 153), which it treats as handicaps inversely proportional to their prior probability values. Jeffrey defends the last p or posterior probability difference explication, which is one that I believe can be used as a basis for the types of considerations urged in the present chapter; it seems both formally and intuitively reasonable.

5.14.7 *Where Might the Numbers Come from in a Bayesian Approach to Global Evaluation?*

In the earlier part of this chapter where I discussed local evaluation and statistical hypothesis testing, as well as in appendixes 1 and 2, appeals were made to various theoretical models that statisticians term *distributions*. For classical statisticians, these function in likelihood determinations, and for Bayesians they can function in both likelihood and prior probability assessments. The selection of a distribution is based on a judgment that the experimental and theoretical information available warrants the choice of that distribution. For well defined and typically local forms of evaluation, good reasons can be offered for the selection of a particular distribution. For the more controversial and largely unexplored territory of global theory evaluation, such distributions may not be easily available, and some of the existing alternatives to such a strategy will need to be explored.

One alternative strategy that offers some promise is utilizing relative frequencies. Holloway writes that "Many data-generation processes can be characterized as tests devised to determine some particular property. For example, . . . medical tests are aimed at diagnosing particular problems. Often the tests are calibrated by trying them on particular populations and obtaining relative frequency information. In some cases these data can be used to calculate likelihoods" (1979, 327). This approach might involve a historical or sociological data-gathering project, wherein investigators would seek to determine the frequency with which laboratory reports and review articles appearing in recognized scientific literature defending a particular theory reported experiments as confirming or disconfirming. This tack has not to my knowledge been tried, even by Bayesian-oriented commentators on experimentation such as Franklin (1986), and it may be difficult to determine how to ask the right questions. It has the attraction of being more "objective" than the third alternative to which I turn in the next paragraph, but it may be much more difficult to implement.

A standard third alternative to obtaining the likelihoods needed in a Bayesian application is to ask the scientists involved to provide "subjective" assessments, or to do this for them in a speculative manner, as I do below. The same approach can be taken for determination of the prior probabilities of hypotheses. This strategy *has* been worked out in considerable detail, along with applications to examples in science, in the Bayesian literature, for example in McGee 1971. The scientist is first asked to provide prior probabilities for the hypotheses that are being tested. There is no reason that a conjoined set of hypotheses, such as constitute the CST and the IT examples above, cannot be employed; neither is there any reason why more focused assessments, along the lines of the τ test assumption discussed in section 5.14.4, could not be obtained. Thus Burnet might have been asked for such a determination and offered $P(CST \mid b) = 0.8$ and $P(IT \mid b) = 0.2$, whereas Haurowitz might have proposed the reverse or even a more extreme difference, such as 0.01 and 0.99.

In addition to the prior probabilities, subjective assessments can be obtained for the likelihood of different experimental results on the assumption of the competing theories. These numbers will also differ between proponents and opponents of a particular theory but will have to cover the range of possibilities, and then *experience in the laboratory* chooses which of the likelihoods actually is employed in Bayes's theorem to update the probability of the competing theories. Thus we might speculate that for Burnet P(recovery of structure outcome of Buckley et al. experiment | CST) = 0.9, whereas Haurowitz might temper his judgment and offer a 0.7. It is likely that a less biased assessor would provide a fairly high likelihood for this assessment, say 0.85, and a correspondingly low likelihood for the actual outcome on the assumption of the IT. Similar likelihoods could be obtained from scientists for additional experiments, such as the Koshland and Engleberger (1963) results. This permits the use of the reiterative form of Bayes's theorem to operate and drive the successive posterior probabilities toward high probability for the CST.

The actual calculations for determining either posterior odds or posterior probability are facilitated in the general case by using the "evidence form" of Bayes's theorem, which is stated in the Bayesian literature as:

$$\text{ev}\,(T\,|\,e\&b) = \underset{\substack{\text{prior} \\ \text{evidence}}}{\text{ev}\,(T\,|\,b)} + \underset{\substack{\text{increment or decrement} \\ \text{in evidence}}}{10\,\log_{10}\,[P(e\,|\,T\&b)/\;P(e\,|\,{\sim}T\&b)]}\,.$$
$$\underset{\substack{\text{posterior} \\ \text{evidence}}}{\phantom{\text{ev}\,(T\,|\,e\&b)}}$$

(This is obtained from the odds form by taking the logarithm of both sides of the equation and rearranging terms — see McGee 1971, 298 for proof.) Tables have been calculated to obtain posterior probabilities, odds, and evidence values (e.g., McGee 1971, Appendix I, 366 was used for this calculation). Application of this form to the unbiased assessor who might choose priors of 0.5 and 0.5 for the competing theories yields a posterior probability of 0.85, which would have been anticipated on intuitive grounds. The more complex calculations for our hypothetical Burnet and Haurowitz examples are left to the reader. They will converge toward increased probability for the CST, but for Haurowitz very slowly because of his strong prior against the CST.

5.15 Conclusion

In this chapter I have sketched the outlines of an application of the Bayesian approach to the issue of global evaluation, extending it from the more local, statistical hypothesis analysis provided in chapter 5. Before concluding, however, we should consider the extent to which such an inductive logic comports with the manner in which scientists actually reason. As Davidson, Suppes, and Siegel (1957) and subsequently Tversky and Kahnemann (1974) noted, people do not in general behave in a Bayesian manner. This raises the question of how a normative analysis such as that sketched above can be defended as a reasonable explication of scientific practice.

Howson and Urbach (1989, 292–295) address this question and cite other research on human problem solving indicating that in a number of circumstances people make clear mistakes in reasoning. Additional support for this point can be obtained from the work of Stich and Nisbett (1980). Just as we do not require that the measure of logical reasoning be based on all-too-human informal fallacies of deductive reasoning, it is inappropriate to reject a Bayesian perspective because many individuals do not reason in a Bayesian manner. But more can be said, I think, namely that we have in the Bayesian framework not only a powerful apparatus for comprehending the testing (in the evaluational sense) of statistical hypotheses but also a plausible application of *extensions* of that analysis in the examples presented above and in the extensive and burgeoning Bayesian literature cited throughout this chapter. Whatever form the foundations of statistics may ultimately take, it is reasonably certain it will be different from contemporary views. Savage himself wrote, toward the end of his career, "Whatever we may look for in a theory of statistics, it seems prudent to take the position that the quest is for a better one, not for the perfect one" (1977, 7). It is a recurring thesis of this book that the Bayesian approach is currently the best and most general foundation from which to search for such a theory.

In sum, then, we seem to have a defensible notion of global evaluation which is a generalization of the Bayesian approach to statistical hypothesis testing. The account sketched is clearly a *framework*, and at a number of points I have indicated that further research, both of a logical and of an empirical nature, will be required to determine the ultimate adequacy of this account. I think, however, because of its considerable internal structure, its fidelity to the historical case considered, and its conformity to other historical cases both in biology and physics, it represents one of the more promising analyses of global theory competition and scientific rationality.

APPENDIX 1

A Mendelian Example Illustrating the Concepts of "Significance" and "Power."

Our first rather elementary example involves testing the Mendelian hypothesis of dominant and recessive genes in the context of data about pea plants.[104]

For two contrasting traits or "unit characters" represented by pea color, namely yellow peas and green peas, Mendelian genetics predicts that yellow seed color (albumen color) will dominate the green color. On the basis of the simple dominance observed in Mendel's classical experiments, Mendel's theory predicts that random segregation of the factors or "genes" will yield four hybrid classes with the genotypes yy, yg, gy, gg that display a phenotypic $3 : 1$ ratio of yellow to green seeded progeny in the F_2 generation. We represent a test of the hypothesis that the ratio of a pea selected at random will be yellow as a test of the hypothesis $H_0 : p = 3/4$. Our sampling procedure yields 70 yellow and 30 green peas. We wish to know if this data supports the Mendelian hypothesis, H_0 i.e., since $70/100 = .70$, we want to know if this value is *sufficiently close* to .75 to support the theory. This notion of "sufficiently close" requires us to consider two types of error and their consequences.

There are two ways in which errors can arise in acceptance or rejection of a hypothesis. First, we may mistakenly *reject* a *true* hypothesis; second, we may mistakenly *accept* a *false* hypothesis, or, in other words, *fail to reject* a *false* hypothesis. These are usually called errors of the first kind (or type I errors) and errors of the second kind (or type II errors), respectively. These two types of errors can be made clearer by introducing another interesting and crucial feature of the Neyman-Pearson theory, namely that an evaluation or "test" is not made solely in terms of *one* hypothesis and the experimental data but is made comparatively: in addition to the primary hypothesis H_0 (often this is called the "null" hypothesis), an *alternative hypothesis*, H_1 (or a *class* of alternative hypotheses) must be proposed. (The term "null" arises from the discipline of statistical medical testing, an investigator often wishes to compare two treatments, say A and B, and a hypothesis asserting there is no difference between treatments — the difference is null — is called the "null hypothesis.") The Neyman-Pearson theory refers to the two (or more) hypotheses to be tested as the set of admissible hypotheses. The table presented below indicates the nature of the two types of error in connection with H_0 and H_1.

	H_0 accepted	H_1 accepted
H_0 true	correct decision	type I error (α)
H_1 true	type II error (β)	correct decision

When both the primary hypothesis H_0 and the alternative hypothesis H_1 are "simple," that is, when their *specific* values are given (such as p = 5/8 say), the test situation is straightforward. When, on the other hand, H_1 is either nonsimple or composite, for example, say $H_1 : p/4$, the situation can become quite complicated. Our first two examples will involve simple hypotheses, but we will briefly discuss tests of composite hypotheses further below. As an alternative hypothesis in our Mendelian example, we will fancifully suppose that the *gy* genetic class (but not the *yg* class) has half yellow and half green progeny, yielding a prediction of $H_1 : p = 5/8$, as an example of a bizarre maternal dominance hypothesis — see the discussion earlier in this chapter for the rationale for this alternative.

The Neyman-Pearson theory suggests that type I error is the most important kind to control. The control is exercised by making a decision, on *non-statistical grounds,* as to how serious an error might be committed by rejecting a "true" hypothesis. This decision fixes a *level of significance,* which is expressed in terms of a number such as 0.05, 0.01, 0.001 and the like. A significance level, sometimes called the "P value" and sometimes the *size* of the test, indicates what the chances are of rejecting a true hypothesis, H_0. The level of significance is usually denoted algebraically by the Greek letter α. Thus if a significance level of 0.05 is chosen, the chances are about one in twenty of rejecting a hypothesis which is in fact true. The specific nature of the test situation is then investigated to determine a *critical region* compatible with the chosen level of significance. The critical region is that set of outcomes of a (series of) test(s) which allows one to reject the hypothesis tested, H_0. Formally, one can write this, using the notation $P(X \in A | H_0)$, to read the probability that the observed random variable X will fall in the critical region A, assuming the truth of H_0 as:

$$P(X \in A | H_0) = P(X \in A) \leq \alpha.$$

To clarify these notions of level of significance and of critical region, as well as the relation of type I and type II errors, let us return to the Mendelian example introduced above.

Statistical theory utilizes a number of theoretical models termed *distributions,* which it borrows from the theory of probability.[105] Statistics also make use of certain approximations relating actual data to the theoretical distributions. In the Mendelian case, we are dealing with a "binomial distribution" which, because the sample is fairly large, approximates a "normal distribution." (I shall discuss a specific example involving the binomial distribution later.) As such we can assume that p under H_0 or H_1 is a normal variable with means of $3/4 = 0.75$ and $5/8 = 0.625$ respectively, and normal spread or "variance."

Statisticians prefer to measure the "spread" of samples in terms of the square root of the variance, termed the standard deviation, σ. For a proportion such as is involved in our example, the standard deviation is given by:

$$\sigma = \sqrt{(p)(1-p)/n}$$

where n is the number of entities observed (here n = 100). It should be obvious that if σ is small the experimental results are precise or sharply peaked and therefore are more discriminating.

In our example I have graphed the theoretical distributions of $\hat{p}$ for H_0 and H_1 with n = 100 in figure 5.2.[106] I have also noted in figure 5.2 where the observed proportion $\hat{p}$ obs = 0.7 falls. Note that if it is located in the overlap area between the means, it is not strictly excluded as supporting H_0 or H_1 without additional constraints.

Suppose we wish to test H_0 against H_1 at the 0.05 level of significance. On the basis of the known distribution of p, we choose a criti-

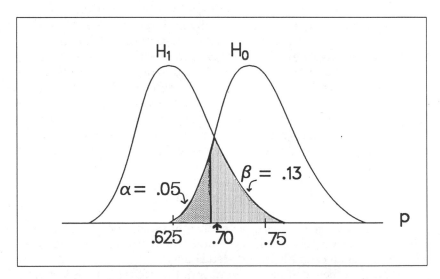

Figure 5.2 Distribution of p under H_0 and H_1 with selected initial region. Drawing is not to scale to allow emphasis of α and β areas.

cal region A which contains those data points signifying equal to or less than 5% probability on the truth of H_0. This is a "one tailed test" — we are only interested in the probability in the left region of H_0 because the comparison here is with competitor H_1.

From any elementary statistics text with tables of the area under different portions of a normal distribution, we can determine that the region containing 5% of the probability is to the left of

$$p - 1.64 \sqrt{(p)(1-p)/n} \quad = \quad 0.75 - 1.64 \sqrt{(3/4)(1/4)/100} \quad = 0.68.$$

Since the observed proportion (= 0.7) does *not* fall into this critical region, H_0 *is significant at the 0.05 level.*

Now we can use the data and figure 5.2 to compute the type II error and ascertain this error in relation to the type I error. In the case of $H_1 : p = 5/8$, and $\sigma = \sqrt{(5/8)(5/8)/100} = .048$, we are interested in computing the lightlyshaded area in figure 5.2. This area represents the probability of the observed data resulting in acceptance of H_0 when H_1 is in fact true, or the type II error. We determine this by consulting a statistics table for a normal variable which will give us the z or standard normal curve value in terms of p, p, (1 - p) and n. This value, subtracted from 0.500 (because of symmetry), will indicate how much probability is in the β area. The determining equation is

$$z = (\hat{p} - p)/\sigma = (0.68 - 0.625)/0.048 \approx 1.1$$

A z table indicates the area between the middle of the z curve and this point is = 0.364. Therefore 0.500 - 0.364 = .13. Thus β is approximately 13%.

Note that if α were chosen at a higher level (i.e., further to the left), the β area would become correspondingly larger. Thus another important feature of the Neyman-Pearson theory is exemplified in figure 5.1, namely that α and β are *inversely* proportional, and an attempt to decrease one type of error will lead to an increase in the other type of error. The value of β can also be used to determine the value of another concept in the Neyman-Pearson theory. This is the *power* of the test. The power of a test is the probability of *not* making an error of the second kind, or the probability that the test will detect the falsehood of H_0 when H_1 is true. It is given by $(1 - \beta)$, and is equal to .87 in our Mendelian example. The concept of the power of a test can be importantly generalized to the concept of a *power function*, referring to a critical region associated with a test of H_0. The power function gives the range of (varying) probabilities of rejecting H_0 with respect to any values of competing alternative H_1's (assuming that H_0 is true), and not merely the single specified alternative H_1.

The example described above should serve to illustrate the clarity and force of the Neyman-Pearson approach to statistical hypothesis testing and to provide some rationale for the extraordinarily broad acceptance that the approach has garnered. There is still more powerful machinery available within this tradition, such as a characterization of the general conditions under which one obtains a *best test* (where for any chosen α, β will be minimized; see Neyman 1950, 304-415. In addition, this notion can be generalized still further to a concept of a "uniformly most powerful" (UMP) test. These generalizations have limitations, however, that lead to serious questions about the ultimate strength of the approach. (See Silvey 1970, 104 and Giere 1977.) Furthermore, the Neyman-Pearson theory seems committed to questionable before-and-after asymmetries and the odd dependence of rejection on sample size (see Howson and Urbach 1989, 162–175 for details).

APPENDIX 2

A Mendelian Example Employing a Bayesian Approach

For a variable p between 0 and 1 and a set of trials in which there are *a* "successes" and *b* "failures," the probability density follows what is termed by the statisticians a beta distribution, given by the expression:

$$\frac{(a+b+1)!}{a!\,b!} \cdot p^{\,a} (1-p)^{\,b} .$$

The binomial probability distribution is a special case of this more general beta distribution. Since in our Mendelian case we used a normal or Gaussian (z) approximation to the binomial distribution, and an exact binomial formula for the clinical case, the beta distribution will suffice for both of our examples, though details will only be provided for the Mendelian case.[107]

If we were to assume a uniform or flat prior distribution representing no preference between probabilities prior to our testing the Mendelian hypothesis, $H_0: p = 3/4$, and the alternative hypothesis, $H_1: p = 5/8$, we could represent this graphically by the curve u on figure 5.3.

On the other hand, if on the basis of theoretical considerations an investigator felt that the probability was likely to be in the region of p = 3/4 and fairly small elsewhere, we could represent this by curve t. Both of these are beta priors, the curve u is obtained by setting a = b = 0, and the curve t represents a = 12, b = 4. (The beta distribution has a mean = $(a+1)/(a+b+2) = .722$ here, and a variance $(\sigma^2) = (a+1)(b+1)/(a+b+2)^2 (a+b+3)$, here ≈ 0.01, so $\sigma \approx 0.1$.)

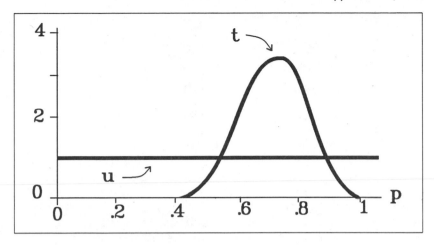

Figure 5.3   Two possible choices for the initial distribution of p. (After Smith 1969, v. 2, p. 364.)

Now if one formed a likelihood ratio *ignoring* prior probabilities for the Mendelian case, remembering $H_0: p = 3/4$ and $H_1: p = 5/8$, one would obtain:

$$\frac{p(H_0 \mid 70 \text{ yellows}; n=100)}{p(H_1 \mid 70 \text{ yellows}; n=100)} = \frac{C_1}{C_1} \cdot \frac{(3/4)^{70}(1/4)^{30}}{(5/8)^{70}(3/8)^{30}} = 1.82$$

where the C_1 is the identical binomial constant.

The posterior probability for a beta distribution of n trials with r successes is given generally by:

$$\frac{(a+b+n+1)!}{(a+r)!(b+n+r)!} \cdot p^{(a+r)}(1-p)^{b+n-r} \ .$$

Since this constant will be identical in our comparison, the *posterior* odds will be:

$$\Omega \text{ posterior}(H_0 : H_1) = \frac{P_0{}^{a+r}(1-P_0)^{b+n-r}}{P_1{}^{a+r}(1-P_1)^{b+n-r}} \ .$$

Now if we use the uniform prior ($a = b = 0$), we obtain the *same* posterior probabilities as the classical likelihood ratio test, that is, odds of 1.82 in favor of H_0 over H_1. If, however, we utilize the prior distribution which reflects the influence of theory (a = 12, b = 4), we obtain:

$$\Omega \text{ posterior}(H_0 : H_1) = \frac{(3/4)^{12+70}(1/4)^{4+30}}{(5/8)^{12+70}(3/8)^{4+30}} = 3.20 .$$

Therefore the effect of the prior is to heighten belief in H_0, which is as expected.

However, if figure 5.4 is examined, one notes the closeness of the two posterior distributions, which indicates that the effect of the prior can be largely "swamped" by the data. The data also sharpen the initially diffuse prior probability, even one already reasonably focused, such as the a = 12, b = 4 prior. For the *posterior* variance of the probability distribution (after the n = 100 trials) is 0.00002, and the standard deviation is 0.004 compared to the initial distribution 0.1.

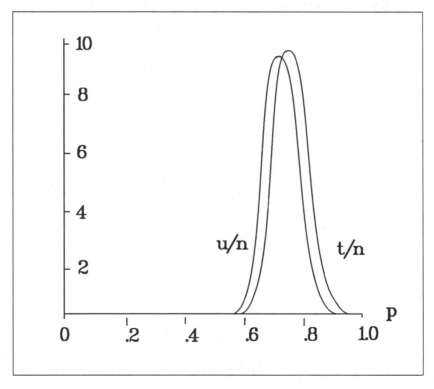

Figure 5.4   Final distributions for p based on a sample of n = 100 using the two initial distributions given in figure 5.3 above. (After Smith, 1969, v. 2, p. 366.)

This illustration demonstrates one way that a Bayesian statistician might approach the subject of hypothesis testing, or what we term local evaluation.[108] A closer comparison is possible, and Barnett, for example, suggests that we might test two hypotheses, H and ¬ H, as follows. Consider a manufacturer who produces biscuits, and who must label his packages with a weight 1/2 ounce less than the mean weight, θ. He aims for 8 oz. packets and prints his labels indicating the contents are 7.5 ounces. He thus wishes to test the hypothesis that H : θ < 8 against the alternative hypothesis ¬ H : $\theta \geq 8$. Barnett writes that:

> on the Bayesian approach we have a direct evaluation of the probabilities of H and ¬ H, in the form
>
> $$P(H \mid x) = \int_H \pi(\theta \mid x) = 1 - P(\neg H \mid x) \ .$$
>
> [Here $\pi(\theta \mid x)$ is a posterior distribution representing the manufacturer's current knowledge of θ.] If $P(H \mid x)$ is sufficiently small we will want to reject H, and this can again be expressed in terms of 'significance levels' if required. Thus a 5 percent Bayesian *test of significance* rejects H if $P(H \mid x) \leq 0.05$; similarly for other significance levels. (1982, 202)

Barnett adds that "the direct expression of the result of the test in the form $P(H \mid x)$ eliminates the asymmetric nature of the test observed in the classical approach. In particular there is no need to distinguish formally between the *null (working)* and the *alternative* hypotheses" (1982, 202).[109]

Jeffreys (1961, chapter 5) has proposed a Bayesian method for testing a point hypothesis of the form H : $\theta = \theta_0$. The essence of the approach is to compute the posterior "odds in favor of H," and on this basis to accept or reject H. This proposal and Savage's similar approach to the King Hiero's crown problem (Savage et al. 1962, 29–33) have been criticized as lacking generality (see Pratt 1976 and Bernardo 1980). At present there is no *general theory* of Bayesian hypothesis testing which might be used to resolve these controversies, though, as mentioned earlier, Bayesians may find that many of these problems are vestigial in nature, and relics from classical considerations that will vanish in the light of a strong and consistent Bayesian orientation (see Kadane and Dickey 1980).

In spite of the lack of a general theory, the Bayesian approach, as a treatment of the examples above shows, seems general enough to encompass all the precise and powerful results of classical statistics, and to place it in a flexible inferential context that permits generalization to more global contexts, as was shown in the later parts of this chapter.

CHAPTER SIX

Explanation and Causation in Biology and Medicine: General Considerations

6.1 Introduction

WITH THIS CHAPTER we begin an inquiry which will continue through several chapters to the end of the book. There are a cluster of issues intertwined with "explanation" in biology and medicine, including prediction, causation, historicity, teleology, organization, and the autonomy of biology. In this chapter I shall focus on the problem of explanation in rather general terms, though in the context of biology and medicine, and in subsequent chapters, I shall consider more specific types of explanation, such as historical, functional, and teleological explanations.

From the inception of this book we have been implicitly considering explanation. For example, in the discussion of discovery we dealt with new hypotheses' and theories' ability to *account* for the data, and that issue was reconsidered in connection with the topics of theory structure and evaluation. It is now appropriate to make explicit some of the assumptions latent in the earlier discussion concerning explanation. *Webster's Dictionary*[1] can be cited to indicate the everyday aspects of the term *explanation*, defining it as "the act or process of explaining"; the verb *to explain* as is in turn defined as "1: to make plain or understandable . . . 2: to give the reason for or cause of" and "3: to show the logical development or relationships of." Each of these three facets will play a role in the account(s) of explanation to be developed in the remainder of this book.

An explanation is usually given in response to a question or a problem, whether this be implicit or explicit. It will be useful to mention some typical questions that arise in biology and medicine as a prelude to an analysis of explanation. Consider the following queries:[2]

(1) Why does the presence of lactose in *E. coli*'s environment result in the bacterium's synthesis of the enzyme β-galactosidase?[3]

(2) Why does the "sea hare," *Aplysia californicum*, develop a heightened response to touch stimulation when subjected to a simultaneous noxious stimulus?[4]

(3) Why does the pattern of color coats in mice in the F2 generation, whose grandparents are both agouti (a grayish pattern) with genotype AaBb, follow a 9:3:4 ratio (9/16 = agouti ; 3/16 = black; 4/16 = albino)?[5]

(4) Why do 2–6 percent of African-Americans living in the northern United States have a sickle-cell gene?[6]

(5) What is the function of the thymus in vertebrates?[7]

These are representative types of requests for explanations in biology and medicine. The first example admits of a causal microlevel deterministic explanation and has already been discussed extensively in chapters 2, 3, and 4. The second example is an illustration from recent neurobiology and will be discussed in some detail later in this chapter. The third example involves a partially stochastic or statistical explanation but in addition has causal components involving biosynthetic pathways, and it will also be discussed later in this chapter. The fourth example is a typical request for an evolutionary explanation and will be considered extensively in chapter 7. The last example is a request for a functional analysis with an explanatory capacity; these types of explanations are the subject matter of chapter 8. Each of these examples has an explanation which involves the general issues on which I shall focus in this chapter. Some of the examples, however, will require further analysis for a *complete* account of the types of explanation associated with them.

Analyzing "explanation" in science has been a major concern of the past forty years of the philosophy of science.[8] In the past ten years there have been significant additional developments on this topic. My approach to explicating "explanation" in biology and medicine will begin with an overview of some of this history, including recent developments, and will then move to more specific analysis of these general problems in the context of biological explanation.

Before I turn to this historical overview, however, it will be useful to indicate the direction in which I want to take this discussion, so as to provide a set of pointers toward the model of explanation developed in this chapter and then used in the remaining chapters of this book. The recurrent theme will be the appeal to (possibly probabilistic) *causal model systems which instantiate generalizations of both broad and narrow scope of application.* I will argue that both the Hempel model of scientific explanation and Salmon's earlier S-R account suffered from defects that an appeal to causation could remedy. I will also indicate by means of an extended example from the neurosciences how such causation is appealed to by working scientists and how complex and interlevel are their various explanatory sentences. In order to ground the causal/mechanical features of the model developed below, I will examine logical, epistemological, and metaphysical components of causation and in the process will argue that an intertwined mechanism and generalization "overlap" model of explanation, which is heavily indebted to Salmon's recent theory, is the most defensible. Finally, I will touch on some recent alternative accounts of explanation, including Kitcher's unification view and van Fraassen's pragmatic analysis, and will also provide several arguments, in part based on Railton's notion of an ideal explanatory text, that viable aspects of those models can be conceived of as congruent with my preferred approach.

The account of explanation that will be elaborated below has six components worth distinguishing, which I will term E1 through E6.

(E1) *The Semantic (BMS) Component*: Relying on the conclusions of chapter 3, I will reintroduce the notion of a theoretical model as a type of system whose characteristics are given by an explicit definition comprising a series of generalizations Σ, where $\Sigma_i(\Phi(_1 \ldots _n))$ represents the ith generalization, and

$$\prod_{i=1}^{n} \sum_i (\Phi(\eta_1 \ldots \eta_n))$$

is the conjunction of the assumptions (that we term Π) constituting a "biomedical system" or BMS. Any given system that is being investigated or appealed to as *explanatory of some explanandum* is such a BMS if and only if it satisfies Π. We will understand Π, then, as implicitly defining a kind of abstract system. There may not be any actual system which is a realization of the complex expression "Π." The claim that some particular system satisfies Π is a theoretical hypothesis which may or may not be true. If it is true, then the BMS can serve as an explanandum of a phenomenon. If the theoretical hypothesis is potentially true and/or supported to a greater or lesser degree, then it is a potential and/or well-supported explanation.

(E2) *The Causal Component.* This I will develop as two sub-components: (a) deterministic causation and (b) probabilistic causation. I will argue that explanations in biology and medicine are typically causal, and the Φ's appearing in a BMS involve such causal properties as "phosphorylation" and "secretion" as well as statements that a process "causes" or "results in" some event. Causation will be analyzed in depth in terms of its logic, epistemology, and metaphysics. The concept of causation will be further explicated as licensing a "probabilistic" aspect, which can be based on (possibly occult) variation or on "stochastic bedrock" (only in quantum mechanics). I will illustrate the relation between the deterministic and the probabilistic aspects using the examples of neurotransmitter release at the neuromuscular junction and of color coat determination.

(E3) *The Unificatory Component.* Though appeals to causation are frequently (and typically) involved in explanation, some BMSs might involve generalizations which are statements of co-existence (i.e., indicating quantities which vary together). We also need to keep open the possibility of appealing to some fundamentally indeterministic system (such as one involving quantum mechanical assumptions). In such cases it seems reasonable to appeal to another aspect of explanation and accept as scientifically legitimate BMSs which "unify" domains of phenomena. In general, I will view these explanations as provisional surrogates for deeper causal explanations, though with an acceptance of (rare) quantum mechanical limitations on such "deeper" explanations.

(E4) *The Logical Component.* Connections between a BMS and an explanandum will frequently be recastable in terms of *deductive logic* (with the proviso that the generalizations in the BMS will typically be causal and thus that the explanandum may be construed as following as a "causal consequence" from the premises in the BMS). In addition, where the BMS involves some probabilistic assumption and the explanandum is a singular (or a collection of singular) event(s), the logical connection will be one of inductive support.

(E5) *The Comparative Evaluational Inductive Component.* In conformity with the personal probability perspective developed in chapter 5, any inductive support (whether of the type described in (E4) or more general inductive support) appearing in explanations will be viewed in Bayesian terms. The notion of support will also be construed as "doubly comparative," in van Fraassen's sense (to be described in more detail toward the end of this chapter): for a given explanation one compares (often implicitly) an explanandum with its contrast class in terms of the support provided, and one also (perhaps only implicitly) compares rival explanations for that explanandum. This, we shall see, introduces evaluational components into explanations.

(E6) *The Ideal Explanatory Text Background Component.* Explanations that are actually given are partial aspects of a complete story, and those aspects that are focused on are frequently affected by pragmatic interests. Following Railton, I will accept the notion of an "ideal" explanatory text background from which specific explanations are selected.

In the three chapters that follow, this model of explanation, involving assumptions (E1)–(E6), will be further elaborated and applied to examples from evolutionary theory and Mendelian and molecular genetics and to issues arising in the context of requests for "functional" explanations in immunology.

6.2   General Models of Explanation in Science

I will begin with a brief summary recalling several of the extant *classical* models of scientific explanation. Basically these fall into three categories: (a) the deductive nomological or D-N model, (b) the deductive-statistical or D-S model and the inductive statistical or I-S model, and (c) the statistical-relevance or S-R model.

6.2.1   *The Deductive-Nomological Model*

The deductive-nomological or D-N model has been seen as the ideal form of scientific explanation.[9] There are foreshadowings of it in Aristotle's *Posterior Analytics* and *Physics*, and it is discussed, though not under that name, in Mill's *A System of Logic*. Sir Karl Popper discussed this type of explanation in his *Logik der Forschung* (The Logic of Scientific Discovery, 1959 [1934]). Today it is closely associated with the names of Oppenheim, who about forty years ago argued for it in an extremely clear and influential article (1948) and of Hempel, who has been its principal elaborator and defender (see his 1965).

Schematically, the deductive-nomological model can be presented as

$$L_1 \ldots L_n$$
$$C_1 \ldots C_k$$

$$\therefore E$$

where the Ls are universal laws and the Cs represent initial conditions, together constituting the "explanation" or "explanans," while E is a sentence describing the event to be explained, called the "explanandum." In this model, E follows *deductively* from the conjunction of the laws or nomological premises (from the Greek *nomos*, law) and the statements describing the initial conditions. E may be a sentence describing a specific, particular event; on the other hand, if the initial conditions are interpreted in a suitably general way, for example as boundary conditions, E may be a law, such as Snell's law in optics or the Hardy-Weinberg law in population genetics.[10]

Hempel and Oppenheim (1948) proposed that an adequate D-N explanation must satisfy three logical requirements: that the explanandum be deduced from the explanans (R1), that the explanans contain at least one law (R2), and that the explanans have empirical content (R3). In addition, the following empirical condition was specified: the sentences constituting the explanans must be true (R4) (see Hempel 1965 [1948], 247–249).

Hempel and Oppenheim (1948) defended this strong truth requirement (R4) on the grounds that an explanation should be timelessly adequate, but Hempel (1965) later relaxed the condition. In this later essay, Hempel introduced the notion of a "*potential* explanation" in which "the sentences constituting its explanans need not be true" (1965, 338). The laws in the explanans will in such a situation be "law*like*," since they *may* be false. Hempel suggested, however, that these lawlike sentences still be "referred to as *nomic* or *nomological*" (1965, 338). This relaxation is important to us, inasmuch as the discussion concerning truth and realism (in chapter 5) assumes weaker requirements for hypotheses and theories than "truth."

The D-N model of explanation has generated a number of criticisms which do not need to be rehearsed here (see Hempel 1965, chap. 12, for the extensive criticisms and a response). Many of the criticisms are developed by citing various counterexamples. For instance, in Scriven's "barometer" example, Scriven (1959) noted that, though we could *predict* a storm from a dropping barometer reading, we would not want to say that the falling barometer reading *explained* the storm. The storm *is* explained, however, by the falling air pressure associated with a low pressure weather front, which also causes the barometer reading to drop. As I shall argue later, an appeal to causation is usually an adequate response to such criticisms and counterexamples.

Adequate deductive-nomological explanations can be found in biology and medicine, and certain limiting notions of causal explanations are instances of this type of explanation. Because of the number and variability of initial conditions, as well as the genetic and environmental variations discussed in chapters 3 and 4, however, partially or completely stochastic processes are widespread in biology and medicine. In such cases the premises will involve one or more statistical "laws."

6.2.2 *Deductive Statistical and Inductive Statistical Models*

When the premises of an explanation involve *statistical* generalizations, the type of logic in the model may change. If the generalizations deductively yield an explanandum sentence, as in population genetics with infinite populations, for example, we have an instance of deductive statistical or D-S explanation, and the logic is still deductive. There will be those situations, however, in which we wish to explain an event in which the sentence describing that event only follows *with probability* from a set of premises. For example, to use one of Hempel's illustrations, if we wish to explain John Jones's recovery from a streptococcus infection, we might be told that he had been given penicillin. There is, however, no general, universal, exceptionless law that requires *all* individuals who have been given penicillin to recover from such an infection.

We can schematize the logical relations involved in the John Jones case as follows:

> The statistical probability of recovery from severe streptococcal infections with penicillin administration *is close to 1.*
>
> John Jones has severe streptococcal infection and was given penicillin.
>
> ═══
>
> John Jones recovered from the infection.

Here the double line does not stand for a *deductive* inference but rather means "makes practically certain (very likely)."[11] The double line accordingly represents *inductive* support, whence the appellation "inductive statistical (or I-S) model" for this type of explanation.

The general form of the I-S model is schematized as follows, using the probability formalism employed in previous chapters:

$P(R \mid S \& P)$ is close to 1
$S_j \& P_j$
$$\overline{\qquad\qquad\qquad\qquad\qquad\qquad} \quad \text{[makes practically certain (very likely)]}$$
R_j

Most readers will realize, for reasons already mentioned, that a reasonably large percentage of explanations in biology and medicine will have this inductive statistical character. The I-S model has several peculiarities not usually associated with the D-N model. For example, it should be obvious that, were John Jones severely allergic to penicillin, the probability of his recovery would not have been close to 1 — he might well have died due to anaphylactic shock. This consideration points us toward the need to place John Jones, or any individual entity that is named in an I-S explanation, into the *maximally specific* reference class about which we have available data (Hempel 1965, 394–403). Hempel maintains that any "information . . . which is of potential explanatory relevance to the explanation event" must be utilized in "formulating or appraising an I-S explanation" (1965, 400).

6.2.3 *The Statistical Relevance Model*

Reflection on some of these considerations and on certain counterexamples to the D-N model led Wesley Salmon in the late 1960s to propose an alternative to the models discussed thus far. For example, Salmon noted that the following argument fulfills Hempel's requirements (Rl)–(R4): "John Jones avoided becoming pregnant during the past year, for he has taken his wife's birth control pills regularly, and every man who regularly takes birth control pills avoids pregnancy" (1970, 34). It is clear, however, that the above is *not* an explanation — men simply do not become pregnant.

Salmon's first approach to explicating explanation developed his novel thesis that an explanation is *not an argument* and thus does not require us to appeal to either deductive or inductive logic in analyzing the relation between premises and conclusion (1970, 10–11). Rather, according to Salmon, an explanation of the sentence "Why does this X, which is a member of A, have the property B" is "a set of probability statements." These represent the probability of members of various *epistemically homogeneous subclasses* having a particular property A, say A & C_1, A & C_2, . . . , also possessing another property B. Additionally necessary to the explanation is "a statement specifying the compartment to which the explanandum event belongs" (1971, 76–77). Thus this model is really a partition of a class into epistemically homogeneous subclasses, made on the basis of any available statistically relevant information. A property C_i "explains" because it is *statistically relevant* to X having the property B if it has A. Salmon's approach here is accordingly called the Statistical-Relevance or S-R model of explanation.

In addition to differing with Hempel over the argumentative status of an explanation, Salmon also contended that there was no reason why a probabilistic statement involving a *very low* probability could not be utilized in an explanation. Even if the statistically relevant class, for example, the class of atoms of radioactive ^{238}U that will decay into lead, is such that the probability of the event (the decay) is very low, that is all that can be said in response to an explanation of why a particular atom of ^{238}U decayed into lead. This assumes, of course, that the class of atoms of radioactive ^{238}U that will decay into lead is statistically homogeneous.

The S-R model possessed several attractive features. First, it provided an answer to the birth control pill counterexample: John Jones' taking of his wife's birth control pills is not an explanation of his failure to become pregnant because the ingestion of such pills by males is *not relevant* to their pregnant/ nonpregnant condition. Second, the S-R model offered a way of handling the barometer counterexample in terms of "screening off" —a concept that was originally introduced by Reichenbach and that also has more general utility than as an adjunct to the S-R model. This notion is defined by Salmon as follows:[12]

D screens off C from B in reference class A iff:
$$P(B \mid A\&C\&D) = P(B \mid A\&D) \neq P(B \mid A\&C),$$

where $P(\mid)$ represents the conditional probability expression we encountered earlier in chapter 5 (Salmon 1970, 55). Intuitively, a "screened off" property "becomes irrelevant and no longer has explanatory value" (Salmon 1971, 55). Applied to Scriven's barometer example, the drop in air pressure screens off the drop in the barometer reading from being statistically relevant to explaining the storm.

I shall return to the S-R and I-S models again later, but for the moment let us turn to a consideration of the D-N model in the context of the important issues of causal explanation and causal series explanation. This will permit a better understanding of the limits of the S-R model.

6.3 Recent Debates Concerning Explanation: The Role of Causal Explanation

In the past fifteen or so years, a number of philosophers of science have reconsidered the role of causal notions in connection with explanations. Van Fraassen (1977), for example, in his review article foreshadowing certain aspects of his influential book *The Scientific Image* (1980), argued that we need to return to a more Aristotelian-like causal explication of explanation to remedy defects with the various received models of Hempel and Salmon.[13] The views of Salmon himself have evolved and now mainly stress causal explanations, suggesting that these lie behind and are more fundamental than S-R explanations. These views will be considered in more detail later; initially it will be useful to indicate the place of causal explanation in Hempel's analysis, where causal explanations are derivative from the D-N and I-S models.

6.3.1 *Hempel's Analysis*

For Hempel, "causal explanation conforms to the D-N model" (1965, 348). Causal connection can be represented in general laws, for example as in Lenz's law of the direction of current induced in a wire near a moving magnet. Initial conditions, the Cs cited earlier, can function as the causal *antecedents* in a D-N schema, so that, in light of the Ls, the Cs constitute a sufficient condition for an effect, the explanandum E.

Hempel has also applied his models of explanation to sequences of events, sometimes referred to as "genetic explanations" (to be distinguished from "genetic" in the sense of "Mendelian genetics" — here "genetic" refers to a developmental sequence of events, a *genesis*). Hempel provided an illustration in the form of a historical explanation of why popes and bishops came to offer indulgences. This type of explanation is "basically nomological in character" (1965, 448). "In a genetic explanation each stage must be shown to "lead to" the next, and thus to be linked to its successor by virtue of some general principles which make the occurrence of the latter at least reasonably probable, given the former" (1965, 448–449). A genetic explanation, then, for Hempel, is a chain of either D-N or I-S sub-explanations, the explanandum of the previous explanation functioning as one of the premises in the next sub-explanation. In my view, genetic explanation is best seen as a kind of causal-sequence explanation, and I will examine the import of genetic explanation in biology and medicine in depth in chapter 7. The inclusion of statistical premises in causal explanations raises an interesting question, however, namely whether causality is purely deterministic or whether some probabilistic characterization of causality can also be provided. I shall return to this question and discuss it in section 8.

6.3.2 *Brody's and van Fraassen's (Initial) Aristotelian Approach*

In his 1972, Brody argued that the following type of argument he called example (B) met all of Hempel's conditions for a D-N explanation:

(1) If the temperature of a gas is constant, then its pressure is inversely proportional to its volume

(2) at time t_1, the volume of the container c was v_1 and the pressure of the gas in it was p_1

(3) the temperature of the gas in c did not change from t_1 to t_2

(4) the pressure of the gas in container c at t_2 is $2p_1$

---

(5) the volume of x at t_2 is $1/2\ v_1$. (1972, 21)

This purported explanation, to Brody, was a clear counterexample to Hempel's account since his (Brody's) "intuitions are that (B) is no explanation at all" (1972, 21). What is required, Brody argued, is supplementation of Hempel's conditions (Rl)–(R4) above with an additional, Aristotelian type of sufficient condition:

> . . . a deductive-nomological explanation of a particular event is a satisfactory explanation of the event when (besides meeting all of Hempel's requirements) its explanans contains (sic) essentially a description of the event which is the cause of the event described in the explanandum. If they do not then it may not be a satisfactory explanation. And similarly, a deductive-nomological explanation of a law is a satisfactory explanation of that law when (besides meeting all of Hempel's requirements) every event which is a case of the law to be explained is caused by an event which is a case of one (in each case, the same) of the laws contained essentially in the explanans. (1972, 23)

In addition to adding a *causal* requirement, Brody also suggested that an alternative way of repairing Hempel would be to require an *essentialist* assumption (see his 1972, 26). Brody was aware of objections to essential properties by Duhem and Popper, among others, but believed that these philosophers misunderstood the nature of essences.[14] Brody also argued that his approach permitted a natural solution to criticisms of Hempel's D-N model by Bromberger (1961) and Eberle, Kaplan, and Montague (1961).

Brody's account was initially supported by van Fraassen (1977), who argued that only a model such as Brody's could explicate the *asymmetries* that have plagued Hempelian and other analyses of explanation.[15] Van Fraassen argues provocatively that there are no explanations *in* science and that explanations are ultimately pragmatic in character: "which factors are explanatory," he writes, "is decided not by features of the scientific theory but by concerns brought from the outside" (1977, 149). (A similar view is developed in his 1980, 156 — see p. 314). Nonetheless, there are conditions for an adequate pragmatic account of explanations, and these, van Fraassen maintained in 1977, were to be sought in large part by returning to Aristotle.[16]

In my view, Brody and the earlier van Fraassen focused attention on some important questions concerning explanations but falsely saw the solution in a superseded Aristotelian philosophy. Science has not found the search for "essence" either experimentally or theoretically fruitful. A better way to approach this type of question would be to look at explanations which involve well confirmed scientific theories and generalizations, as well as at recent investigations of the concepts of causality and causal explanation. I also believe, however, that Brody (and to a lesser extent the earlier van Fraassen) somewhat overstated the argument for a *purely* causal model of explanation. Bracketing the problems with asymmetries until later, the purported counterexample (B) above is, in my view, a counterexample that requires qualification and further analysis. Generalizations that are laws of coexistence and not laws of succession *can* provisionally explain, and they themselves can in turn be *further* explained. One construal of explanation, which is defensible in some contexts, is that it is provided by an underlying pattern given by the generalizations that hold in this world, supplemented by the individualizing initial conditions. This approach is represented in the Hempel account, but it is also one favored by Kitcher and other unificationists, who will be examined in more detail later. Brody's intuition would presumably also exclude, as in any sense legitimate, the explanation of refraction by Snell's law, which seems to be a paradigm of explanation in optics texts.

This said, however, I want to add that, in the account to be defended in this book, non-causal explanations are (with the rare exception of quantum mechanics) best seen as provisional surrogates for deeper causal explanations. This is a theme which will be developed in more detail in the next several sections, but the two examples of the general gas law and Snell's law just cited support this "surrogate" view. The general gas law was subsequently explained by statistical mechanics which, in spite of its stochastic elements, is still a causal theory. Snell's law was later explained by Maxwell's theory (and again by quantum electrodynamics). Causal explanations, it would seem, also deserve a more important place than is provided for in Hempel's approach. In addition to explicating asymmetries and blocking counterexamples, such as Bromberger's flagpole example,[17] an appeal to causal explanations also turns out to be required if we conduct a deeper examination of the S-R model.

6.3.3 *Salmon's Later Emphasis on the Role of Causal Explanations in the S-R Model*

In elaborating the S-R model, Salmon (1976) found that he had to amplify it to accommodate theoretical explanations. Further reflection on theoretical explanation appears to have led him to consider the appropriateness of *causal* explanations of the statistical generalizations that constituted the explanans of the original S-R model. In his (1978) turning point essay,[18] Salmon wrote:

> If we wish to explain a particular event, such as death by leukemia of GI Joe, we begin by assembling the factors statistically relevant to that occurrence—for example, his distance from the atomic explosion, the magnitude of the blast, and the type of shelter he was in. . . . We must also obtain the probability values associated with the relevancy relations. *The statistical relevance relations are statistical regularities, and we proceed to explain them. Although this*

differs substantially from things I have said previously, I no longer believe that the assemblage of relevant factors provides a complete explanation—or much of anything in the way of explanation. We do, I believe, have a bona fide explanation of an event if we have a complete set of statistically relevant factors, the pertinent probability values, *and* causal explanations of the relevance relations. Subsumption of a particular occurrence under statistical regularities—which, we recall, does not imply anything about the construction of deductive or inductive arguments—is a necessary part of any adequate explanation of its occurrence, but *it is not the whole story. The causal explanation of the regularity is also needed.* This claim, it should be noted, is in direct conflict with the received view, according to which the mere subsumption—deductive or inductive—of an event under a lawful regularity constitutes a complete explanation. One can, according to the received view, go on to ask for an explanation of any law used to explain a given event, but that is a different explanation. I am suggesting, on the contrary, that if the regularity invoked is not a causal regularity, then a causal explanation of that very regularity must be made part of the explanation of the event. (1978, 699; my emphasis)

Salmon subsequently went on to develop this insight into a mainly causal approach to scientific explanation in his book (1984) as well as in his lengthy, historically oriented essay on scientific explanation (1989). I shall return to these views of his later in this chapter after I have illuminated his current view with the aid of an illustration from the neurosciences.

For a variety of reasons, then, causal explanation has assumed (or perhaps *re*assumed) a central role in the analysis of scientific explanation. The pervasiveness of causal components in the six representative examples outlined above indicates that these recent developments may be quite relevant to our inquiry. In order to provide an additional example of a complex causal mechanism that I believe will help us see how explanation and causation go hand in hand, let me now turn to an area of biology which we have not as yet examined. This is the area known variously as the neurosciences or neurobiology. The subject has developed extraordinarily vigorously over the past twenty years, and one of its major investigators, Eric R. Kandel, has with his colleagues been responsible for the proposal and elaboration of a set of complex causal mechanisms that explain learning in the comparatively simple organism *Aplysia californicum*. This research program is the source of the answer to our second question raised at the beginning of this chapter:

(2) Why does the "sea hare," *Aplysia californicum*, develop a heightened response to touch stimulation when subjected to a simultaneous noxious stimulus?

It is to an account of Kandel's program that I now turn.

6.4   Short-Term and Long-Term Learning in *Aplysia*

In a series of extraordinarily influential papers in neurobiology, Kandel, Schwartz, and their colleagues have been deciphering the complex neurobiological events underlying the primitive forms of learning which the marine mollusc *Aplysia* exhibits.

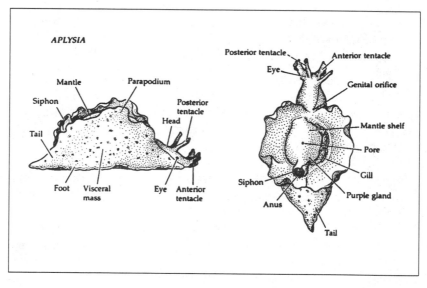

Figure 6.1   *Aplysia californica,* the sea hare, as viewed from the side and from above, with the parapodia retracted in order to show mantle, gill, and siphon (from Kuffler et al., 1984, modified from Kandel, 1976, with permission from publisher and original author).

This invertebrate organism, sometimes called the "sea hare" (*Lepus marinus* after Pliny; see figure 6.1 for a diagram of its gross structure and note its similarity to it) exhibits simple reflexes which can be altered by environmental stimuli. The nervous system of *Aplysia* is known to consist of discrete aggregates of neurons called ganglia, which contain several thousand nerve cells. These nerve cells are large enough to be visualized under a microscope and to have microelectrodes inserted into them for monitoring purposes. Individual sensory as well as motor nerve cells have been identified and are essentially identical from organism to organism, permitting the tracing of the synaptic connections among the nerve cells as well as the identification of the organs which they innervate. "Wiring diagrams" of the nervous system have been constructed from this information.[19]

It has been a surprise to many neuroscientists that such simple organisms as crayfish, fruit flies, and shellfish can be shown to exhibit habituation, sensitization, classical conditioning, and operant conditioning.[20] Both short-term and long-term memory can be demonstrated in these organisms and can provide a model for understanding the molecular basis of learning and memory. Though it is not expected that a single, universal mechanism will be found to underlie learning, one holding for all organisms including humans, it is felt that basic mechanisms will have certain fundamental relationships to one another, such as reasonably strong analogies.

6.4.1 Sensitization and Short-Term Memory

There is a simple form of learning, termed *sensitization,* in which an organism develops a more vigorous and longer lasting reflex response as a result of the presentation of a strong stimulus. In laboratory experiments *Aplysia* learns to respond to a usually noxious stimulus (e.g., a squirt of water from a water pik or an electric shock) with a strengthening of its defensive reflexes against a previously neutral stimulus. A well-known defensive reflex in *Aplysia*, the *gill-siphon withdrawal reflex,* has been studied intensively by Kandel and Schwartz and their colleagues. When the siphon or mantle shelf of *Aplysia* is stimulated by light touch, the siphon, mantle shelf, and gill all contract vigorously and withdraw into the mantle cavity (see figure 6.1 for these struc-

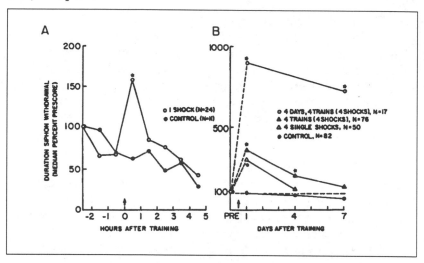

Figure 6.2   Short- and long-term sensitization of the withdrawal reflex in *Aplysia*. A: Timecourse of sensitization after a single strong electric shock to the tail or neck of *Aplysia* (arrow). B: Sensitization in groups of animals receiving varied amounts of stimulation. From Kandel, E., Castellucci, V., Goelet, P., and Schacher, S. (1987) in Kandel, E. (ed.) *Molecular Neurobiology in Neurology and Psychiatry*. New York: Raven Press. Pp. 111–132. With permission.

tures). Short-term and long-term sensitization of the withdrawal reflex is shown in figure 6.2 A and B (from Kandel et al. 1987). Short-term sensitization (like other forms of short-term memory) persists over minutes to hours; long-terms sensitization occurs or periods lasting from a day to years (in some organisms). Figure 6.2A shows the results of experiments in Kandel's laboratory of short-term sensitization, specifically the time course of sensitization after a single strong electric shock to the tail or neck of *Aplysia* (arrow). The reader will note the increased duration of the siphon withdrawal in the shocked animals in contrast to the control group, and also that this heightened response fades over the course of two to four hours, returning to the controls' level after that time. Figure 6.2B shows sensitization in groups of animals receiving varied amounts of stimulation over the course of days.

The nerve pathways that mediate this reflex are known, and a simplified wiring diagram of the gill component of the withdrawal reflex is shown in figure 6-3.[21] The sensitizing stimulus

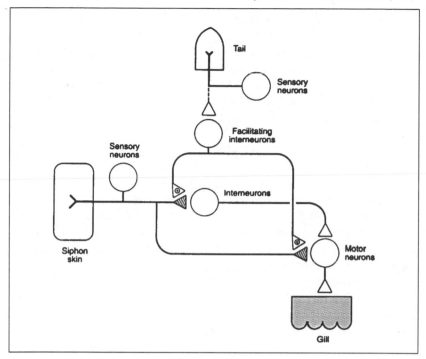

Figure 6.3   Simplified diagram of the gill component of the withdrawal reflexes in *Aplysia*. From Kandel E., Schwartz, J. and Jessell, T.(eds.) (1991) *Principles of Neural Science*, 3d ed. New York: Elsevier Science Publishing Co.; assigned to Appleton & Lange, Norwalk, CT. Page 1013, with permission of publisher and Dr. Kandel.

applied to the sensory receptor organ (in this case the head or the tail) activates *facilitatory* interneurons that in turn act on the follower cells of the sensory neurons to increase neurotransmitter release. In figure 6.3 these facilitating interneurons, some of which use serotonin (= 5 H T), end on the synaptic terminals from the siphon skin where they increase neurotransmitter release through presynaptic facilitation. This explains sensitization at the cellular level to some extent, in the sense that an increase in the amount of the neurotransmitter can be expected to heighten the reaction of the cell to which it is chemically linked. Kandel and his colleagues, however, have pushed this investigation to a deeper level, that of the molecular mechanisms involved.

For short-term sensitization, all the neurotransmitters have a common mode of action: each activates an enzyme known as adenylate cyclase, which increases the amount of cyclic AMP—a substance known as the "second messenger"—in the sensory neuronal cells. This cyclic AMP then turns on (or turns up) the activity of another enzyme, a protein kinase, which acts to modify a "*family* of substrate proteins to initiate a broad cellular program for short term synaptic plasticity" (Kandel et al. 1987, 118). The program involves the kinase that phosphorylates (i.e., inserts a phosphate group into) a K^+-channel protein, closing one class of K^+ channels that normally would restore or repolarize the neuron's action potential to the original level. This channel closing increases the excitability of the neuron and also prolongs its action potential (or active state), resulting in more Ca^{++} flowing into the terminals and permitting more neurotransmitter to be released. (There may also be another component to this mechanism involving movement of a C-kinase to the neuron's membrane, where it may enhance mobilization and sustain release of neurotransmitter.) The diagram in figure 6.4 should make this sequence of causally related events clearer.

6.4.2 *Long-term Memory in Aplysia*

A similar type of explanation can be provided for long-term memory for sensitization, but I will not go into it in any detail here, save to point out that the mechanism can best be described as exhibiting important *analogies* with short-term memory. Suffice it to say that the long-term mechanism is somewhat more complex, though it shares similarities with the short-term mechanisms such as the adenylate cyclase—cyclic AMP—protein kinase cascade. Since there are strong indications that protein synthesis occurs in connection with long-term memories (Kandel et al. 1987, 127), different, additional mechanisms need to be invoked, almost certainly involving genetic regulation that would permit genes to be turned on and new protein synthesis to occur. Figure 6.5 provides us with one of at least two possible overviews of this more complex—and at present more speculative—mechanism.

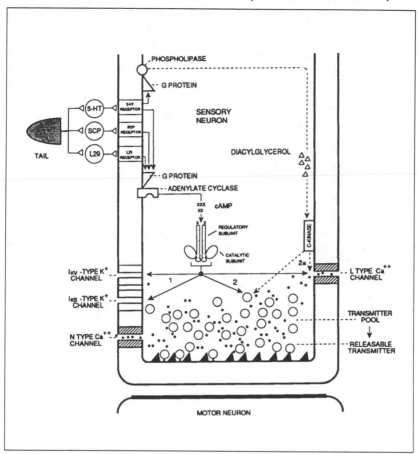

Figure 6.4   Molecular model of short-term sensitization. See text for discussion and explanation. Updated from Kandel, E., Castellucci, V., Goelet, P., and Schacher, S. (1987) in Kandel, E. (ed.) *Molecular Neurobiology in Neurology and Psychiatry*. New York: Raven Press. Pp. 111–132. With permission

6.4.3 *Additional Complexity and Parallel Processing*

The above description of Kandel and his associates' work focuses on an account that has "had the advantage of allowing a relatively detailed analysis of the cellular and molecular mechanisms underlying one component important for both short- and long-term memory for sensitization" (Frost, Clark, and Kandel

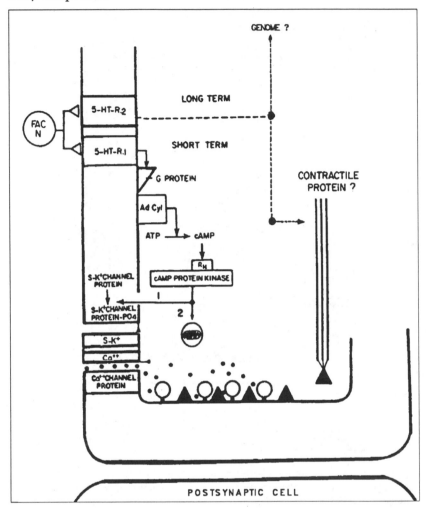

Figure 6.5   A speculative model of how long-term memory may operate in "parallel." From Kandel, E., Castellucci, V., Goelet, P., and Schacher, S. (1987) in Kandel, E. (ed.) *Molecular Neurobiology in Neurology and Psychiatry*. New York: Raven Press. Pp. 111–132. With permission.

1988, 298). As these authors note in this more recent analysis, however, "the siphon withdrawal response exhibits a complex choreography with many different components." Further work on both the gill component and the siphon component of this reflex has suggested that memory for sensitization in *Aplysia*—as well as other organisms—appears to involve "parallel processing," an expression which Frost, Clark, and Kandel (1988, 298) state is "similar" to a "view . . . called 'parallel distributed processing,' . . . [which] has emerged from theoretical studies in artificial intelligence and cognitive psychology and is based on the idea that common computational processes occur at many sites within a network."

TECHNICAL DISCUSSION 9

Parallel Processing in Aplysia

In this chapter I will not have an opportunity to explore the complex interactions which Kandel and his colleagues have found even in this comparatively simple form of short-term memory. Suffice it to say that they have found it involves at least four circuit sites, each exhibiting a different type of neuronal plasticity (which are shown in figure 6.6):

(1) presynaptic facilitation of the central sensory neuron connections, as described earlier in this section; (2) presynaptic inhibition made by L30 onto circuit interneurons, including L29, as shown; (3) posttetanic potentiation (PTP) of the synapses made by L29 onto the siphon motor neurons; and (4) increases in the tonic firing rate of the LFS motor neurons, leading to neuromuscular facilitation (Frost, Clark, and Kandel 1988, 299).

Frost, Clark, and Kandel (1988) anticipated such complexity but were also surprised to find that, though the PTP discovered at L29 was a homosynaptic process, the other three components appeared to be coordinately regulated by a common modulatory transmitter, serotonin, and that the common second-messenger system, cyclic AMP, was involved in each (1988, 323–324). Additional modulatory transmitters and other second-messenger systems are not explicitly ruled out, however (see 1988, 324).

In some other recent work, Kandel has in fact reported that tail stimulation in *Aplysia* can lead to transient inhibition (in addition to prominent facilitation). Studies of this inhibitory component indicate that the mechanism is presynaptic inhibition, in which the neurotransmitter is the peptide FMRFamide, and that the "second messenger" in this component is not cyclic AMP; rather, inhibition is mediated by the lipoxygenase pathway of arachidonic acid. This "unexpected richness," as Kandel has characterized the existence of the

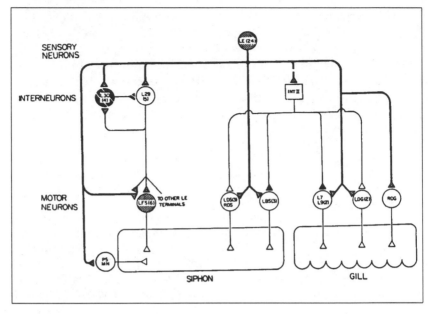

Figure 6.6   The gill- and siphon-withdrawal reflex circuit showing the sites found to be modified by sensitizing stimuli (shaded structures). See technical discussion 9 for details of these modifications. After Frost, Clark, and Kandel (1988) *Journal of Neurobiology*. Copyright © 1988 and reprinted by permission of John Wylie & Sons, Inc.

two balancing pathways, constitutes still further evidence for the philosophical views about theory structure discussed in chapter 3.

6.5   What Does this Example Tell Us about Explanation in Neurobiology?

6.5.1 *Causal Generalizations of Varying Scope Are Prevalent in Neurobiology*

There are several important points to note in the above account, which gives a *molecular* explanation of a *behavioral* explanandum. First, we do not have anything quite like the "laws" we find in physics explanations.[22] There are some generalizations of fairly broad generality — for example, that protein kinase enzymes act by phosphorylating molecules and that cAMP is a (second) messenger — that we could extract from the account, though they are typically left implicit. Such generalizations are, however, introduced explicitly in introductory chapters in neuroscience texts. In addition, however, there are usually also generalizations of prima facie quite narrow scope, such as the "two balancing pathways" found in Kandel's very recent work and perhaps the C-kinase mechanism depicted in figure 6.4.[23] Further, these generalizations are typically borrowed from a very wide-ranging set of models (protein synthesis models, biochemical models, etc.). The set of models in biology is so broad it led Morowitz's (1985) committee to invoke the notion of many-many modeling in the form of a complex "matrix."[24] But even when such generalizations, narrow or broad, are made explicit, they need to be supplemented with the details of specific connections in the system in order to constitute an explanation, such as the linkage of a three-fold L-29–SCP–5-HT receptor to the G protein shown in figure 6.4. Are these connections playing the role of "initial conditions" in traditional philosophy of science? I think this is not quite the case because we do not have a set of powerful generalizations such as Newton's laws of motion, to which we can add rather minor details concerning the force function and the initial position and momentum and generate explanations across a wide range of domains. The generalizations we can glean from such molecular mechanisms as are found in neurobiology have a variable scope and typically need to be changed to *analogous* mechanisms as one changes organism or behavior. The brief account I gave of the relation between short-term mechanisms and long-term mechanisms for sensitization in *Aplysia* is a case in point, as is the further complexity found in the account of classical conditioning described by Kandel (in Kandel and Schwartz 1985, chap. 62) as well as in short-term sensitization in the more recent "parallel processing" account above.

What we appear to have are rather intricate *systems* to which apply both broad and narrow *causal generalizations* that are typically framed not in purely biochemical terminology but rather in terminology that is characteristically *interlevel* and *interfield*.[25] This point is a feature of biological explanation importantly stressed by Darden and Maull in their 1977 that I think has not been sufficiently appreciated outside of a somewhat limited group of philosophers of biology. In chapter 3, I reemphasized the interlevel feature of typical biological theories and also suggested that such theories often explain by providing a temporal sequence as part of their models (also see Schaffner 1980a, 1986); now it is appropriate to emphasize that this temporal sequence is actually a *causal* sequence.

An interlevel causal sequence[26] is what we seem to have in the example from Kandel above. As an explanation of a phenomenon like sensitization is given in molecular terms, one maps the initially behavioral phenomenon into a neural and molecular vocabulary. Sensitization is not just the phenomenon shown earlier in figure 6.2 but is *reinterpreted as* an instance of neuronal excitability and increased transmitter release, or in other words, as *enhanced synaptic transmission.*[27]

Is this explanation also in accord with explanation by *derivation* from a theory? I think the answer is yes, but with some important qualifications and elaborations. We do not have, I have argued above, a very general set of sentences (the laws) that can serve as the premises from which we can deduce the conclusion. Rather what we have is *a set of causal sentences of varying degrees of generality,* many of them quite specific to the system in question. It may be that in some distant future all of these causal sentences of narrow scope, such as "This phosphorylation closes one class of K^+ channels that normally repolarize the action potential,"[28] will be explainable by general laws of protein chemistry, but this is not the case at present, in part because we cannot even infer the three-dimensional structure of a protein, like the kinase enzyme or the K^+ channels mentioned, from a complete knowledge of the sequence of amino acids that make up the proteins. Fundamental and very general principles will have to await a more developed science than we will have for some time. Thus the explanans, the explaining generalizations in such an account, will be a complex web of interlevel causal generalizations of varying scope and will typically be expressed in terms of an idealized system of the type shown in figure 6.4, with some textual elaboration on the nature of the causal sequence leading through the system.

This, then, is a kind of partial model explanation with largely implicit generalizations, often of narrow scope, licensing the temporal sequence of causal propagation of events through the model. It is not unilevel explanation in, for instance, bio-chemical terms, but it *is* characteristically what is termed a *molecular biological explanation*. The model appealed to in the explanation is typically interlevel, mixing different levels of aggregation, from cell to organ back to molecule, and the explaining model may be still further integrated into another model, as the biochemical model is integrated into or seen as a more detailed expansion of the neural circuit model for the gill-siphon reflex. The explanation is thus typically *incomplete* at the strictly molecular level; it is, however, not therefore (necessarily) *causally* incomplete.[29] The model or models also may not be robust across this organism or other organisms; it may well have a narrow domain of application, in contrast to what we typically encounter in physical theories.

In some recent discussion on the theses developed in the present chapter, Wimsatt (personal communication) has raised the question, why not simply refer to the explanation as being accomplished by "mechanisms," in the sense of his 1976a and 1976b, and forget about the more syntactic attempt to examine the issues in terms of "generalizations"? Though I view Wimsatt's suggestion (and his position) as fruitful and correct as a first approximation,[30] I do not wish to take "mechanism" as an unanalyzed term. It seems to me that we do have "generalizations" of varying scope at work in these "molecular biological explanations" that are interlevel and preliminary surrogates for a unilevel explanation (a reduction), and that it is important to understand the varying scope of the generalizations and how they can be applied "analogically" within and across various biological organisms. This point of view relates closely to the question of "theory structure" in biology and medicine discussed in chapter 3.[31] In addition, as I shall argue below, "mechanisms" are significantly intertwined with "laws of working," which they instantiate, and thus will not suffice per se.

All this said, however, there is no reason that the *logic* of the relation between the explanans and the explanandum cannot be cast in deductive form. Typically this is not done because it requires more formalization than it is worth, but some fairly complex engineering circuits, such as the full adder shown in figure 6.7, can effectively be represented in the first-order predicate cal-

The full adder shown in figure 6.7 is an integer-processing circuit consisting of five subcomponents called "gates." There are two exclusive "or" (*xor*) gates, x_1 and x_2, two "and" gates, a_1 and a_2, and an inclusive "or" gate o_1. There are input ports on the left side of the box and output ports on the right, as well as ports into and out of the subcomponents. The universe of discourse thus consists of 26 objects: 6 components or subcomponents and 20 ports.

The structure and operation of this circuit can be captured in first order predicate logic (FOL) and a theorem-prover used with the logical formulas to generate answers to questions about the device's operations. A full treatment is beyond the scope of this paper (but can be found in Genesereth and Nilsson's 1987, 29–32 and 78–84). Here we will give only a few of the axioms used to characterize this circuit in FOL. After the vocabulary is introduced, some 30 logic sentences are needed for the full description.

Vocabulary examples: Xorg(x) means that x is an *xor* gate; I(i,x) designates the ith (1, 2, or 3) input port of device x; Conn (x,y) means that port x is connected to port y; V(x,z) means that the value on port x is z; 1 and 0 designate the high and low signals respectively.

Connectivity and behavior of components examples:

...

(7) Conn (I(1,F1),I(1,X1))
(8) Conn (I(2,F1),I(2,X1))

...

(26) $\forall x \ (Org(x) \land V(I(n,x),1) \Rightarrow V(O(1,x),1))$

...

(30) $\forall x \forall y \forall z \ (Conn \ (x,y) \land V(x,z) \Rightarrow V(y,z))$

(As noted, these assumptions represent only 4 of the 30 needed.)

culus and useful deductions made from the premises, which in the adder example number about 30 (see text box). [32]

The picture of explanation that emerges from any detailed study of molecular biology as it is practiced is not a simple and elegant one. A good overall impression of the complexity of the subject of molecular biology and of its explanations can be obtained if one will browse through such a text as Watson et al.'s

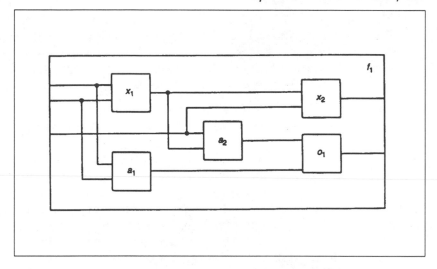

Figure 6.7   A full adder. See textbox on page 288 for a description of the operation and logic of the full adder. (From Genesereth, M. and Nilsson, N. (1987) *Logical Foundations of Artificial Intelligence*. Los Altos, CA: Morgan Kaufmann, p. 29, with permission.)

recent (1987) version of the classic *Molecular Biology of the Gene* or Lewin's recent (1990) *Genes IV*. Alternatively, a similar impression can be gotten from inspecting those intermediary metabolism charts that hang on many laboratory walls, displaying wheels and cycles of complex reactions feeding into still more cycles and pathways of additional reactions. This material plays the role of the explaining theories and initial conditions of molecular biology and biochemistry. A nonbiologist encountering such material, as in the examples given in this and the previous chapters, might feel a spirit of kinship with Pierre Duhem, who expressed his reaction to "English" science thusly:

> The employment of mechanical models, recalling by more or less rough analogies the particular features of the theory being expounded, is a regular feature of the English treatises. . . . Here is a book intended to expound the modern theories . . . and to expound a new theory. In it there are nothing but strings that move around pulleys, which roll around drums, which go through pearl beads,

which carry weights, and tubes which pump water while others swell and contract; toothed wheels which are geared to one another and engage hooks. We thought we were entering the tranquil and neatly ordered abode of reason, but we find ourselves in a factory. (1914, 70–71)

Duhem was writing about "English *physics*," but the impression he would have of contemporary international molecular biology would surely be similar.

This material (the multiple and complex "mechanisms" I am referring to here) plays the role of the explaining theories and initial conditions for molecular biology and biochemistry. As already remarked, in these fields it is not possible usefully to separate out a small core of general laws and add a list of initial conditions to the core in order to generate an explanation. In the following section, I will attempt to generalize this point and relate it to scientific explanation in biology and medicine outside of molecular neurobiology. As noted, causal explanation in biology and medicine is complex, and causal and (re)interpretative connections are found at a number of loci. Before we close this section, however, it would be well to introduce one additional point of clarification to guard against the misinterpretation of *interpretative* connections as *causal* connections.[33]

6.5.2 *Causal versus Perspectival Sequences*

An examination of the system studied by Kandel and his associates indicates that the *behavioral* level of analysis (represented by figures 6.1A and 6.1B) deals with such entities as shocks administered to organisms, gross reflex descriptions, and a time course of hours or days. Comparison with the *neural network* level indicates that these entities are, at this "cellular" level, viewed in a greater degree of detail; this degree of detail is further increased at the *biochemical* level. As one descends levels from the behavioral to the biochemical, however, one does not traverse a causal sequence in reverse, with behavior viewed as effects and biochemical mechanisms as causes; rather, one traces a *perspectival* sequence. Causal sequences can be found at any level of aggregation and between levels of aggregation, but a description of a set of parts of a whole does not automatically entail a causal account relating the parts as causes to the whole as an effect.

What frequently is the case is that the causal sequence between cause and effect is *best understood* at the biochemical level. Thus stimuli can be *interpreted* as propagating action potentials, and neurotransmitters can be construed as chemical messengers. Biochemical cascades can be examined as fine-structure connecting networks ultimately leading to the event to be explained, which can be *reinterpreted* so as to be identified with an original explanandum. What should not be done, however, is to conflate perspectival reinterpretation with causation, for it can only lead to confusion in an already extraordinarily complex set of relations. (I should perhaps add that a perspectival reinterpretation *can*, however, be associated with a causal interpretation *if* we are examining the causes of *perceptions*. *This* causal language, however, is focused on such causal sequences as photons impacting on rods and cones, the translation of chemical pigment (rhodopsin, opsin) changes into electrical impulses, and the like. Thus, if perspectival or "level" analyses are to be construed as causal, one must be careful to disentangle two different dimensions of putative causal sequences (causes of perceptions versus a noncausal difference in perspective) in an explanation (or, as we shall see in chapter 9, in a reduction).)

6.6 What Does this Example Tell Us about Scientific Explanation in General?

In the (comparatively) simple example from Kandel and his associates' analysis of learning in *Aplysia*, we appear to encounter a paradigm case of a scientific explanation. This suggests the question how the account of explanation given in association with the Kandel example relates to extant models of scientific explanation discussed earlier.

I think that the most useful approach will be to continue with our discussion of Salmon's position, but now to refer to a contrast between two very general analyses of scientific explanation noted by Salmon in his more recent work. In his *Scientific Explanation and the Causal Structure of the World* (1984), Salmon contrasts the "epistemic" approach to explanation with the "ontic" approach. The former, in its "inferential" interpretation, is best represented by the Hempel-Oppenheim model of explanation. The "ontic" approach, on the other hand, is one which

Salmon has articulated and defended under the rubric of the "causal/mechanical" tradition. Salmon believes that the epistemic approach also characterizes the "theoretical unification" analyses developed by Michael Friedman (1974) and Philip Kitcher (1981, 1989), about which I shall have more to say later.

Though favoring a causal/mechanical analysis, Salmon was unwilling to yield completely the valuable feature of "unification" to the epistemic approach, and he suggested how this feature could be accommodated within the causal/mechanical tradition. In his (1984) book he wrote:

> The ontic conception looks upon the world, to a large extent at least, as a black box whose workings we want to understand. Explanation involves laying bare the underlying mechanisms that connect the observable inputs to the observable outputs. We explain events by showing how they fit into the causal nexus. Since there seem to be a small number of fundamental causal mechanisms, and some extremely comprehensive laws that govern them, the ontic conception has as much right as the epistemic conception to take the unification of natural phenomena as a basic aspect of our comprehension of the world. *The unity lies in the pervasiveness of the underlying mechanisms* upon which we depend for explanation. (1984, 276)

In a more recent essay, Salmon introduces two briefly characterized biomedical examples to illustrate his approach. He mentions that "to understand AIDS, we must deal with viruses and cells. To understand the transmission of traits from parents to offspring, we become involved with the structure of the DNA molecule. . . . When we try to construct causal explanations we are attempting to discover the mechanisms — often hidden mechanisms — that bring about the facts we seek to understand" (Salmon 1991, 34).

In this recent essay, Salmon adds that, despite the contrast between the two major traditions, in "an important respect" these two traditions "overlap":

> When the search for hidden mechanisms is successful, the result is often to reveal a small number of basic mechanisms that underlie wide ranges of phenomena. The explanation of diverse phenomena in terms of the same

mechanism constitutes theoretical unification. For instance,
. . . [t]he discovery of the double-helical structure of
DNA . . . produced a major unification of biology and
chemistry. (1991, 34)

Biology and medicine in general, and the neurosciences,
AIDS virology, and molecular genetics in particular, tend, with a
few important exceptions, to propose what Salmon terms
causal/mechanical explanations.[34,35] The Kandel example detailed above offers clear evidence to support this point. As such,
the appeal to "a small number of basic mechanisms that underlie
wide ranges of phenomena" is the way both explanation and reduction is achieved, though an important caveat, suggested earlier but worth further emphasis in this context, is in order. The
caveat has to do with the expression "small number of mechanisms." In point of fact, close analysis of biology and medicine
discloses an extensive variety of mechanisms, some with comparatively narrow scope and some with almost universal scope.
In a number of areas, a range of mechanisms which bear close
analogies to each other are found. This, given the evolutionary
backdrop, is not unexpected, but the subtle variation biologists
continue to encounter requires them to be attentive to changes in
biological processes as they analyze different types of organisms
or even as they analyze different structures in the same organism. Thus though the genetic code is (almost) universal, messenger RNA is processed quite differently in prokaryotes (such as
bacteria) in contrast with eukaryotes (multicellular organisms
such as *Aplysia*). Furthermore, variation can be found in the same
organism; in the human, for example, the actions of muscle fibers
in skeletal muscle are regulated importantly differently than in
cardiac muscle, and serious errors can result if the differences are
not kept in mind.[36]

Thus biology and medicine display a rather complex and
partially attenuated theoretical unification: some mechanisms
are nearly universal, many have evolutionarily fixed idiosyncra-
sies built into them, and some are highly individualized. The
scope of explanatory devices encountered in the diversity of the
life sciences ranges across a broad spectrum, from extremely narrow to almost all-encompassingly broad. Nevertheless, generalizations and mechanisms are available to be used in explanations
and to be tested in different laboratories; the variable breadth of

scope does not negate the nomic force of the generalizations and the mechanisms.[37]

This picture of generalizations of variable scope instantiated in a series of overlapping mechanisms is congruent with the account of theory structure developed in chapters 3 and 6. We can, as in chapter 3, employ a generalization of Suppes's set-theoretic approach and also follow Giere (1984) in introducing the notion of a "theoretical model" as "a kind of system whose characteristics are specified by an explicit definition" (1984, 80). Here entities $\eta_1 \ldots \eta_n$ will designate neurobiological objects such as neurotransmitters and the Φ's such *causal* properties as "phosphorylation" and "secretion," while the scientific generalizations $\Sigma_1 \ldots \Sigma_n$ will be of the type "This enzyme phosphorylates such and such a type of K^+ channel."[38] Then $\Sigma_i(\Phi(\eta_1 \ldots \eta_n))$ will represent the ith generalization, and $\prod_{i=1}^{n} \Sigma (\Phi(\eta_1 \ldots \eta_n))$ will be the conjunction of the assumptions (which we will call Π) constituting a "biomedical system" or BMS. As I have stated earlier, any given system that is being investigated or appealed to as *explanatory of some explanandum* is such a BMS if and only if it satisfies Π. We can understand Π, then, as implicitly defining a (abstract) kind of natural system though there may not be any actual system that is a realization of the complex expression Π. To claim that some particular system satisfies Π is a theoretical hypothesis which may or may not be true, but if it is true, then the BMS can serve as an explanandum of a phenomenon, such as "sensitization." (If the BMS is potentially true and well confirmed, then it is a "potential and well-confirmed explanation" of the phenomenon it entails or supports.)

Explanation on such a view thus proceeds by identifying the system under investigation with the theoretical system and exhibiting the explanandum as the causal consequence of the system's behavior. Laws or (perhaps better) *generalizations* will appear as the Σs in the system's definition, and *deduction* (or *inductive support* in the case of particular event descriptions) will be one means of obtaining or verifying the causal consequences. As such, this is akin to Hempelian explanation with a causal interpretation of the explanans. Explanation (and, as we shall see later, reduction) in biology and medicine accordingly can be located in that "overlap" range discussed by Salmon where (comparatively) few "hidden" mechanisms account for a (comparatively) wide range of phenomena by exhibiting (complex) causal pathways leading to the phenomena. I have already noted that, in his recent essay on scientific explanation (1989), Salmon indicates that an "overlap" existed between the causal/mechanical approach and the unification analysis (see p. 292). Further in that same essay, Salmon poses the interesting question as to whether any type of consensus or emerging rapprochement might exist among those philosophers of science defending prima facie divergent views about scientific explanation. Salmon first suggests that

> the unification approach as defended recently by Watkins [1984] and pursued . . . by Kitcher [1989] is, I believe, viable. In Kitcher's terminology, it is a "top-down" approach. It fits admirably with the intuitions that have guided the proponents of the received view, as well as those that inspire scientists to find unifying theories. This is the form in which the epistemic conception of scientific explanation can flourish today. (1989, 182)

Then, in comparing the theoretical unification view with the causal/ mechanical approach, Salmon adds "These two ways of regarding explanation are *not incompatible* with one another; each one offers a reasonable way of construing explanations."[39]

After relating a story that provides both causal molecular and "principle of equivalence" explanations of an event,[40] Salmon suggests that perhaps there are *two* concepts of scientific explanation: explanation$_1$ (causal/mechanical) and explanation$_2$ (explanation by unification). The former, Salmon speculates, may be primarily concerned with local explanations—particular causal processes and their interactions—though even here provision must be made for causal/mechanical explanations of general regularities (1989, 184). In addition, Salmon notes: "This does not mean that general laws play no role in explanations of this kind, for *the mechanisms involved operate in accordance with general laws of nature*" (1989, 184, my emphasis). In contrast, though, Salmon sees explanation$_2$ as global, as relating to the structure of the whole universe. This is "top-down" explanation.

We can find both types of explanation in biology and medicine, and for reasons indicated we must allow for something like a Hempelian aspect to explanation, in terms of the deductive consequences of causal generalizations and perhaps also where laws of coexistence may be found.[41] As argued above, however, it seems to me that the explanations that are characteristically biological (as well as biomedical) will be "causal/mechanical" more frequently than not. For these types of explanations it is difficult, and may even be counterproductive, to provide anything more than a very general model, such as that of the semantic BMS described above, to which they must conform. These causal/mechanical explanations are of the type that Kandel and his colleagues provided for sensitization in *Aplysia*. The nature of the explanation consists in recounting the causal story, using the best science available. Explanation$_2$, explanation by unification, however, *may* profit from a somewhat more detailed structural model, and we shall in section 9 return to and reconsider this issue in connection with Kitcher's (1989) and van Fraassen's (1980) accounts.[42]

6.7 Causality and Causal Explanation

In his 1984 monograph, Salmon argued that his "frequent reference to the role of causality in scientific explanation" required him to provide "an account of causality adequate for a causal theory of scientific explanation" (1984, 135; also 135, n.1). Since I have accepted important elements of Salmon's "causal/mechanical view," I will also sketch in the present section an account of causality that I believe provides a background for the "overlap" but largely causal model introduced in the previous section.[43] I will not follow Salmon, however, in developing an analysis of causality using his conceptual apparatus of "marks" and "forks," though I will agree with some elements of his account, including the emphasis on a process rather than an event ontology.

The account of causality I favor owes less to Reichenbach (1956) — whose approach Salmon develops — and much more to the analyses of Collingwood (1940), Mackie (1974), and Hart and Honoré (1985 [1959]). Since the problem this section is intended to address arose out of Hume's penetrating critique of causation, however, it will be useful to begin with a few brief remarks about the nature of the problem as Hume originally saw it.

6.7.1 *Hume on Causation*

It has been pointed out a number of times in the philosophical literature that Hume's analysis of causation was not univocal. For example, Mackie, following Robinson (1962), distinguished two definitions of cause in Hume's writings: (1) causation as regular succession, and (2) causation as regular succession plus a "psychological" overlay, "association." Exactly how the two accounts are to be related is not obvious (see Mackie 1974, chap. 1). In addition to these two definitions, moreover, Hume also added a third, *conditional* type of definition. In his *Enquiry*, immediately after offering the first regularity definition ("we may define a cause to be an *object, followed by another, and where all objects similar to the first are followed by objects similar to the second"*), Hume adds "or in other words *where, if the first object had not been, the second never had existed"* (1927 [1777], 76).[44]

Hume's problem has been insightfully dissected by Mackie, who suggests that Hume conflated several different senses of "necessity." The root issue in causation is just what licenses our causal claims, and Hume's general answer is constant conjunction coupled with psychological habit. It is the unsatisfactory character of this Humean reply that shook Kant from his "dogmatic slumber" and that has exercised philosophers ever since. Mackie argues that Hume inappropriately sought a warrant for an a priori inference, that is, for a *power* in C which would clearly show that it would bring about E. Mackie termed this search for a support for an a priori inference a quest for a sense of necessity, necessity$_2$ in Mackie's notation. Mackie distinguished this necessity$_2$ from a different, weaker sense, necessity$_1$, which is the "distinguishing feature of causal as opposed to noncausal sequences" (1974, 12). Mackie still further distinguished a necessity$_3$ which would license causal inference, but not in an a priori manner. Much of Mackie's (1974) monograph is taken up with the working out of an account of causation that provides an analysis of the first and third types of necessity, while contending that an adequate characterization of necessity$_2$ cannot and need not be given.

I take these distinctions to be useful ones and Mackie's suspicions about the effective characterizability of necessity$_2$ to be sound. These Humean preliminaries aside, however, we still have to develop an account of causation which will justify its central place in scientific explanation. To do this I now turn to some other historical figures whose analyses of causation will be used in part to construct this account.

6.7.2 *The Heterogeneous Character of Causation*

A review of the various approaches to causation that have been taken by philosophers over the past two millennia suggests that the concept of causation may not be unitary. In Aristotle we find four different senses of the term, and post-Humean analyses comprise such diverse approaches as regularity and conditional accounts, the activity or manipulability view, the (rationalist) logical entailment theory, a nonlogical entailment version, and the more recent possible world accounts (Lewis 1973, Earman 1986).[45] In my view, several of these diverse approaches need to be drawn on and intertwined to constitute an adequately robust analysis of causation for biology and medicine. Though it will not be possible in this book to provide an extensive discussion of the various elements that I want to incorporate into my preferred analysis, I believe that enough can be said to make the view plausible. I will begin by indicating the outlines of the analysis, then will discuss each of its components in somewhat more detail.

In my view, an analysis of causation adequate to the account of scientific explanation offered above will require three components. The first is what might be termed *logical*: an explication of what type of conditional (e.g., necessary, sufficient, etc.) is to be used to distinguish causal from noncausal sequences. Here I shall draw heavily on Mackie's view that "necessity-in-the-circumstances" is the most appropriate approach.[46] Second, I think that we may make some important progress in understanding our causal language by examining how we come to have ideas about causation. This component might properly be termed *epistemological*, since it characterizes the generation as well as the evaluation of our causal notions. The approach here involves a partially historical or psychological sketch, with both "phylogenetic" (the development in history) and "ontogenetic" (the development in the individual) aspects of the various heterogeneous sources of our concept of causation. For this I rely on the work of Hart and Honoré and R. G. Collingwood, though I do not accept the latter's activity theory as the primary sense of causation, and I also include some suggestions from Mackie on this topic. This will prepare the basis for the third element of causation, this one perhaps best describable as the *metaphysical* component, where I will briefly discuss the role of a process metaphysics as undergirding causation. Here I find myself in sympathy with Salmon, but aspects of the view I defend can also be found in Collingwood and Mackie. I think it is the confluence of these three strands, the logical, the epistemological, and the metaphysical, that constitutes an adequate notion of causation.

The Conditional Component

Necessity in the circumstances. The extent to which causation can and should be analyzed in terms of necessary and/or sufficient conditions has been a topic of considerable debate in the philosophical literature (e.g., see Sosa 1975). I think that a persuasive case can be made for taking the view that Mackie (1974, chap. 2) defends: "the distinguishing feature of causal sequence is the conjunction of necessity-in-the-circumstances with causal priority" (1974, 51).[47] What this means is that "X is necessary in the circumstances for and causally prior to Y provided that if X were kept out of the world in the circumstances referred to and the world ran on from there, Y would not occur" (1974, 51). This notion of "necessary in the circumstances" is sufficiently strong that it will support a counterfactual conditional of the sort Hume cited in his third definition of causation.[48] Because of the "in the circumstances" addendum, it is also strong enough to block counterexamples that are quite pervasive in biology and medicine because of parastasis — the ability of organisms to accomplish the same end by a variety of means.[49] However, "necessity in the circumstances" is not so strong that epistemologically plausible accounts cannot be provided, in both formal and informal ways, to indicate how the notion can be empirically supported.[50] Basically, Mackie sees Mill's method of difference as involved in the more formal way of empirically grounding the notion — a point I shall readdress further below. Several comments on the meaning of the phrase "in the circumstances" are needed at this point to clarify the relation of a "necessity" view to a "sufficiency" account.

Mackie argues that the notion of "sufficiency in the circumstances" is "of no use for our . . . purpose of finding the *distin-*

guishing feature of causal sequences; every cause is sufficient in the circumstances for its effect, *but so are many non-causes for events which are not their effects*" (1974, 39; my emphasis). Mackie adds that this is a weak sense of "sufficiency in the circumstances," but that a stronger sense of the phrase is available:

> This would be that given the circumstances, if Y [in the expression X caused Y] had not been going to happen, X would not have occurred. This is a possible sense, and what we recognize as causes *are in general sufficient in the circumstances* in this strong sense as well as in the weak one. (1974, 39–40; my emphasis)

Mackie adds that "it looks as if the strong counterfactual sense of 'sufficient in the circumstances' will distinguish causal from noncausal sequences, though the weak sense does not," but believes that further analysis is needed to determine whether "necessity in the circumstances" or "sufficiency in the circumstances" or both captures the primary feature of causation (1974, 40).

It is at this point that Mackie introduces his famous (or infamous) three different shilling-in-the-slot candy bar machines and argues that a consideration of his two "indeterministic" slot machines indicates that "necessity in the circumstances" is the primary feature of our causation concept, though outside of the realm of such (rare) machines, "sufficiency in the circumstances" in the strong counterfactual sense will generally hold as well.[51]

This, then, seems to be the crux of the issue: there can be causal explanations in which the constituent causes are "necessary in the circumstances," and these will produce (with probability) their effects.[52] In those (frequent) cases where the constituent causes are *also* "sufficient in the circumstances" in either sense of the term, the result will be guaranteed, though perhaps *explained* in a deterministic manner only if the sense of "sufficiency" is the counterfactual one.[53] This account then permits us to locate probabilistic causal explanation as well as deterministic causal explanation within a general schema, interpreting probabilistic causal sequences as *explanatory* but in a weaker sense than a sufficiency view. (See endnote 52 as well as section 6.8; also see chapter 8.)

"Inus" conditions and gappy generalizations. Our discussion of conditionals provides the opportunity to introduce another refinement, also developed by Mackie, of the traditional notion of a causal condition, showing it to be more complex than just "necessary" or "sufficient." This refinement is based on the notion of an *inus* condition. Mackie introduces this notion on the basis of his reflections on Mill's discussion of the plurality of causes problem. Mill recognized the complication of a plurality of causes, by which several different assemblages of factors, say ABC as well as DGH and JKL, might each be sufficient to bring about an effect P. Let us now understand these letters to represent types rather than tokens. Then if (ABC or DGH or JKL) is both necessary and sufficient for P, how do we describe the A in such a generalization? Such an element is for Mackie an *insufficient but nonredundant [necessary] part of an unnecessary but sufficient condition*—a complex characteristic for which Mackie forms the acronym an *inus* condition from the first letters of the indicated words. Using this terminology, then, what is usually termed a cause is an *inus* condition.

But our knowledge of causal regularities are seldom *fully* and completely characterized: we know some of the *inus* conditions but rarely all the possible ones.

Causal regularities are, according to Mackie, "elliptical or gappy universal propositions" (1974, 66). One can represent this using Mackie's formalism after first invoking (following Anderson 1938) *a causal field* of background conditions, F, which focuses our attention on some specific area and/or subject of inquiry, and noting that:

In F, all (A . . . $\bar{\text{B}}$ or D . . . $\bar{\text{H}}$ . . . or . . .) are followed by P
and,
in F, all P are preceded by (A . . . $\bar{\text{B}}$ or D . . . $\bar{\text{H}}$ . . . or . . .).

The bar above B and H indicates that these types are functioning as negative causes in this generalization.

Though such an account of causal regularities looks on the surface quite unhelpful, Mackie argues, and I agree with him, that such "gappy universal propositions [or] incompletely known complex regularities, which contribute to . . . [causal] inferences will sustain, with probability, the counterfactual conditionals that correspond to these inferences," and also that the gappy universal will "equally sustain the subjunctive conditional that if this cause occurred again in *sufficiently similar* circumstances, so would the effect" (1974, 68; my emphasis).[54] Mackie leaves open what the notion of "sufficiently similar circumstances" might mean. In light of the theses about theory structure developed in chapter 3, I would interpret the notion as referring to fairly narrow subclasses of organisms functioning within a range of narrowly prescribed initial conditions, the range being in large part a pragmatic matter.

The only points of emendation I would want to make to Mackie's "elliptical or gappy universal propositions" are (1) to change "universal" to "general," so as to permit the use of statistical generalizations which may be excluded by connotations associated with the term "universal" (but see Mackie 1974, chap. 9), and (2) to stress that the generalizations which may be cited as potential elements of an explanans are likely to be of narrow scope and polytypic character in the senses discussed in chapter 3.

Comparative Causal Generalizations. In part because of the complexity of systems encountered in biology and medicine and also in part because of their variation, scientists working in biological and medical domains will frequently resort to what might be termed "qualitative" or "comparative" generalizations. These terms "qualitative" and "comparative" are distinguished from "quantitative" in the sense that Newton's law, F = ma, allows precise determination of one quantity if the others in the equation are known. An example of one such generalization from the Kandel example above is:

neurotransmitter $\uparrow$ → adenyl cyclase activity$\uparrow$ →
endogenous cAMP $\uparrow$ →   protein kinase activity $\uparrow$.[55]

The Epistemological Component

In a search for a general, flexible, yet empirical basis for the notion of causation, I think we may find some assistance if we look at several thinkers' speculations about how the concept *arises*. For Hart and Honoré, the central notion in causation is a generalization of our primitive experiences in the world:

Human beings have learnt, by making appropriate movements of their bodies, to bring about desired alterations in objects, animate or inanimate, in their environment, to express these simple achievements by transitive verbs like push, pull, bend, twist, break, injure. The process involved here consists of an initial immediate bodily manipulation of the thing affected and often takes little time. (1985, 28)

These experiences lead to a realization that secondary changes as a result of such movements can occur, and for such (a series of) changes "we use the correlative terms 'cause' and 'effect' rather than simple transitive verbs" (1985, 29). The root idea of cause for Hart and Honoré arises out of the way human action intrudes into a series of changes and *makes a difference* in the way a course of events develops (1959, 29 — also compare Mackie 1974 as quoted below, pp. 303, 305). Such a notion of "making a difference," these authors maintain, is as *central to causation* as is the notion of constant conjunction or invariable sequence stressed by Hume and by Mill. The concept of cause is also generalized by analogy to include not only active elements, but also static, passive, and even negative elements, such as the icy condition of the road causing an accident or the lack of rain causing a crop failure (Hart and Honoré 1985, 30–31).

This position bears some similarities to the work of Michotte (1963) on our basic "perception of causality" as well as to that of Anscombe (1971) and R. F. Holland (unpublished but cited by Mackie 1974, 133) on the way we come to learn to use common transitive causal verbs. Mackie also offers a like view when he discusses the source of the "causal priority" element of his analysis, noting:

It seems undeniable that this notion arises from our experience of our own active intervention in the world. If I *introduce* the change X into an apparent static situation and then the other change Y occurs, I not only see X as in the weak sense sufficient in the circumstances for Y, but also see X as causally prior to Y. (1974, 56–57)

Perhaps the most complex account of how our experiences give rise to our concept(s) of causation can be found in the work of R. G. Collingwood (1940). Collingwood developed a theory involving all of human history as a backdrop to his analysis of causation. For Collingwood, the most primitive notion of cause (sense I) involves those *human actions* by which we *cause another to act* by providing a *motive*. A second notion of cause (sense II) is equivalent to Mackie's interventional story quoted immediately above. Sense II, Collingwood contends, is the sense that "cause" has in "practical science," such as in medicine. It involves "manipulation" of nature, and is both anthropocentric and anthropomorphic, the latter because it resembles Collingwood's first sense of cause, where we manipulate other human beings.

A still third sense of cause for Collingwood (sense III) is that encountered in *theoretical* science (as distinguished from practical science). This sense requires both simultaneity of cause and effect and some form of spatial continuity.[56] Sense III appears to be related to the anthropomorphic aspects of the first two senses through the idea of God as bringing about (semianthromorphically) certain things in nature. Collingwood refers to Newton's approach to causation in physics, noting that, for Newton,

> it is perfectly clear that . . . the idea of causation is the idea of force, compulsion, constraint, exercised by something powerful over another thing which if not under this constraint would behave differently; this hypothetical different behavior being called by contrast 'free' behavior. This constraint of one thing in nature by another is the secondary causation of medieval cosmology. (1940, 325–326)

Collingwood believed that there was an important *developmental* relation among these three senses of cause: "the relation between these three senses of the word 'cause' is an historical relation: No. I being the earliest of the three, No. II a development from it, and No. III a development from that" (1940, 289). Though suggestive, I believe that Collingwood has gotten it wrong here, and that Hart and Honoré (and Mackie, Anscombe, and Holland) are closer to the truth in basing our notion of causation on simple primitive experiences of interaction with the world. I am prepared to accept the view that different notions of causation may be required to make sense of human interactions,[57] but I would still tend to side with Hart and Honoré and Mackie that it is Collingwood's second sense of causation that constitutes *the* root sense of this notion.

It should also be noted at this point that Mackie places much emphasis throughout his (1974) book on the need to utilize Mill's methods to establish empirically various causal sequences. For Mackie, Mill's method of difference has a special role to play in empirical warrants of causation. Mackie bases his naturalistic analysis of conditionals on the ability to envisage "alternative possible worlds" (1974, 52) using both primitive and sophisticated approaches. Imagination and analogy are primitive ways of grounding conditionals; Mill's method of difference is a sophisticated variant of this. This method has a certain type of priority for Mackie because "It is a contrast case rather than the repetition of like instances that contributes most to our primitive *conception* of causation." [58]

The upshot of this somewhat tangled set of suggestions that I have grouped under the *epistemological* component of my approach to causation is that the concept includes a number of differing senses, and that some of its senses and the warrants for its use are dependent on a complex set of learnings that may well have both social and historical as well as individual developmental aspects.

The Ontic Component and Process Metaphysics

In his (1984) monograph, Salmon writes: "One of the fundamental changes that I propose in approaching causality is to take processes rather than events as basic entities." Though Salmon explicitly states that he will not provide any rigorous definition of a "process," he does analogize his notion to Russell's "causal line," a "persistence of something" (Russell 1948, 459; Salmon 1984, 140). Salmon then goes on to develop his distinction between causal processes and pseudoprocesses, employing the "mark" method, and to introduce his "at-at" theory of causal propagation. (For Salmon, who follows Reichenbach on this point, a causal process is distinguished from a pseudoprocess because the former can be "marked" or altered and the causal process will carry (or more accurately is "capable" of carrying) this mark forward in time. Salmon's "at-at" theory characterizes the continuous process of a motion, e.g., a moving arrow is *at* a particular point of space *at* a paticular moment of time.)

Though Salmon's theory is attractive, I do not think that his "mark" method will suffice for us. There are a number of processes in biology and medicine for which we have not yet developed a means of "marking" the process but of which we nonetheless conceive as causal processes. A good example is to be found in the early stages of the development of the concept of the repressor (see chap. 4, p. 160).[59]

This notion of causation as being in some important sense associated with a *continuous* process is an element that can be found in rather different approaches to causation; it can be found, for example, in the writings of Collingwood.[60] A somewhat similar approach can be seen in Mackie's account of causation *in the objects:*

> We can now, at last, reply to the skeptical suggestion . . . that necessity$_1$, the distinguishing feature of causal sequences, cannot be observed. . . . [W]e can now offer a revised account of what causation is in the objects. If our speculations are correct, a singular causal sequence instantiates some pure law of working which is itself a form of partial persistence; the individual sequence therefore is, perhaps unobviously, identical with some process that has some qualitative or structural continuity, and that also incorporates the fixity relations which constitute the direction of causation. . . . This is the answer to the question, 'What is the producing that Hume did not see?' (1974, 229)

Mackie elaborated on this theme, writing: "What is called a causal mechanism is a process which underlies a regular sequence and each phase in which exhibits qualitative as well as spatio-temporal continuity" (1974, 222). Mackie also notes that "these continuities and persistence are an empirical counterpart of the rationalists' necessity." This natural necessity is exhibited or implemented by "laws of working" which, however, require induction and hypothesis testing in order to determine them; they cannot be found in any a priori manner. And Mackie adds that "laws of working are, in part, forms of persistence" (1974, 221). He holds:

> The natural necessity that does . . . the marking off of causal from noncausal regularities . . . we have located . . . first in the distinction of basic laws of working from collocations and mixed laws which involve collocations, and secondly in the qualitative and structural continuity which processes

that obey those basic laws seem to exhibit, in the fact that they are forms of partial persistence. (Mackie 1974, 228)

It is important to note that, just as Salmon (1989, 335) found that causal mechanisms and natural laws (or generalizations) cannot be completely sundered one from another, and that a process ontology was a key element in our understanding of causation, so Mackie also perceives the intertwining of mechanisms, laws, and processes:

> What is called a causal mechanism is a process which underlies a regular sequence and each phase in which exhibits qualitative as well as spatio-temporal continuity.... [Earlier] ... we considered the possibility that some causal mechanism or continuity of process might help to constitute causation in the objects; we have now found a place for it, particularly as constituting a sort of necessity that may belong to basic laws of working. (1974, 222–223)

Mackie thus links this process metaphysics back to his counterfactual analysis: inductive evidence is seen as supporting the laws which then justify the use of counterfactuals. He also links this view to the epistemological aspect of causation, suggesting that these "objective aspects of causation" are sometimes observed, citing the work of Michotte on our basic "perception of causality" as well as Anscombe's and Holland's views on the way we come to learn to use common transitive causal verbs (see above, p. 303).[61]

6.8 Probabilistic Extensions of Causal Explanation

In the sections immediately above I have stressed what might be termed more "deterministic" systems and the types of causal influences one might encounter in such systems. Biology and medicine, however, also encompass systems that exhibit probabilistic or stochastic behavior, and it will be important to extend the account above to cover such systems. This will also permit us to introduce some terminology that will be useful when we encounter "probabilistic causes" in our discussion of evolutionary theories in chapter 8.

The notion of probabilistic causation originated in Reichenbach's work (1956), but other philosophers of science such as

Good (1961, 1962) and Suppes (1970) have developed similar ideas, and still others have provided extensive criticism of such concepts, among them Salmon (1980). Suppes's approach to probabilistic causation is perhaps the most widely known and is worth a few comments. Suppes introduces his notion of a probabilistic cause through the idea of a *prima facie* cause defined in the following way:

The event $B_{t'}$ is a prima facie cause of the event A_t if and only if:
1) $t' < t$
2) $P(B_{t'}) > 0$
3) $P(A_t | B_{t'}) > P(A_t)$
where t denotes time. (Suppes 1970, 12)

Further elaboration of the notion is required so that "spurious" causes occasioned by some common cause producing an artifactual association between two variables are eliminated, and such extensions of the concept can be found in Suppes (1970). Both Reichenbach's and Suppes's proposals still encounter a number of problems, however, including that of the improbable alternative causal path—an issue about which I cannot comment at present but about which I have written elsewhere (in my 1983). There are also other conceptual difficulties associated with probabilistic causation—for an incisive review of these, see Salmon (1980) as well as Cartwright (1980), Skyrms (1980), Otte (1981), Eels and Sober (1983), and Sober (1984b, chap. 7).

I want to introduce a somewhat different approach to the notion of probabilistic causation which I believe is clearer and ultimately more coherent than Suppes's account. My approach will begin from some useful suggestions made by Giere (1980) concerning the relationship between determinism and probabilistic causation in populations. (Also see Sober 1982, Giere 1984, and Mayo 1986.) There are some distinctions that appear in Giere's account which are not explicit in most discussions of probabilistic causation. First, Giere differentiates between deterministic and stochastic systems but permits both types to exhibit probabilistic causal relationships. This is important since it distinguishes two different ways in which determinism may fail to hold for populations, for reasons described in the next paragraph. This is useful for the present inquiry because it licenses a more coherent fit between causation in deterministic, physiologically characterized biological systems and those which we might encounter in evolutionary situations (or in risk factor analysis), though it does not exclude stochastic components in physiological processes. Giere also invokes a "propensity" interpretation of probability for stochastic systems, maintaining that this gives a means of directly attributing probabilistic causality to individuals rather than to populations. In my view, the propensity interpretation is needed only for irreducible, singular, nondeterministic causation, which, though it may have much to recommend it in quantum mechanical situations, is less clearly demanded in biomedical contexts.

In Giere's analysis of deterministic systems, a causal relation between C and E is not necessarily a universal relation. The entities in Giere's account are individual deterministic systems that *can differ in their constitution* (though we may not be aware of all of their differences), so that different individuals in a class with the same causal input C may or may not exhibit E. Furthermore, since E may come about from a different cause than C, some individuals may exhibit E without having had C as a causal input. An example that Giere often uses is the relation between smoking and lung cancer, but one could imagine any biological population in which a causal factor(s) was involved and in which there was a nondeterministic outcome; evolving populations subject to varying, environmentally based influences (or "forces") are a natural application for Giere's approach.

For a population of deterministic systems, some number of individuals with input C will manifest E, and some will not. An actual population can be examined to yield a relative frequency, #E/N, where N is the number of the individuals in the population and #E the number of individuals exhibiting effect E. This fraction has the properties of a probability (though not a propensity). This is because, for any given individual in the (deterministic) population, a universal law L(C) = E is either true or false, depending on their individual constitutions.

Giere prefers to use "counterfactual populations" for which outcomes are well defined. This raises some complexities of interpretation, but these are not issues that will concern us in this book.[62] Thus, by hypothesis, two populations that are counterfactual counterparts of an actual population of interest are envis aged, and one is provided with causal factor input C and the other with input C. Each counterfactual population will exhibit some number of effects #E which will be less than its N. On the basis of this definition, Giere further defines a positive causal factor:

C is a positive causal factor for E in [population] U if and only if:

$P_C(E) > P_{\sim C}(E)$. (1980, 264)

Here P_C and $P_{\sim C}$ refer to the probability in the sense of a relative frequency. A reversed inequality will yield a definition of a negative causal factor, E, and equality will indicate causal irrelevance.

Note that this notion of a positive causal factor is almost identical to the definition given earlier for a prima facie cause in Suppes's system. What is different is the interpretation in the context of explicitly *deterministic* systems and an explicitly *counterfactual* account.

Giere also introduces a measure of effectiveness of C for E in population U,[63] namely:

$Ef(C,E) = Df. P_C(E) - P_{\sim C}(E)$.

These notions, developed in the context of deterministic systems, can be extended to stochastic systems, where Giere notes that "the interesting thing about stochastic systems is that we can speak of positive and negative causal factors for individual systems and not just for populations" (1980, 265). Giere's counterfactual definition (again we say counterfactual because system S may or may not *actually* have C or C as input) is:

C is a positive causal factor for E in S if and only if:

$Pr_C(E) > Pr_{\sim C}(E)$

where now Pr refers to a probability in the sense of a propensity (an inherent objective tendency) of the stochastic individual system. For nonquantum mechanical-level systems (which includes just about any biomedical system discussed in this book), we should not have to invoke the somewhat obscure concept of a propensity, and we can utilize Reichenbach's (1949) notion of a "weight" as a means to apply a relative, frequency-based probability to a stochastic individual system.

We can now generalize the notion of the semantic biomedical system (BMS) introduced earlier in connection with explanation (see p. 294), and extend the more traditionally causal properties to include probabilistically causal influences. I think that the clearest way to do this is to show the need for the extension by introducing an example from neurobiology which *explains* how nerve stimulation *causes* muscular contraction.

Suppose we want an account of how a nerve can stimulate a muscle on which it impinges to contract. The standard view accepted by all neurobiologists is that the signal for contraction is carried by chemical neurotransmitter molecules that are *probabilistically released* from the nerve endings in packets or "quanta," and that these quanta diffuse across the neuromuscular junction space and cause the opening of microscopic channels on the muscular side, resulting in an electrical signal that causes muscle contraction. Furthermore, "fluctuations in release [of the quanta] from trial to trial can be accounted for by binomial statistics . . . [and w]hen the release probability p is small . . . the Poisson distribution provides a good description of the fluctuations" (Kuffler, Nicholls, and Martin 1984, 257). If this is the case, "release of individual quanta from the nerve terminal . . . [is thus] similar to shaking marbles out of a box" through a small hole (1984, 254). Such a model of a probabilistic process yields excellent agreement with what is observed in a variety of micro-experiments at the neuromuscular junction, involving neural signals that cause muscular contractions. It also illustrates how well-characterized, probabilistically causal generalizations can be appealed to in explanations. Thus (partially) stochastic BMSs involving Σs specifying release probabilities for neurotransmitters can be invoked as explanations of such phenomena as neuromuscular contraction. Such BMSs represent a natural extension of the simpler causal BMSs introduced on page 294.

This is as much of an introduction to probabilistic causation as we need when we encounter the concept again in chapter 8. The important thing to realize is that the account given above is coherent with the causal analysis and with the Salmonian orientation elaborated in the earlier sections of this chapter. "Probabilistic causality" does not introduce a *new* notion of causation, and the expression is not an oxymoron. The notion is complex, however, and has generated a large literature to which the reader must be referred for additional details.[64]

6.9 Unification and Pragmatic Approaches to Explanation

In this section I want to examine fairly briefly two significant competitors to the overlap causal/mechanical account I defended in sections 6 and 7. In my discussion of Salmon's search for consensus and rapprochement earlier (p. 295), I briefly referred to Friedman's (1974) and Kitcher's (1981; 1989) views that scientific explanation is best conceived of as unification, and it is to Kitcher's recent extensive account of this position that I now turn.

6.9.1 *Kitcher on Unification*

For Kitcher:

> successful explanations earn that title because they belong to a set of explanations, the *explanatory store*, and . . . the fundamental task of a theory of explanation is to specify the conditions on the explanatory store. Intuitively, the explanatory store associated with science at a particular time contains those derivations which collectively provide the best systematization of our beliefs . . . and I shall suppose that the criterion for systematization is unification. (1989, 430 and 431)

This approach is derivational in a Hempelian sense, but with additional constraints. The main constraint is based on the intuition that explanation yields scientific understanding by somehow *reducing the number of facts that one needs to take as brute* (Friedman 1974, 18). The difficulty lies in just how one can formally specify a criterion for the number of facts (or laws) that is not subject to facile counterexamples (see Kitcher 1976). Kitcher, as part of his response to this problem, appeals to the notion of an "argument pattern," which we have already seen constitutes a part of his metascientific unit of a "practice."[65]

In his 1989, Kitcher spells out in considerable detail what are the general features of these argument patterns and also provides a number of specific examples of such patterns. I find this approach suggestive and consistent with certain aspects of theory structure and explanations in biology and medicine. I do not, however, find enough fine structure in Kitcher's notion of "practice" (or its component "argument patterns") to enable it to account for the complexity of interlevel interactions and detailed case-based scientific progress. In contrast to the temporally extended version of the account of theory structure I elaborated in earlier chapter 5, I find it lacks sufficient detail in its present schematic form to account for "high fidelity" historical case development.[66] I do not doubt that Kitcher's account could be extended to provide such additional fine structure, but I also believe that, in his overly positivistic attempt to avoid the metaphysics which the alternative causal/mechanical approach to explanation requires (see section 7), Kitcher is deflected away from a causal model and thus captures only a small part—though a very important part—of the explanatory structures in biology and medicine.

6.9.2 *Van Fraassen's Analysis of Explanations as Answers to "Why-Questions"*

Earlier I discussed some of van Fraassen's concerns with the traditional Hempelian model of explanation and cited van Fraassen's view that perhaps something like a modified Aristotelian approach would indicate a way out of those problems. In his book, published about three years after the article developing those Aristotelian speculations, however, van Fraassen (1980) largely went in a different, more pragmatic direction.[67] He does nonetheless continue to subscribe to the view that explanations should not be conceived of as not part of science proper but rather as reflecting various pragmatic interests and desires of humans. He writes, reiterating this pragmatic theme:

> Scientific explanation is not (pure) science but an application of science. It is a use of science to satisfy certain of our desires; and these desires are quite specific in a specific context, but they are desires for descriptive information. . . . The exact content of the desire, and the evaluation of how well it is satisfied, varies from context to context. It is not a single desire, the same in all cases, for a very special

> sort of thing, but rather, in each case, a different desire for something of a quite familiar sort. (van Fraassen 1980, 156)

More specifically:

> An explanation is not the same as a proposition, or an argument, or list of propositions; it is an *answer* ... An explanation is an answer to a why-question. So a theory of explanation must be a theory of why-questions. (1980, 134)[68]

In van Fraassen's model:

> The why-question Q expressed by an interrogative in a given context will be determined by three factors:
>
> The *topic* P_k
> The *contrast-class* $X = \{P_1, \ldots, P_i, \ldots\}$
> The *relevance relation* R
>
> and, in a preliminary way, we may identify the abstract why-question with the triple consisting of these three:
>
> $Q = (P_k, X, R)$
>
> A proposition A is called *relevant to* Q exactly if A bears relation R to the couple (P_k, X). (1980, 142–143)

Here the topic is what Hempel and others have called the explanandum (or a description of the event to be explained), and the contrast class is understood, following the unpublished work of Hanson which van Fraassen cites, to be the set of alternatives, fixed by the context, from which the topic is being selected. For example, when one asks "Why did a sample of heated copper placed in cool water reach equilibrium at 22.5°C?" contrast case can be at any other temperature than 22.5°C (though the contrast *could* in some different context be with reading *equilibrium* rather than, say, oscillating about a mean temperature). According to van Fraassen, a direct answer to the why-question Q is of the form "P_k *in contrast to* (the rest of) X *because* A" (1980, 143). It should be noted that, for van Fraassen, P_k is *true*, and that all P_i, where $i \neq k$, are *false*.

The relation R is not explicitly well defined by van Fraassen, a point that has convinced Kitcher and Salmon (1988) and Salmon (1989) that there is a fatal flaw in van Fraassen's account. R is clearly more than statistical relevance, since van Fraassen writes "*the context . . . determines relevance* in a way that goes well beyond the statistical relevance, about which our scientific theories give information" (1980, 129).

Presumably, relevance may be partially unpacked in van Fraassen's evaluation procedure (though, since he accepts Belnap's erotetic logic—a formal "logic of questions"—which contains a characterization of erotetical relevance, a partially erotetic logical elaboration of relevance is not to be completely excluded). I suggest that the evaluation process may help us generally triangulate on relevance because it is through evaluation that one more formally takes into account the comparative strengths of competing explanations, though I agree with Kitcher and Salmon (1988) that without a more developed set of restrictions on the relevance relation the account is seriously incomplete.

For van Fraassen, the evaluation of answers is an important part of a theory of explanation. Explanation evaluation is demanded according to van Fraassen because "[t]he main problems of the philosophical theory of explanation are to account for legitimate rejections of explanation requests, and for the asymmetries of explanation." Evaluation involves three judgments. The first is an evaluation of a preferred answer, say A, in the light of a background theory and background information K. K itself is determined (at least in part) by the context in which the question arises. (This, however, seems to me to give too much to context, for, as noted in chapter 2, the discipline in which a new theory is developed as a solution to a problem is quite generally and objectively significantly constrained by the recent history and current state of that discipline. These constraints involve much of van Fraassen's K, but they are largely independent of subjective interests and exercise considerable constraints over acceptable answers.)

Van Fraassen's second and third components of evaluation involve comparative assessments.[69] Van Fraassen introduces these components as follows:

The second concerns the extent to which A *favors* the topic B as against the other members of the contrast class. (This is where Hempel's criterion of giving reasons to expect, and Salmon's criterion of statistical relevance may find application.) The third concerns the comparison of *Because A* with other possible answers to the same question; and this has three aspects. The first is whether A is more probable (in view of K); the second whether it favours the topic to a greater extent; and the third, whether it is made wholly or partially irrelevant by other answers that could be given. (To this third aspect, Salmon's considerations about *screening off* apply.) Each of these three main ways of evaluation needs to be made more precise.

The first is of course the simplest: we rule out *Because A* altogether if K implies the denial of A; and otherwise ask what probability K bestows on A. (1980, 146–147)

Each of these points is elaborated on further by van Fraassen. I shall comment on only a few of his suggestions. First, the notion of favoring is one which admits of a probabilistic interpretation. Specifically, some subset of K is constructed which deletes the topic's (and the contrast core's) truth (and falsity) predicate(s). (This is to eliminate begging the question and thus trivializing the explanatory scheme. The problem is reminiscent of the difficulty with using old evidence in Bayesian conformation, encountered in chapter 5, and may well involve an appeal to counterfactual considerations. Exactly how to specify K(Q) — the background knowledge associated with the why-question Q — generally is not indicated by van Fraassen.) Then we examine how well answer A supports topic B in comparison with its contrast class C,D, . . . , N by evaluating the prior and posterior probabilities:

Let us call the probability in the light of K(Q) alone the PRIOR probability (in this context) and the probability given K(Q) plus A the POSTERIOR probability. Then A will do best here if the posterior probability of B equals 1. If A is not thus, it may still do well provided it shifts the mass of the probability function toward B; for example, if it raises the probability of B while lowering that of C, . . . , N; or if it does not lower the probability of B while lowering that of some of its closest competitors. (1980, 147–148)

Note that this way of proceeding is congruent with the comparative Bayesian approach developed above in chapter 5.

Finally, we compare various answers, and it is here that some complex problems of "screening off" may arise. Van Fraassen points out that a simple and straightforward application of the screening-off criterion may do a disservice and is cautious about the use of the criterion.[70] Van Fraassen's view then seems to suggest that explanation is *doubly comparative:* for a given answer A one compares the probability of P_k to its alternatives, and one compares answers A, A', and soon in connection with P_k *and* its alternatives. This is a useful suggestion and it is one that has implications for difficulties some philosophers of biology have detected with evolutionary explanations, as I shall discuss in chapter 7.

This doubly comparative component of explanation has, I think, some evidence that will support it. An inspection of scientific research papers developing explanatory models (see, for example, Jacob and Monod 1961 and Frost, Clark, and Kandel 1988) will disclose frequent reference to van Fraassen's third evaluational component, and occasional (perhaps largely implicit) use of his second comparative evaluational component.

Though I am in agreement with van Fraassen that scientific explanation often has pragmatic elements, I believe that there are deductive and inductive structures *intrinsic* to science which represent explanatory relations. The search for causal mechanisms and for generalizations (even though they may have a narrow scope in biology and medicine) that organize and unify (in either Salmonian or Kitcherean senses) their sciences seems sufficiently central to scientific inquiry that I cannot fully subscribe to van Fraassen's position, which denies that explanations exist *within* basic science. I also find van Fraassen's attempt to develop his model only in terms of "why-questions" insufficiently defended (also see Salmon 1989, 141–142 for specific problems with "why-questions"). What is useful in the van Fraassen account is what may also be its weakness: its generalization of the relevance relation so that causal, statistical, or (appropriately interpreted) deductive (or even intentional) connections may satisfy it, as, for example, in the Tower and the Shadow story (1980, 132–134). (In this brief story, van Fraassen indicates how different contexts will determine different explanations, specifically showing how an account which does explain the height of an object in terms of its shadow can (contra Bromberger) be devised.) Also attractive and, I think, defensible is its more general account of evaluation; I see this account as in good accord with the Bayesian perspective developed in chapters 5 and 6.

Van Fraassen's approach, particularly when interpreted as an important pragmatic aspect of the causal generalization model of explanation argued for earlier, offers answers to several traditional conundra in the area of scientific explanation. As van Fraassen notes, the famous Scriven paresis example becomes explicable if one understands that the contrast cases may vary so that syphilis *is* an explanation of paresis in one context with one set of contrast cases (nonsyphilitic) but not in another context (where the comparison is with other syphilitics) (see van Fraassen, 1980, 128). The causal element in van Fraassen and also in the causal generalization model proposed earlier yields the types of asymmetries that block such counterexamples as those concerning Scriven's barometer and also Bromberger's flagpole.[71] The issue of how best to understand the pragmatic aspect in scientific explanations is one of the concerns underlying van Fraassen's theory. It seems to me, however, as I believe it does also to Kitcher (1989) and Salmon (1989), that a proposal developed by Railton can handle this problem better than a thoroughgoing pragmatic analysis.

6.9.3 *Railton's Concept of the "Ideal Explanatory Text"*

Railton (1980) has proposed that we distinguish between an "ideal explanatory text" and "explanatory information." For some explanandum, the ideal explanatory text would provide *all* the causal and nomic connections that are relevant to its occurrence—it tells the "whole story" (Railton 1980, 247). This text would be, in Salmon's words, "brutally large and complicated" but would contain "all of the objective aspects of the explanation; it is not affected by pragmatic considerations" (1989, 159 and 161). In contrast, when we consider "explanatory information," pragmatic considerations become supremely relevant: here context, interests, and background knowledge govern what aspects of the ideal explanatory text *will be selected*. This suggestion of Railton's, then, would appear to offer a means of achieving a "rapprochement" between an objective construal of explanation and that which has been characterized by the pragmatic theories such as van Fraassen's.

In addition, Salmon (1989) usefully suggests that the "ideal explanatory text" might provide a means of effecting a similar rapprochement between the causal/mechanical approach and the unification approach to explanation. Either top-down or bottom-up approaches can be taken in selecting different aspects of the "ideal explanatory text." In the context of biology and medicine, we can frequently see something like this happen when there are different theories that can capture the same phenomenon at different levels of detail. As I have pointed out above, however, a higher-level vocabulary can also represent a causal sequence.

6.9.4 *The Meshing of Different Levels of Detail in the Ideal Explanatory Text*

This capture of the same phenomenon at different levels of detail in point of fact is what frequently happens in the area of genetics. Recall question (3) posed at the beginning of this chapter:

(3) Why does the pattern of color coats in mice in the F2 generation, whose grandparents are both agouti (a grayish pattern) with genotype AaBb, follow a 9 : 3 : 4 ratio (9/16 = agouti; 3/16 = black; 4/16 = albino)?[72]

The answer to this question that can (and has) been given in genetics texts involves a phenomenon known as epistasis, in which one gene par can "hide" the expression of another, thus causing a deviation from the (simpler) Mendelian phenotypic ratio of 9 : 3 : 3 : 1, which holds for pairs of independently assorting genes in the absence of gene interactions. This 9 : 3 : 3 : 1 ratio is widely known as Mendel's second law (see Watson et al. 1987, 10–11). The "Mendelian" explanation is "probabilistic" and assumes independent assortment of the gene pairs, but with the added assumption that one gene pair in a homozygous recessive state is epistatic to the other. Thus a probability distribution in which aa is expected (where A is any color dominant over albino [a] and B is the agouti color dominant over black [b]) four out of the 16 times will account for the 4/16 albino ratio.[73] If we examine the 16 possible combinations of two gene pairs ranging from AABB through aabb, the phenotypes associated with pairs aaBB aaBb and aaBb will be found to be albino, in addition to the expected albino double pair aabb. This is explained by the fact that the aa pair blocks the appearance of any color controlled by the B (or b) genes. Strickberger provides a simplified developmental schema for this type of epistatic interaction:

> In developmental terms, we may envisage the appearance of color in this example as arising from two sequential processes, the first of which is controlled by gene A and the other by gene B. When the first process is inhibited (by aa), the second process cannot occur.
>
> original   A gene ↓   intermediate   B gene ↓
> substance ——————————> substance ——————————> color
>   1st process   2nd process

(Strickberger 1976, 204)

The other color distributions follow similarly. Though a probabilistic distribution is used here, geneticists viewed the color distributions as being "caused" by genes, and in addition viewed the probabilistic distribution of the genes to progeny as a consequence of the causal sequences involved in meiosis, which can be treated as resulting in a partially random segregation of genes. This view of probabilistic causation is coherent and is an instance of the probabilistic extensions of causation discussed in section 8.

Such an explanation as given did not long satisfy geneticists, however, who set about providing a more detailed molecular level biosynthetic pathway (and also a molecular causal sequence) account of such patterns. Figure 6.8 depicts an example of the effects of different color coat genes in the mouse that are thought to act on pigment cells, showing a series of biosynthetic pathways in which an epistatic gene blocks further melanin synthesis. The explanation provides additional, deterministically causal details in a process that continues to be described as partially stochastic and partially deterministic.

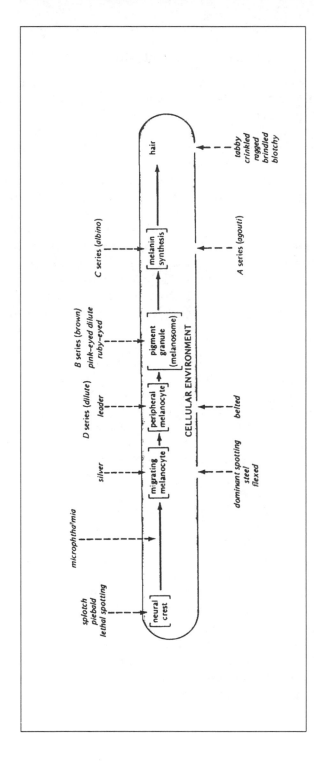

Figure 6.8.   Developmental stages at which coat color genes in the mouse are believed to act. The upper part of the figure shows genes that probably act directly on the pigment cells, and the lower part shows genes that may act on the environment of these cells. Reprinted from Strickberger, 1976, after Searle, 1968.

6.10 Summary and Conclusion

In this chapter I have discussed a number of features that have been couched in terms of a detailed example of explanation in biology; in subsequent chapters this approach will be applied to additional domains and examples, both to test it and to illustrate it within other contexts. The recurrent theme regarding explanation in this chapter has been the appeal to (possibly probabilistic) *causal model systems which instantiate generalizations of both broad and narrow scope of application*. We found that both the Hempelian model of scientific explanation and Salmon's earlier S-R account suffered from defects which an appeal to causation could remedy. We also showed, by means of an extended example from the neurosciences, how such causation is appealed to by working scientists and how complex and interlevel the explanans may be in various biological contexts. In order to ground the causal/mechanical type of model, we examined logical, epistemological, and metaphysical components of causation, in the process showing that an intertwined mechanism and generalization "overlap" model of explanation, which was heavily indebted to Salmon's recent theory, was the most defensible. Finally, we touched on some recent alternative accounts of explanation, including Kitcher's unification view and van Fraassen's pragmatic analysis, providing several arguments, in part based on Railton's notion of an ideal explanatory text, that viable aspects of those models could be conceived of as congruent with our preferred approach.

The account of explanation I have developed in this chapter can also be summarized in terms of a model with six components, E1 through E6:

(E1) represents the *Semantic (or BMS) Component*: In conformity with the analysis of scientific theory elaborated in chapter 3, I introduced the notion of a theoretical model as a type of system whose characteristics were given by an explicit definition comprising a series of generalizations Σ, the conjunction of these assumptions was termed Π, and this constituted a "biomedical system" or BMS. Any given system that is being investigated or appealed to as explanatory of some explanandum, say some sentence describing an experimental result, is such a BMS if and only if it satisfies (in the logical sense of "satisfies") Π. We understand Π then as implicitly defining a kind of natural system. There may not be any actual system which is a realization of the complex expression Π. To claim that some particular system satisfies Π is a theoretical hypothesis which may or may not be true. If it is true, then the BMS can serve as an explanandum of a phenomenon. If the theoretical hypothesis is potentially true and/or supported to a greater or lesser degree, then it is a potential and/or well-supported explanation. This component thus yokes an account of explanation fairly tightly to a semantic conception of scientific theory.

(E2) I developed the *Causation Component* as two subcomponents: (a) deterministic causation and (b) probabilistic causation. I argued that explanations in biology and medicine are typically causal, and the predicates that appear in a BMS involve such *causal* properties as "phosphorylation" and "binds to," as well as statements that a process "causes" or "results in" some event. Probabilistic causation was illustrated in the example describing neurotransmitter release at the neuromuscular junction and also in the example of color coat determination.

(E3) *The Unificatory Component.* Though appeals to causation are frequently (and typically) involved in explanation, some BMSs might involve generalizations that are statements of "coexistence" or generalizations which indicates that certain quantities vary together without specifying clearly a causal direction. In such cases it seems reasonable to appeal to another aspect of explanation and accept as scientifically legitimate BMSs which "unify" domains of phenomena. In general, I viewed these explanations as provisional surrogates for deeper causal explanations.

(E4) *The Logical Component.* I suggested that connections between a BMS and an explanandum will frequently be recastable in terms of deductive logic (with the proviso that the generalizations in the BMS will typically be causal and thus that the explanandum would be construable as following as a "causal consequence" from the premises in the BMS). In addition, where the BMS involves some probabilistic assumption and the explanandum is a singular (or a collection of singular) events(s), the logical connection will have to be one of inductive support.[74]

(E5) *The Comparative Evaluation Inductive Component.* In conformity with the personal probability perspective developed in chapter 5, I view any inductive support appearing in explanations in Bayesian terms. The notion of support outlined in this chapter was also construed as "doubly comparative," in van Fraassen's sense: for a given explanation one compares (often implicitly) an explanandum with its contrast class in terms of the support provided, and one also (perhaps only implicitly) compares rival explanations for that explanandum.

(E6) *The Ideal Explanatory Text Background Component.* Following Railton, I accepted the notion of an "ideal" explanatory text from which specific explanations were selected. In general, explanations that are actually given are but partial aspects of a much more complete story, and those aspects that are focused on are frequently affected by pragmatic interests.

In the three chapters that follow, this model of explanation involving assumptions (E1)–(E6) will be further elaborated and applied to examples from evolutionary theory and molecular genetics and to issues in the context of requests for "functional" explanations in immunology.

CHAPTER SEVEN

Historicity, Historical Explanations, and Evolutionary Theory

7.1 Introduction

IN THE PREVIOUS CHAPTER a general model of explanation which would cover both probabilistic and deterministic systems was elaborated. As I noted at the beginning of chapter 6, there are several different types of "why questions" to which different kinds of explanations might be provided. In this chapter I examine "historical" explanations which have been claimed to have a distinctive character, permissible in the biomedical sciences, but not of the type characteristically found in the physical sciences.

A number of biologists and philosophers of biology have maintained that there is something logically and explanatorially idiosyncratic about the role of both history and the historical explanations which one finds in the biomedical sciences. For example, the molecular geneticist Max Delbruck claimed:

> The complex accomplishment of any one living cell is part and parcel of the first-mentioned feature, that any one cell represents more an historical than a physical event. These complex things do not rise every day by spontaneous generation from the non-living matter—if they did, they would really be reproducible and timeless phenomena, comparable to the crystallization of a solution, and would belong to the subject matter of physics proper. No, any living cell carries with it the experiences of a billion years of experimentation by its ancestors. You cannot expect to explain so wise an old bird in a few simple words. (In Blackburn 1966, 119)

325

The evolutionary theorist G. G. Simpson associates a historical process with complexity and consequently nonmechanistic *uniqueness*:

Physical or mechanistic laws depend on the existence of an immediate set of conditions, usually in rather simple combinations, which can be repeated at will and which are adequate in themselves to determine a response or result. In any truly historical process, the determining conditions are far from simple and are not immediate or repetitive. Historical cause embraces the *totality* of preceding events. Such a cause can never be repeated, and it changes from instant to instant. Repetition of some factors still would not be a repetition of historical causation. The mere fact that similar conditions have occurred twice and not once would make an essential difference, and the materials and reagents (such as the sorts of existing organisms in the evolutionary sequence) would be sure to be different in some respects. (1964, 186)

The important role of history in assessing the nature of evolutionary theory has also been recently emphasized by Burian:

in assessing the directions in which evolutionary biology is headed, I will emphasize a characteristic of evolutionary theory which I think is of great importance in thinking about its future: namely its peculiarly *historical* character. I claim that a full appreciation of the nature of historical theories, historical reasoning, and their role in evolutionary biology ought to shape much of our thinking about the relation of evolutionary biology to other branches of biology and to the sciences more generally. (1989, 149)

Ernst Mayr, a distinguished scholar of evolutionary biology, approvingly cites the arguments of Goudge (to be elaborated below) and seems to believe that the lack of attention to the special features raised by historicity and historical processes in biology are part of a general insensitivity of philosophers steeped in the physical sciences. Mayr holds:

Philosophy of science, when first developed, was firmly grounded in physics, and more specifically in mechanics, where processes and events can be explained as the consequences of specific laws, with prediction symmetrical to causation. History-bound scientific phenomena, by contrast, do not fit well into this conceptualization. (1982, 71)

Moreover, he adds:

Philosophers trained in the axioms of essentialistic logic seem to have great difficulty in understanding the peculiar nature of uniqueness and of historical sequences of events. Their attempts to deny the importance of historical narrative or to axiomatize them in terms of covering laws fail to convince. (1982, 72)

Mayr wishes to introduce a distinction between a "proximate cause" and an "evolutionary cause." Generally, he suggests, "biology can be divided into the study of proximate causes, the subject of the physiological sciences (broadly conceived), and into the study of ultimate (evolutionary) causes, the subject matter of natural history" (1982, 67). Mayr tends to identify the proximate causes with physicochemical causes, and evolutionary causes with nonmechanistic explanations (see his 1982, 67–73). Interestingly, other philosophers of biology have discerned even in some examples of proximate causes a nonmechanistic historicity (or more accurately, a historicity that requires modes of explanation that are acceptable in biology but weaker than the deductive-nomological type of explanation characteristic of the mechanistic sciences). Considerable discussion has occurred concerning "historical" types of explanations in embryology, specifically whether this kind of "historical" development is similar to or different from evolutionary or "phylogenetic" explanations. Philosophers such as Woodger, Gallie, and Beckner have taken different positions on the issue. Woodger, like Mayr, perceives a difference between embryological and phylogenetic explanations. Gallie does not, but Beckner does. Beckner, however, sees the problem differently from Woodger (and possibly from Mayr). It is to these debates that I shall turn in a moment.[1] Before examining the details of these arguments, however, it will be useful for the reader to have a brief overview of how the main thesis of this chapter will be developed.

The main thesis of the present chapter is that historical explanations are logically embraced by the account of explanation given in the previous chapter, but that epistemologically they are typically *weak* explanations. This is because they are empirically *data-deficient* in comparison to other forms of explanation we encounter in biology and medicine. I extract what I argue are the defensible elements in the work of Gallie, Goudge, and Beckner with respect to their classical discussions of this type of explanation and then develop one of the best-supported examples to be found in evolutionary biology, concerning the shift in prevalence of the sickle-cell trait in African-Americans in comparison with their African ancestors. I then consider the nature of the empirical weakness of this explanation and compare and contrast the position in this chapter with older views of Scriven and more recent accounts of Sober, Horan, and Brandon, locating the thesis of this chapter within the spectrum of views about historical and evolutionary explanations in contemporary philosophy of biology.

7.2   Models of Historical Explanation in Biology

The logical core of the debates over "historical" explanations in the biomedical sciences resides in two theses, one of which has two subtheses. Each or all of these theses have been held by at least one of the proponents to be discussed below. (It should be added here that these "historical" explanations are often referred to as "genetic" explanations—not in that they relate to a theory of the gene, but rather because they cite a *genesis* or a developmental process.) The two core theses are that "historical" explanations or "genetic" explanations are:

(1) *nonnomological*, in that they do not utilize laws and initial conditions. This thesis can be further analyzed into (a) a weak nonnomological claim, to wit, that a genetic explanation is not *deductive*-nomological, or into (b) a stronger thesis, namely that a genetic explanation is *not analyzable as any species of "covering law" explanation*, for example as an inductive statistical or a statistical relevance explanation.

(2) *nonpredictive*, in that one can have a good explanation which nonetheless would not permit the explained event to be predicted. Sometimes this is further explicated by maintaining that the explanation explains by identifying a *necessary* condition but not one that is *sufficient* for an effect.

In analyzing these theses I will work backward from the positive claim that explanation occurs by virtue of necessary conditions toward the more global but negative claims that nonpredictability and nonnomologicality characterize explanations in the biomedical sciences.

7.2.1 *Gallie's Account*

In introducing his arguments for a distinctive model of explanation of historical events, the philosopher W. B. Gallie noted that: "historians . . . sometimes explain events . . . by referring to one or a number of temporally prior *necessary* conditions" (Gallie 1955, 161). These necessary conditions are events which, together with certain persistent factors, account for some temporal whole. Gallie believed that these historical explanations were found in evolutionary theory and also in embryology. For example, he cites Woodger's illustration of an explanation of "the tortuous course taken by a nerve or artery." "Such a course," Woodger wrote, "may strike us as strange and we seek an explanation . . . and we find one if it can be shown that in the course of individual development this state of affairs has been brought about by a shifting of the neighboring parts" (Woodger 1929, 394). This type of explanation is in point of fact found pervasively in embryological texts and in other areas of biology as well. For example, in accounting for the location of the phrenic nerves which innervate the diaphragm, Langman wrote in his *Medical Embryology*:

> Initially the septum transversum [which forms part of the diaphragm] lies opposite the cervical somites [near the head end of the embryo], and nerve components of the third, fourth, and fifth cervical segment of the spinal cord grow into the septum. At first the nerves, known as the phrenic nerves, pass to the septum through the pleuropericardial folds . . . this explains why, with the further expansion of the lungs and descent of the septum [as the embryo matures] they are located in the fibrous pericard[ium (i.e., in the fibrous sac surrounding the heart)]. . . . Hence, in the adult the phrenic nerves reach the diaphragm via the fibrous pericard[ium]. (1981, 148)

Such explanations are not restricted to "high levels of organization," as in this embryological example. In cytogenetics, for example, the central and critically important processes of mitosis (and meiosis) are similarly presented as a "genetic" sequence with successive, fairly well-defined stages termed prophase, metaphase, anaphase, and telophase, where the level of description oscillates between cell and organelle levels. Likewise, with respect to DNA and cell duplication in *E. coli*, though there are additional molecular and chemical levels that have been at least partly characterized, the *logic* of the genetic sequence is not fundamentally different.[2] (*Some* of the causal transitions in this last example do approach mechanistic sufficiency explanations, but not *all* transitions are so well understood.)

In Gallie's account of genetic or historical explanations a continuous development through time also plays an important role:

> The first prerequisite of a characteristically genetic explanation is that we shall recognize the *explicandum* as a temporal whole whose structure either contains certain persistent factors or else shows a definite direction of change or development. Thereupon we look for an antecedent event, the *explicans*, which can be accounted a *necessary condition* of the *explicandum, on ordinary inductive grounds (observations of analogous cases)* but more specifically on the ground of a probable continuity—in respect either of persistent factors or of direction of change—between explicans and explicandum. (1955, 166; my emphasis)

Gallie added that this temporal order often "has to be inferred . . . [e.g.,] certain aspects of an ovum's development are such that they cannot all be observed in any one particular instance" (1955, 16).

A common objection to Gallie's view of explanation as accounted for by necessary conditions is that necessary conditions per se generally do not explain. For example, as Ruse points out, if it is a necessary condition that I take a specific course for a college degree, this condition does not by itself explain my getting the degree. Furthermore, it has also been argued that *sets* of necessary conditions constitute more adequate explanations only insofar as they move toward sufficiency types of explanations (see Ruse 1973, 75–76 and Montefiori 1956 for further discussion on this objection). In fact, a close inspection of Gallie's account seems to suggest that *additional* "persistent factors are assumed," which may well constitute a movement toward a sufficiency explanation (though, as we shall see, Gallie denies this). Interestingly, Goudge's approach, which has a number of similarities to Gallie's, disavows the necessary condition thesis of historical explanation and substitutes a nonnomological *sufficiency* view of such explanations.

7.2.2 *Goudge's Integrating and Narrative Explanations*

In characterizing historical explanations in evolutionary theory, Goudge draws a distinction between (1) *integrating explanations,* in which homologies and vestiges are explained and integrated with a doctrine of descent, and (2) *narrative explanations,* in which singular events of evolutionary importance are analyzed. In my view, the similarities in logic between both types of explanation are more critical than whether such a nonnomological and non-predictive model of causal explanation is applied to individual cases or to general cases. In my treatment of Goudge, I shall focus on his account of narrative explanations, and readdress the issue of the "integrating explanation" later in this chapter.

In evolution, according to Goudge, narrative explanation

> consists not in deducing the event from a law or set of laws, but in proposing an intelligible sequence of occurrences such that the event to be explained 'falls into place' as the terminal phase of it. The event ceases to be isolated and is connected in an orderly way with states of affairs which led up to it. Thus the explanation is an historical one. . . . We can consider [the reasoning] as formulating by means of a pattern of statements a complex sufficient condition of the event to be explained. (1961, 72–73)

Goudge characterizes a "complex sufficient condition" as follows:

> Each of certain factors n_1, n_2, n_3, . . . , is a necessary condition of E_1, and each of C_1, C_2, $C3$, . . . , is a contingent contributory condition of E. The complete set of necessary conditions together with at least one contingent contributory condition, constitute a sufficient condition of E. That is to say there are several different *complex sufficient conditions* S_1, S_2, S_3 of E or as it is usually put, a plurality of causes of E. (Goudge 1961, 63; my emphasis)

Goudge cites Romer's 1941 explanation of amphibian development of limbs and adoption of terrestrial life as an example of this type of reasoning. This example and others like it constitute speculative "likely stories," constrained by the gappy evolutionary fossil record but open to diverse imaginative scenarios.[3] Romer wrote:

> Why should the amphibians have developed these limbs and become potential land-dwellers? Not to breathe air, for that could be done by merely coming to the surface of the pool. Not because they were driven out in search of food, for they were fish-eating types for which there was little food to be had on land. Not to escape enemies, for they were among the largest animals of the streams and pools of that day.
>
> The development of limbs and the consequent ability to live on land seem, paradoxically, to have been adaptations for remaining in the water, and true land life seems to have been, so to speak, only the result of a happy accident. . . .
>
> The Devonian, the period in which the amphibians originated, was a time of seasonal droughts. At times the streams would cease to flow. . . . If the water dried up altogether and did not soon return . . . the amphibian, with his newly-developed land limbs, could crawl out of the shrunken pool where he might take up his aquatic existence again. Land limbs were developed to reach the water, not to leave it.
>
> Once this development of limbs had taken place, however, it is not hard to imagine how true land life eventually resulted. Instead of immediately taking to the water again, the amphibian might learn to linger about the drying pools and devour stranded fish. Insects were already present and would afford the beginnings of a diet for a land form. Later, plants were taken up as a source of food supply. . . . Finally, through these various developments, a land fauna would have been established. (Romer 1941, 47–48, quoted by Goudge 1961, 71.)

One can see several necessary conditions proposed in the above scenario, such as seasonal droughts, and also contributory conditions, such as the availability of food was available on dry land. Note that the explanation constitutes a temporal sequence which selects as relevant certain specific necessary or contributory conditions. Like Gallie (1955) and Dray (1957) before him, Goudge is providing an account of what he calls a "narrative explanation" in which no *laws* are presented, and yet (for Goudge) one in which a complex sufficient condition makes the explanandum intelligible.

The question raised by Goudge's account (and his example from Romer) is whether this explanation actually constitutes a *sufficiency* explanation. To Gallie, who employs a similar example (also cited by Woodger) from Darwin's On the *Origin of Species*, the answer is no. It will be instructive to look at his argument on this point.

7.2.3   Gallie and Goudge Redux

Gallie was aware that his model of genetic explanation might be turned into a sufficient condition explanation and in his essay termed such a metamorphosis misleading and fallacious, even though the fallacy was committed by a number of scientists. He wrote that the fallacy arises because scientists, adhering consciously or unconsciously to the view that only predictive or "sufficiency" explanations genuinely explain, are tempted to believe when they arrive at a perfectly good, characteristically genetic explanation that it must be, or ought to be, or anyhow — if valid and useful — can easily be translated into an explanation of predictive or quasi-predictive pattern (1955, 168).

Gallie disagrees that this translation can be done, offering as support for his view an example from Darwin. This same example was also discussed by Woodger as an illustration of a historical explanation (Woodger 1929, 401–402). In On the *Origin of Species*, Darwin proposed the following explanation of the long necks of giraffes:

> That the individuals of the same species often differ slightly in the relative lengths of all their parts may be seen in many works of natural history, in which careful measurements are given.

Darwin then goes on to point out that, although these differences are of no importance to most species,

> it will have been otherwise with the nascent giraffe, considering its probable habits of life; for those individuals which had some one part of several parts of their bodies rather more elongated than usual, would generally have survived. These will have intercrossed and left offspring, either inheriting the same bodily peculiarities, or with a

tendency to vary again in the same manner; whilst the individuals, less favored in the same respects, will have been most liable to perish.

. . . the individuals which were the highest browsers and were able during dearths to reach even an inch or two above the others, will often have been preserved; for they will have roamed over the whole country in search of food. (Woodger 1929, 400–401, quoting Darwin 1906, 277)

This is, both Woodger and Gallie point out, an extraordinarily speculative explanation, and Gallie agrees with Woodger that "no one in fact knows the detailed characters of the environments within which possession of longer and longer necks is supposed to have been advantageous" (Gallie 1955, 169). However, there is much more that would be required in order to obtain a *sufficiency* explanation from the giraffe example, and Gallie suggests:

Perhaps more pertinent is the fact that variations in this respect must in all cases have called for a vast number of minute adjustments in other organs, without which this variation—or rather this more or less single direction of a great number of successive variations—would have proved, and perhaps in many cases did prove, disastrous rather than advantageous. The truth is that in this kind of spurious 'sufficiency' explanation *everything* is assumed that needs to be assumed to get our alleged explanation to do its appointed work. (1955, 169)

This is a strong objection to a *complete* sufficiency explanation, but I think it is misdirected. Gallie seems to believe that Darwin was in point of fact offering an adequate, characteristically genetic explanation. Further below I will contrast this illustration (as well as Romer's cited by Goudge above) with a more contemporary evolutionary example (see p. 339). Suffice it to say for now that exactly what needs to be done to turn a necessary condition explanation into a sufficiency explanation is not entirely clear, and the question whether we need more historical detail or need general laws will be investigated later.

One possible strategy for moving to a sufficiency explanation (which incidentally would also permit predictions) seems to follow from a generalization of Goudge's "complex sufficient condition" explanation. In fact Goudge anticipated this move, the force of which would have been to generalize his complex sufficient condition and its consequent into a *law*. Such a move can be rationalized in part by recalling Gallie's comment above that we utilize "inductive grounds (observations of analogous cases)" to support a claim of a *necessary* condition. Why not then allow such inductive methods to yield generalizations which would be logically equivalent to the types of laws we find in physics, for example to Snell's law of refraction or to the general gas law? Woodger, in fact, seemed to understand *embryological* explanations as just so generalizable, though he argued against such generalizations in *phylogenetic* contexts because of the "uniqueness" of the phylogenetic sequence. Goudge employs a similar argument, depending on evolutionary uniqueness.

Since, in Goudge's view, the historical or "narrative" explanations involve complex sufficient conditions, why not, whenever one has a sufficient condition S for E, generalize to a sentence "whenever there is a condition of kind S, there will be an event of kind E"? Then, why not utilize this generalization as a premise on a deductive nomological species of explanation? Goudge considered this move and replied:

> Whenever a narrative explanation of an event in evolution is called for, the event is not an instance of a kind but is a singular occurrence, something which happened just once and which cannot recur. It is, therefore, not material for any generalization or law. (1961, 77)

It seems that Goudge's position, which as noted mimics Woodger's, is based on several confusions. First, it is not at all evident that a similar pattern *cannot* recur in evolution. Goudge *could* argue that location in time and space are individuating characteristics which make it impossible to compare the causes of an evolutionary process in two different populations, but this position is not accepted in the physical sciences and has no obvious rationale in the biological sciences. Second, and perhaps more importantly, even in situations which are *compositively* unique, where the bringing together of various parts only happens once (to the best of our knowledge), it is often possible through abstraction and analogies to distinguish between *individual* initial conditions and generalizations which apply to those initial conditions, and thus to explain a "unique" event. (To be sure, this possibility is tempered in the biomedical sciences, as noted in chapters 3 and 6, where the narrowness of scope of many generalizations was stressed, but the distinction between initial condition and generalization can still be made within this narrowed scope; see chapter 4.) An example from the mechanistic sciences may make the point clearer. Nagel (personal communication) has noted that though a particular steam locomotive may be unique, nonetheless engineers can explain its behavior by applying general principles from mechanics and thermodynamics to its structure.

The argument from the uniqueness of the evolutionary process, then, does not seem to support a claim that there can be no generalizations which can be applied to explain aspects of the process. Much of the foregoing discussion, it seems to me, turns on two types of mistakes. One mistake is to assume that all "laws" worthy of that term are like Newton's laws or those found in Maxwell's theory in physics. A more sensible position would be to permit a continuum of generalizations from rough tendency statements, perhaps of the type found in the more descriptive parts of embryology, such as the explanation of the path of the phrenic nerves cited above, to more general principles of the type found in physiology, such as the Frank-Starling law (i.e., that "within limits, an augmentation of the initial volume of the [heart] ventricle . . . results in an increase in the force of ventricular contraction" [Rosenwald, Ross, and Sonnenblick 1980, 1027]), to the most general principles of molecular and population genetics. A second type of error includes assuming that one cannot explain *general* features of a biological organism or a population and that any adequate explanation requires immensely detailed knowledge. Gallie's position concerning sufficiency explanations seems to fall prey to such errors.

Such a position, however, is not even defensible in the physical sciences. We can adequately explain a simple billiard ball collision in Newtonian terms without taking into account the color of the balls or the atomic interactions. Similarly, in embryology we might explain the types of cell differentiation in adjacent areas by a general gradient theory without knowing the underlying molecular genetics (see Wolpert 1978), or we might account for the rate of a genetic change in a population, such as the rates of a sickle-cell gene's disappearance, without requiring all the *details* of the population's breeding behavior (more on this example below).[4]

7.2.4 *Beckner's Genetic Analyses and Genetic Explanations*

Morton Beckner, in his (1959) account of genetic explanation, does seem to escape these confusions. Beckner's account is, I think, generally correct and only requires that some of the prima facie sharp distinctions he introduces be relaxed to permit a more graded typology of genetic explanations. This relaxation will be congruent with the analysis of conditionals in causation, developed in chapter 6, that largely followed the work of Mackie (1974).

Basically what Beckner suggests is that we distinguish between genetic *analyses* on the one hand and genetic *explanations* on the other. In a genetic *analysis* an analysandum E is shown to be

> the outcome of a set of chains of events. . . . Each link in each claim is causally connected with the previous link and is either contiguous with it or temporally overlaps it. . . . E is the last event, a spatiotemporal part of it, or a property of it or its spatiotemporal parts. (1959, 82)

These events can be and often are on a "high level of organization." Though the events are causally connected we do not have causal explanation in such an *analysis*, since for Beckner, *explanation* is a term reserved for those situations in which conditions like those of the deductive-nomological model of explanation are satisfied—for instance, "the connection is stated in the form of a set of laws [and] the initial and boundary conditions are shown, with the help of the laws, to be sufficient for the occurrence of the explanandum" (1959, 84). In genetic analysis, however,

> it is neither presupposed . . . nor stated that any link in a chain from beginner-event to E is sufficient for the occurrence of the next link. On the contrary it is usually assumed and in most cases known, on rough inductive grounds, that any link in the chain is jointly caused by a set of factors, only some of which are included in the previous link. (1959, 84)

Beckner's distinction between genetic analysis and genetic explanation affords me an opportunity to return briefly to my examination of the type of conditionals involved in causation, a topic originally pursued in chapter 6. Recall that the analysis of the causation conditional defended there was Mackie's "necessity in the circumstances." As noted earlier, there can be causal explanations in which the constituent causes are "necessary in the circumstances," and thus will produce their effects with a certain probability.[5] In those (frequent) cases where the constituent causes are *also* "sufficient in the circumstances" in either sense of the term, the result will be guaranteed, though perhaps *explained* in a deterministic manner only if the sense of "sufficiency" is the counterfactual one.[6] This account, then, permits us to locate probabilistic causal explanation as well as deterministic causal explanation within a general schema, interpreting genetic analyses as *explanatory* but in a weaker sense than a sufficiency view. As we shall see further below, it also permits us to construe some of what Beckner would characterize as genetic *explanations* as of questionable explanatory force, because of the weak evidence provided in support of needed "subsidiary hypotheses."

Interestingly, though Beckner maintains that genetic *explanations* are "sufficiency" explanations, he asserts that "in general they are not predictive." This, he suggests, is due to their "model character." For Beckner, much explanation in biology has this "model character," which involves *having false* premises (false in the sense of being idealizations), termed *subsidiary hypotheses*, together with existential statements of idealized and abstract initial and boundary conditions, which Beckner terms "simplifying assumptions."[7] In genetic explanations "just those subsidiary hypotheses are assumed which will enable the deduction of the explanandum . . . [and] often . . . there is no independent evidence that the subsidiary hypotheses are indeed exemplified in the system" (1959, 108). I shall discuss just such an example from population genetics in the next section.

The line between genetic *analyses* and genetic *explanations* for Beckner, in contrast with Gallie, can be easily crossed. Beckner notes that "genetic analyses . . . do not pretend to be sufficiency explanations, although they can be easily converted into genetic explanations by the use of a model, i.e., by the introduction of subsidiary hypotheses and simplifying assumptions" (1959, 109).

To return to Beckner's general views, I want to note that Beckner is content to apply his distinction between genetic analysis and genetic explanation to *both* ontogeny (embryology) and to phylogeny. Thus he disagrees with Woodger (and implicitly with Goudge's later work), arguing that phylogenetic explanations are possible but that in such cases we must invoke general laws describing a mechanism of heredity, such as Mendelian or population genetics.

A key notion, then, in clarifying the nature of historical or genetic explanations is the nature of those features of ontogenetic or phylogenetic explanations that might function as analogues of laws in physics and that might thus give us a better purchase on this recurrent problem of predictability. At this juncture we have examined the contrasting claims regarding necessary condition explanations, complex unique sufficient condition explanations, and the claim of the uniqueness of phylogenetic explanations. Further clarification regarding these notions will, I submit, not come until we have examined a representative though somewhat restricted example of a contemporary phylogenetic (evolutionary) explanation, which will be done in section 7.3. Subsequently, I will return to these general issues and reconsider the problem of predictability.

7.3 A Historical Explanation of the Frequency of the Sickle-Cell Gene in African-Americans

In chapter 6 (p. 262) one of the typical questions in the biomedical sciences for which an explanation is sought was:

> Why do 2–6 percent of African-Americans living in the northern United States have a sickle-cell gene?[8]

It was noted at that point that this is usually construed as a request for an evolutionary explanation, and I am in this section going to present this explanation in some detail. It can be taken as a prototype of historical, evolutionary, or genetic explanations in the biomedical sciences, and close attention to its logic and its strengths and defects should do much to clarify some of the problems with such explanations, as discussed above.

7.3.1 *Sickle-Cell Trait and Sickle-Cell Disease*

One of the virtues of this example is that we understand Mayr's proximate cause(s) of the phenotypes "sickle-cell disease" and "sickle-cell trait" fairly well down to the molecular level. (The difference between normal + or "A" hemoglobin (Hb^A) and sickle-cell hemoglobin (Hb^S) is due to a point mutation in the gene which alters the 6th amino acid in the chain from glutamine to valine.[9] Individuals with sickle-cell *trait* have one normal and one sickle-cell hemoglobin gene; individuals with the *disease* are homozygous for the sickle-cell gene.) In addition, extensive population data has been gathered both for the disease and the trait. Though the population data is by no means complete, the type of data that *is* available can be used to indicate quite clearly what the limitations of such historical explanations are. The example is perhaps atypical since the relevant data is so close to our time period, in contrast to the examples concerning the limb development of mammals and the evolution of the giraffe. I believe, however, that there are sufficient similarities among these illustrations such that the logical lesson need not be lost due to the near-contemporary character of the example.

7.3.2 *Evolutionary Theory and Population Genetics*

Further below I shall reintroduce the characterization of evolutionary theory presented in chapter 3, where Sewall Wright's model for evolutionary change was discussed. Before I do so, however, some justification needs to be provided for using this approach rather than, say, Williams's (1970) more general selective theory.

As noted in chapter 3, the role of population genetics in evolutionary theory is somewhat controversial among philosophers of biology. In the earlier discussions on this matter, Ruse (1973) defended population genetics as the core of evolutionary theory against Beckner's (1959) "family of theories" view of evolutionary biology. Biologists appear to view population genetics as "an essential ingredient" (Lewontin 1974, 12; also see the treatments in Dobzhansky 1971 and Dobzhansky, Ayala, Stebbins, and Valentine 1977). Beatty (1981) and Rosenberg (1985), however, have argued that evolutionary theory does not require Mendelian genetics, and, moreover, that Mendel's laws are the *outcome* of an evolutionary process and not a constituent part of the process. Rosenberg also adds, further, that the principles of Mendelian genetics (and a fortiori their application to populations as found in the Hardy-Weinberg law) "imply the absence of evolution" (1985, 135).

Rosenberg argues for an alternative, suggesting that we utilize Williams's (1970) axiomatization, which is neutral on the mechanism of heredity as a basis for understanding evolutionary theory. I think this is an appropriate proposal for certain contexts. Certainly, in those situations in which Mendelian inheritance is not present, it would be inappropriate to appeal to its principles. A good example would be in the "RNA world" of molecular evolution (see Watson et al. 1987, chapter 28). However, Williams's axiomatization is too weak—eschewing a specific hereditary mechanism—to substitute for contemporary theories of evolution which incorporate population genetics, *if* we wish to examine the strongest *explanans* candidates.[10] Accordingly it seems suitable to look to a current theory such as Wright's to examine the nature of the evolutionary explanation of the sickle-cell trait.[11]

7.3.3 *Wright's Model*

It will be useful to consider in more detail what conditions are assumed in Wright's model. A clear summary of the model is presented in Jacquard.

The assumptions made in this model are as follows:

1. We consider a locus with two alleles whose frequencies are p and q.
2. Mutations occur at constant rates, $u(A_1 \to A_2)$ and $v(A_2 \to A_1)$.
3. Selection occurs: the selective values are constant and the values for different genotypes are close to one another.
4. The effective population size N_e is finite and constant.
5. Mating is not at random, but can be characterized by a coefficient of deviation from panmixia (random interbreeding), δ, which is assumed to remain constant from one generation to another.
6. A constant proportion *m* of the population consists of migrants from another population, whose genic structure remains constant throughout, with gene frequencies $\pi(A_1)$ and $1 - \pi(A_2)$.

Let the selective values[12] be $w_{11} = 1$, $w_{12} = 1 + hs$, $w_{22} = 1 + s$. Also, let the generation number be denoted by *g*. Of the various parameters listed above, only p and q are functions of *g*. (Jacquard 1974, 389)

These assumptions suffice for the derivation[13] of Wright's general equation of evolutionary change, given as in chapter 3 as:

$$\Delta p + \delta p = -\mu p + \lambda (1 - p) + p (1 - p) (t + wp) + \delta p \qquad (*)$$

Jacquard's development of Wright's general equation on the basis of the above assumptions makes use of several simplifications. These involve both empirical simplifications and notational changes (changes of variable), as well as approximations (e.g., dropping higher order terms if their effects are comparatively small). I will not explicitly trace all of Jacquard's steps but will point out two of his simplifications in order to show the connection between the general equation and its more complex component parts.

First, in Jacquard's derivation, mutation and migration are combined into the first two terms of equation (*) above. This involves a simple change of variable which allows Jacquard to write:

$$\Delta p \text{ mutation and migration} = -\mu p + \lambda(1 - p)$$

This expression is obtained (via the substitution which lumps together in parameters μ and λ the effects of mutation and migration) from two more explicit equations of separate effects:

$$\Delta p \text{ mutation} = -up + v(1 - p)$$

and

$$\Delta p \text{ migration} = (1 - m)p + \pi m - p = -m(1 - \pi)p + m\pi(1 - p).$$

These equations are simple algebraic renderings of assumptions (1) and (6) above. In my discussion of the sickle-cell anemia case I will be ignoring mutation effects, which are very low and inconsequential, but I will be consider the effects of migration. Accordingly, we may drop further consideration of mutation, but it will be useful to look at a slightly different form of the migration equation. If one multiplies out the second form of the migration equation and collects terms, the expression simplifies to $m(\pi - p)$. Now, this reflects an effect on allele A_1. We could have looked for a similar effect on allele A_2, with frequency q receiving a migratory contribution from a population whose frequency of A_2 was Q. Simple substitution yields $\Delta q = m(Q - q)$ for this allele's change. I use these two forms of the same expression because of Livingstone's argument (which I shall draw on below), which uses this type of formalism.

What Jacquard does[14] in his further development of the general equation is to make several assumptions involving mathematical approximation, such as "s^2 can be neglected compared with s." On the basis of these simplifying assumptions, he obtains the equation of motion of the population in successive generations. The key idea in such an account is to explain the changes in the frequencies, p and q, of two alleles due to the operation of the evolutionary forces and to genetic drift.

Now we could proceed directly from Wright's general equation of motion and either (1) introduce available values of the parameters based on empirical investigation or (2) make additional simplifying assumptions, such as holding a parameter constant, so that it would drop out of the equation. We would then apply the equation successively to the requisite number of generations or turn it into a different equation, integrate it, and apply it to the problem. For our purposes, however, it will be more useful to present an *alternative* and more accessible (though perhaps less mathematically elegant) representation than Wright's, which will capture the same empirical and theoretical content as does the more formal representation. This alternative formalism is closer to the standard textbook presentations of population genetics, and it also coheres better with the standard form of the sickle-cell example to be developed below.[15]

7.3.4 *A Standard Account of Balanced Polymorphism*

Let us first take a very simple situation of one genetic locus with two alleles, A (which is the dominant allele) and a (the recessive allele). (A = A_1 and a = A_2 in Jacquard's notation.) We then introduce initially just *one* "evolutionary force," natural selection. (Later we will return to the role of migration.) Natural selection, in genetic terms, is represented by an increase or decrease of a gene (A or a) or genotype (AA, Aa, or aa) due to the "differential fertility of the differential survival of its bearers" (Levitan and Montague 1971, 765). If the allele or genotype is selected against, it has a selective disadvantage (in that environment), which is conventionally represented by the letter s. This s is a fraction less than or, if s is lethal, equal to 1. We could speak of the adaptive value or "fitness" W of the allele or genotype which is set, again by convention, equal to 1 – s; this s captures the percentage of surviving bearers of a gene. Again, if s is lethal, we have a fitness equal to zero.

With these ideas in mind, the population geneticist can represent the relative contribution of three genotypes, the two homozygous, A/A and a/a, and the heterozygote, A/a, to the next generation, where there is a selective disadvantage of one of the genotypes. If A/A is "less fit" than either of the two alternatives A/a or a/a, the "standard manner of diagramming the effect of selection" (Levitan and Montague 1977, 767) is in the form of table 7.1.

TABLE 7.1 GENERAL FITNESS TABLE

	A/A	A/a	a/a	Total
Old population	p^2	$2pq$	q^2	1
Selective disadvantages	s	0	0	
Relative adaptive value (W)	$1-s$	1	1	
Relative contribution to new population	$(1-s)p^2$	$2pq$	q^2	$1-sp^2$

A little algebra will show that in the new population the frequency of A (= p′) will be

$$p' = \frac{(1-s)\, p^2 + pq}{1 - sp^2}$$

and a similar expression can be calculated for q′ from the table. From this expression we can also calculate the *change* in p (or in q), that is, Δp (or Δq), as $\Delta p = -sp^2 (1-p)/ (1-sp^2)$, which if s is small $-sp^2(1-q)$, and if p is small $-sp^2$. This representation is equivalent to using the general Wright equation given above under the simplified assumptions of no mutation, no migration, random mating, and an infinite population (which eliminates genetic drift).

Now let us complicate this situation slightly by assuming that the heterozygote A/a has an advantage over *both* homozygous genotypes A/A and a/a. This is in fact the case in the sickle-cell example under certain conditions I shall indicate below. First let us look at the general representation and examine the relative contribution of each genotype to the next generation. This situation is shown, following Levitan and Montague (1977, 777), in table 7.2.

TABLE 7.2 SICKLE CELL FITNESS TABLE

	A/A	A/a	a/a	Total
Old population	p^2	$2pq$	q^2	1
Selective disadvantage	t	0	0	
Relative fitness [W]	$1-s$	1	1	
Relative contribution to new generation	$(1-t)p^2$	$2pq$	$(1-s)q^2$	$1-tp^2-sq^2$

Again, inspection of the table will show that:

$$p' = \frac{pq + (1-s)\,q^2}{1 - sp^2} = \frac{q - sq^2}{1 - tp^2 - sq^2}$$

using the fact that $p = 1 - q$, since we are dealing with only two exclusive alleles, and thus that $p + q = 1$.

The change then in q (or Δq) is given by

$$\Delta q = q' - q = \frac{q - sq^2}{1 - tp^2 - sq^2} - q,$$

which by algebraic simplification is

$$\Delta q = \frac{pq\,(tp - sq)}{1 - tp^2 - sq^2}.$$

Now this change can be shown to be identical in successive generations, or, in other words, that for any n in q_n, the change Δq in the next generation q_{n+1} is given by the same expression derived for one generation (again assuming only selective forces operating). This evolving population will *cease* evolving, or come to equilibrium when there is no *further* change, that is, when q = 0. Inspection of the numerator, pq (tp - sq), shows immediately that this will occur if p = 0 or q = 0 (which are trivial solutions), or if (tp - sq) = 0. Equivalently this requires that

$$tp = sq$$

$$t(1 - q) = sq.$$

Thus $\hat{p}$ and $\hat{q}$, the equilibrium values, are given by

$$\hat{q} = t/(s + t)$$

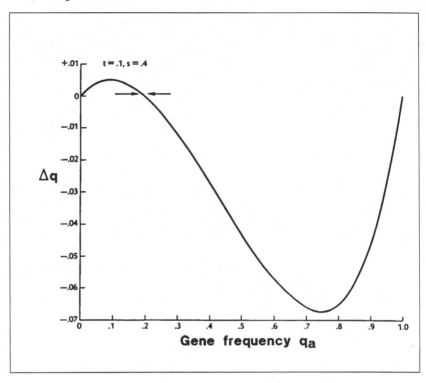

Figure 7.1 A stable equilibrium point showing changes in the frequency of *a* (Δq) when the selective disadvantage of the *A/A* is 0.1 and that of the *a/a* is 0.4. Note that the changes stop when q = 0.2. At other values of q the changes push it toward 0.2 (arrows), so this is a stable equilibrium point. Figure and caption from Levitan and Montague (1977) *Textbook of Human Genetics*, p. 779, © Oxford University Press. With permission.

and

$$\hat{p} = s/(s + t).$$

This situation is termed a state of *balanced polymorphism* in which neither gene is lost. The equilibrium frequencies of a and A in this situation will depend on the relative magnitude of the selective forces against the two homozygous genotypes. Following Levitan and Montague, who use the representative values of t = 0.1 and s = 0.4 for the two coefficients of selective disadvantage against A/A and a/a (these are *not* values for a sickle-cell allele), a graphical representation of Δq as a function of q_a can be sketched showing the three equilibrium points (where $\Delta q = 0$); see figure 7.1.

It is now generally accepted that in those regions where malaria is hyperendemic, the heterozygous condition of sickle-cell hemoglobin gene/normal hemoglobin gene, represented as Hb^s/Hb^A, with the Hb^s/Hb^s genotype, confers a selective advantage over the Hb^A/Hb^A genotype. Individuals with the genotype on the other hand have a severe disease, one which can be lethal at a comparatively early age.[16] Only about forty years ago, however, such a heterozygote advantage was thought "absurd," almost as unlikely as the drastically high mutation rate of 1×10^{-1} which would have had to be involved to explain the prevalence of the Hb^s gene in some parts of Africa (see Levitan and Montague 1977, 801).

7.3.5 *Allison's and Livingstone's Research on the sickle-cell Gene*

In a series of investigations (beginning in the early 1950s), A. C. Allison (1955, 1964), showed that those individuals bearing a sickle-cell gene are less likely to be infected with a severe form of malaria (caused by the parasite *Plasmodium falciparum*) than normals, or that, if infected, the infection was less likely to be less serious. The net result is that there is a significant difference (generally $p \leq 0.05$) in mortality in the two populations. (A number of studies subject to chi square analysis — see tables 17-7 and 19-8 in Levitan and Montague 1977, 806-807 — support this claim.)

The specific frequencies of the Hb^A/Hb^s genotype do vary with the distribution of falciparum malaria. The main evolutionary agent invoked to explain the frequency of the Hb^s gene in these populations is selection, and the structure of the explanation follows that outlined above for heterozygote equilibrium. A specific example is given by C. C. Li for the Baamba population in Africa (Li 1961, 161–163).

Li's reasoning is actually given in two stages: (1) he infers the selective value of Hb^A/Hb^A assuming $Hb^A/Hb^s = 1$ and $Hb^s/Hb^s = 0$ from population data, and (2) he cites this value as explanatory of the stability. Specifically, Li shows that the observed 40% prevalence of the heterozygous sickle-cell trait can be accounted for by a set of fitness values (.75, 1.00, 0 for Hb^A/Hb^A, Hb^s/Hb^A, Hb^s/Hb^s). Li computes values for the gene frequencies given a prevalence of 40% adult heterozygous individuals in the population: here p — the frequency of the Hb^A gene — will be 0.8, and q will be 0.2 (see any standard population genetics text for the formulas needed to compute these values, e.g., Mettler and Gregg, 1969, p. 32). Li then assigns a fitness of 1 to the heterozygote and a fitness of 0 to the homozygous sickle-cell genome. On these assumptions the frequencies of births in the next generation will be 0.64, 0.32, and 0.04 for the three genotypes Hb^A/Hb^A, Hb^S/Hb^A, and Hb^S/Hb^S. The adult frequencies will be 0.64 (1 – s) [where s is the selection coefficient related to deaths by malaria of individuals lacking the protection of the sickle-cell gene], 0.32, and 0, respectively. The equilibrium condition will be met if s satisfies the equation:

$$\frac{0.32}{0.64\,(1-s)+0.32} = 0.4 \,.$$

Solving for s yields a value of 0.25, and thus the set of fitness values given above. Li notes that "mutation plays very little role in this type of equilibrium because the selection coefficients are so many times larger than the mutation rates" (1961, 163).

When it comes to explaining the *change* of the percent of the heterozygous (Hb^A/Hb^S) condition, selection is normally not sufficient. Livingstone's explanation of the percentage of sickle-cell trait in African-Americans is illustrative:

> The Negroes of the northern United States also have lower frequencies of hemoglobin S, but this appears to be due to greater white admixture. Using [see below for equation] . . . we can estimate how the hemoglobin S frequency should have changed in American Negro populations. Assuming m = .02 from the White population, s = 1.0, and Q = 0, then if the American Negro arrived with a hemoglobin S gene frequency of .12, in 10.7 generations the frequency would be .045, which it is on the average today. If the population started instead with a hemoglobin S frequency of .1, then in 9.3 generations it would be .045. Although many simplifying assumptions were necessary to apply the model, it seems to be a reasonable approximation to the hemoglobin S change in the American Negro. (1967, 100)

The equation (14) cited is an expression which is obtained from the equilibrium condition:

$$\Delta q = -sq^2 + m(Q - q) = 0 .$$

(This equation, which represents the effect of selection against q by the approximation $-sq^2$, is of questionable validity since s is not small.) This equation is written as a differential equation, that is, Δq is divided by Δt and the limit assumed. Then it is put into integral form,

$$\int dt = \int dq/(-sq^2 - mq + mQ)$$

and integrated to yield Livingstone's equation (14):

$$t\Big|_{t_1}^{t_0} = \left| -\frac{1}{\sqrt{m^2 + 4msQ}} \ \log \frac{2sq + m - \sqrt{m^2 + 4msQ}}{2sq + m + \sqrt{m^2 + 4msQ}} \ \right|_{q_1}^{q_0}$$

Note that, as complex as this solution appears, it is still the consequence of approximations and ignores genetic drift, mutation, and the mating system of the population. Furthermore, the values which were used for m, q_0, Q, and s are rather speculative. Livingstone is one of the most meticulous gatherers of such information, and yet his comment on the inaccessibility of much relevant genetic data is almost nihilistic:

> In many areas of the world, human mating behavior is such that it is impossible to divide the people into several discrete, exclusive groups. This indicates that our theory is only a rough approximation to reality, and raises the question as to how much the process of approximation has affected our conclusions. However, all sciences make simplifying assumptions and thus in a sense are only approximations to actuality. Mathematical theories are models of actuality, and those in population genetics are no exception. To indicate that any particular application of mathematics does not "fit the facts" is an irrelevant criticism. None do. It must be shown how the differences between the model and the data it is attempting to interpret affect the conclusions of the application and result in wrong ones. Nevertheless, the interaction between new measurements and old theories is the progress of science.

This aside into the philosophy of science can be considered either the rationalization or the rationale of the approach used in this book. *All the interpretations of the gene frequency differences can be dismissed as not proven.* This is true because many of the parameters necessary to predict future gene frequencies or interpret present ones are simply estimated and not measured from concrete data on human populations. Such data do not exist and, more importantly, I think never will. Data on the amount of gene flow among prehistoric populations or the amount of natural selection by malaria are gone for good. But this does not mean that historical problems are not valid ones for "science." The choice of one interpretation over another will not result from its being "proven" but from its being able to explain a greater array of data. (1967, 23; my emphasis)

It is clear that such explanations will be speculative ones, with much uncertainty involved in the "initial conditions." It also appears that the problem in the present case does not arise from the difficulties associated with the dispositional aspects of the notion of fitness but rather is a consequence of the difficulties of empirically obtaining differential survival data. Such an explanation also appears (at least in part) to fit Beckner's description of a "model explanation" discussed earlier, in which "just those subsidiary hypotheses are assumed which will enable the deduction of the explanandum . . . [and] often . . . there is no independent evidence that the subsidiary hypotheses are indeed exemplified in the system" (1959, 108). This problem of empirically obtaining differential survival data also affects the larger issue of the confirmation of evolutionary theory in all of its many forms—an issue which has generated extensive comment and one that I will not be able to pursue in any detail in this book. Suffice it to say that though laboratory investigations into evolutionary mechanisms appear to lend strong support to the theory (see Rosenberg 1985, 169–174 and Lloyd 1988), the relevance of these investigations has been questioned (Sober 1984b). Other means of support for the theory (or better, theor*ies*), such as appeals to the variety of the evidence, seem to provide stronger bases (see Rosenberg 1985 and Lloyd 1987b). In the example of sickle-cell trait polymorphism presented above, I believe we have an example that is reasonably representative of the *best* type of data outside of laboratory situations that is likely to be available to support a strong theory of evolution. As we have seen, it is somewhat fragmentary and importantly incomplete but nevertheless significant. It now remains to see what this fairly lengthy excursion into population genetics and one of its *explananda* tell us about "historical" or "genetic" explanations.

7.4 Evolutionary and Embryological Historical Explanations as Data-deficient Causal Sequence Explanations

In this section I want to generalize from the sickle-cell example and several other illustrations cited earlier and discuss the issues of nomologicality, sufficiency, and predictability once again.

It should be evident from our review of the explanation of the changes in the sickle-cell trait that even some of the best-understood instances of evolutionary change rely on critically incomplete data. Even in those areas where biological laws are available that are close analogies of mechanistic laws, a number of conjectural assumptions must be made to generate an explanation. In many cases, only grosser generalizations of a qualitative sort will be available, yielding a correlatively less precise type of explanation.

7.4.1 *Mechanistic Historical Explanations*

These features, however, do not logically distinguish the biomedical disciplines from the mechanistic or physicochemical sciences. Similar problems arise, for example, in explaining accidents such as a DC-10 airplane crash. A combination of precise and gross generalizations are brought to bear on insufficient data — data which are incomplete and partially inaccessible due to the circumstances of the airplane accident. When the physicist performs and accounts for the results of an experiment in the laboratory, many potentially interfering factors can be measured and controlled.[17] When, on the other hand, a critically placed bolt shears in an airplane due to previously applied weakening stresses whose magnitudes were not recorded, the engineer must make certain plausible assumptions about the magnitude of those stresses based on similarities to accessible systems and his general knowledge of materials.

The same situation can be found in the sickle-cell example. An explanation for genetic change can be constructed by assuming (1) a well-confirmed set of general laws, (2) a set of plausible initial conditions, and (3) a group of simplifying assumptions, for example, that we can ignore inbreeding in the mating system, that genetic drift need not be invoked, that mutation can be disregarded, and the like. When such general laws are not available we often rely on grosser generalizations that are less secure, since we are ignorant of possible interfering factors. For example, to expand on the phrenic-nerve diaphragm example, the diaphragm normally develops and separates the peritoneal and pleural cavities. However, in approximately one case out of two thousand, the closure fails to occur and a "diaphragmatic hernia" results, with accompanying entry of the abdominal viscera into the pleural cavity. The cause(s) of this "relatively common" malformation is not known, but the point to be stressed here is that in most cases the sequence of normal development can be predicted with a high degree of certainty, probably with a higher degree of precision than in many mechanistic areas. In most cases of embryological development we do not know the underlying genetic-physicochemical mechanisms, just as for centuries the Maxwellian mechanism underlying Snell's law of refraction was not known. In both cases, however, explanations and predictions could be and are made with a high degree of accuracy.

In my view, there is also no logical difference in kind between explanations accounting for a *specific* historical sequence and for a *set* of sequences. Thus the sickle-cell example could be generalized as it is in hemoglobin genetics to account for other hemoglobinopathies. These other hemoglobinopathies include the thalassemias (where the mutation is not a point mutation but a deletion mutation) and hemoglobin Lapore (which results from deletion due to a chromosomal crossover error). Thus what Goudge terms "integrating explanations" are in my opinion the application of the same logical model of explanation applied to *similar* processes.

Though there is, I want to argue, no logical difference between historical explanations in the biomedical sciences and similar explanations in the physical sciences, there are, nonetheless, many situations in the biomedical sciences where explanation does not seem to carry a high degree of predictability. The critical question is whether this indicates a difference in the logic of explanation between the two kinds of sciences.

7.4.2 *From Scriven to Sober, Horan, and Brandon*
on Evolutionary Explanation

Scriven

A number of years ago, Michael Scriven (1959) marshalled several arguments why we should not expect predictability in evolutionary theory. Specifically, Scriven asserted that "evolutionary theory . . . shows us what scientific explanation need not do. In particular it shows us that one cannot regard explanations as unsatisfactory if they do not contain laws or when they are not such as to enable the event in question to have been predicted" (1959, 477). Scriven based his views on what he believed to be five features of the evolutionary process whereby explanations can be provided but where predictions are impossible. Scriven noted, first, that *environmental* changes could not have been predicted, so that at best one could have had hypothetical or probabilistic predictions. Second, Scriven referred to *accidental deaths* as interfering with predictability. Third, he noted that unpredictable *catastrophes* might eliminate whole species. Fourth, Scriven cited the fact that *mutations* are random and thus not specifically predictable. Fifth, and finally, he referred to the fact that there may be *accidental* and maladaptive *survivals* — in a sense the converse of his second point above.

These points of Scriven have some force but it is unclear that they characterize correctly the type of explanation which is actually provided by contemporary evolutionary theory. Scriven's arguments succeed, if at all, by implicitly sketching a largely unattainable ideal — an evolutionary analogue of a deterministic mechanistic system — with which real evolutionary explanations are contrasted and found wanting. Since "real" (real at least in Scriven's eyes) evolutionary explanations are "good science" and yet do not and could not conform to this mechanistic straw man, the fault for Scriven lies with the *desiderata for explanation* commonly found in mechanistic science.

In point of fact, as we have seen in the sickle-cell example, the form of explanation provided for many evolving populations is quite different than Scriven envisions. Predictability is hypothetical and based on the assumption that certain initial conditions were realized. In other cases, such as in the examples of Darwin's giraffe and Romer's amphibian limb, we find very weak explanations. There the empirical constraints are the available fossil records. Genetic initial conditions are not available, and even if they were, our current knowledge of genetic interactions is insufficient to characterize what could be the specific sequence of viable modifications or to tell a complete story. What are constructed by Darwin and others are plausible naturalistic accounts that have weak explanatory power. Nonetheless, these accounts employ general principles such as selection, gross generalizations about feeding patterns of herbivores, and implicitly, if not explicitly, gross nutritional generalizations.

Sober

To some extent, the position I want to defend here against Scriven's straw man account is congruent with Elliot Sober's (1984b) suggestion that population genetics can provide good explanations even if knowledge concerning the forces of evolutionary change is fragmentary. Sober suggests that, in addition to "causal" explanations we embrace the notion of an "equilibrium explanation," in which we only need know some constraints to see why a specific gene distribution arises in a population (see his 1983 and 1984b, 140–142). The problem I see with Sober's suggestion is that the sickle-cell example discussed above *is* just such an example of an equilibrium explanation, and we have seen in connection with Livingstone's comments quoted earlier the seriously incomplete nature of the data supporting the explanation.

Horan

Barbara Horan, in several recent articles (1988, 1989), has examined some of the differences between physicists' and biologists' use of models and argues that there are important trade-offs between realism (which she views as a necessary condition for explanatory power) and predictability. In Horan's analysis, which employs some distinctions developed by Richerson and Boyd (1987) that echo similar views developed by Levins (1966), the use of theoretical models in evolutionary biology should give way to the practice of natural history and the use of inductive methods. This is a strategy that she believes will yield explanatory power as well as as much predictive power, via *robust* theories that can be obtained in biology. The difficulty with this diagnosis is that it conflates two domains of biological theorizing. I think Horan is quite correct in her analysis of biological complexity and the limitations it imposes on simple and generalizable theories, but I see the resolution of *this* problem as lying in the direction recommended in chapter 3. For *historically* oriented biological explanations, however, I am skeptical of the likelihood that sufficient empirical data will be forthcoming to provide the basis for such explanations as Horan would prefer to see developed using natural history and inductive methods.

Brandon

Recently, Robert Brandon (1990) proposed an account of what he terms "complete adaptation explanations," in which he recognizes the problem of obtaining adequate data for evolutionary explanations. Such complete adaptation explanations have 5 components, each of which "has a historical dimension" (1990, 179). Brandon characterizes a complete adaptation explanation in the following terms:

> An ideally complete adaptation explanation requires five kinds of information: (1) Evidence that selection has occurred, that is, that some types are better adapted than others in the relevant selective environment (and that this has resulted in differential reproduction); (2) an ecological explanation of the fact that some types are better adapted than others; (3) evidence that the traits in question are heritable; (4) information about the structure of the population from both a genetic and a selective point of view, that is, information about the patterns of gene flow and patterns of selective environments; and (5) phylogenetic information concerning what has evolved from what, that is, which character states are primitive and which are derived. (1990, 165)

Brandon illustrates this notion by discussing as an example the evolution of heavy-metal tolerance in plants, which he states is "perhaps the most complete explanation extant in evolutionary biology" (1990, 174). In Brandon's account, this example is used to illustrate the *ideal* character of such explanations, and, though it is not flawed by its strong atypicality, it does misrepresent evolutionary explanations by its extremely unrepresentative character. Brandon contends that even empirically weaker adaptation explanations are satisfactory ones, however, and moreover that this type of explanation has important implications for teleological explanation in biology. This latter point is one that I will defer until the next chapter, where I discuss functional and teleological explanations in depth, suffice it to say at this juncture that Brandon does not conceive of adaptation explanations as representing a specific type of formal model of explanation. He does, however, see them as consistent both with Salmon's causal/mechanical and Kitcher's unification approaches to explanation; a complete adaptation explanation has aspects of both forms of explanation (1990, 159-161 and 185–186). To this extent Brandon's views about explanation in general, formal terms agree with the views developed in the preceding chapter. However, Brandon does note that his "ideal" conditions for an evolutionary explanation are "rarely, if ever, realized in practice because of the severe epistemological problems one encounters in trying to gather the requisite information" (1990, viii). Nevertheless, Brandon continues to maintain that largely conjectural explanations, which he terms "how-possibly" explanations in contrast to his ideal explanations (characterized by contrast as "how-actually" explanations, 1990, 176–184), are legitimate and testable explanations; he disagrees that they are equivalent to "just-so" stories (1990, 183). I am prepared to grant him this point, as long as it is realized that, in the absence of his difficult-to-obtain empirical information, such explanations are extremely weak ones, bordering on the metaphysical.

One way to identify better the weakness in the type of explanations we have been considering is to point out the existence of *alternative explanatory accounts* that are *not excluded* by the available data and background knowledge. Thus a thesis proposed in the previous chapter about the essentially comparative nature of explanation might be usefully reconsidered here.[18]

7.4.3 *Evaluation and Explanation*

Recall that in chapter 6 I suggested that, in evaluating an explanation, one should look for support for (1) the *explanandum*, as against other members of its contrast class, and (2) the *explanans*, as against other, incompatible rival explanantia which account for the explanandum. Darwin's and Romer's examples allow for a very large number of different scenarios, whereas Allison's and Livingstone's accounts of the establishment of the stability and change of the sickle-cell allele (as well as Brandon's metal tolerance example) are more constrained by a well-confirmed population genetics mechanism. (Note that only two or three rival explanations are provided in the literature for the establishment of this balanced polymorphism. The mutationist versus selectionist explanations, together with a migrationist component, are fairly exhaustive. Curiously, I have not seen any sustained discussion of a genetic drift factor in this case, though its possibility is mentioned by Dobzhansky et al. 1977, 109.) The contrast class of explananda in the sickle-cell example are also fairly well defined: They are the hemoglobin genes in other human populations. In the Darwin and Romer examples, the classes of contrasting explananda are much more vague.

The weakness of many historical explanations also joins with the incompleteness of data and the incompleteness of our knowledge of potentially interfering factors to permit, if not necessitate, ad hoc historical explanations which have very weak associated prediction capability. To see how this occurs, let us represent a historical explanation diagrammatically (using the relatively well-understood sickle-cell example) as:

where S and M represent the Livingstone equation expressions for selection and migration pressures on the frequency q of Hb^S and U is an unknown (set of) factor(s) affecting the frequency of the allele. (This diagram can in point of fact be used to construct a formal partial regression equation that represents the contribution of the various input elements to the determination of q. This is a technique known as "path analysis." For an exposition of the fundamental tenets that follows approaches developed by Wright and Li, see my 1983, 98–105. The fact that a logarithmic function is involved in Livingstone's equation is not a problem since we could use a transformation to linearize the system.) Explicitly left out of Livingstone's system was the variable U, which nonetheless implicitly is involved in "accounting for" any unexplained variance in such a system.

Now in less well understood systems the value of U will be rather large. One way to decrease the amount of unexplained variance in historical systems is to decrease U by unpacking it (using background knowledge) into a more complex set of factors which are rather specific to the process in question. Thus some of Scriven's "accidents" might be exported out of U and made explicit, for example when a set of idiosyncratic explanatory factors is applied over time to an evolving species. Such a strategy may also be what Horan (1988) is recommending when she urges that we make use of natural history to strengthen evolutionary explanations. This results in a trade-off between explanatory power in one case and general applicability and, a fortiori, predictive power in a broader class of cases. Often, as Beckner indicated, *just* those specific features are assumed which are necessary *in this case* to warrant the explanandum.

In my view this represents not inadequate science or an inadequate explanation but rather a *weak explanation* in comparison to *other* sciences. Evolutionary biology and developmental biology *do as well as they can* given the incompleteness of their data. The *pattern* of the explanation is not different, but an evaluation of individual explanations indicates a good deal of incompleteness in knowledge of initial conditions as well as of general principles. In such circumstances we *expect* low predictability. Though we could express this as also representing a tolerance for correlatively *weak* explanations, this would conflate the concepts of explainability and predictability which, as we saw in chapter 6, are better distinguished.[19] Genetic explanations are sufficiency explanations, but weak ones, since, given an explanandum, a sufficient number of factors are postulated to operate, either explicitly by hypothetical assumption or implicitly in the "U" term to account for the explanandum.

Thus, in my view, Gallie had the situation backwards: we do move to sufficiency explanations, but weak ones. On the other hand, Goudge was correct in his claim that complex sufficient conditions explain but wrong in his view that no generalizations were operative to connect and make intelligible stages in a genetic sequence. Scriven was correct in his arguments about the low degree of predictability in such explanations, but wrong seeing it as a strength rather than a weakness due to incomplete knowledge. Beckner was right in many of his arguments concerning the weakness of genetic analyses and explanations, but misleading in implying that these are features of the biomedical as opposed to the more physicalistic sciences. I also think Beckner was too stringent in his contrast between traditional nomological types of explanations, which he termed Humean, and his "model" type of explanations, which he found fairly pervasive in biological systems and in genetic explanations. Brandon's views in this regard seem much more plausible and comport well with the account I developed in chapter 6, though I view the model articulated there as probably going beyond what Brandon would be prepared to accept. Even if one were committed to explanation that is paradigmatically deductive-nomological, which I am not, it could be noted that such explanations have many of the features involving idealizations and ceteris paribus assumptions that model explanations have.[20] Our elimination of the need for literal truth, which Beckner attributed to Humean explanation (see chapter 6), decreases the sharpness of this contrast, and a tolerance for a continuum of laws varying in precision, scope, and degree of predictive power also blurs the distinction between Humean and "model" explanation. Furthermore, our acceptance of a spectrum of explanatory approaches (though with an emphasis on causal explanation) and the recognition of the distinction between prediction and explanation deflect Beckner's criticism by interpreting it partially as a category mistake.

As we shall see in the next chapter, speculative evolutionary explanations have *important unifying roles* in the biomedical sciences. I shall argue in chapter 8 that the evolutionary process provides a background naturalistic framework theory at a nearly metaphysical level of generality and testability, permitting heuristically useful functional and teleological language to be applied to organisms. This is the case because evolution provides a set of mechanisms by which we can understand the natural development of hierarchically organized systems, which are conveniently described in terms of systems and subsystems. As such, one can attribute to an entity within a subsystem (or to a subsystem per se) a role of preserving the larger system of which it is a part, if one can provide a naturalistic sketch of why it is that a system containing subsystems exists and persists in a changing environment.

7.4.4 *Conclusion*

In conclusion, I do not discern in historical or genetic explanations any logically distinct pattern of explanation, only a set of explanations which involve less available data—they are "data-deficient"—than we perhaps characteristically find in some areas of physics and chemistry (and in physiology). This weakness is, however, not something which is characteristically *biological*; it is also found in the physical sciences where data are poor and mechanisms conjectural. This thesis, however, should not be taken as attributing a second-rate status to the biomedical sciences. They have a greater need to deal with historical materials, and this necessitates dealing with incompletely specified information. Important specific knowledge and generalizations have been articulated by evolutionary and developmental biology. In this chapter I have dealt with some of the characteristics of, and examples from, these disciplines.

APPENDIX: THE HIERARCHICAL TURN IN EVOLUTIONARY THEORIZING AND NEW TECHNIQUES FOR OBTAINING DATA ON EVOLUTION

In the past decade, there has been an explosion of interest in what have been termed "hierarchical expansions" of the evolutionary theory of natural selection (Arnold and Fristrup 1982; Damuth and Heisler 1988). The perspective on the theory of evolution and population genetics developed in the chapter above is essentially what can be termed the "received" or "traditional" view of evolution. This "received view" is often referred to as "Darwinism," "Neo-Darwinism," the "synthetic theory," or the "modern synthesis." It developed out of a welding together of Darwinian assumptions with genetics in the 1940s. Though there were some modifications of this approach in Mayr's work on speciation, including development of the notion of the "founder effect," even the early work on molecular genetics did nothing to call it into question.

These newer, hierarchical interpretations of evolution include essays and monographs targeted toward a number of overlapping issues in evolutionary theory and in the philosophy of biology, such as the "units of selection" controversy (Lewontin 1970; Wade 1978; Wimsatt 1980 and 1981; Sober 1981 and 1984b; Lloyd 1986 and 1988; Griesemer and Wade 1988), the theory of punctuated equilibria (Eldredge and Gould 1972; Gould and Eldredge 1977; Gould 1980; Gould 1982; Eldredge 1985), and the ontological status of species as "individuals" (Ghiselin 1966, 1974; Hull 1976; Hull 1978; Kitcher 1984; Mishler and Brandon 1987).[21]

One of the more visible critiques of the traditional "Darwinian" perspective in recent years has been the theory of Gould and Eldredge, who have emphasized a series of problems with the more traditional approach to evolution (including the apparent gappiness of the fossil record) and in particular have focused on species formation. They have proposed, in a still rather speculative and tentative form, their alternative "punctuated equilibrium" approach, so-called because it envisions the evolutionary record as one with long periods of "stasis" punctuated by short periods of rapid speciation.

Gould suggests that this hierarchical model should have significant consequences for our understanding of evolution:

> The hierarchical model, with its assertion that selection works simultaneously and differently upon individuals at a variety of levels, suggests a revised interpretation for many phenomena that have puzzled people where they explicitly assumed causation by selection upon organisms. In particular, it suggests that negative interaction between levels might be an important principle in maintaining stability or holding rates of change within reasonable bounds. (1982, 385)

These considerations of Gould's reflect significant developments in contemporary evolutionary theory and, in addition, indicate the diversity of positions found in evolutionary studies today. However, these alternative approaches do not provide the type of data that evolutionary explanations would require to counteract the conclusion reached in the present chapter.

One approach that appears to offer more promise in this regard is the application of recent molecular biological techniques to the DNA of both living and extinct species. The advent of the powerful DNA-amplifying technique using the polymerase chain reaction (PCR) now permits the amplification of minute amounts of DNA from the genes of contemporaneous organisms as well as DNA recoverable from preserved tissues of extinct organisms (see Innis 1990 for details). Analysis of the molecular sequences of these specimens, as well as comparison of the DNA and protein sequences of contemporaneous organisms, can yield new data that may provide important empirical controls for evolutionary speculations. Though the use of DNA sequence analysis is based on certain yet-to-be-proved assumptions regarding evolutionary rates and rates of nucleotide substitution (see Martin, Naylor, and Palumbi 1992, 153), this approach does provide information about the likely evolutionary trajectories of species not otherwise available. (Also see Hillis and Moritz's 1990 volume for various examples.) DNA data has also been used together with Sober's recent parsimony approach (Sober 1988) to construct phylogenetic trees, but this strategy is fraught with a number of practical and methodological problems (see Stewart 1993). These molecular approaches are also likely to facilitate integration of evolutionary research with developmental biology; in this regard see Marx (1992) for an overview, Ruddle and his associates' model (Murtha, Leckman, and Ruddle 1991), and Holland's (1991) analysis of the importance of work on homeobox genes.

CHAPTER EIGHT

Functional Analysis and Teleological Explanation

8.1 Introduction

BIOLOGY AND MEDICINE DIFFER, at least on a prima facie basis, from sciences such as chemistry and physics in that the former make extensive use of "functional language." Though most claim to eschew teleological explanations, contemporary investigators in the biomedical sciences clearly continue to refer to the "roles" and "functions" of organs, cells, subcellar entities, and even molecules. Such functional ascriptions also appear to convey some explanatory force.

One type of important advance in biology and medicine has been the discovery of the "function" of a major biological entity such as a macromolecule or an organ. For example, the discoveries of the immunological functions of the thymus (in vertebrates) and the bursa of Fabricius (in birds) in the late 1950s and early 1960s laid the ground for much of the research explosion that has been termed immunology's "second golden age" (Nossal 1977). Also in the late 1950s, Francis Crick's (1958) theoretical prediction of the existence and function of an adaptor RNA intermediate in protein synthesis (later termed transfer RNA) was an important advance in the rapidly developing discipline of molecular biology.

In addition to serving ascriptions as discoveries or descriptions, such functional ascriptions also seem to be at least protoexplanations. For example, one of our sample questions posed in chapter 6 was "What is the function of the thymus in vertebrates?" On one interpretation, this can be construed as equivalent to "Why do vertebrates have a thymus?" Two types of answers to this latter question would be recognized as legitimate: (1) a (not yet available) detailed evolutionary answer along the lines of the sickle-cell anemia example sketched in the previous chapter, and (2) a (possibly covertly evolutionary but) more explicitly *functional* explanation which points out the immunological role of the thymus (see chapter 3, p. 84 and chapter 4, p. 150 for earlier discussions about the immunological role of the thymus, and also p. 385 below).

Thus it appears that functional ascriptions carry some explanatory force. Functional language seems natural enough in biology and medicine, but importantly it is not employed (in the same senses) in the physical sciences. We might consider, for instance, the emission of a photon of frequency v from a hydrogen atom, associated with an electron transition between energy levels E_1 and E_2: it would be inappropriate to use the sentence "The function of the electron transition between E_2 and E_1 is to provide photons of frequency v" to describe this event. I do not believe that it is simply the absence of a background evolutionary theory here that accounts for the impropriety, since theories of chemical evolution and stellar evolution do not appear to license functional language.[1] Some other factor or factors are involved, to be discussed later in this chapter.

Another feature of biology and medicine that must be considered in any philosophical analysis of those disciplines is the apparently *goal-directed* nature of the systems studied. Such phenomena as the complex developments in morphogenesis and embryogenesis, the sensitive regulation of glucose and pH levels in the blood of higher organisms, and the healing wounds (including limb regeneration in lower organisms) have led many biologists and philosophers to discern distinctive principles at work in such systems that require nonmechanistic modes of explanation.

The early parts of this chapter will be concerned with some of the analyses that have been offered to explicate goal-directed systems and teleological explanations. Later in the chapter I shall discuss several attempts to elucidate the structure of functional ascriptions and the explanatory force such ascriptions have in biology and medicine. I will return again toward the end of the chapter to teleological explanations. My general strategy is to review a series of three different classes of approaches that have been taken toward analyzing functional and teleological language in biology and medicine. From this review I attempt to extract a primary but empirically weak sense of functional ascription and a secondary but empirically stronger notion (see p. 389). Both senses share two components—a causal component and a goal ascription component—to be elaborated on in the course of the discussion. I begin with a few remarks about an "intentional" approach, then turn to the influential "cybernetic" type of analysis. After that the "evolutionary" approach is discussed, and finally what I term the "anthropomorphic" type of account is reviewed.

In this chapter I have not attempted to avoid words such as "teleology" or "teleological" or replace them with alternatives such as Pittendrigh's (1958) term "teleonomy" or Mayr's expression "teleonomic" (see his 1961 and especially his 1988, chapter 3). The analysis that I develop below does distinguish various senses of function as used in the teleological context, but I did not see any advantage to introducing new terminology.

8.2 Intentional Analysis of Teleology

In his comprehensive monograph *Teleology*, Andrew Woodfield (1976) introduced what he termed a "unifying theory of teleological description." For Woodfield, our teleological notions, whether they be ascribed to biological organisms or to "cybernetic" machines (to be discussed below), are extensions of a "core concept" associated with "mental goal-directedness." Rather than attempt to begin with a general approach neutral to the distinction between human intentional acts and automata, Woodfield suggests that "the best way to approach the task of analysis [of teleology] is to *hypothesize* that there is a core-concept and a broadened concept, such that the core concept of having G as a goal involves the concept of wanting G, and such that the broadened concept involves the concept of either wanting G, or being in our internal state analogous to wanting G" (1976, 163–164). More succinctly, "the core-concept of a goal is the concept of an intentional object of desire." A *teleological description* is then explicated as follows:

> S did B because S wanted to do G and believed that B ⇒ G, and this desire-belief pair initiated and sustained a desire to do B, which after joining forces with a belief that the time was ripe gave rise to an internal state that controlled the performance of B. (1976, 182)

This analysis is generalized to Woodfield's "unifying" theory, in which "the theme is, to put it simply, the idea of a thing's happening *because it is good*" (1976, 205). "The essence of teleology," Woodfield claims, "lies in welding a causal element and an evaluative element to yield an explanatory device" (1976, 206).

Though, as will be argued later, there is an element of truth in Woodfield's approach, it is, in the opinion of this author, both mislocated and misused. On Woodfield's account we would have to attribute intention, belief, and evaluation *analogues* to unconscious organisms such as plankton and even to inanimate systems such as thermostats and torpedoes. Such ascription would extend these notions to the point of vacuousness and would obscure a number of useful distinctions between conscious beings, living systems, and inanimate devices. Analogical or metaphysical panpsychism is more confusing than enlightening.[2]

The most generally accepted alternative to Woodfield's approach, namely a "cybernetic" attempt to provide a more neutral analysis,[3] appears prima facie more plausible. I shall argue that it is in point of fact incomplete, but that a somewhat different form of intentional component than Woodfield's can rectify this. Let us consider this influential alternative, also sometimes referred to as the "systems view" of goal-directedness.

8.3 Cybernetic or Systems Analyses of Goal-Directed Systems

Over forty years ago, the distinguished mathematician Norbert Weiner, writing with his colleagues A. Rosenbleuth and J. Bigelow, proposed an explication of purposive or goal-directed behavior (Rosenbleuth, Weiner, and Bigelow 1943). The explication relied on one of the fundamental concepts — "negative feedback" — involved in the then-developing field of communication and control which Weiner later christened "cybernetics" (Weiner 1948).[4]

To Rosenbleuth, Weiner, and Bigelow, any instances of purposeful behavior could be considered essentially to involve a process of negative feedback. Such a process, appropriately implemented, would obtain information from the environment and correct any perturbations in a system moving toward (or remaining in) a goal state. The authors believed that this construal of purpose could result in an increase in the epistemic and scientific status of the concept. They wrote:

> [Our analysis] . . . emphasizes the concepts of purpose and teleology, concepts which, although rather discredited at present, are shown to be important. . . . It reveals that a uniform behavioristic analysis is applicable to both machine and living organism, regardless of the complexity of the behavior. (Rosenbeluth, Weiner and Bigelow 1943, 14)[5]

Further amplification of the Rosenbleuth, Weiner, and Bigelow (RWB) analysis need not be offered here since their general approach has been accepted and developed in considerable detail in different directions by Sommerhoff (1950) and by Braithwaite (1953), Beckner (1959), and Nagel (1961). In his (1988), Mayr suggests that "Purely logical analysis helped remarkably little to clear up the confusion [about teleology]. What finally produced the breakthrough in our thinking about teleology was the introduction of new concepts from the fields of cybernetics and new terminologies from the language of information theory" (1988, 39). In this chapter we shall primarily consider Nagel's (1961) approach. This detailed and influential reconstruction of goal-directed systems bears reasonably strong analogies with the other cybernetic and system accounts in the literature.

Nagel believed that a logical analysis of the term "directively organized" could be provided which "is neutral with respect to assumptions concerning the existence of purposes or the dynamic operation of goals as instruments in their own realization" (Nagel 1961, 410). He cited the influence of cybernetics and the language of negative feedback on our perceptions of goal-directed behavior and referred to the RWB account and to Sommerhoff's analysis (1950) before presenting an account that is analogous to but much more developed than these earlier RWB types of approaches.

It is not necessary to present all the details of Nagel's analysis; a summary of its salient points will indicate the type of analysis offered and can be used to argue for the theses proposed in this chapter. For Nagel, a goal-directed system operating in some environment, E, consists of several components which can be described by different state variables. The variables can change, and some subset of the system's possible states is stipulated as being a goal- or G-state. The system is directively organized if changes in the environment or in two or more of its independent or "orthogonal" state variables cause compensatory changes in the remaining variable(s), tending to keep (or bring) S in (into) a G-state, i.e., the system would be self-regulating. A homeostatic temperature regulatory system, either in an animal (involving blood vessels, sweat glands, etc.) or in a thermostatically controlled furnace system, would be a realization of Nagel's analysis. The logical analysis is made in the cybernetic spirit of Rosenbleuth, Weiner, and Bigelow, and prima facie does amount to a neutral analysis as regards teleology and reduction. Nagel does not in his account, however, present any criteria for goal states. Accordingly, though his account, with its emphasis on the orthogonality of state variables, may characterize an internally necessary condition, it is not sufficient since it provides no noncircular means of identifying a goal state in nongoal terminology.

If we turn to two other philosophers in this cybernetic tradition, namely Braithwaite and Beckner, we find that goal states are roughly characterized as termini which are achieved under a variety of conditions. Braithwaite explicitly defines purposive behavior as "persistence towards the goal under varying conditions" and subsequently characterizes functional analysis and explanation in terms of his account of teleological explanation. Beckner, in his (1959) monograph, attempts to unpack this behavioristic idea by using the earlier analyses of *purpose* by R. B. Perry (1921) and by A. Hofstadter (1941). Beckner states that an action is purposive if and only if:

(1) there is a goal;

(2) the system shows persistence in reaching that goal; and

(3) the system shows sensitivity to the conditions which support and/or impede the reaching of that goal. (1959, 143)

Beckner goes on to note that "the reader might object that the behavioristic analysis is faulty because it involves a logical circle; we are trying to define goal-directed behavior, yet the *definitions* begin with the statement 'There is a goal.'"

He replies that:

this difficulty can be overcome in practice—and these are intended as practical criteria—by the method of successive approximation. The goal, the persistence, and the sensitivity to conditions are so to speak discovered together in any particular case. If, e.g., we find an animal's behavior with the look of persistence about it, we can tentatively locate a goal and thus confirm our location by the presence of persistence and sensitivity. . . . By using the criteria, we may get successively closer to a correct identification of the goal. (1959, 143–144)

I do not think that this is an appropriate reply to the issue at hand, though Beckner's suggestions are valuable from a methodological point of view. The important philosophical problem is the introduction of the goal *concept*, expressed in goal language. Neither Nagel nor Braithwaite provides an argument for the introduction of a preliminary, rough identification of a goal except by postulate. Insofar as this is the case, introduction of the goal state by postulate, these authors have not provided a full analysis that is "neutral" to distinctions between conscious, animate, and inanimate systems. Without the introduction of the goal, the account generates an infinite regress, since any system in which a goal state is not defined needs to be embedded in an inclusive system in which the same consideration, defining a goal concept, holds. I shall argue further below that the postulation of a goal state in directively organized systems is analogous to defining an "end-in-view" with respect to human intentional actions. In contradistinction with Woodfield, however, I suggest that teleological descriptions and functional analyses are *heuristic* and do not constitute assignment of intentional analogues to nonconscious organisms and inanimate systems. An elaboration of this position must wait on further exposition.

8.4 Nagel's Account of Functional Analysis

I have claimed that Nagel's account of directively organized systems is incomplete. Nonetheless, it would be useful at this point to indicate how it is employed in connection with the closely related notion of functional analysis. Nagel's explication has been influential and contains, in my view, importantly correct elements which will be incorporated into an analysis to be further developed below.

Nagel's analysis offers a translation schema, or general guidelines for replacing functional statements by standard causal statements located in a special context. Specification of this context, which is that of the directively organized systems considered above, is important in Nagel's view, since it constitutes the reason why one does not find functional language in the physical sciences: in general one does not find directively organized systems in those sciences.

Nagel suggests that we construe a statement of the form "the function of X is to do Y" as equivalent to the statement "X is a (relatively) necessary condition of Y." The relativization is to real systems and is proposed to meet the following type of objection: Suppose we analyze the statement "the function of chlorophyll in plants is to enable plants to perform photosynthesis." We would reformulate it in accordance with the Nagel translation schema as "plants perform photosynthesis only if plants contain chlorophyll," that is, chlorophyll is a necessary condition for photosynthesis in plants. It may be objected that this necessary sentence is *stronger* than the functional statement since it is at least *logically* possible that there exists a class of plants which could perform photosynthesis without chlorophyll. Moreover, it would appear that the existence of such a plant would *falsify* the necessary condition translation but *not* falsify the weaker functional statement. Most thinkers feel that, if the translation schema is adequate, it should not strengthen or weaken a statement by translation.

Nagel replied that one must not deal with logical possibilities but with the "actual function of definite components in concretely given living systems." Moreover, functional statements must "articulate with exactitude both the character of the end product and the defining traits of systems manifesting them" (1961, 401). Thus, by relativizing the functional statement to a well-defined class of systems, it will be the case for *those* systems behaving in *that* manner that the functional role of component X is a necessary condition for Y. (It is of interest that this appears equivalent to Mackie's "necessary in the circumstances" explication of causality discussed above in chapter 6. Recall that in this explication "the distinguishing feature of causal sequence is the conjunction of necessity-in-the-circumstances with causal priority" [1974, 51].[6] What this means is that "X is necessary in the circumstances for and causally prior to Y provided that if X were kept out of the world in the circumstances referred to and the world ran on from there, Y would not occur" [1974, 51]. This notion of "necessary in the circumstances" is sufficiently strong that it will support a counterfactual conditional of the sort Hume cited in his third definition of causation. Because of the "in the circumstances" addendum, it is also strong enough to block counterexamples that are quite pervasive in biology and medicine because of parastasis — the ability of organisms to accomplish the same end by a variety of means — which is exactly what Nagel is attempting to do here.)

Nagel also considered another pertinent objection. Though it may perhaps be said that a teleological functional statement entails a nonfunctional statement, the converse is not true. For example, it does not appear that necessary condition statements in the physical sciences are appropriately translated into functional statements. Nagel's reply to this objection is to agree that biological systems are prima facie different and that this difference consists in their being "directively organized" or self-regulating in accordance with his analysis as outlined above.

Thus Nagel's analysis of functional sentences of the form "the function of X is to do Y" can be summarized into two components:

(1) An assertion of a necessary condition: X is a necessary condition of Y (in this system . . .), and

(2) A claim that X and Y refer to properties or activities of a directively organized system involving a specific set of goal states G.

The fact that there are *two* distinguishable components to the analysis, a *causal* component, sentence (1), and what I will refer to as the *goal state* component, sentence (2), is important for later discussion.

8.5   Evolutionary Analyses of Functional Explanation

The cybernetic or systems approach to directive organization and functional analysis has not been the only strategy for analyzing these notions. Several philosophers and biologists have seen in the process of Darwinian evolution or natural selection a basis for accounting for functional and teleological language and explanation in biology and medicine. The approach is initially plausible and appealing. Let us examine two such analyses, and some of the criticisms which have been raised against them.

8.5.1 *The Canfield, Ruse, and Brandon Analyses*

John Canfield (1964) proposed a translation schema which he develops out of a preliminary analysis of construing a function as *useful* to an organism:

> FA is a correct functional analyses of *I* [an item] *if and only if* FA has the linguistic form of a functional analysis, and FA states that *I* does *C* in [system] S, and what *I* does is useful to S. (1964, 288)

The amplification of "useful" is developed in his more specific translation schema:

> a function of *I* (in *S*) is to do *C* [some specific action] means *I* does *C*; and if *ceteris paribus*, *C* were not done in an *S*, then the probability of that *S* surviving or having descendants would be smaller than the probability of an *S* in which *C* is done surviving or having descendants. (1964, 292)

Somewhat later, Michael Ruse (1972) provided an analysis which is similar in approach to Canfield's account. For Ruse, though he accepted Nagel's general account of directively organized systems, a *cybernetic* schema like Nagel's approach to functions cited above missed the essential *evolutionary* aspect of functional statements. Ruse suggested that we explicate or translate a sentence of the form: "the function of x in z is to do y" as equivalent to (1) "z does y by using x" and (2) "y is an adaptation," meaning "y is the sort of thing which helps in survival and (particularly) reproduction" (Ruse 1973, 186–187).[7]

Canfield's and Ruse's evolutionary analyses of functional statements occasioned a number of objections by Lehman (1965), Frankfurt and Poole (1965), Wright (1972), and Munson (1971). It would take us beyond the scope of the present chapter to discuss these objections and Ruse's (1972) rejoinder, though I will in subsequent pages discuss problems with these analyses. Suffice it to note for our purpose that both the Canfield and Ruse translation schemas also possess the dual structure noted above in the discussion of Nagel's more cybernetic analysis, namely a straightforward causal component and a component which refers to a "goal." We can perhaps see this more clearly if I elaborate on these schemas.

As regards the first component, it should be remarked that Canfield does not appear to interpret his "determinable" action word—"does"—in the necessary condition form as did Nagel. Ruse, in turn, is quite explicit on this point in wishing to eliminate reference to a necessary condition, preferring to translate the causal aspect of Nagel's chlorophyll example as a simple action statement: "plants perform photosynthesis by using chlorophyll" (Ruse 1973, 183). The second component, namely that adaptation as it is being used here involves specification of a *goal* state, is a more controversial claim on my part, and requires some argument.

Recently (in his 1990 book), Robert Brandon further developed his (1981) account of functional analysis and teleological explanation in his (1990) book. In the previous chapter, I introduced his account of "ideally complete adaptation explanations" as paradigms of "historical explanation." Brandon adds, however, that adaptation explanations have important functional and teleological features, writing "adaptations seem to be *for* something, they seem to have some special consequences, called *functions*, that seem to help explain their existence," and he asks "are adaptation explanations teleological?" (1990, 186). His reply to his rhetorical question is affirmative:

> Whenever we hypothesize that some trait is an adaptation, it makes sense to inquire about its function. I will call this sort of question a *what-for question*. A complete adaptation explanation, in particular the component that gives the ecological explanation of the relevant course of selection, answers this question. (1990, 188)[8]

For Brandon these "what-for" questions are apparently teleological and can be asked both of "small" and "big" adaptations (1990, 188). This type of question asked about adaptation A is answered by "citing the effects of past instances of A (or precursors of A) and showing how these effects increased the relative adaptedness of A's possessors (or possessors of A's precursors) and so led to the evolution of A." Brandon adds that these effects are the *function* of A:

> More fully, A's existence is explained in terms of effects of past instances of A; but not just any effects: we cite only those effects relevant to the adaptedness of possessors of A. More fully still, adaptation A's existence is explained by a complete adaptation explanation that includes not only the ecological account of the function of the adaptation, but

also the other four components detailed [in the analysis quoted on p. 355]. (1990, 188)

Brandon thus sees adaptation explanations as teleological in the sense that they answer *what-for* questions, but he also construes them as "perfectly good causal/mechanical explanations" to the extent that one is able to meet the requirements of ideally complete adaptation explanations as described in the previous chapter. However, Brandon also writes that "in a sense, adaptations are explained in terms of *the good* they confer on some entities" (1990, 189; my emphasis). As I shall indicate below, I view this comment as revealing the implicit evaluative character contained in evolutionary analyses of function and teleology — a feature which is not licensed by evolutionary theory per se but only by what I term a "vulgar" interpretation of evolutionary theory that importantly begs the question whether an adaptationist account can be provided for functional analysis. Brandon's account nonetheless has a simplicity and directness that makes it most attractive as an explication of why biological and medical sciences employ such language, and, if interpreted as I urge below along heuristic lines, is compatible with the thesis advanced in the present chapter. The next few sections develop the evidence for this approach to evolutionary explications of functional analysis.

8.5.2 The Ateleological Character of Evolutionary Theory: The Views of Stebbins and Lewontin

I want to argue for the following claims: (1) that evolutionary theory cannot per se be used to infer a goal state or purpose, and (2) that "evolutionary" *explications* of functional analysis covertly introduce, by postulate, a goal state. If these two claims can be established, *purely* evolutionary explications of functions can be shown, like the cybernetic analysis above, to be necessarily incomplete.

Traditionally, there have been two general approaches to evolutionary theory: Lamarkian types of theory, which attributed directionality in a strong sense to the evolutionary process, and Darwinian, which did not. I will assume that the Lamarkian approach has been discredited, though the approach does continue to have a remarkable resiliency, and from time to time aspects of the approach, such as the inheritance of acquired characteristics, reappear in speculative hypotheses in disciplines such as immunology (see J. M. Smith 1982, 91–93 for examples).

My argument for the claim that Darwinian evolutionary theory cannot be used to infer a goal state, even in the weak sense which I shall specify below, is based on the fact that the theory involves essentially three processes: (1) genetic mutation (change of genes) and variation (reshuffling of genes), (2) natural selection, and (3) genetic drift (see chapter 7 for details).[9] The first and third processes are essentially random and directionless, and those thinkers who have attributed purposes in the sense of functions to evolution have focused on the second process, natural selection. George C. Williams, in his stimulating monograph, *Adaptation and Natural Selection* (1966) maintains:

> Any biological mechanism produces at least one effect that can properly be called its goal: vision for the eye or reproduction and dispersal for the apple. . . . Whenever I believe that an effect is produced as the function of an adaptation perfected by natural selection to serve that function, I will use terms appropriate to human artifice and conscious design. The designation of something as a *means* or *mechanism* for a certain *goal* or *function* or *purpose* will imply that the machinery involved was fashioned by selection for the goal attributed to it. (1966, 8–9)

It is one of the subsidiary theses of this chapter that such attribution of goals to evolutionary consequences represents a category mistake—a confusion of two modes of discourse which, though they exhibit strong analogies, are fundamentally different. I think that the fallacy involves a kind of "reverse Darwinian" move. Darwin inferred the concept of "*natural* selection" by analogy with the "*artificial* selection" of breeders. I suspect that the term "natural selection" still has some of these "selective" connotations. Interestingly, the term more preferred by biologists such as Lewontin (1969), namely "differential reproduction," lacks those connotations and is, I believe, an aid to clearer thinking in these areas, as we shall see later on.[10]

Natural selection accounts for genetic dissemination, for genetic equilibrium, and for genetic extinction, depending on the environmental conditions and rates of reproduction. I would argue that natural selection characterizes a natural process in complex ecosystems, and only through abstraction and *a focus on certain special consequences by conscious beings*, do we "infer" goals or purposes in evolving populations. Let me try to put the points as starkly as possible and then offer some arguments for my position.

I want to contend that:

(1) Evolutionary theory understood according to a gross general sense of genotypic/phenotypic change occurring in organisms in a direction approaching "optimality" is a version of the theory which is commonly, uncritically, and unwarrantedly held by many, including some biomedical scientists, and it is this version which licenses functional ascriptions in biology and medicine, but

(2) Evolutionary theory understood in its fully developed, fine-structured, sophisticated and "mechanistic" sense is a purely efficient causal theory and cannot per se warrant the goal ascriptions which are required in my account of functional analysis.

I have already outlined a defense of point (2), but let me further argue for this point before offering a rationale for (1).

The argument for (2), that evolutionary theory does not entail any goal, is based on certain features of contemporary population genetics and also on the evolutionary record. The general idea is that there is overall no direction in evolution and that no properties are univocally maximized. There is a famous theorem derived by Sewall Wright and based on his theory as discussed in the previous chapter, holding that natural selection will act so as to maximize the mean fitness of a population. This theorem holds, however, for only certain simplified cases, and as I will note below, does *not* hold in certain well-characterized cases.[11] Other theorists have argued that a sign of directionality can be found in increasing complexity. If there were such evolutionary sequences representing clearly increasing complexity, *perhaps* their termini could be identified as goal states, though I doubt it for reasons developed in later parts of this chapter.

In point of fact, one evolutionary theorist, in attempting to deal with apparent evolution toward increasing complexity, has noted that

organisms like bacteria and blue-green algae have perpetuated their evolutionary lines for at least three billion years without evolving into anything more complex. Moreover, even in those phyla which we regard as progressive, the

> proportion of species which have evolved into more complex adaptational types is minuscule compared to those which either became extinct or evolved into forms not very different from themselves. . . . Looking at the whole sweep of evolution, one sees not progressive trends, but rather successive cycles of adaptive radiation followed by wholesale extinction, or by widespread evolutionary stability. (Stebbins 1968, 33–34)

Thus any clear directionality in the evolutionary record is extremely doubtful. If one averages over the full record, such directionality is just not present.

Other arguments for evolutionary goal-directedness are based on the notion that *fitness* is maximized. However, a more precise analysis of the nature of evolutionary directionality, based on arguments from theoretical population genetics provided by Lewontin (1965) in the context of a discussion of intrademe and interdeme evolution, does not support any such clear directionality. Lewontin noted that "the principle of maximization of fitness must be stated as follows: The population will change its gene frequency in a way that leads the population to *one* of many local maxima of fitness" (Lewontin 1965, 307). And Lewontin further added that:

> An important exception to the role of maximization arises when the fitnessess of genotypes are functions of the commonness or rarity of those genotypes. There are many experimental examples and a few natural ones known of such frequency dependence. In such cases the fundamental law breaks down, and it is easy to construct simple cases in which the population evolves to a point of minimum rather than maximum fitness. (1965, 307)

As noted in the previous chapter, the information needed to apply models like Sewell Wright's in a historical evolutionary context is usually not forthcoming, except perhaps in the sketchiest form. Lewontin in his 1977 is possibly even more pessimistic. He writes "such information is difficult enough to get under controlled laboratory conditions and virtually impossible to acquire in nature" (1977, 6). As a consequence of this information scarcity, population biologists interested in natural ecological communities have resorted to a quite different methodology. It is worth quoting Lewontin on this methodology *in extenso*:

Since none of the genetic information exists for natural populations, evolutionary ecologists have had to resort to a form of reasoning that is a short-cut attempt to predict community evolution. This is the use of *optimality* arguments, as distinct from *dynamical* arguments. A dynamical theory of the evolution of a community uses the machinery of expressions (1)–(4) [which are generalizations of the equations used in Sewall Wright's model as outlined in chapters 3 and 7] to predict the evolutionary trajectory of the community ensemble on a purely mechanical basis. The differential equations and the initial conditions are sufficient to predict the outcome or direction of community evolution based on a general maximization principle. Optimality arguments begin by postulating a "problem" to be solved by organisms. The "problem" may be heat expenditure of energy, avoiding predators, and so on. Sometimes the problem is asserted to be that of leaving the most genes in future generations; but that is never the actual problem set in the optimality argument itself, since it would require the very genetic information that optimality arguments are designed to dispense with. Rather the "problem" of leaving more genes in future generations is always converted immediately into one of the more specific "problems" of finding mates, heat regulation, food search, and such. Having set the "problem" that the organism is to solve, the evolutionary ecologist then uses an explicit or implicit engineering analysis to prescribe what morphology, physiology, or behavior would "best" "solve" the "problem." It is then asserted that the species or the community will evolve so as to establish that phenotypic manifestation. (1977, 6–7)

Lewontin adds:

But optimality arguments are useful only to the extent that they are truly short cuts to the result of the dynamical process and not simply plausible stories that may or may not predict the actual evolutionary events. (1977, 7)

More importantly, Lewontin sees a number of serious problems with optimality arguments, such as "problem" recognition, extensive use of ad hoc modification of extensive ceteris paribus conditions, as well as the possibility of restrictions on required genetic variation. These objections are all the more worrisome for optimality proponents given Lewontin's additional arguments against this methodology. It would take us beyond the scope of this book to analyze these in depth, but the salient conclusions can be cited. First, the argument mentioned above concerning maximization is elaborated by Lewontin on the basis of two hypothetical but reasonable examples and yields the conclusion that "there is nothing in the process of selection that implies optimization or improvement," or more generally that

> the dynamics of natural selection does not include foresight, and there is no *theoretical* principle that assures optimization as a consequence of selection. If, then, we are to have any faith in optimality arguments as a substitute for the actual mechanics of natural selection, we will have to reach for *empirical* generalizations in the actual world of organisms. That is the domain of experimental ecological genetics. (Lewontin 1977, 12)

Turning then to the experimental area, Lewontin reports the results of a series of experiments on *Drosophila*. The results were equivocal: in one case the process of natural selection does not appear to support optimization, in the other there is such support. Lewontin's general conclusion is quite clear:

> I must reiterate, then, that the consequences of natural selection of genotypes, for the life history of populations and species, depends in detail on the particular biology of the species and its form of interaction with others. No empirical generalizations seem possible, and, in the absence of theoretical generalizations, optimality arguments are quite dangerous. At the very least, we must say that the price of optimality arguments is eternal vigilance. (1977, 21)

This cautionary note of Lewontin's is also supported by more recent criticisims of optimality approaches. Emlen (1987), for example, argues that genetic and ecological constraints on optimization lead to extreme difficulties in identifying optima and that connections between adaptedness and optimality are virtually impossible to confirm. Kitcher (1987) is somewhat less pessimistic, but even he views optimality as a strategy that can be utilized only under very special conditions. Horan, in her 1988 and also in her recent review of much of the recent literature on optimality (1992), believes that optimality analysis "actually makes it *less likely* that the correct functional description will be found" (1992, 94).

Now I have suggested in point (1) above (p. 375) that evolutionary theory does, however, license the use of functional language. I think it does so because (a) in its gross general sense it has a prejudice for optimality interpretations built into it, and (b) in either gross or sophisticated interpretations, it offers a mechanism by which the development of complex systems involving parts, which act in concert to produce systematic ("holistic") properties, can be accounted for.[12] But the choice of a system property as a *goal*, and not as an *effect*, requires another element, which on my analysis is *added by analogy* with human purposive situations. In sum, evolutionary theory accounts for the development of entities for which we can extrinsically provide goals, but per se evolutionary theory does not provide any goals.[13]

I suspect that the reasons why neither cybernetic systems nor dynamically construed natural selection processes can be utilized to infer goals have affinities and analogies with the argument in value theory known, after G. E. Moore, as the naturalistic fallacy. Moore contended that the property "good" was "simple" and could not be defined or identified with naturalistic properties or entities such as pleasure. According to Moore (1960 [1903], 14–21), such an identification could not be argued nor be proven, and it could always be questioned.[14] I think that such queryings of identities are appropriate at some points in the development of a science, and at present I believe that no naturally occurring causal *consequence* can be shown by language involving *only causal terms* to be a goal or purpose. A natural consequence has to be *chosen* as a goal or purpose on analogies with intentions or ends-in-view in human design situations. Until we have a powerful and general reductionistic theory of human learning and action which would license very complex identities, I think that a functional analysis will be irreducible to causal analysis. This, however, is *not* an argument for *in principle irreducibility*.

The issue between the view argued for here and those accounts of evolutionary or adaptational explications of function such as Brandon's (1990) may turn on the definability of *function* in terms of adaptation (= natural selection processes). In the view defended in this chapter, such an identification is at the least a "synthetic identity," for which evidence must be marshalled, and I have given my reasons why I do not believe that such evidence on the basis of nonvulgar evolutionary theory is available.[15] That adaptational definitions are not simple identities of an analytic sort can be supported by the fact that they fail standard logical criteria for definitions; specifically they do not meet the criteria of *eliminability* and of *noncreativity*. Eliminability means that a defined symbol should always be deletable or replaceable from any sentence in a theory; noncreativity means that "a new definition does not permit the proof of relationships among the old symbols which were previously unprovable" (Suppes 1957, 153). (See Suppes 1957, 154 for formal statements of these criteria.) The possibility of adaptational explications of function does raise the profound question whether there are "values" in the world, and relatedly, whether something like an Aristotelian teleology can be defended on the basis of such adaptational explications of functional language so pervasive in biology and medicine.[16] This is a topic which I cannot address in the present volume, but an important literature does exist to which the interested reader can be directed.[17]

8.5.3 *Aptation, Adaptation, and Exaptation*

In two insightful essays on evolutionary theory, Gould, writing with Lewontin (1978) and with Vrba (1982), has provided a forceful critique of the "adaptationist programme." This adaptationist interpretation of evolution, which appears to lie behind the optimality approach, generally proceeds in two steps:

(1) An organism is atomized into "traits" and these traits are explained as structures *optimally designed* by natural selection for their functions. . . .

(2) After failure of part by part optimization, interaction is acknowledged via the dictum that an organism cannot *optimize* each part without imposing expenses on others. The notion of "trade-off" is introduced, and organisms are interpreted as *best* compromises among competing demands. (1978, 256)[18]

Gould and Lewontin argue that this program is unfalsifiable (at least as practiced by its proponents) and that it does not, contrary to popular beliefs, even carry Darwin's endorsement. In addition, they present examples from biology (1978, 261–626) in which both adaptation and selection are completely lacking (genetic drift accounts of polymorphisms, allele fixation in spite of selection against, and allele loss in spite of selection in favor) or are lacking with respect to the part at issue (byproducts of such processes as rapid or truncated maturation, as in the case of arthropods). Gould and Lewontin argue for the decoupling of selection and adaptation using both a hypothetical and a real example, the latter being the case of sponges that "adapt" to the flow regions they inhabit probably because of *phenotypic* inductions by the ocean currents. Furthermore, the existence of "multiple adaptive peaks" suggests that there may be no answer to the question of why one "solution" is better than another. Finally, there are cases in which the "adaptation" is more properly described as a "secondary utilization of parts present for reasons of architecture, development or history" (1978, 264). This latter issue is one which subsequently was taken up in Gould and Vrba 1982, to which I now turn.

Gould and Vrba draw our attention to a gap (as of 1982) in our language used to describe evolutionarily generated features of organisms. They begin by noting that the term *adaptation* has at least two meanings in the literature on evolution. One is a narrow definition proposed by G. C. Williams, who claims we should speak of an adaptation only when we can "attribute the origin and perfection of this design to a long period of selection for effectiveness in this particular role" (1966, 6). The other construal is defended by Bock, who holds: "An adaptation is . . . a feature of the organism, which interacts operationally with some factor of its environment so that the individual survives and reproduces" (1979, 39). This broad definition runs the risk of conflating historical genesis with current utility, so to clarify the terminology Gould and Vrba suggest that

> such characters, evolved for other usages (or for no function at all), and later "coopted" for their current role, should be called *exaptations*. They are fit for their current role, hence *aptus*, but they were not designed for it, and are therefore not *ad aptus*, or pushed toward fitness. They owe their fitness to features present for other reasons, and are therefore *fit (aptus) by reason of (ex)* their form, or *ex aptus*. . . .The general, static phenomenon of being fit should be called aptation not adaptation. (1982, 6)

Exaptation can also account for the development of birds' flight capabilities after the development of feathers, which adaptively evolved for insulation or warmth and were subsequently coopted for flight. Feathers are thus both an adaptation and an

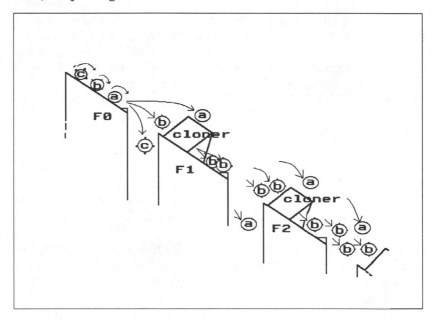

Figure 8.1 The "cloner." See text for a description.

exaptation. Gould and Vrba argue that given the current state of knowledge about genetics and evolutionary theory such a clarifying terminology is sorely needed. Here they refer to the weakness of the adaptationist program in accounting for "neutralism" — the type of examples raised by Gould and Lewontin above — as well as for the "substantial amounts of DNA [that] may be nonadaptive at the level of the phenotype," citing Orgel and Crick's (1980) and Doolittle and Sapienza's (1980) investigations (Gould and Vrba 1982, 6–7).

These essays of Gould and his coauthors add further support to the *fundamental ateleologicality of evolution.* In addition, these suggestions for a new terminology can help us understand better both the strength and weakness of the use of functional language in biology and medicine. They can also assist us in dealing with some counterexamples developed by philosophers who have been critical of an evolutionary explication of "function." In connection with these issues, I shall return to the "aptation" and "exaptation" again later in this chapter.

8.5.4 *The "Cloner" Example*

In an attempt to clinch the argument that evolutionary theory is not per se sufficient to license functional language, let me introduce a rather fanciful example. This example is so constructed that it has the essential features of an evolving population cited by Lewontin (1969), namely phenotypic variation, a phenotypic correlation between "parent" and "offspring," and differential reproduction. Lewontin notes (1969, 41) that if these three features are satisfied "there will be unavoidable evolutionary change in the population." Nonetheless, because the example I will introduce is a blatantly mechanical example, I do not believe we would find it appropriate to use functional language to describe it.

Imagine a set of ball bearings of at least three types, a, b, c, with different degrees of surface roughness. This population is found in its "first generation" rolling down a plane towards a gulf. On the other side of the gulf, somewhat below the termination of the first plane, a second plane commences. Near the edge of the gulf on the second plane is a row of "cloner" machines into which a bearing may roll, and out of which come two "second generation" bearings identical to the bearing which entered the cloner. There are planes 3, 4, and so on with "cloners" as well. A diagram is presented in figure 8.1. The type a bearings are smoothest with no surface indentations, their coefficient of rolling friction being $f < 0.05$. The type c bearings are roughest, with deep surface indentations, their coefficient of rolling friction being $f > 0.1$. Type b bearings have $0.05 < f < 0.1$, with "gentle" surface indentations.

Now the c bearings are quickly eliminated: they do not roll fast enough to cross the first gulf. Type a bearings do jump the gulf, but they move so quickly they typically pass over rather than through the row of cloners — they move so fast they do not replicate frequently. Type b bearings jump the gulf and pass through the cloners, doubling, accordingly, in number on each plane or in each "generation." After a sufficient number of generations the gentle surface indentations trait is fixed in the population (the coefficient of rolling friction is $0.05 < f < 0.1$ for all the bearings present).

If this example of pure natural selection were sufficient to license a functional ascription, we should say that "the function of the gentle surface indentations is to permit the proper velocity required for cloning." I submit that this is not the way a scientist would describe the coefficient of rolling friction of the bearings. The reason is because we have a transparently mechanical account of the dissemination of the trait of possessing rolling friction between 0.05 and 0.1, and, as noted earlier in connection with the Bohr atom electron transition example, we do *not* find functional language appropriate in the mechanical sciences. However, from a *formal* point of view this example has all of the properties of a biologically evolving population. Our inclination not to use functional language therefore indicates that natural selection accounts, and a fortiori evolutionary theory per se are not sufficient to license functional ascriptions. It also suggests that a functional ascription may be found less useful or less appropriate if we can provide a complete mechanistic explanation, a point of view once defended by Braithwaite (1953) and by Charles Taylor (1964).

Suppose, however, we were unaware of the mechanical explanation for the restricted range of the coefficient of friction. We can imagine an individual encountering a population of ball bearings of approximately uniform smoothness but possessing gentle surface indentations, wondering why they had that property, and conjecturing that perhaps the smoothness *served some function*. Such a conjecture involves an overt or covert postulation of a preferred state (having the property generally fixed in the population) and a hypothesis which suggests how the possession of the property (by a part of the population) leads to that preferred state. This way of analyzing the system allows one to introduce functional or teleological language which will not, perhaps contra Taylor, be entirely appropriate (1965, chapter 1) once a complete mechanical explanation is available, becoming at that time an odd and "more primitive," less scientifically appropriate way of characterizing the system.[19]

8.5.5 Functional Ascriptions Appear to Be Licensed by a "Vulgar" Form of Evolutionary Theory

Biomedical scientists frequently use explicit functional and teleological language, and though they seem to view it implicitly as licensed by evolutionary theory, usually not even the slightest of details required by an evolutionary explanation is developed. The general strategy of the typical scientist is to postulate that health, survival, or reproductive fitness is a G-state, and that the "purpose" of various systems is to contribute to that state.[20] This also seems to be a helpful heuristic in both organizing existing knowledge and seeking further effects and interconnections.[21]

The following quotation from Milnor's (1980) essay on "The Cardiovascular Control System," in Mountcastle's *Medical Physiology*, is illustrative:

> *Teleologically*, the *purpose served* by the response to the hypoxia [low oxygen] is only partly clear. The *propriety* of the increased respiratory effort is obvious, and with moderate degrees of hypoxia the cardiovascular responses may do little more than *meet the needs* incident to the increased work of breathing. On the other hand, the bradycardia [slow heart beat] of severe anoxia, like the "diving response" described earlier . . . , resembles a move toward a much lower metabolic state in which hypoxia could be *better* tolerated. (1980, 1081; my emphasis)

It may be important to stress that the teleological language here is not just a consequence of working at a supramolecular level of organization, one that would disappear if a molecular explanation were provided for an organism's response to hypoxia. Functional explanations are applied in molecular biological contexts pervasively. As an example, consider Lewin's account of the operon model of genetic regulation, which we have encountered at a number of points in previous chapters. In describing "enzyme induction," Lewin writes:

> It has been best characterized in bacteria and in particular in *E. coli*, where the lactose system provides the paradigm for this type of control system. When cells of *E. coli* are grown in the absence of a β-galactoside, they contain very few molecules of the enzyme β-galactosidase—say fewer than five. The *function* of the enzyme is to break the β-galactoside into its component sugars. (Lewin 1985, 221; my emphasis)

8.5.6 *Miller's Discovery of the Immunological Function of the Thymus*

The type of investigation that leads to the *discovery of a function* is perhaps the clearest indication of what type of information is needed to warrant a functional ascription. I have already, in chapters 3 and 4, touched on the discovery of the immunological function of the thymus and also on its later elaborated role in the immune response. At this point I want to draw together some of that earlier discussion in the context of our concerns with functional analysis and functional explanation. As noted in chapter 3, there were two and possibly three independent lines of investigation that led to the discovery of the immunological role of the thymus. For simplicity's sake I am going to cite only one line here, due to J. F. A. P. Miller.

Miller's (1961) paper, entitled "Immunological Function of the Thymus," stated that "Mortality in the thymectomized group (of mice) was . . . higher between the 1st and 3rd month of life and was attributable mostly to common laboratory infections. This suggested that neonatally thymectomized mice were more susceptible to . . . such infections than even sham-thymectomized littermate controls" (1961, 748). Miller found that if the two groups (thymectomized and sham-thymectomized controls) were isolated in a germ free environment that "the mortality in the thymectomized group was significantly reduced" (748).

Miller also examined the absolute and differential white cell counts of his mice and found that the thymectomized mice had a "significantly" decreased lymphocyte to polymorph production ratio compared to the control. (See chapter 4, figure 4.1, for a graphical presentation of Miller's results.) Histological evidence from the lymph nodes and spleens of the thymectomized mice confirmed immune deficiency in these immunologically related organs. Finally, skin grafting between unrelated strains demonstrated that the thymectomized mice tolerated the grafts for much longer periods than either the controls, intact mice, or even thymectomized mice which had had a thymus grafted to them three weeks after thymectomy. Thus evidence on cellular, histological, and epidemiological levels suggested that the thymus has a significant effect on the immune response of the mouse, and that neonatal removal of the thymus will result in a marked increase in morbidity and/or mortality in comparison with normal controls. Note that *no* evolutionary argument is offered here. It is virtually certain, however, that if Miller had been pressed, he would have said that he had identified a vital role for the thymus which offered significant evolutionary advantages for animals with the organ in contrast to similar animals without the organ. In their account of the generation of immunological specificity, Watson et al. (1987) state what I believe to be a (nearly) universal view[22] of the immune system by biologists in the following way:

The immune response is a highly sophisticated defense system of vertebrates that *evolved to* combat invading pathogenic microorganisms and certain forms of cancer. Without it we would quickly die from bacterial, viral, or fungal infections. (1987, 832–833; my emphasis)

The evidence obtained by Miller was deemed sufficient to establish "the immunological function of the thymus," though of course these and related experiments had to be confirmed in other laboratories. (As noted in chapter 2, a sufficient number of research programs in Good's and Waksman's laboratories were under way that such confirmation occurred nearly simultaneously with Miller's announcement. A conference organized by Good and his colleagues in 1962 [see Good and Gabrielsen 1964] brought all participants together and the immunological function of the thymus was accepted by the scientific community within two years of its discovery.)

I have argued above that sophisticated evolutionary theory is not *sufficient* to provide goals or functions. What we see, however, in the type of thinking represented in the quotation from Watson et al. (1987) above, is a kind of "vulgar" or "common" and unsophisticated way of conceiving of evolution in association with functional ascriptions. I think this vulgar view of evolution has strong analogies with the "optimality" approaches to evolutionary theorizing criticized by Lewontin above. In both cases holders of such views direct their attention at a problem to be solved — sometimes this is even described explicitly as a "need" of an organism[23] — and elaborate on the function of the organ or mechanism as the solution to the problem or need. This way of thinking makes good sense if we can view evolution as a designer or problem solver. But the strategy is not that of a typical human designer; rather, "blind variation and selective retention"[24] is the way in which one writer has described the way of evolution. I mentioned earlier, in what I termed a "reverse Darwinian" move, that Darwin inferred the concept of "natural selection" by analogy with the "artificial selection" of breeders. The term *natural selection* still has these "selective" connotations, and I think that it is these connotations which support the vulgar view of evolution and which license functional ascription by analogy with human purposive problem solving situations.

I have argued above that sophisticated evolutionary theory is not *sufficient* to provide goals or functions, but that a vulgar form of evolutionary theory *can do so*, though only by an implicit appeal to an unsubstantiated optimality interpretation or by analogy with human purposes. Some other philosophers, such as Cummins (1975), whose analysis we will examine further below, have proposed that evolutionary theory is, however, *not necessary* to license functional attributions in biology. Cummins provides the following counterexample: even if flying behavior in pigeons became *evolutionarily dysfunctional*, or led to a decrease in long-term fitness, the *function* of wings on pigeons, he asserts, would still be to permit flying.

I think that this argument does not really succeed, and believe it depends on a subtle equivocation between (1) a function ascribed at a stage of pigeon population development when wings were presumably of long-term evolutionary advantage,[25] and (2) a function ascribed at the currently postulated evolutionary dysfunctional stage, where pigeons still use the wings for some short-term advantages.[26] Just as we noted at least two senses of adaptation in the literature, it seems to me that there are (at least) *two* biological senses of function, though one is primary and the other secondary. Consider the following example.

8.5.7 *Two Senses of "Function"*

Suppose that, as a result of a mutational reversion, a human individual is born in the near future in the vicinity of Three Mile Island with a functioning bursa of Fabricius.[27] Suppose, in addition, that the bursa can be shown to increase remarkably the efficiency of that individual's immune system so that the individual is not susceptible to any viral infections, but that, unfortunately, the individual is also sterile.

I would submit that we would ascribe *a* sense of biological function to the human bursa even though it (1) was not selected for evolutionarily, and (2) could have no role in increasing future fitness. The systemic property of being immune to viral infections can be conceived of as a G-state. Such a sense of function is, however, *not* what most biologists mean when they make "functional" ascriptions.

My suspicion is that some form of evolutionary role is a necessary condition for attributing the *primary* sense of natural function.[28] Thus, when it is discovered that the putative "function" is either (1) an accident or, possibly, (2) a consequence of a "cooptation," that is, an exaptation, the primary sense of functional ascription found in biology and medicine loses its appropriateness. However, I have also argued above that sophisticated mechanistic evolutionary theory will not license functional ascription. Thus I come to the conclusion that the *primary* sense of function as biologists employ it is based on an unsubstantiated optimality interpretation of evolutionary theory or it is based on a covert analogy with human purposive situations in which we characterize decreased morbidity and or mortality as a G-state. From an empirical point of view, functional ascription in this primary sense is extraordinarily *weak*. This weakness is just what is expected given the basis of the explanations which support it— they are the type of "historical" explanations discussed in detail in the previous chapter.

Now there is, as noted, a *secondary* sense of function where we have reason to believe that some organ, mechanism, or process is "useful" to the organism in the sense that it keeps it alive and/or allows it to thrive. Conjecturally, this would permit it to leave more descendants, but no *evidence* is offered as such in connection with this sense. Paradoxically, this sense of function can obtain *strong* empirical support in the laboratory or in fieldwork investigation; the Miller example of the thymus described above provided just this type of strong ("statistically significant") support. Even fieldwork investigations have a limited empirical import for determinations of evolutionary fitness, however, in terms of the development of new organs or new species. The *primary* sense of function, then, becomes (from an empirical point of view) *parasitic* on the established *secondary* sense of function. Were one to be able to construct and verify a sophisticated evolutionary explanation of the entity to which a function in the primary sense is being ascribed, the primary sense of functional ascription could be markedly and directly *strengthened*.[29] However, such strengthening would *not*, in my view, license teleological language of the form to which proponents of adaptational explications of functions seem to be committed. Paradoxically again, however, the appropriateness of functional language in such situations decreases as the role efficient cause explanation increases (if my "cloner" example and its conclusions are accepted).

What these arguments and examples demonstrate is that evolutionary explications of functional ascriptions (1) are not sufficient (unless we accept a gross optimality interpretation of evolutionary theory) but (2) are necessary, though empirically weak to the point of becoming almost metaphysical. I also have argued that if and when we achieve a *complete and simple* dynamical or mechanistic explanation, the need for a "designer" interpretation becomes attenuated, and with it the appropriateness of functional language. What, then, accounts for the extraordinary pervasiveness of functional language in biology and medicine? As suggested at several points above, it seems to me that such language has important heuristic roles in focusing our attention on entities that satisfy the secondary sense of function and that it is important for us to know more about for both practical and theoretical aspects of research program development. This point about the "heuristic" difference of functional language has been made by others (see Mayr 1988, 53–55, though I think my sense of heuristic might be different than his). I would now like to comment briefly on why postulation of goals for goal-directed systems is explanatory and illuminating, and how explanation by goals is used in purposive human situations.

8.5.8 *Why Goal Postulation Is Explanatory: A Heuristic Approach*

In human situations, purposes, aims, goals, or ends-in-view, plus a knowledge of circumstances and sensitivity to the circumstances, allow one to build up a chain of conditionals *backwards*, in *conceptually reversed time order* from the end-in-view, and then to actualize the end by implementing the antecedents of the conditionals. Outside of human situations,[30] one can impute in an "as-if" manner, a goal or, what I will term, a *"virtual cause,"* in order to systematize behavior.[31] Nevertheless, unless the presence of an intentional end-in-view can be argued for,[32] teleological explanation and functional analysis have *heuristic* use only. Evolution would have to have a clear purpose, an end, something that was maximized by the process for one to obtain a purely evolutionary explication of functional analysis.[33] If my argument is sound, evolution does not. It is very easy to slide back and forth between discourse that is appropriate for human situations and descriptions of complex systems analyzable in part-whole relations, in which the part "plays a role" in maintaining the "whole."[34] My point is that there *is* an important contextual shift in such situations and that evolutionary theory per se cannot be used to define a purpose — only *we* define purposes.

(I think this position has some analogies with Rosenberg's views that are distributed through several chapters of his 1985, though there are some significant differences in our positions. I do not think that Rosenberg would *ever* want to say that functional language can lose its appropriateness or utility, even if we were to achieve a *complete and simple* dynamical or mechanistic explanation of a biological feature. Further, his account of functional ascription seems to rely on Cummins's analysis, with which I disagree [p. 399]. Finally, Rosenberg's views about the relation of teleological language and causal language are somewhat more complex than mine. He seems to see *some* of the more complex forms of teleological language as involving a Brentano-like intentionality [1985, 256], rather than the "ends-in-view" metaphor which I favor.[35] For a discussion on this latter point, see p. 402.)

Functional ascriptions, because they are based on investigations into entities and processes that play vital roles for *currently existing* populations, focus scientists' attentions on biologically important features of organisms. Thus functional discoveries can energize a field, as the discovery of the immunological function of the thymus did, leading to a number of research programs on cellular and molecular aspects of immune response regulation. Thus the heuristic power of functional ascriptions lies not only in the economy of thought that a problem-solving or optimality interpretation might bring to biological inquiry, whereby we can systematize an organism's behavior with the help of an identified G-state; there is also this focusing role which such ascriptions can play in biology and medicine.

Let me in closing this section briefly argue for another point made above, namely that evolutionary explications such as Canfield's and Ruse's do in point of fact covertly introduce goals. An examination of Canfield's and Ruse's translation schemas, as well as Brandon's (1990) explication, discloses that "survival," "reproduction," and "having descendants" are proposed as end states which an item possessing a function is supposed to assist. Thus "survival," and so on behave as ends or goals. Now I have argued above that evolutionary theory does not license a selection of goals. If this argument has been successful, then it follows that the introduction of "survival" in the translation schema is by postulate, which is what I intended to prove.

8.6 Anthropomorphic Accounts of Functional Analysis

Having argued now that both cybernetic and evolutionary analyses of function covertly utilize human purposes, it seems very appropriate that in my last type of functional analysis I consider various explications that are frequently *explicitly* claimed to be irreducible to standard causal analysis. Whereas both the cybernetic and evolutionary approaches to functional analysis propose to provide complex translation schema for "naturalizing" functional claims, the accounts in this last type explicitly invoke evaluational or purposive aspects in their explications. It is partly for this reason, and partly because these analyses are quite close to the human sense of purpose and involve a concept of design, that I refer to this type as "anthropomorphic."

8.6.1 *Hempel's Analysis*

In 1959, C. G. Hempel published an article on "The Logic of Functional Analysis" (reprinted in his 1965 to which references are keyed). Hempel did not confine his inquiry to biology and medicine, and specifically noted that "functional analysis . . . has found extensive use in biology, psychology, sociology, and anthropology" (Hempel 1965, 297). He drew his examples from the works of Freud, Merton, Radcliff-Brown, and Malinowski, as well as from the domain of physiology.

Hempel construed a functional analysis as representing an *explanation* of rather weak import. His account is significant and most useful for the clarity it brings to the area; it is also of special interest to us because of its explicit appeal to *evaluational* criteria of proper or "adequate" functioning. Hempel ultimately interpreted functional analysis as follows:

(a) At time t, system s *functions adequately* in a setting of kind c

(b) s functions adequately in a setting of kind c *only if* requirement n is satisfied

(c′) I is the class of *empirically sufficient* conditions for n, in the context determined by s and c; and I is not empty

(d′) Some *one* of the items included in I is present in s at t. (Hempel 1965, 313; my emphasis)

On his analysis, (d') is the weak conclusion that follows deductively from premises (a), (b), and (c'); that is, the premises *explain* the presence, not of a specific item *i*, but only of a *class* of items *I*. Hempel accordingly broadened the necessary condition formulation of Nagel, for example, which is still contained in premise (b), by explicitly adding premise (c'), which specifies *alternative means* of satisfying the necessary condition. This is important because it points out a critical weakness of such forms of explanations; as was argued in the previous chapter and again above in the discussion of Lewontin on optimality, we often do *not* have the requisite information to identify a specific entity or process as the only "solution." I will return to this point again near the end of this chapter.

Hempel also explicitly introduced a notion of *adequate* functioning. Later in his essay he noted:

> For the sake of objective testability of functionalist hypotheses, it is essential, therefore, that definitions of needs or functional prerequisites be supplemented by reasonably clear and objectively applicable criteria of what is to be considered a *healthy state* or a *normal working order* of the systems under consideration; and that the vague and sweeping notion of survival then be construed in the relativized sense of survival in a healthy state as specified. Otherwise, there is definite danger that different investigators will use the concept of functional prerequisite—and hence also that of function—in different ways, and with valuation overtones corresponding to their diverse conception of what are the most "essential" characteristics of "genuine" survival for a system of the kind under consideration. (Hempel 1965, 321; my emphasis)

Hempel, then, argued that it is (in some place) essential to specify particular states representing *preferred* goal states, selecting them out of a much broader class of causally possible states. It would also be to the point to note that one can locate in premises (b) and (c') what I have referred to as the *causal* component of a functional analysis.

Lehman (1965) later criticized Hempel's account and suggested that the explication had to be supplemented with a proviso excluding "normal" but dysfunctional entities and processes such as blood vessel blockages in aging humans. In other respects, however, he admitted that Hempel's account was "basically correct" (Lehman, 1965, 10).

Two other accounts of functional analysis exist in the literature which fall essentially into this "anthropomorphic" class of analyses. Let us first consider Wimsatt's (1972) explication and then turn to Wright's (1976) account. As earlier, the general thrust of the comments which I shall make concerning these variant analyses is to underscore the two components inherent in the explications.

8.6.2 *Wimsatt's Analysis*

Wimsatt's account attempts to make explicit all of the relevant aspects of a functional ascription of the preliminary form "the function (f) of item i is to do c." Wimsatt argues that the item i is actually redundant, since its behavior $B(i)$ has to be specified, and that this is the crucial aspect of i. In addition, he maintains it is necessary to refer (1) to the system S to which $B(i)$ is relevant, (2) to the environment E, since functions vary in different environments (say in an E'), (3) to the theory (or theories) concerning the items i and T, and (4) to the causal consequences of the item's behavior (C), since consequences are dependent on the theory. In an important but somewhat controversial move, Wimsatt also introduces a variable P which is the purpose, end, or goal of some item (or of its behavior). Wimsatt notes that the need to introduce a purpose is "most easily and ambiguously seen in nonbiological contexts" such as in human design situations (Wimsatt 1972, 20). He also believes, however, that it is necessary to specify a purpose in all functional analyses, and in biology he suggests that the theory of evolution can be appealed to as a source of the basic or *primary purpose* in biology. As I have argued above, I do not agree that evolutionary theory can provide such a purpose. For Wimsatt the primary purpose is "increasing the fitness (or long-term survival) of an evolutionary unit." Once a primary purpose is chosen, a functional hierarchy can be introduced with subsidiary purposes.

Wimsatt is aware that the introduction of a purpose variable is a "singularly important step" and argues for it on the ground that cybernetic analyses such as Nagel's and Braithwaite's are inadequate to infer functions. These various considerations are summarized in what Wimsatt refers to as a "normal form" for "teleological" functional statements, which is to be read "according to theory T, a function of behavior B of item i in system S in environment E related to purpose P is to do C" (Wimsatt 1972, 32). This constitutes a *logical* analysis of a function statement; Wimsatt next proposes a *meaning* analysis of functional statements. The analysis is intended to clarify what Wimsatt discerns are two distinctive *senses* of function: the teleological and the evaluative. In both cases the kernel of his meaning analyses is that $B(i)$ helps promote the attainment of a goal state P. The actual analysis is elaborated in more detail to include probabilistic functioning. These senses are introduced in somewhat formalistic terms.[36] At this point we will not discuss the details of these senses except to point out that a proper subsystem is conceived on the analysis with a proper subset in logic and that a simple, primary purpose is a purpose which (1) has only one logically independent criterion for its attainment and (2) is the highest order purpose in a given functional hierarchy (see Wimsatt 1972, 22-26).

Behind its prima facie complexity designed to accommodate the variety of examples in which one utilizes functional language, it would appear that Wimsatt's explication is consistent with the theses so far advanced in this chapter. Wimsatt is clearly committed to a purpose P which is tantamount to what I have termed a specified goal state. He also introduces a (probabilistic) causal component via his reference to $B(i)$ doing C (with probability or frequency r ($0 < r \leq 1$). Wimsatt's account is more sophisticated on this second aspect than those explications examined earlier since he explicitly allows for probabilistic consequences and has also introduced a parameter T which specifies the "causal" laws regulating the production of C. Thus Wimsatt's account can interdigitate well with the model of explanation developed in chapter 7.

Perhaps the most interesting and distinctive feature of Wimsatt's analysis, as was remarked on earlier, is the introduction of a purpose into the logical and meaning forms of analysis of functional statements. Wimsatt believes that this does not introduce a nonnaturalistic element into his analysis, since for him a purpose can be said to appear in any system subject to a differential selection process. He speculates that teleological systems involving purposes and systems subjected to differential selection processes may be logically identical, but he is willing to settle for the weaker claim that they are causally related, that it is proper to talk of purpose in any case in which differential selection has operated. The selection processes can be biological or psychological (a result of human choice), and presumably physical and sociological as well. Wimsatt believes, as noted above, that "purpose associated with biological adaptive function is to be derived from the structure of evolutionary theory — in particular from the mode of operation of natural selection."

I think Wimsatt's basic mistake lies in this aspect of his generally excellent analysis of functional statements. The problem is based on the argument given above in section 8.5.2, that it is improper to construe natural selection as per se purposeful and thus as providing the P value in Wimsatt's analysis.

8.6.3 Wright's Analysis

In a series of essays later gathered together into a monograph, Larry Wright (1973, 1976) has argued for an explication of functional sentences which is both simple and general. Wright was apparently strongly influenced by Charles Taylor's (1964) analysis of teleological behavior and his account shows analogies with Taylor's approach. Wright in addition provides an analysis of goal-directed behavior which is similar to his account of function. Wright maintains that his analysis unifies both "natural and conscious functions" by applying to the two species "indifferently" (Wright 1973, 164).

The Etiological Translation Schema

Wright sets forth his position by criticizing several of the standard accounts by Canfield (1964) and by the later Beckner (1969) and then arguing that one of the main aspects of functionality which extant accounts have missed is its "etiological" character, with respect to how items expressing functions "*got there*." He states:

> Functional explanations, although plainly not causal in the usual, restricted sense, do concern how the thing with the function *got* there. Hence they *are* etiological, which is to say "causal" in an extended sense. (Wright 1973, 156)

According to Wright's translation schema, "the function of X is Z *means*: (a) X is there because it does Z, (b) Z is a consequence (or result) of X's being there," to which he adds "the first part, (a), displays the etiological form of functional ascription-explanations, and the second part, (b), describes the convolution which distinguishes functional etiologies from the rest" (Wright 1973, 161). Wright argues that this schema will apply both to conscious functions involving human artifacts such as snow fences — they are there because they keep snow from drifting across roads, and the elimination of drifting snow is a consequence of their being there — and to natural functions, such as the heart's pumping of blood. In the latter case the etiology involves natural selection.

It will not be possible in these pages to discuss Wright's objections to alternative explications, nor to say much about his own defense of his schema against potential counterexamples. Wright's account has elicited extensive comment and criticism and it will be worth citing some of these. The criticisms range from broad critiques, such as Ruse's (1973) comment that Wright's explication was *too* general and unilluminating, as compared to Ruse's own evolutionary analysis of natural functions, to more specific objections raised by Boorse (1975), Achinstein (1977), Enç (1979) and Brandon (1990, 189, n. 26).

Criticisms of Wright's Analysis

Achinstein argues that Wright's account is neither sufficient nor necessary. Achinstein's examples are complex, and his argument against necessity had already been anticipated by Wright and rejected as being "nonstandard." Enç criticized Wright's account as not being necessary since if "cells had fallen together purely by chance . . . to produce the creatures we know today . . . it would still be true that the function of the heart is to pump the blood" (1979, 362). What this counterexample does is to question the etiological connection in Wright's analysis. The point, however, is obscured by the unnatural or miraculous character of the counterexample, and I also think the general objection is questionable if we remember that there may be two distinct senses of biological function. Wright's account would apparently eliminate any "accidentally" arising structure which nonetheless might then obtain what most scientists would characterize as a function, albeit it not in the most important sense. Still, given the prospect that genetic drift may be as important in evolution as is natural selection, the etiological link is almost certainly too strict to capture *all* senses of "function." As noted earlier in my discussion of Lewontin and of Gould, possibly important roles of random mutations and cross-over genetic duplications also de-emphasize the place of natural selection. Finally, we might note that on a *strict* interpretation of Wright's account we could not attribute a function to a *new* organ (such as the example given earlier of an efficient bursa in the hypothetical individual born in the vicinity of Three Mile Island) that kept an individual in better health than usual, if it were not subsequently selected for. This appears to be too strong and would certainly be in violation of such usage as would be employed by a physician in describing the function of the bursa for the so-endowed human.

Though Wright's schema places too much emphasis on etiology and also implicitly on the inferability of a goal state from natural selection, it is still a very helpful analysis. It should be noted that Wright's schema possesses the two components of functional analysis discussed earlier. Wright claims that his part (a) represents the etiological aspect of his analysis. In the context of application to artifacts, it is clearly meant to refer to the *purpose* of the (human) designer. In the context of natural functions, however, we are forced to attribute something like an optimal survival or reproductive aspect, or a *value*, to the item X (or more precisely to its activity Z). I have argued above that this involves postulating purposes just as much as artifacts involve postulating ends. It should also be noted that the evolutionary theory invoked here is extraordinarily crude and does not even begin to approach the (still incomplete) detail given in the sickle-cell example in the previous chapter. This is in fact exactly what we would expect, since if I am correct, to give a detailed, mechanistic evolutionary answer would cause the teleological feature to become less appropriate.

As regards Wright's part (b), it should first be noted that this represents a straightforward efficient causal claim: the thrust of (b) is to assert that X has causal consequence Z. Second, I must also confess that I do not detect any "convolution" in part (b) per se; at most a "convolution" arises out of the conjunction of (b) with (a). Part (a), however, simply represents the specification of a goal state on my analysis. Accordingly, on the account argued for in these pages, Wright's analysis possesses the two components specified in the various models, and without the necessity to introduce any special "convolutions."

Wright's account is unabashedly teleological. Many other accounts also have this feature (Wimsatt's, for example), but

Wright's is one criticized by Cummins. Though Cummins's account is not explicitly anthropomorphic, I believe that it covertly uses a notion of "needs" or an interpretation of "significant," such as in Cummins's expression "biologically significant capacities" (1975, 403), that it is tantamount to an anthropomorphic account.

8.6.4 *Cummins' Containment Account*

Cummins's (1975) analysis of functions makes a number of useful observations. Among them are that (almost?) all philosophical explication of functional analysis has implicitly made the following two assumptions:

(A) The point of functional characterization in science is to explain the presence of the item (organ, mechanism, process, or whatever) that is functionally characterized.

(B) For something to perform its function is for it to have certain effects on a containing system, which effects contribute to the performance of some activity of, or maintenance of some condition in, that containing system.

(Cummins 1975, 386)

Cummins thinks that "adherence to (A) and (B) has crippled the most serious attempts to analyze functional statements and explanations" (1975, 387), and he proposes his own account which eliminates dependence on (A).

One of Cummins's arguments against the need to invoke an evolutionary background etiology has already been cited and criticized (p. 388). The pigeon-wings counterexample, which, it seems to me, proves just the reverse of what Cummins is attempting to argue for, is part of Cummins's general strategy to replace a dependency on *etiology* with an "inference to the best explanation" (see chapter 2, p. 17, for a discussion of this notion). He writes that once we clearly perceive this distinction we can reanalyze Nagel's chlorophyll-photosynthesis example:

It becomes equally clear that (A) has the matters reversed: given that photosynthesis is occurring in a particular plant, we may legitimately infer that chlorophyll is present in that plant because chlorophyll enters into our best (only) explanation of photosynthesis. (1975, 392)

But this view clearly cannot be sufficient as an analysis. If we have any inferences to the best explanation, we have them in physics where functional language of the type used in biology is inappropriate. Moreover, this part of Cummins's analysis does not support our intuitions about the primary sense of function not being ascribable to the Three Mile Island bursa example.

In his full positive account, Cummins eschews thesis (A) but stresses (B) above, elaborating on it to emphasize the dispositional *capacity* inherent in functional analyses. For Cummins, "To ascribe a function to something is to ascribe a capacity to it which is singled out by its role in an analysis of some capacity of a containing system" (1975, 407). His more precise explication is:

> x functions as a φ in s (or: the function of x in s is to φ) relative to an analytical account A of s's capacity to ψ just in case x is capable of φ-ing in s and A appropriately and adequately accounts for s's capacity to ψ by, in part, appealing to the capacity of x to φ in s. (1975, 405)

In my view there is a significant gap here: the choice of ψ as in some sense a "biologically significant capacity." Here the "analytical account A" provides the background account of some containing property ψ of s which, as I see it, amounts to covertly specifying the *useful* effects of x's φ-ing. Cummins does not tell us how to identify what he takes to be "biologically significant capacities" (1975, 403), nor does he provide any account, other than that it "sounds right" (1975, 404), for distinguishing *insignificant* capacities from *significant* capacities.[37] Neither dispositional capacity nor a containment relation are sufficient per se to license functional ascriptions in the physical sciences, and they do so in Cummins's account, I submit, only because of an implicit appeal to "useful" properties (in the "vulgar" but still evolutionarily secondary sense discussed earlier) through Cummins's use of standard biological examples. Thus I believe that Cummins's account, and a fortiori Rosenberg's (1985, chapter 3) analysis of functional terminology in biology and medicine, is wanting.[38] I also believe that the same holds of Bechtel's (1986) helpful generalization of Cummins's type of account from a two-level analysis to a multiple-level account. It seems to me that both Cummins and Rosenberg, as well as Bechtel, mistake the need for discourse at higher levels of organization and the utility of part-whole analysis for an argument for functional language (compare Rosenberg 1985, 59). [39]

8.6.5 *Rosenberg's Intentional Account of Complex Teleological Language*

It remains to return to Rosenberg's views mentioned briefly above (p. 391) and to attempt to disambiguate a potential confusion between Rosenberg's recent (1985) argument about the "intentionality" of teleological language and my own approach. In his (1985) Rosenberg provides a splendid example of teleological and other anthropomorphic language utilized by a standard biochemistry textbook (Stryer's *Biochemistry*) in describing molecular interactions:

> These enzymes are highly selective in their *recognition* of the amino acids and of the prospective tRNA acceptor. . . . tRNA molecules that accept different amino acids have different base sequences, and so they can be readily *recognized* by the synthetases. A much more demanding *task* for these enzymes is to *discriminate* between similar amino acids. For example the only difference between isoleucine and valine [two amino acids] is that isoleucine contains an additional methyl group. . . . The concentration of valine *in vivo* is about five times that of isoleucine, and so valine would be *mistakenly* incorporated in place of isoleucine 1 in 40 times. However, the observed *error* frequency *in vivo* is only 1 in 3000, indicating that there must be a subsequent *editing* step to enhance fidelity. In fact the synthetase *corrects* its own *errors*. Valine that is *mistakenly* activated is not transferred to the tRNA specific for isoleucine. Instead, this tRNA promotes the hydrolysis of valine-AMP, which thereby prevents its *erroneous* incorporation into proteins. . . . How does the synthetase *avoid* hydrolyzing isoleucine-AMP, the *desired* intermediate? Most likely, the hydrolytic site is just large enough to accommodate valine-AMP, but too small to allow the entry of isoleucine-AMP. . . . It is evident that the high fidelity of protein synthesis is critically dependent on the hydrolytic *proofreading action* of many aminoacyl-tRNA synthetases.

(Rosenberg 1985, 255 quoting Stryer 1981, 644–5; emphasis added by Rosenberg)

Rosenberg has argued that this type of language is clearly "intentional." He claims:

> Cognitive or intentional states have a logical property that distinguishes them from all other states and especially from merely physical, or even goal-directed, states of nonintentional teleological systems, plants, thermostats, organs of the body, or simpler forms of biological life or macromolecules. It is a property that hinges on their representative character, on the fact that they "contain" or are "directed" to propositions about the way things are or could be. The property they have is this: When we change the descriptions of the states of affairs they "contain" in ways that seem innocuous, we turn the attributions of functional states into false ones. (1985, 256)

Rosenberg gives some examples of changes in truth value of sentences involving "beliefs" when the same entity is characterized by different descriptions, such as Oedipus's beliefs about Jocasta as "queen" and Jocasta as "mother of Oedipus." Similar points can be made about other propositional attitudes such as "desiring."

The subject of "intentionality" in this sense is a deep philosophical problem.[40] In the nineteenth century, Brentano first raised the problem and viewed it as posing considerable difficulties for any explication of the "mental" in terms of the "physical." Putnam underscored the difficulty of the problem when he entitled a subsection in one of his recent essays "Why Intentionality Is So Intractable" (1978, 13). Putnam also has argued that "there is no scientifically describable property that all cases of any particular intentional phenomenon have in common" (1988, 2), suggesting that Rosenberg is raising a particularly arduous problem when he ascribes intentionality to biological language.

Rosenberg's conclusion of his analysis of intentionality—I need not in these pages indicate how he gets there (see his 1985, 257–261)—is that "regularities employing the intentional description of mental states can never be theoretically linked up with neuroscience . . . [and] must therefore remain isolated from the remainder of natural science" (1985, 261). For Rosenberg, molecular biology can employ such intentional terms legitimately only if they are redefined so that the intentional metaphorical component is eliminated and replaced by strictly causal language. This is what he believes occurs in such research programs as Kandel and Schwartz's analysis of learning in *Aplysia* (see Rosenberg 1985, 263–264). Rosenberg sees intentional language as *irreducible in principle* to any type of causal language, regardless of the progress that the neurosciences may make.

This irreducibility of intentional language is a radical thesis, and it has been explored in depth by, among others, Patricia S. Churchland in her recent book *Neurophilosophy* (1986). Paul M. Churchland considers ways that the problem might be approached by eliminativist materialism in his 1981 essay. My discussion of it here is intended, not to assess this thesis of the irreducibility of intentional language, but primarily to point out that it is a much stronger thesis than the one I am arguing in this chapter, namely the indefinability of "goal" language in either cybernetic or evolutionary terms. Nevertheless, it also seems to me that the type of goal language that is employed in biology and medicine *borrows on* human intentional language (in the Brentano sense), and thus the difficulties with reducing "intentionality" in this stronger Brentano sense lend some support to my weaker thesis.

I have now concluded my fairly long account of four general types of explications of functional analysis: the intentional, the cybernetic, the evolutionary, and the anthropomorphic. It now remains to draw some general conclusions from this review. I have argued that all extant explications of functional analysis involve two components: a goal ascription and a causal claim. I have contended that the choice of a goal is extrinsic to functional explications, that it cannot be reduced, at least by the available models, to standard causal language, and that goals cannot be provided by a sophisticated dynamical evolutionary theory. As noted above, I suspect that the reasons why neither cybernetic systems nor dynamically construed natural selection processes can be utilized to infer goals have affinities and analogies with the argument in value theory known, after G. E. Moore, as the naturalistic fallacy.

My general point, then, is that in a very important sense functional language is irreducible (at present and probably for the foreseeable future) to nonfunctional language. However, because organisms and their subsystems possess strong analogies with human artifacts, such as, for instance, the eye and the camera, it is, however, *heuristically valuable* to use functional language in biological contexts. Purposes, such as survival, are often proposed in vague language, and subsidiary purposes can in turn be specified in somewhat sharpened language. Because of common experiences and common background knowledge, intersubjective agreement about the subsidiary purposes and the mechanisms which serve these purposes or functions is often obtainable. G. C. Williams, whose views on natural selection were cited earlier, thinks this is the case, but he also pointed out in this concluding chapter that we might do better:

> In this book I have assumed as is customary, that functional design is something that can be intuitively comprehended by an investigator and convincingly communicated to others. Although this may often be true, I suspect that progress in teleonomy will soon demand a standardization of criteria for demonstrating adaptation, and a formal terminology for its description. (Williams 1966, 260)

I think we can use the notion of some *general goal property*, G, such as survival of the systems or reproduction of the system (to obtain the principle sense (my earlier "secondary" sense) of function in biology and medicine) and/or a further, more *specific goal property(ies)*, g (related to the general goal property in some specific way), as part of any general explication of functional analysis. This, however, is with the proviso that it is *we* who choose these consequences as goal input. We only have to add, to a specified goal property, a causal claim involving an aspect A of item i (entity or process) that promotes it, either universally or in a significant probabilistic way, in order to attribute a function to A(i). Thus to claim that i has a function in system s is to claim:

(1) System S has a goal G (or g) property, and

(2) i, via A(i), results in or significantly promotes G (or g).

This, it seems to me, yields the most general sense of function and would permit ascribing functionality to the Three Mile Island bursa. To obtain the *primary biomedical science* sense, we need to restrict the G (or g) property to something like species (or deme or "subclan") survival. Thus if the "bursa-endowed" individual were not sterile, his *descendants'* bursas could have a "function" in this sense, though the "first" human bursa would only have a "function" in the more general sense—as a Gould-Vrba "exaptation."

I think that the conditions (1) and (2) just given are severally necessary and jointly sufficient for functional attribution. Condition (2) is consistent with and can be further analyzed in terms of the (probabilistic) causal model of explanation developed in chapter 6.

8.7 Teleological and Functional Explanations

Having gotten clearer about the nature of functional analysis, let me return to a discussion of the relation of this explication to an analysis of goal-directed systems and also comment on the relation of the account to *explanation*.

8.7.1 *The Relation of Goal-Directed Behavior to Functional Analysis*

A number of commentators have stressed the distinction between teleological and functional language. Thus, though Nagel admits that "some biologists use the words 'goal' and 'function' interchangeably," he contends both that there are distinctions linguistic usage recognizes, and more importantly, that "the analyses of what constitutes goal-directed behavior is different from the analysis of what counts as a function, and secondly the structure of functional explanations in biology differs from the structure of explanations of goal-directed behavior" (Nagel 1977, 227–278). Beckner (1969) similarly argues that there is a three-fold distinction between function ascriptions, goal ascriptions, and intention ascriptions. He points out that one can imagine cases of functionless goal direction, such as "an ingenious mechanism regulated by feedback that pumped sea water out of and back into the sea at a constant rate," in which "the activity of the machine would be goal-directed," but where "achievement of the goal serves no function." Further, Beckner notes that there are processes which serve functions without being goal-directed, for example, the blink reflex of the eye.

Wright also distinguishes function from goal-directed behavior and notes that:

> Even when goal-directed behavior has a function, very often its function is different from the achievement of its goal. For example, some fresh water plankton diurnally vary their distance below the surface. The goal of this behavior is to keep light intensity in their environment

> selectively constant . . . but the *function* of this behavior is to
> keep the oxygen supply constant, which normally varies
> with the sunlight intensity. (Wright 1976, 74)

The distinctions are useful but they should not obscure a deeper
structural identity between goal-directed behavior and functional analysis. Lack of attention to this deep structural identity
is, I think, both (1) the source of incompleteness in the analysis of
goal-direction or the missing element which provides the cessation of the infinite regresses in the system-necessary condition
account of Nagel and (2) the missing rationale for partially successful natural selection explication accounts of functional analysis.

Fundamentally, the ascription of both goal-directed behavior and functional analysis is "forward looking." This term is unfortunately vague but captures the important point that, in
ascriptions both of goal-directedness and function, something is
done or something exists *for the sake of* a distinguishable state or
system, which is seen as somehow *special*. This special state or
system is what I have termed in the account of functional analysis above the goal property. In behavioral patterns in which attainment (whether actual or inferred) of the goal property by the
system occurs after some finite time, a form of explication in
terms of purposiveness, goal-direction, or teleology is appropriate. In those situations in which the process itself results contem-
poraneously in the general or specific goal property, such as
"survival/reproduction" or "circulating the blood," a functional
analysis form is suitable.

8.7.2 *Explanation in Functional Analysis and*
Goal-Directed Behavior

On the basis of the above discussion of functional analysis and
goal-directed behavior, I want to argue first that functional ascriptions have a rather weak explanatory role in biomedical inquiry, though they are heuristically important. A number of
philosophers, for example Wimsatt and Wright, have suggested
that functional ascriptions do explain. According to Wimsatt,

> attributions of function play an explanatory role in tele-
> ological explanation. . . . They help to explain why the
> functional entity is present and has the form that it does.
> Performance of the functional consequence is *why* it is

there, for this is the property responsible for its selection, and past performances by the corresponding functional entities of ancestors are partially causally responsible, through selection, for the presence and form of the functional entity under consideration. (1972, 70)

Wimsatt criticizes Hempel among others for misinterpreting the nature of this type of explanation. For Hempel:

[functional analysis'] explanatory force is rather limited; in particular, it does not provide an explanation of why a particular item rather than some functional equivalent of it occurs in system S. And the predictive significance of functional analysis is practically nil—except in those cases where suitable hypotheses of self-regulation can be established. (1965, 324)

Wimsatt construes this as too sweeping. Though Hempel's judgment may be a valid one in the social sciences, Wimsatt proposes that:

it would seem possible to construct a valid *teleological* schema for functional explanations if population genetic and Mendelian genetic laws are assumed as premises, together with assumptions concerning the introduction of mutations in ancestors of the organisms in question and the magnitude of selection forces since their introduction. (Wimsatt 1972, 72, n. 121)[41]

Another vigorous defender of teleological explanations in biology, who views their legitimacy as underwritten by evolutionary theory, is Ayala (1970). Ayala maintains that "the presence of organs, processes and patterns of behavior can be explained teleologically by exhibiting their contribution to the reproductive fitness of the organisms in which they occur" (1970, 10). Moreover, the teleological character of the explanation captures the notion that the system in which it applies is "directively organized." Ayala thus views the use of teleological explanations so conceived as "not only acceptable but indeed indispensable" in biology (1970, 12).

Let us consider one of our representative biomedical explanation questions raised earlier in chapter 6, namely

(5) What is the function of the thymus in vertebrates?

to help sort out the truth in such claims as Wimsatt and Ayala make. I noted in chapter 6 that this is usually conceived of as a request for a functional analysis with an explanatory capacity. In the account of Miller's research leading to the discovery of the immunological function of the thymus (p. 385), we have an example that we may use to see exactly how this question is answered in the biomedical literature and how this answer relates to the present discussion, including Wimsatt's, Ayala's, and Hempel's divergent views. In somewhat oversimplified but I think accurate terms, an examination of the evidence for the thymus's immunological "function" shows the following:

(1) The thymus (item i) importantly contributes to the health of the mouse (and other vertebrates) in normal environments (the G-state) (though it can be ablated after the neonatal period without an immediately discernible effect).

(2) The thymus acts via the immune system, aspect A(i), composed of lymphocytes, lymphoid tissue, and a subspecies (strain) recognition system (graft rejection mechanism).

Neither functional alternatives to the thymus (though lower order organisms do not have one) nor any evolutionary process whereby the thymus was developed is indicated by the evidence. No laws of population genetics need be assumed in order to attribute function; in fact, if the arguments introduced earlier are correct, such a mechanistic explication might argue against a functional characterization. It thus seems sufficient for the attribution of a natural function in its primary sense (1) to introduce, vaguely, evidence for a major reduction in morbidity and/or mortality (the G-state) as an effect which the item (i) in question causes via A(i), and (2) *to conjecture* a significant difference in differential reproduction between a population without (i) and another (control) population with (i).

The *explanatory* capacity of such a functional ascription is quite weak. Because of a background evolutionary theory we (most likely by using the gross optimality interpretation) *suspect* that the thymus confers a selective evolutionary advantage (the primary sense of function discussed earlier), but we do not know what alternatives there were (nor what the environment was) against which (or in which) the "advantage" was exercised. All we have evidence for at this point in evolutionary time is that the thymus is important for the health of those organisms possessing it (the secondary sense of function). Because of this effect on health we *hypothesize* that an evolutionary account (presumably using the laws of population genetics *if such were ever available*) would yield an etiological explanation, but this hypothesis, if our thesis in chapter 7 is correct, is probably only a promissory note collectable in metaphysical currency. Furthermore, I would argue, if we ever got a *complete and dynamical* account of the etiology of the thymus, the appropriateness of a *functional* characterization of it would be attenuated, though not eliminated. This is because of the heuristic power that such functional language has in biology and medicine.[42]

Accordingly, I tend to side with Hempel and against Wimsatt on the explanatory force of functional ascriptions. I also think that Ayala's (1970) indispensability thesis and Rosenberg's (1985) similar claims are too strong in principle, though in practice they reasonably reflect the situation in biology and medicine. Such functional ascriptions are a combination of a causal assertion regarding current effects and a (probably metaphysical) hypothesis regarding etiology. Metaphysics is, however, not to be construed as useless or as antiscientific, since yesterday's metaphysics is often today's science (recall Democritus's atomism, and see Popper 1959, 277–278). In point of fact the metaphysical etiology claims point the way to comparative biomedical investigations that can have beneficial heuristic consequences. The focus on the important consequences (the G-state) and the aspect A(i) under which the entity (i) produces its consequences can also have powerful heuristic results for a research program. The explosive growth in immunology, resulting in the discovery of a multiplicity of thymus-derived (T) cells (helpers and suppressors) as control elements in the immune response, is a case in point. Such heuristic results, however, do not usually disclose more sound evidence for any detailed dynamical etiological or evolutionary account; the heuristic results rather are elaborations of the causal claim within a functional assumption. In sum, well-founded functional ascriptions explain weakly but are often of considerable heuristic power.

The situation is similar with respect to the explanatory force of teleological or goal-directed explanations. One can give a teleologically-oriented account of a thermostat or a torpedo and one can, *pace* Braithwaite (1953, chapter 9), even organize knowledge and make predictions in terms of such accounts. Still, for most purposes, the causal account in terms of the inner workings of the system in question will be more powerful and hence, if available, will be preferable to the teleological account other than for heuristic reasons.

Teleological explanations and predictions depend for their force on what Hempel has characterized as an established hypothesis of self-regulation. Such a hypothesis he characterizes as

> within a specified range c of circumstances, a given system S (or any system of a certain kind S, of which s is an instance) is self-regulating relative to a specified range R of states; i.e., that after a disturbance which moves S into a state outside of R but which does not shift the internal and external circumstances of S out of a specified range C, the system s will return to a state in R. (1965, 324)

Hempel notes that "biological systems offer many illustrations of such self-regulation," e.g., the regenerative ability of a hydra. Such explanations are important in a number of areas of biology and medicine where detailed and complete efficient causal accounts are not yet available. Presumably, in addition, subject to the concerns and empirical assumptions discussed by Lewontin (1977), evolutionary optimality methodology will stand in the same relation to underlying dynamical explanations. Such teleological and optimality-based accounts do not (and cannot) contradict these deeper level explanations; behaviorially, the teleological optimality and the efficient cause(s) of dynamical explanations lead to the same result. This convergence, however, does not entail that teleological explanations in which goal properties are used are definable in nonteleological terms.

In summary, the position taken in this chapter has been that functional teleological language is of heuristic value in biology and medicine, that it is sui generis in the sense of not being reducible to causal language, but that it is in principle, though perhaps not in practice, eliminable as these sciences progress.

CHAPTER NINE

Reduction and Reductionism in Biology and Medicine

9.1 Introduction

AS NOTED IN THE PREVIOUS CHAPTERS, several biomedical scientists and philosophers have argued that biology (and a fortiori, medicine) involves types of concepts and forms of explanation which are *distinct* from those employed in the physical sciences. The reductionistic alternative is to view these concepts and modes of explanation as only prima facie distinct and really definable in terms of (or fully explainable and perhaps replaceable by) concepts and modes of explanation drawn only from the physical and chemical sciences. The issues of reduction and reductionism in the biomedical sciences often provokes vigorous debate, as witness the claims and counterclaims made in chapters 7 and 8. There are a number of differing senses of reduction and reductionism, as well as the latter's opposite counterparts such as antireductionism, emergentism, and holism, which it will be useful to disentangle prior to a detailed examination of these topics. (I will use the term 'reductionism' to describe generally a disposition that favors reduction and believes reduction(s) can be carried out; the term 'reduction' will be defined and distinguished into various senses in the pages below.)

The discussion in this chapter will be primarily concerned with biology and medicine, where there are special problems for reduction, as foreshadowed by the material reviewed in the previous two chapters. It will also be useful to develop an extended example to help focus our discussion, and because of the considerable attention that the relation of classical (Mendelian-Morganian) genetics to molecular genetics has received from philosophers of biology in recent years, I shall concentrate on that exemplar. (I now explicitly add T. H. Morgan's name to

Mendel's to characterize classical genetics in this chapter since, as will be discussed below, Morgan's cytological extensions of Mendel's discoveries are key issues in discussions about reduction in genetics.) However, a number of the issues associated with reduction have broad import, and much of the philosophical literature on the topic has employed examples from the non-biomedical sciences — from physics in particular — to make certain points clear, so some brief examples from those sciences will be cited from time to time.

Reduction and reductionism, as well as the opposing antireductionistic positions, can, at least to the first approximation, be usefully distinguished into ontological and methodological claims. In table 9.1 the essential features of these positions are set out in brief summary form and representative scientists and philosophers who hold these views listed. (I hasten to add that, as with all classifications, there are individuals who do not easily fit into a classification or who span two categories.)

TABLE 9.1 REDUCTIONISTIC AND ANTIREDUCTIONISTIC
APPROACHES IN BIOLOGY AND MEDICINE

Type of Approach	Reductionistic	Antireductionistic
Ontological: Strong	"Nothing but" chemistry and physics: Loeb	Vitalism: Driesch
Ontological: Weak	De facto emergence: Nagel	Emergentism-in-principle: Bernard, Weiss, Polanyi, Oparin, Elsasser
Methodological: Strong	Sound biological generalizations or explanations are molecular: Kandel	Biological explanations *must* involve higher levels: Weiss, Simpson, Mayr, Grene
Methodological: Weak	For the present, we must appeal to interlevel or interfield features: Grobstein, Simon, Kitcher, Darden and Maull, Bechtel, Wimsatt	For the present *and future* we must appeal to related but not-fully-connected higher levels: Fodor, Hull, Rosenberg

Reductionism, to a number of biomedical scientists, often has the connotation that biological entities are "nothing but" aggregates of physicochemical entities; this sort of approach can betermed *ontological* reductionism of a strong form. A weak form of ontological reductionism is represented by the de facto emergentism of Nagel. The contrary of the first ontological position is the antireductionist view, which often is further distinguished into a strong *vitalistic* position and a second, weaker *emergentist-in-principle* view. From the perspective of both of these antireductionist views the biomedical sciences not only are autonomous at the present time but always will be so. Emergentism, including the "in-principle" type, should probably be distinguished from the strong vitalistic thesis, championed earlier in this century by Hans Driesch, that proposed the existence of special forces and irreducible causes which were peculiar to living entities. The vitalist thesis led to no testable hypotheses and is essentially moribund in contemporary biology.[1]

A *methodological* counterpart to strong ontological reductionism holds that sound scientific generalizations are available only at the level of physics and chemistry. I view the work of Kandel and his associates, discussed in chapter 6, as representing this type of position. The contrary of the *methodological* reductionist position is a kind of methodological emergentism. It too can be distinguished into a strong position, such as that taken by Weiss (1969), Mayr and Grene in various writings, and Simpson (1964). I will discuss this type of position in detail in section 9.2. There is also a weaker form of antireductionist methodological emergentism represented in the writings of Fodor, Hull, and Rosenberg, maintaining that for the present and the future we will have to appeal to related but not-fully-reducible higher levels. These authors do not accept *ontological* antireductionism, but they parse the problem in a way that will not permit the satisfaction of methodologically useful reductionistic approaches in biology and (in Fodor's case) psychology. The views and arguments of these authors will receive extended treatment later in this chapter. Finally, there is what might be termed a pragmatic, holistic, but in-principle reductionistic approach (to use Simon's 1981 terminology) of the weak metholodological sort that attributes the necessity of working with higher-level entities to current gaps in our knowledge. I interpret a number of authors' positions as falling into this classification, as noted in the table above, and myself favor this view; I see it as resonating strongly with the construal of theories in biology and medicine as essentially (for the present and forseeable future) interlevel, a position developed in detail in chapters 3 and 5. In later sections of this chapter the views of these and other authors will be presented in detail.

It will be useful to develop some of the emergentist arguments as a prelude to a philosophical account of reduction. Readers who are familiar with the extensive philosophical literature on reduction will note the absence in the table of any explicit reference to "intertheoretic" reduction, about which much of the debate in recent years has been focused. That is because I view the "intertheoretic" perspective as a second-order position in terms of which the various positions in table 9.1 can be usefully reformulated. I view that reformulation as best developed after the reader has been familiarized with the antireductionist positions of both ontological and methodological form, thus it is to that task that I now turn. (I shall defer until later in this chapter consideration of several arguments for emergentism which have been offered on the basis of quantum mechanical considerations and a generalization of the principle of complementarity, since these arguments raise rather specific issues.)

9.2 Arguments for In-Principle Emergentism

By the expression "in-principle emergentism" I mean the claim that the biomedical sciences are incapable, regardless of progress in biology and the physicochemical sciences, of being reduced to physics and chemistry. Generally this type of position is based on what its proponents perceive to be certain general timeless *logical* features of biomedical entities and modes of explanation. In this section I will distinguish two types of arguments, which I shall call "structural" and "evolutionary." The two types of arguments are not completely independent, and I view the second, "evolutionary" type of argument as parasitic on the first, "structural" argument for emergence. However, some defenders of emergence, such as Oparin and Simpson, have stressed in different ways the evolutionary rationale for their theses, and I shall follow them in providing a discussion which accepts this distinction, at least for the purposes of exposition. In a later section of this chapter, I shall argue that evolutionary considerations *are* important in providing an answer to the question of emergence, but that, contrary to the views of Oparin and Simpson, evolution underwrites a reductionist position.

9.2.1 *Structural Arguments*

Quite frequently, defenders of in-principle emergentism appeal to special properties of a combination that are not predictable on the basis of the component parts of the combination. For example, Ernst Mayr has suggested that one of the reasons for the differences in determinancy and predictability in biology, as contrasted with the physical sciences, might well be the presence of emergent properties. Mayr noted that one of several factors responsible for the relative lack of predictability was "*Emergence* of new and unpredictable qualities at hierarchical levels" (1982, 59). Mayr further claimed:

> Systems almost always have the peculiarity that the characteristics of the whole cannot (even in theory) be deduced from the most complete knowledge of the components, taken separately or in other partial combinations. This appearance of new characteristics in wholes has been designated as *emergence*. (1982, 63)[2]

(Also see Mayr 1988, 15 and 34–35, for a recommitment to this view.)

The locus classicus of this view can be found in John Stuart Mill's *Logic*, where Mill cites "the chemical combination of two substances produces, as is well known, a third substance with properties different from those of either of the two substances separately or of both of them taken together. Not a trace of the properties of hydrogen or of oxygen is observable in those of their compound, water" (1973 [1843], 371). This view of Mill's is echoed in the work of Claude Bernard, who wrote:

> As we know, it happens that properties, which appear and disappear in synthesis and analysis, cannot be considered as simple addition or pure subtraction of properties of the constituent bodies. Thus, for example, the properties of oxygen and hydrogen do not account for the properties of water, which result nevertheless from combining them. . . .
>
> It follows also, in physiology, that analysis, which teaches us the properties of isolated elementary parts, can never give us more than a most incomplete knowledge of all the institutions which result from man's association, and which can reveal themselves only through social life. In a word, when we unite physiological elements, properties appear which were imperceptible in the separate elements.

We must therefore always proceed experimentally in vital synthesis, because quite characteristic phenomena may result from more and more complex union or association of organized elements. All this proves that these elements, though distinct and self-dependent, do not therefore play the part of simple associates; their union expresses more than addition of their separate properties. (l961 [1865], 90–91)

Bernard then offers the following injunction:

Physiologists and physicians must therefore always consider organisms as a whole and in detail at one and the same time, without ever losing sight of the peculiar conditions of all the special phenomena whose resultant is the individual. (1961 [1865], 91)

This position is frequently referred to by the term "holism" (sometimes spelled "wholism"), introduced by Smuts in 1926 to describe a general philosophical approach in which the "whole" is an active irreducible factor, though it is obvious from the claims by Bernard that the thesis precedes Smuts. Sometimes the emergentist thesis focuses on the *organization* encountered in biological systems as the source of the emergence. For example, von Bertalanffy maintained:

Since the fundamental character of the living thing is its organization, the customary investigation of the single parts and processes, even the most thorough physicochemical analysis, cannot provide a complete explanation of the vital phenomena. This investigation gives us no information about the co-ordination of the parts and processes in the complicated system of the living whole which constitutes the essential 'nature' of the organism, and by which the reactions in the organism are distinguished from those in the test-tube. But no reason has been brought forward for supposing that the organization of the parts and the mutual adjustments of the vital processes cannot be treated as scientific problems. Thus, the chief task of biology must be to discover the laws of biological systems to which the ingredient parts and processes are subordinate. (1933, 64–65)

The distinguished embryologist Paul A. Weiss has argued in a similar vein that a holistic, supramolecular approach must be taken in analyzing biological systems. Weiss distinguished between the "two opposite extremes of reductionism and holism," noting that the former finds currently its most outspoken advocates in the field of so-called molecular biology (1969, 10). In an exegesis of the phrase "the whole is more than the sum of its parts,"[3] Weiss contends that he takes a middle position between reductionism and holism:

> the 'more' than the sum of parts in the above tenet does not at all refer to any measurable quantity in the observed systems themselves; it refers solely to the necessity for the observer to supplement the sum of statements that can be made about the separate parts by any such additional statements as will be needed to describe the *collective behavior* of the parts, when in an organized group. In carrying out this upgrading process he is in effect doing no more than *restoring information content* that has been lost on the way down in the progressive analysis of the unitary universe into abstracted elements. (1969, 11)

In Weiss's view, the organism is a set of hierarchically subordinated structures which are not reducible to lower level constituents: "In the cell," he writes, "certain definite rules of order apply to the dynamics of the *whole* system, in the present case reflected in the orderliness of the overall architectural design, which cannot be explained in terms of any underlying orderliness of the constituents" (1969, 23). In addition, Weiss adds, "the overall order of the cell as a whole does not impose itself upon the molecular population directly, but becomes effective through intermediate ordering steps delegated to subsystems such as organelles, each of which operates within its own, more limited authority" (1969, 23).

Weiss argues that the molecular constituents are not precisely determined, but that, in spite of this, macro-level patterns persist with a considerable degree of regularity. He believes that, though the physical sciences have been able to abstract and isolate microentities and treat the sum of a group of such entities' interactive behavior by "recombinatory methods," these methods have only limited applicability and cannot be used to understand the "integrality of a living system" (1969, 32). The thrust of these claims goes beyond any de facto gaps in our knowledge about the chemical properties and relationships among physico-chemical entities, and thus his is an argument for a timeless and *in-principle* emergentism.

One of the clearest antireductionist arguments defending this view can be found in the theses developed by Michael Polanyi (1968). In certain ways Polanyi's position is synergistic with Weiss's views as outlined above, in the sense that Weiss wishes to underscore the at least equal importance of the cell's control over its parts, in comparison to the direction exerted by the parts (organelles and molecules) over the whole cell. Weiss is careful in his writings not to argue for an explicit antireductionist position, whereas Polanyi is an unabashed antireductionist. In Polanyi's view, not only do, say, cells exert control over molecules, but the "mind" exerts control over corporeal parts, and the mind itself is constituted by an ascending sequence of principles in which "responsibility" harnesses the principles of "appetite" and "intellect." Polanyi's thesis stresses the *structure* of living things and argues that this structure is not reducible to physics and chemistry. (I am sympathetic with a rather different interpretation of the impact of biological structure, and will defend it in the present chapter in a later section on the distinction between structural and ultimate reductionism. For now, however, let us look at Polanyi's interpretation of biological organization.)

Polanyi argues that the structure of living organisms constitutes a set of "boundary conditions":

> Its structure serves as a boundary condition harnessing the physical-chemical processes by which its [the organism's] organs perform their functions. Thus, this system [the living organism] may be called a system under dual control. These boundary conditions are always extraneous [to the processes] which . . . they delimit. . . . Their structure cannot be defined in terms of the laws which they harness. (1968, 1308)

Polanyi contends that a similar situation holds for "machines" as well as for living organisms, for

> a machine as a whole works under the control of two distinct principles. The higher one is the principle of the machine's design [that is, presumably, the "structure" of the interrelated parts] and this harnesses the lower one

which consists in the physical-chemical processes on which the machine relies. (1968, 1308)

Polanyi explicitly considers the role that DNA plays in the production of living organisms. He claims that the nucleotide sequence:

> can function as a code only if its order is not due to the forces of potential energy. It must be as *physically* indeterminate as a sequence of words is on a printed page. As the arrangement on a printed page is extraneous to the chemistry of the printed page, so is the base sequence in a DNA molecule extraneous to the chemical forces at work in the DNA molecule. (1968, 1309; my emphasis)

The implication here is that there is some higher, nonchemical force that encodes the DNA.

Polanyi admits that DNA acts as a blueprint for the organism, but he harbors doubts about the translation of the DNA information without the aid of some higher operative principles, principles analogous to Driesch's *entelecheia morphogenetica* and to an irreducible version of Spemann's and Weiss's "field" that guides the growth of embryonic fragments. In Polanyi's words:

> Growth of a blueprint into the complex machinery that it describes seems to require a system of causes not specifiable in terms of physics and chemistry, such causes being additional both to the boundary conditions of DNA and to the morphological structure brought about by the DNA. (1968, 1310)

Polanyi's philosophy of biology is, accordingly, a clear claim of the irreducibility of biology. It suggests that a hierarchy of controlling principles that are additional to and unspecifiable in terms of physics and chemistry must be taken into account, and as just indicated, seems to suggest that a neo-Drieschian vitalism may be the correct answer as regards embryological development.

As I have indicated above, in addition to the "structural" arguments for in principle emergence, some scholars have suggested that "evolutionary" types of considerations license an antireductionist position. It is to these arguments that I now turn.

9.2.2 *Evolutionary Arguments*

The distinguished Russian biologist A. I. Oparin has argued, based on his investigations into the origin of life, that *new, biological laws* are required to explain the evolution of living systems. It should be noted that Oparin does assert that the laws of physics and chemistry are sufficient to account for the very earliest stages of chemical evolution, during which some complex compounds arose spontaneously in the hypothesized prebiotic "soup" or "primaeval broth" present billions of years ago on the earth. Experimental evidence by Miller (1953) and Fox (1965) indicates that amino acids and proteinaceous structures will form naturally in such an environment if suitable energy sources, such as lightning bolts or volcanic erruptions, are provided. Oparin proposed and was able to demonstrate in the laboratory that proteinaceous molecules would form droplets, which he termed "coacervates." He conjectured that these droplets could contain active enzymes and nucleic acids, though he noted in a text written in the early 1960s that "in view of the extreme complexity of the phenomenon . . . the theory of coacervation cannot be considered as fully worked out" (1962, 69). Further developments of origin-of-life theories will be considered later; suffice it for now to note that Oparin believed that, when the first complex self-sustaining (in that environment) and replicating systems appeared, *newly emergent laws* also appeared. He stated:

> Once life has come into being, however, the laws of physics and chemistry alone are not enough to determine the course of further evolution of matter. An understanding of this course can now only be achieved on the basis of new biological laws which developed concurrently with life. (1962, 97)

Oparin went on to explain how these "new biological laws" arise and what their function is in biological inquiry:

> Each essential link in the metabolic chain can, from the purely chemical point of view, be brought about by a very large number of related chemical processes none of which would, in any way, violate the laws of physics or chemistry. In the process of the development of life, however, natural selection has preserved for further development only a few individual combinations of reactions out of all these numerous chemical possibilities. These were then trans-

ferred from one generation to the next. We are far from always able to understand why this happened to one particular combination or chemical mechanism, as a purely chemical approach would always show that other combinations were equally good. In such cases the matter is clearly determined by some historic necessity, some specific biological adaptation. It is, however, important, that the further uses of these particular biologically selected collections and mechanisms, rather than any others which were chemically possible, became as obligatory in the whole subsequent development of the living world as the constancy of chemical reactions or physical processes is in the world of inorganic things.

We can now find, in particular metabolic sequences, sets of reactions which appear to be common to all organisms without exception, that is, a certain constancy of biological organization . . . This constancy of biological organization cannot be determined by the general laws of chemical kinetics or thermodynamics alone. It is the expression of a form of organization which could only have been elaborated historically in the process of the development of living material.

Thus the property of living bodies which we have noticed takes on the character of a specific biological law. An understanding of this law will enable us to use increasingly detailed comparative biochemical analysis of the metabolism of modern organisms as a basis for tracing the evolutionary paths followed by the living world many hundreds of millions of years ago, just as we use the general laws of physics and chemistry in trying to understand the process of development of organic material which preceded the appearance of life. (1962, 97–98)

There is much in these passages that calls for further comment and I shall analyze Oparin's reasoning in more detail in a later section. Oparin is not alone in appealing to origin of life considerations in defending an emergentist thesis; a more recent defense of this type of position can be found in the (1964, 1968) monograph by John Koesian, *The Origin of Life*, which cites Oparin as well as the British biologist J. D. Bernal on evolution and then develops an emergentist thesis.

In a rather different type of argument, the evolutionary biologist G. G. Simpson has maintained that explanations involving evolution force us beyond reductionistic positions. Simpson's claim is not focused on the issue of emergent laws but rather asserts that there is a different type of explanation that evolutionary theory demands and provides which is antireductionist. Simpson claimed:

> A second kind of explanation must be added to the first or reductionist explanation in terms of physical, chemical, and mechanical principles. This second form of explanation, which can be called compositionist in contrast with reductionist, is in terms of the adaptive usefulness of structures and processes to the whole organism and to the species of which it is a part, and still further, in terms of ecological function in the communities in which the species occurs. (1964, 104)[4]

This quotation from Simpson completes for the moment my summary of a number of the antireductionistic positions which have been advanced by biologists and philosophers. I hope to have shown through these summaries and quotations that the issues of reduction and emergence have a number of facets as well as that differing points of view have been taken in regard to them.

In a later section of this chapter I shall return to both the structural and the evolutionary arguments for emergence and present arguments against their claims. As already noted earlier, however, a major aspect of recent discussions about the concept of reduction has revolved around what has been termed *intertheoretic* reduction, though I think the term is somewhat misleading. In order to develop adequate answers to the antireductionist arguments presented thus far in this chapter, I will need to employ some of the distinctions developed under this rubric. Essentially, intertheoretic reduction is the *explanation* of a theory initially formulated in one branch of science by a theory from another discipline. I shall develop a notion of intertheoretic or branch reduction from a core sense of intertheoretic reduction, and then discuss it in the context of the various senses of reduction and emergence outlined above. I shall also respond then to the specifics of antireductionist arguments developed in the present section.

9.3 Intertheoretic and Branch Reduction

Before we can determine whether the above emergentist arguments carry validity or, alternatively, if reductionist counterarguments are sound, it is necessary to examine in some detail exactly what constitutes a successful reduction. Philosophers of science have attempted to specify certain criteria for reductions in science generally. With appropriate augmentation these will also prove useful for examining reduction in biology and medicine.

As noted earlier in this chapter, a major component of the concept of reduction to be elucidated is often referred to as *intertheoretic* reduction. Much of the discussion by scientists and philosophers has focused on this notion, though I think the term is somewhat misleading since occasionally theories are eliminated but, more often, a preexisting domain or *branch* of science is (at least partially) reduced.[5] Sometimes, for example by Kemeny and Oppenheim (1950), this type of reduction is referred to as *branch* reduction when it is felt that emphasis on *theories* is not appropriate. This I think is a useful corrective, since, as was argued in chapter 3, what can be captured by general, high-level abstract theory in biology and medicine is often considerably different from what can be so represented in physics.

The most succinct way to introduce several approaches which have been developed by philosophers of science will be to present schemata or models of reduction. I shall develop several of these fairly formally and mention some others less formally; they will be useful as initial vantage points from which to examine the classes of models themselves as well as problems concerning biomedical reductions.

The first of the models that I wish to consider is primarily due to Ernst Nagel (1949, 1961) and is congruent with similar views developed by J. H. Woodger (1952) and W. V. Quine (1964). Following what has become standard usage I will refer to it as the Nagel model.

9.3.1 *The Nagel Model*

This account of reduction can be characterized as *direct* reduction, in which the basic terms (and entities) of one theory are related to the basic terms (and entities) of the other, assuming that the reduced theory is an adequate one and that the axioms and laws of the reduced theory are derivable from the reducing theory. The last assumption must be expanded somewhat, for quite often in intertheoretic explanation terms appear in the reduced theory which are not part of the reducing theory — for instance, the term "gene" does not appear in organic chemistry. Thus we have to conjoin additional sentences to the reducing theory which associate these terms of the reduced or secondary theory with combinations of terms from the vocabulary of the reducing or primary theory. The exact logical and epistemic natures of these associating sentences will be discussed later.

A precondition of the Nagel model is its assumption that the reduced and reducing theories can be *explicitly* characterized. Nagel recognized that this was an "ideal demand" rather than one satisfied in the normal course of scientific reductions (1961, 347). In addition, Nagel suggested that it would be useful to distinguish the most general statements of a theory from others — these would typically be the fundamental "laws" of the theory[6] — and to cast the reduced and reducing theories into *axiomatic form*, in which deductive systematization was disclosed. Further, Nagel felt that the theoretically primitive terms of a theory should be explicitly noted, distinguished from the branch's observational vocabulary, and that the terms of the theories under consideration should have stable meaning, fixed by the procedures of the science from which they were drawn (1961, 346–352).

These are "preliminary" assumptions and constitute background for Nagel's model, which I shall introduce shortly. It should be noted, however, that even though these preliminary assumptions are recognized as "ideals" by Nagel, philosophers of science have largely drifted away from subscribing to them. As I have noted in chapter 4, the sharp separation of scientific vocabulary into "theoretical" and "observational" has essentially been dismissed by philosophers of science. Also, Nagel's preference for representing a theory as a small collection of general statements or laws is of questionable applicability in biology and medicine, as I have noted in chapter 3. The requirement that we represent the theory in terms of general laws has been criticized by Wimsatt (1976a; 1976b) and Kitcher (1984), and is an issue to which I shall return later.

The Nagel model for intertheoretic reduction essentially contains two formal conditions:

1. *Connectability*, such that "assumptions of some kind must be introduced which postulate suitable relations between whatever is signified by 'A,' a term appearing in the reduced science but not in the reducing science, and the traits represented by theoretical terms already present in the primary [or reducing] science."
2. *Derivability*, such that "with the help of these additional assumptions, all the laws of the secondary [reduced] science, including those containing the term 'A,' must be logically derivable from the theoretical premises and their associated coordinating definitions in the primary discipline" (1961, 353–354).

As we shall see in more detail below, connectability later came to be best seen as representing a kind of "synthetic identity," such as gene = DNA sequence, (Schaffner 1967, Sklar 1967, Causey 1977). For an example of this type of reduction, see Nagel's (1961, 338–345) illustration of the reduction of thermodynamics by statistical mechanics, which occurred in the latter half of the nineteenth century.

9.3.2 *The Kemeny-Oppenheim Model*

J. G. Kemeny and P. Oppenheim developed what might best be termed a model of *indirect* reduction, since one does not obtain a second theory, T_2, from the original, T_1, as in the usual case of reduction, but rather identical observable predictions from both theories (though T_1 may predict more).[7] We shall bring out the implications of this assertion in discussion below. This model can be articulated in more formal terms (see Kemeny and Oppenheim 1957), but this will not be required for my purposes here. An example of this type of reduction might be the explanation by Lavoisier's oxidation theory of all the observable facts which the phlogiston theory explained. Notice in this case we would not be able to define "phlogiston" in terms of the oxidation theory.[8]

9.3.3 *The Suppes-Adams (Semantic) Model*

An interesting alternative third model (and more semantic approach to reduction) was developed by Suppes and Adams. According to Suppes:

Many of the problems formulated in connection with the question of reducing one science to another may be formulated as a series of problems using the notion of a representation theorem for the models of a theory. For instance, the thesis that psychology may be reduced to physiology would be for many people appropriately established if one could show that, for any model of a psychological theory, it was possible to construct an isomorphic model within physiological theory. (1967, 59)

Another example of this type of reduction is given by Suppes as follows:

To show in a sharp sense that thermodynamics may be reduced to statistical mechanics, we would need to axiomatize both disciplines by defining appropriate set-theoretical predicates, and then show that given any model T of thermodynamics we may find a model of statistical mechanics on the basis of which we may construct a model isomorphic to T. (1957, 271)

This model-theoretic approach provides a somewhat complementary but essentially equivalent way to approach the issues, to which I shall return shortly.

9.3.4 The General Reduction Model

Suppes and Adams excepted, and thus also later work by Sneed (1971), Stegmuller (1976), and Balzer and Dawe (1986), most writers working on reduction have dealt with the more syntactic requirements of Nagel's connectability and derivability. The derivability condition, as well as the connectability requirement, was strongly attacked in influential criticisms by Popper (1957), Feyerabend (1961, 1962), and Kuhn (1962). Feyerabend, citing a personal communication from Watkins, seemed to suggest that perhaps some account of reduction could be preserved by allowing approximation, but he never developed the thesis (1962, 93). In my 1967, I elaborated a modified reduction model designed to preserve the strengths of the Nagel account but flexible enough to accommodate the criticisms of Popper, Feyerabend, and Kuhn. That model, which I termed the *general reduction paradigm*,[9] has been in turn criticized (Hull 1974; Wimsatt 1976a, 1976b; Hooker 1981), defended (Schaffner 1976; Ruse 1976), further developed (Wimsatt 1976a, 1976b; Schaffner 1977; Hooker 1981), and recriticized recently (Kitcher 1984; Rosenberg 1985). A somewhat similar approach to reduction was developed by Paul Churchland in a several books and papers (1979, 1981, 1984).[10] In a form close to that of the original general reduction model, such an approach has quite recently been applied in the area of neurobiology by Patricia Churchland (1986). Churchland's account is one of the most concise statements of that general model, as follows:

> Within the new, reducing theory T_B, construct *an analogue* T^*_R of the laws, etc., of the theory that is to be reduced, T_R. The analogue T^*_R can then be logically deduced from the reducing theory T_B plus sentences specifying the special conditions (e.g., frictionless surfaces, perfect elasticity). Generally the analogue will be constructed with a view to mapping expressions of the old theory onto expressions of the new theory, laws of the old theory onto sentences (but not necessarily *laws*) of the new. Under these conditions the old theory reduces to the new. When reduction is successfully achieved, the new theory will explain the old theory, it will explain why the old theory worked as well as it did, and it will explain much where the old theory was buffaloed. (1986, 282–283)

Churchland goes on to apply this notion of reduction to the sciences of psychology (and also what is termed folk psychology), which are the sciences *to be reduced*, and to the rapidly evolving neurosciences, which are the *reducing sciences*. In so doing she finds she needs to relax the model to accommodate, for example, cases not of full reduction but of partial reduction or replacement. She never explicitly reformulates the model to take such modifications into account, however, and it would seem useful, given the importance of such modifications, to say a bit more as to how this might be accomplished.

9.3.5 *The General Reduction-Replacement Model*

The *most* general model of reduction must also allow for those cases in which the T_R is *not* modifiable into a T_R^* but rather is *replaced* — but with preservation of the empirical domain — by T_B or a T_B^*, a "corrected" reducing theory. Though not what occurred historically, a reduction of phlogiston theory by a combination of Lavoisier's oxidation theory and Dalton's atomic theory would be such a replacement. Replacement of a demonic theory of disease with a germ theory of disease but with retention, say, of the detailed observations of the natural history of the diseases and perhaps preexisting knowledge of syndrome clusters as well, would be another example of reduction with replacement (see Schaffner 1977). (Later I shall discuss a detailed example of replacement-reduction of the generalized induction theory by the operon theory of genetic regulation—see p. 482 ff. below.)

In the simplest replacement situation, we have the essential *experimental arena* of the previous T_R (but not the theoretical premises) directly connected via new correspondence rules associated with T_B (or $T_B{}^*$) to the reducing theory. A correspondence rule is here understood as a telescoped causal sequence linking (relatively) theoretical processes to (relatively) observable ones. (A summary of this approach can be found in chapter 4, and a more detailed account of this interpretation of correspondence rules is given in Schaffner 1969a.) Several of these rules would probably suffice, then, to allow for further explanation of the experimental results of T_R's subject area by a T_B (or $T_B{}^*$).

In the more complex but realistic case, we also want to allow for partial reduction, that is, the possibility of a partially adequate component of T_R being maintained together with the entire *domain* (or even only part of the domain) of T_R. (The sense we give to domain here is that of Shapere 1974, as discussed in chapter 2: a domain is a complex of experimental results which either are accounted for by T_R and/or *should be* accounted for by T_R when, and if, T_R is or becomes completely and adequately developed.) Thus, there arises the possibility of a continuum of reduction relations in which T_B (or $T_B{}^*$) can participate. (In those cases where only one of T_B or $T_B{}^*$ is the reducing theory, we shall use the expression $T_B(*)$.) To allow for such a continuum, T_R must be construed not only as a completely integral theory but also as a theory dissociable into weaker versions, and also as associated with an experimental subject area(s) or domain(s). Interestingly, the Suppes-Adams model might lend some additional structure, through the use of model-theoretic terminology, to this notion of partial reduction, though the original schema will need some (strengthening) modifications.

We may conceive of "weaker versions of the theory" either (1) as those classes of models of the theory in which not all the assumptions of the theory are satisfied or (2) as a restricted sub-

GENERAL REDUCTION-REPLACEMENT (GRR) MODEL

T_B — the reducing theory/model
T_B^* — the "corrected" reducing theory/model
T_R — the original reduced theory/model
T_R^* — the "corrected" reduced theory/model
(In those cases where only one of T_B or T_B^* is the reducing theory, we shall use the expression $T_B(*)$.)

Reduction in the most general sense occurs if and only if:

(1)(a) All primitive terms of T_R^* are associated with one or more of the terms of $T_B(*)$, such that:
(i) T_R^* (entities) = function ($T_B(*)$ (entities))
(ii) $T_R(*)$ (predicates) = function ($T_B(*)$ (predicates))[†]
or
(1)(b) The domain of T_R^* be connectable with $T_B(*)$ via new correspondence rules. (Condition of generalized connectability.)

(2)(a) Given fulfillment of condition (1)(a), that T_R^* be derivable from $T_B(*)$ supplemented with (1)(a)(i) and (1)(a)(ii) functions.
or
(2)(b) Given fulfillment of condition (1)(b) the domain of T_R be derivable from $T_B(*)$ supplemented with the new correspondence rules. (Condition of generalized derivability.)

(3) In case (1)(a) and (2)(a) are met, T_R^* corrects T_R, that is, T_R^* makes more accurate predictions. In case (1)(b) and (2)(b) are met, it may be the case that T_B^* makes more accurate predictions in T_R's domain than did T_R.

(4)(a) T_R is explained by $T_B(*)$ in that T_R and T_R^* are strongly analogous, and $T_B(*)$ indicates why T_R worked as well as it did historically.
or
(4)(b) T_R's domain is explained by $T_B(*)$ even when T_R is replaced.

[†]The distinction between entities and predicates will in general be clear in any given theory/model, though from a strictly extensional point of view the distinction collapses. See endnote 21.

class of all the models of the reduced and/or reducing theory. The first weakening represents a restriction of assumption, the second a restriction in the applied scope of the theory. As an example of the first type of restriction, consider a set of models in which the first and second laws of Newton are satisfied but which is silent on or which denies the third law. The application to reduction is straightforward, since in point of fact there are models of optical and electromagnetic theories in the nineteenth century which satisfy Newton's first two laws but which violate the third (see Schaffner 1972, 65). As an example of the second type of restriction, consider a restriction of the scope of statistical mechanical models that eliminates (for the purpose of achieving the reduction) those peculiar systems (of measure zero) in which entropy does not increase, such as a collection of particles advancing in a straight line. This second type of restriction is unfortunately ad hoc.

The Suppes-Adams model can be strengthened to require that what Quine has termed a "proxy function" hold—this proxy function is essentially a homomorphic mapping (see Hooker 1981), but it needs to be interpreted semantically as a synthetic identity. It can then be proven that the Suppes-Adams schema is a special case of a Nagel type of reduction (see Schaffner 1967 for a formal proof). For partial reductions, however, the strengthened Suppes-Adams approach still seems (1) to permit an account that is both consistent with the general reduction model (and with its successor, the general reduction-replacement model developed below) and (2) to cohere well with the semantic interpretation of scientific theories, which is a nice additional bonus.[11]

If these considerations seem reasonable, then the general reduction model introduced above should be modified into the general reduction-replacement model (or GRR model), characterized by the conditions given in the textbox. These conditions are of necessity formulated in somewhat technical language, but the concepts involved should be reasonably clear from the discussion above. (The italicized *ors* should be taken in the weak, inclusive sense of "or.")

Such a model has as a limiting case what we have previously characterized as the general reduction model, which in turn yields Nagel's model as a limiting case. The use of the weak sense of *or* in conditions (1), (2) and (4) allows the "continuum" ranging from reduction as subsumption to reduction as explanation of the experimental domain of the replaced theory. Though in this latter case we do not have intertheoretic reduction, we do maintain the "branch" reduction mentioned earlier. This flexibility of the general reduction-replacement model is particularly useful in connection with discussions concerning current theories that may explain "mental" phenomena. It will also be essential to account for the "reduction" of enzyme induction by the operon theory of Jacob and Monod (and the replacement of the "generalized induction theory"—see p. 482). Finally, I should note that the GRR model can be further enriched to accommodate the partial reductions entailed by the use of the multi-level γ, σ, δ distinctions introduced in chapter 6. Further below, where I consider a "complex GRR" approach (see p. 498 ff.), I argue that the GRR model given in the textbox on the previous page is a "simple" interpretation of reduction; a more "complex" GRR account is also constructable, and in certain cases will be more desirable (see section 9.6).

To this point I have treated reduction in terms of explanation and/or replacement but without introducing a directional aspect of reduction which is traditionally very important in reductions involving biology. The directional aspect is sometimes articulated in terms of "levels," according to which reduction is assumed to involve an explanation or replacement of a higher-level theory by a lower-level theory. An example would be the replacement of the traditional theory of Mendelian-Morganian genetics by a molecular biochemical theory involving DNA, RNA, and proteinaceous entities. The general reduction-replacement model as outlined above does not per se involve this "level" directionality, and it is thus capable of encompassing what might be termed unilevel reduction relations, such as can be found in the relation of the optical aether-theoretic and electromagnetic aether-theoretic theories in the nineteenth century.

In biology and medicine, however, the term "reduction" is often taken to have a directional connotation inherently associated with it. This directionality can be construed as a special case of the more general reduction-replacement model when we deal with theories applied to entities involved in a part/whole relation. It would be useful to point out here, however, an additional problem for the reduction-replacement model presented above, namely, that the model can be interpreted in a historically misleading manner. Though the model has a dynamic element built into it through its starred theories or models, actual historical reductions, no matter where they may lie on the continuum from reduction as explanation to reduction as replacement, rarely if ever go to completion in the sense of attaining stasis. The model presented above, with the exception of its explicitly partial aspects, is thus an ideal of finished "clarified" science (to use Putnam's and Hooker's term — see p. 472), or of science that has evolved but has stopped evolving. The science we know today and the science we know from history do not have this characteristic.

Furthermore, it is important to note, as will be developed in a later section, that the reason why reductions are not completed follows from an intrinsic and central component of scientific inquiry. Reductions are not completed because science is constantly changing, and because reductions in a directional sense are only accidentally the aim of science. I will discuss this perhaps provocative thesis later.

Though what I have said thus far constitutes a useful expansion of the traditional model, we have yet to reexamine one of the basic assumptions introduced by Nagel, that reduction is best conceived of as a relation between *theories* (though we have allowed a reduction to occur between a theory and the domain of a previous theory); we also have not yet seriously questioned whether the notion of laws or a collection of laws is the appropriate reductandum and reductans.[12] It is to these issues and to a broad range of other criticisms of intertheoretic models of reduction that I now turn.

9.4 Criticisms and Elaborations of Intertheoretic Reduction Models

As mentioned already, a number of philosophers of science have made contributions to the burgeoning literature on intertheoretic reduction. At this point in my exposition I have only touched on those criticisms and elaborations which were minimally needed to develop the general reduction-replacement model. There are, however, a number of additional interesting issues closely associated with these models and some are crucially connected with reduction in biology and medicine.

9.4.1 *Theory Structure Issues: Are "Laws" Relevant?*

In his 1976a, Wimsatt criticized my earlier approach to theory reduction (Schaffner 1967a, 1969b, 1976) for, among other things, not taking "mechanisms" as the focus of the reducing science. He seems to have been motivated in part by some of Hull's (1976) observations and especially by Salmon's (1971) model of explanation. Wimsatt construes one of Salmon's important advances as shifting our attention away from statistical *laws* to statistically relevant *factors* and to underlying *mechanisms* (Wimsatt 1976a, 488). As I have acknowledged in chapter 6, this focus on mechanisms is to a first approximation a salutary one, and though I believe it still requires references to laws (because of the intertwining of mechanisms and laws — see chapter 6), Wimsatt's suggestions are very much to the point. Their implications are considered further below in terms of the causal gloss placed on reductions as explanations.

The question of the relevance of "laws" in reductions in the biomedical sciences in general, and in connection with genetics in particular, was also raised more recently by Philip Kitcher. In his paper on reduction in molecular biology, Kitcher (1984a) argued that the Nagel model of reduction and all analogous accounts suffered from several problems. One of those problems was that, when one applies such accounts to biology and to genetics, it is hard to find collections of sentences which are the "laws" of the theory to be reduced. In Kitcher's view, any model of reduction of the type proposed by Nagel is committed to a thesis he terms (R1), namely:

(R1) Classical genetics contains general laws about the transmission of genes which can serve as the conclusions of reductive derivations. (1984a, 339)

Kitcher notes (correctly it seems to me) that it is difficult to find many laws about genes in the way that one finds various gas laws peppering the gas literature or to the extent to which there are explicit laws in optics, such as Snell's law, Brewster's law, and the like. Why this is the case is, I think, rather complex (see chapter 3 as well as my 1980a and 1986), but it has some interesting implications for reduction, as well as some important consequences for the ease of fit of the standard model of reduction to the genetics case, as we shall see later in this chapter.

As Kitcher adds, however, there are two sentences extractable from Mendel's work that have had the term "law" applied to them. These are the famous laws of segregation and of independent assortment. They continue to be cited even in recent genetics texts, such as Watson et al.'s 1987 edition of *The Molecular Biology of the Gene*. These authors characterize Mendel's two laws (or principles) as follows:[13]

> *Law of Independent Segregation*: Recessive genes are neither modified nor lost in the **hybrid** (*Rr*) generation, but . . . the dominant and recessive genes are independently transmitted and so are able to segregate independently during the formation of the sex cells. *Law of Independent Assortment*: Each gene pair . . . [is] independently transmitted to the gamete during sex cell formation. . . . Any one gamete contains only one type of inheritance factor from each gene pair. . . . There is no tendency of genes arising from one parent to stay together. (1987, 10-11)

These laws were the subject of a searching historical inquiry by Olby (1966).[14] Olby concerns himself with two questions that are of relevance to the issue of reduction: (1) what are Mendel's laws? and (2) to what extent are they still applicable today? Olby notes that Mendel himself referred to a *law* governing inheritance in the pea plant (*Pisum sativum*) at least seven times. This was what we today term the law of independent assortment, but what Mendel referred to as the "law of combination of different characters." This law, in Mendel's own (though translated) words, was stated as follows:

> there can be no doubt that for all traits included in the experiment this statement is valid: *The progeny of hybrids in which several essentially different traits are united represent the terms of a combination series in which the series for each pair of differing traits are combined.* This also shows at the same time that *the behavior of each pair of traits in a hybrid association is independent of all other differences in the two parental plants.* (1966 [1865], 122)

Later in his paper, Mendel sketched an explanation for his results which appealed to a cytological basis:

> In our experience we find everywhere confirmation that constant progeny can be formed only when germinal cells

and fertilizing pollen are alike, both endowed with the potential for creating identical individuals, as in normal fertilization of pure strains. Therefore we must consider it inevitable that in a hybrid plant also identical *factors* [my emphasis] are acting together in the production of constant forms. Since the different constant forms are produced in a *single* plant, even in just a *single* flower, it seems logical to conclude that in the ovaries of hybrids as many kinds of germinal cells (germinal vesicles), and in the anthers as many kinds of pollen cells are formed as there are possibilities for *constant* combination forms and that these' germinal and pollen cells correspond in their internal make-up to the individual forms.

Indeed, it can be shown theoretically that this assumption would be entirely adequate to explain the development of hybrids in separate generations if one could assume at the same time that the different kinds of germinal and pollen cells of a hybrid are produced on the average in equal numbers. (1966 [1865], 124)

Mendel subjected this hypothesis to experimental test and concluded:

Thus experimentation also justifies the assumption *that pea hybrids form germinal and pollen cells that in their composition correspond in equal numbers to all the constant forms resulting from the combination of traits united through fertilization*. (129)

I view it as most important that Mendel's theory of heredity be understood to involve not only several general laws or principles, but also that these laws are *intertwined* with a cytological and subcytological basis. I shall return again to this point below.

Olby notes that Mendel himself recognized one exception to his law of independent assortment, and also one modification. The former was in the hawkweed *Hieracium*, and the latter in the flower color of *Phaseolus*. (In *Hieracium*, the genetics are quite complex and involve the process of apomixis. In *Phaseolus*, the genetic factors interact—a situation which is now understood to be quite common, as we shall discuss further below.) Biologists also recognize other circumstances which limit the applicability of independent assortment, such as polyploidy, linkage, and extrachromosomal inheritance. To the question whether Mendel's law still holds, Olby answers:

yes, but like any other scientific law, it holds only under prescribed conditions. Mendel stated most of these conditions, but the need for no linkage, crossing over, and polyploidy were stated after 1900. (1966, 140)

In his essay, Kitcher gleans a different lesson from the post-1900 discoveries of the limitations of Mendel's law. It is not that one could not save Mendel's law by specifying appropriate restriction or articulating a suitable approximation, but rather that "Mendel's second law, amended or unamended, simply becomes irrelevant to subsequent research in classical genetics" (1984, 342). If I understand him correctly, what concerns Kitcher is that Mendel's second law is only interesting and relevant if it is embedded in a cytological perspective which assigns Mendelian genes to chromosomal segments within cells. Kitcher writes:

What figures largely in genetics after Morgan is the technique [of using cytology], and this is hardly surprising when we realize that one of the major research problems of classical genetics has been the problem of discovering the distribution of genes *on the same chromosome*, a problem which is beyond the scope of the amended law. (1984, 343)

I think Kitcher is only partially right here and that he was in any event anticipated by Mendel on his point about cytology — see the quotations from Mendel above and also my additional comments on this point further below. An inspection of standard scientific textbooks indicates that Mendel's laws continue to be useful in the sense defended by Olby above. Moreover, Kitcher's views on the relation of Mendelism and cytology are considerably oversimplified in comparison with the historical record, which in my interpretation does not support Kitcher's conclusions.[15] What I do take from Kitcher's discussion is that a focus on the notion of a theory as a collection of general laws may be problematic in the biological sciences, and that a broader embedding of any such generalizations needs to be carried out in order to capture adequately the nature of the science. This view is similar to that urged in other work on theory in biology (see chapter 3 and also my 1980a, 1986, and 1988, as well as Rosenberg's 1985), and we shall see how this works out in further detail shortly.

There is an important point here, however, which it would be well to underscore. This is the notion that genetics (from its inception) is closely associated with cytological mechanisms, and that what we mean by "genetics" is not only a set of general (re-stricted) universal "law" type of statements but also a set of mechanisms which are associated with the hypothesized entities of genetics. Recall that even in his first paper Mendel proposes that "in the ovaries of the hybrids there are formed as many sorts of egg cells, and in the anthers as many sorts of pollen cells, as there are possible *constant* combination forms" (1968 [1865], 136). What this suggests is that theory reduction needs to consider not only rather general summary statements of entities' behavior, which might be said to function at the γ level of theory axiomati-zation, but also to note the significance of the finer-structured elements of a theory—here the cytological, or what I have re-ferred to as the σ level, of specification. I shall reexamine the im-plications of these levels of specification for reduction further below.

9.4.2 *Connectability Problems*

A number of problems with reduction can be grouped under the category of connectability. Recall that this notion is bound up with the problem of how to associate entities and terms in the reduced theory (biology in general or, say, genetics in particular) with entities and terms in the reducing theory (organic chemis-try). For expository purposes, I shall divide these issues into three subcategories: (1) questions concerning the connection of natural kinds in reduction, (2) questions about the nature of the connections as synthetic identities, and (3) problems associated with the approximate or analogical relation between the original reduced theory and the *corrected* reduced theory.

Connectability of Natural Kinds

Are the Connections "Many-Many" in the Hull Sense? David Hull, in a number of articles and in his 1974 book on the philosophy of biology, proposed a thesis which argues for nonconnectability between biological theories and physiocochemical theories and, specifically, between Mendelian classical genetics and molecular genetics. (Hull's views appear logically similar to some later and independent views of Fodor concerning the relation between psychology and the natural sciences which will be commented on further below.) The essence of Hull's view is that connections between classical genetics and molecular genetics are many-many, or that to one Mendelian term (say the predicate "dominant") there will correspond many diverse molecular mechanisms which result in dominance. Further, Hull adds, any one molecular mechanism, say an enzyme-synthesizing system, will be responsible for many different types of Mendelian predicates: dominance in some cases, recessiveness in others. With the increase in precision which molecular methods allow, furthermore, major reclassifications of genetic traits are likely, and when all of these difficulties are sorted out, any corrected form of genetics that can be reduced is, accordingly, likely to be very different from the uncorrected form of genetics. To Hull:

> given our pre-analytic intuitions about reduction . . . [the transition from Mendelian to molecular genetics] *is* a case of reduction, a paradigm case. [However on] . . . the logical empiricist analysis of reduction [i.e., on the basis of the Nagel type of reduction model introduced earlier] . . . Mendelian genetics cannot be reduced to molecular genetics. The long awaited reduction of a biological theory to physics and chemistry turns out not to be a case of "reduction" . . . , but an example of replacement.[16] (Hull 1974, 44)

Hull argues for his influential position by citing numerous phenomena which are explained in Mendelian terms by a form of gene interaction known as "recessive epistasis." These phenomena include coat color in mice, feather color in Plymouth Rock and Leghorn chickens, feathered shanks in chickens, as well as a certain type of deaf-mutism in humans. Hull points out that it is very unlikely that all of these phenomena are produced by a single molecular mechanism; at best several different mechanisms will be involved. Hull goes on to state that each of these different mechanisms is not likely always to produce phenomena that will be characterized as Mendelian "recessive epistasis." The lesson that Hull draws from this example is that even *if* we were able to translate all gross phenotypic traits into molecularly characterized traits, the relation between Mendelian and molecular predicate terms would "express prohibitively complex many-many relations." Hull elaborates on this conclusion as follows:

Phenomena characterized by a single Mendelian predicate term can be produced by several different types of molecular mechanisms. Hence, any possible reduction will be complex. Conversely, the same types of molecular mechanism can produce phenomena that must be characterized by different Mendelian predicate terms. *Hence, reduction is impossible.* (Hull 1974, 39; my emphasis)

Hull admits that some correction and reclassifying might be done to bring about a reduction but believes that this would raise the "problem of justifying the claim that the end result of all this reformulation is reduction and not replacement." He adds: "Perhaps something is being reduced to molecular genetics once all these changes have been made in Mendelian genetics, but it is not Mendelian genetics" (1974, 39).

I believe that Hull has misconstrued the application of the general model of reduction which I outlined earlier in several ways, and that he thus sees *logical* problems where they do not exist. *Empirical* problems do exist, namely, exactly what mechanisms are involved in the cytoplasmic interactions that result in genetic epistasis of the dominant and recessive varieties, but these ought not be confused with the the logical problems of the type of connections which have to be established and with the appropriate manner of derivation of a corrected form of classical genetics from molecular genetics. Let me argue for this position in some detail.

Hull's primary concern is with the reduction functions for Mendelian predicates. Let us briefly recall what predicates are, prior to sketching the way in which they can be replaced in a reduction. In the general model of theory reduction-replacement as outlined above, I implicitly follow modern logicians such as Quine as construing predicates in an extensional manner. From this perspective, the extension of a predicate is simply a class of those things or entities possessing the predicate. This nominalistic position can be put another way by using standard logical terminology and understanding predicates to be open sentences which become true sentences when the free variable(s) in the open sentence are replaced by entities which possess the predicate characterized by the open sentence. Thus the open sentence "x is odd" where x ranges over positive integers, say, introduces the predicate "odd" (or "is-odd"). When the free variable x is replaced by a named object, then the sentence becomes closed and can be said to be true or false depending on whether the named object in fact possesses the predicate. Relations can be similarly introduced by open sentences containing two free variables, for example, the relation of being a brother, by "x is the brother of y." Following Quine (1959), we may then say that "the extension of a closed one place predicate is the class of all the things of which the predicate is true; the extension of a closed two-place predicate is the class of all the pairs of which the predicate is true; and so on" (1959, 136).

The extensional characterization of predicates and relations is important because reduction functions relate entities and predicates of reduced and reducing theories extensionally via an imputed relation of synthetic identity.

Let us examine the predicate "dominant" or "is-dominant" from this point of view. Though the importance of the notion of "dominance" has faded as genetics has developed (see Darden 1990), the concept is a significant one in Mendel's work and in early Mendelian genetics.[17] A molecular account of dominance is required in order to reduce Mendel's laws; further, the notion is useful for illustrating certain aspects of predicate reduction.

First it will be essential to unpack the notion. Though the predicate is one which is ascribed to genes and might prima facie appear to be a simple one-place predicate,[18] in fact the manner in which it is used in both traditional classical genetics and molecular genetics indicates that the predicate is a rather complex relation. The predicate is defined in classical genetics in terms of a relation between the phenotype produced by an allele of a gene in conjunction with another, different allele of the same locus (a heterozygous condition) and that produced by each of these alleles when present in a double dose (a heterozygous condition); the gene exhibiting dominance will be the one whose (homozygous) phenotype is expressed in the heterozygous condition. The predicate "epistatic," which Hull believes to be a particularly troublesome one for the general reduction model, is similarly unpackable as a rather complex relation between different genes and not simply between different alleles of the same gene.

More specifically, suppose that the phenotype of the homozygous condition (aa) of a gene a is A. Similarly, suppose that genotype bb biologically produces phenotype B. (The causal relation of biological production will be represented in the following pages by a single arrow:→.) If a and b are alleles of the same genetic locus, and the phenotype produced by genotype ab is A, then we say that gene a is dominant (with respect to gene b). The predicate "dominant" therefore is in reality a *relation* and is extensionally characterized by those *pairs* of alleles of which the relationship "$(aa \rightarrow A)$ & $(bb \rightarrow B)$ & $(ab \rightarrow A)$ = $_{df}$ a is a dominant (with respect to b)," is true.

Epistasis can be similarly unpacked. If two nonallelic genes, a and c say, are such that $aa \rightarrow A$ and $cc \rightarrow C$ when each genotype is functioning in isolation from the other but genotype $aacc$ biologically produces A, we say that a "hides" c or "is epistatic to" c (A and C here are contrasting phenotypic traits). The gene a may so relate to c that a in its dominant allelic form obscures c (this is "dominant epistasis"). The gene a may also relate to c such that a's absence (or a recessive allele of a, such as b) prevents the appearance of c's phenotype (this is "recessive epistasis"). (See my discussion in chapter 6 of epistasis effects of genes on the color coat of mice for additional information.)

The various interactions between genes, of which the two forms of epistasis mentioned above are but a subset, can be operationally characterized, since they result in a modification of the noninteractive independent assortment ratio of $9 : 3 : 3 : 1$ for two genes affecting the phenotypes of the organisms. (For a survey of these interactions and the specific modifications of the ratios which they produce the reader must be referred to other sources; Strickberger 1976 and 1985, chapter 11, are good introductions.)

Having sufficiently analyzed some of the predicates that appear in classical genetics, I now return to the problem of specifying reduction functions for such predicates. Specification of reduction functions, which are like dictionary entries that aid a translator, can be looked at in two ways, analogous to the two directions of translation: (1) from the context of the theory to be reduced, one must be able to take any of the terms—entity terms or predicate (including relation) terms—and univocally replace these by terms or combinations of terms drawn from the reducing theory; and (2) from the context of the reducing theory, one must be able to pick out combinations of terms which will unambiguously yield equivalents of those terms in the reduced theory which do not appear in the reducing theory. Such sentences characterizing replacement and combination selections must, together with the axioms and initial conditions of the reducing theory, entail the axioms of the reduced theory if the reduction is to be effected.

To obtain reduction functions for Mendelian predicates we proceed in the following manner: (1) The predicate is characterized extensionally by indicating what class of biological entities, or pairs or other groupings of entities, represent its extension. This was done for dominance and epistasis above in terms of genotypes and phenotypes. (2) In place of each occurrence of a biological entity term, a chemical term or combination of terms is inserted in accord with the reduction functions for entity terms. (3) Finally, in place of the biological production arrow which represents the looser or less detailed generalizations of biological causation, we write a double-lined arrow ($\Rightarrow$), which represents a promissory note for a chemically causal account, that is, a specification of various chemical mechanisms which would yield the chemically characterized consequent on the basis of the chemically characterized antecedent. Thus if a reduction function for gene a, say, was "gene a = DNA sequence α" and phenotype A possesses a reduction function "phenotype A = amino acid sequence $\aleph$," then if we represented the Mendelian predicate for dominance as $(aa \rightarrow A)$ & $(bb \rightarrow B)$ & $(ab \rightarrow A)$, we would obtain:

Allele a is dominant (with respect to b) =
(DNA sequence α, DNA sequence α $\Rightarrow$ amino acid sequence $\aleph$) &
(DNA sequence β, DNA sequence β $\Rightarrow$ amino acid sequence $\Im$) &
(DNA sequence α, DNA sequence β $\Rightarrow$ amino acid sequence $\aleph$).

where gene b is identified with DNA sequence β, and phenotype B with amino acid sequence $\Im$. This reduction function for dominance is, as was the characterization of dominance introduced earlier, somewhat oversimplified and for complete adequacy ought to be broadened to include Muller's more sensitive classification and quantitative account of dominance.[19] This need not be done, however, for the purposes of illustrating the *logic* of reduction functions for predicates. I have deliberately left the interpretation of the double-lined arrow in the right-hand side of the above reduction function unspecified. As noted, it essentially represents a telescoped chemical mechanism of production of the amino acid sequence by the DNA. Such a mechanism must be specified if a *chemically adequate* account of biological production or causation is to be given.[20] Such a chemically complete account need not be included explicitly in the *reduction function* per se, even though *it is needed in any complete reduction.*

Such a reduction function (and similar though more complex ones could be constructed in accordance with the above-mentioned steps for epistasis in its various forms) allows the translation from the biological language into the chemical and vice versa. Notice that the relations among biological entities which yield the various forms of dominance and epistasis, for example, can easily be preserved via such a construal of reduction functions. This is the case simply because the interesting predicates can be unpacked as relations among biological entities, and these selfsame entities subsequently identified with chemical entities. The extensional characterization of predicates and relations as classes and (ordered) pairs of entities accordingly allows an extensional interpretation of reduction functions for predicates.[21]

Assuming that we can identify any gene with a specific DNA sequence and that, as Francis Crick (1958) observed, "The amino acid sequences of the proteins of an organism . . . are the most delicate expression possible of the phenotype of an organism," we have a program for constructing reduction functions for the primitive entities of a corrected classical genetics. (A detailed treatment would require that different types of genes in the corrected genetic theory, e.g., regulator genes, operator genes, structural genes, and the recon and muton subconstituents of all these, be identified with specific DNA sequences. Examples of how this is done in practice will be provided further below.)

Substitution of the identified entity terms in the relations which constitute the set of selected primitive predicates, which yields reduction functions for predicates, then, allows for two-way translation, from classical genetics to molecular genetics and vice versa. Vis-à-vis David Hull, molecular *mechanisms* do not appear in connection with these reduction functions *per se*, rather they constitute part of the reducing *theory*.[22] Chemically characterized relations of dominance can be and are explained by a variety of mechanisms. The only condition for adequacy which is relevant here is that chemical mechanisms yield predictions that are unequivocal when the results of the mechanism(s) working on the available DNA and yielding chemically characterized phenoytpes are translated back into the terms of neoclassical genetics. A specific example of how this is done is covered in chapter 6 in my discussion of the epistatic effects of genes on mouse coat color.

What Hull has done is to misconstrue the locus where molecular mechanisms function logically in a reduction, and he has thus unnecessarily complicated the logical aspects of reduction. Different molecular mechanisms can appropriately be invoked in order to account for the same genetically characterized relation, as the genetics is less sensitive. The same molecular mechanisms can also be appealed to in order to account for different genetic relations, but only if there are further differences at the molecular level. It would be appropriate to label these differences as being associated with different *initial conditions* in the reducing theory.

This point is important and is one of the main areas of continued disagreement between Hull and myself. Hull seems to believe that the list of "initial conditions" is likely to be impossibly long. I, on the other hand, believe that molecular biologists are able to identify a (comparatively) small set of crucial parameters as initial conditions in their elucidations of fundamental biochemical mechanisms. These initial conditions are usually discussed explicitly in the body of their research articles (sometimes in the "materials and methods" sections). Specification of the initial conditions, such as the strain of organism, the temperature at which a specific strain of organisms was incubated, and the specific length of time of incubation, is absolutely necessary in order to allow repetition of the experiment in other laboratories whose scientists know the experiment only through the research article. The fact that mechanisms such as the Krebs cycle and the *lac* operon are formulatable in a relatively small set of sentences, with a finite list of relevant initial conditions specifiable, indicates to me that Hull is too pessimistic.

Our concerns with respect to molecular mechanisms and their initial conditions raise an additional but closely related issue about the types of connections between theories, to which I shall return in a moment. At this point, however, I want to note that there are several appeals that I believe can be made to contemporary genetics which will support my position over Hull's. First, traditionally discovered gene interactions, not only epistasis but also suppression and modification, are in fact currently being treated from a molecular point of view. Several textbooks and research papers can be cited in support of this claim.[23] The logic of their treatment is not drastically to reclassify the traditionally discovered gene interactions but rather to identify the genes with DNA and the phenotypic results of the genes with the chemically characterized biosynthetic pathways, and to regard gene interactions as due to modifications of the chemical environments within the cells. Traditional genetics is not radically reanalyzed; it is rather corrected and enriched and then explained or reduced, at least in part. I shall provide extensive evidence from the genetics literature to support this point later on.

Second, I would note that it is sometimes the practice of molecular geneticists to consider what types of genetic effects would be the result of different types of molecular mechanisms. A most interesting case in point, to which I shall return in a broader historical context later in this chapter, is the prediction by Jacob and Monod of what types of genetic interaction effects in mutants would be observable on the basis of different hypotheses concerning the operator region in the *lac* system of *E. coli*.[24] In brief, they were able to reason from the chemical interactions of the repressor and the different conjectures about the operator to infer whether the operator gene would be dominant or recessive and whether it would be pleiotropic or not. The fact that in such a case molecular mechanisms yielded unequivocal translations into a corrected genetic vocabulary is a strong argument against Hull's concerns.

Finally, I should add that, if the relation between modified classical genetics and molecular genetics were one of replacement, then it is very likely that considerably more controversy about the relations of classical to molecular genetics would have infused the literature than did so. Further, it is also likely that those persons trained in classical genetics would not have made the transition as easily as they clearly have, nor would they be able to continue to utilize classical methods comfortably without developing, in a conscious manner, an elaborate philosophical rationale about the *pragmatic* character of classical genetics. Clearly such was the case with the type of historical transitions that are termed replacements and not reductions, such as the replacement of the physics of Aristotle by that of Newton or the astronomy of Ptolemy by that Copernicus and Kepler.

Are There Any Connections between the Classical Gene and the Molecular Gene? I have argued in the previous subsection against Hull that relatively general reduction functions can be constructed which allow us to relate classical and molecular characterizations of genetics. Hull is not alone in his skepticism that such connections can be forged; more recently Philip Kitcher also argued that any such connections as I have suggested exist between classical genetic mapping techniques and molecular techniques are not supported by geneticists' research programs. More specifically, in his characterization of the Nagelian models of reduction, Kitcher suggests that such models are committed to another *false* thesis, which he terms (R2). This (R2) thesis is in addition to (R1) discussed above on p. 433, and is stated by Kitcher as follows:

> (R2) The distinctive vocabulary of classical genetics (predicates like '① is a gene', '① is dominant with respect to ②') can be linked to the vocabulary of molecular biology by bridge principles. (Kitcher 1984, 339)

"Bridge principles" are but another name for the Nagelian connectability assumptions or reduction functions discussed above. Kitcher's claim against (R2) is that, if we construe a bridge principle as something of the sort "(*) (x) (x is a gene ≡ Mx) where 'Mx' is an open sentence (possibly complex) in the language of molecular biology," we shall find that "molecular biologists do not offer any appropriate statement . . . , nor do they seem interested in providing one" that will assist us in filling in the M expression given in (*) (1984, 343). Kitcher further claims that "no appropriate bridge principle can be found."

Here the argument seems to depend on certain empirical claims by Kitcher to the effect that it is not possible to locate any expressed interest (or success) in the molecular biological literature in defining a higher level notion, such as a "gene" unambiguously in molecular terms. I think Kitcher has both misinterpeted and overlooked important parts of the literature on this matter. To some extent Kitcher's argument seems to parallel some of Hull's earlier arguments, as well as Kimbrough's (1978) views, to be considered in more detail below. First let me summarize Kitcher's specific claims, and then I will cite appropriate biological literature that both constitutes an objection against his assertion of the lack of interest and provides evidence of some reasonably successful results from the search for a bridge principle of the (*) form, as defined in the quotation above.

Kitcher's primary objection to attempting to provide a bridge principle between classical and molecular genetics is based on the difficulty of finding any simple identification[25] between the classical gene and the now-known material basis of the gene, namely DNA.[26] Since genes come in different sizes and different sequences, it will not do to attempt to specify a gene by these properties. Kitcher also adds that using initiation and termination codon delimiters will not do, since one could (counterfactually) always envisage some mutation occurring between the delimiters which would obviate such a definition. (I must confess that I do not follow his argument here, since what we would seem to obtain in such circumstances would be described as different, mutant alleles of that gene.) Most importantly, defining a gene as a segment of DNA will not do because there are some "genes" which in point of fact are never transcribed into mRNA.[27] In support of this point Kitcher refers to the operator gene in the *lac* system, which primarily serves as the site of attachment for the repressor molecule. (Kitcher has gotten his facts wrong here — the operator *is* transcribed in the *lac* system, but the promoter is not transcribed. Thus Kitcher could have made his point by varying the example slightly.)

I think this is a fair summary of Kitcher's objections to trying to articulate any simple bridge principle, but, as noted above, I believe that he has ignored biologists' concerns as well as more successful attempts to introduce such bridge principles. In response, I am first going to comment on the historical impact of the Watson-Crick discovery of the DNA structure of the gene and, in particular, the work of Benzer on the gene concept. Then, at the risk of somewhat oversimplifying the discussion, I shall cite some passages from a widely used introductory textbook in the biological sciences. I shall then refer to several recent, more advanced discussions on this topic.

Perhaps the first thing that ought to be said concerning the definition of the gene is that the concept has undergone alteration in some manner or another almost since its inception. This is to be expected in light of the nature of scientific change as described in chapter 6, but it is important to realize that such change does not automatically eliminate interlevel identifications. Early in the development of genetics — in particular in Mendel's work — the gene is understood as a factor functionally (in the sense of causally) responsible for some phenotypic characteristic (in Mendel's words, "factors are acting together in the production of . . . forms"). In the early 1900s the gene was also construed as a unit of mutation. The work of Sutton and Morgan on genetic maps further permitted the gene to be characterized as a unit of recombination. For many years these three ways of characterizing the gene (as a unit of mutation, of recombination, and of function) were thought to pick out the same basic unit, in spite of advances made in the area of biochemical genetics, such as the Beadle-Tatum hypothesis of "one-gene–one enzyme." As organisms such as bacteria and bacteriophages began to become available for use in genetic research in the 1940s, however, some puzzling results concerning the size and properties of the unit of heredity began to surface. Stent (1968) remarks that these early results fueled antireductionist leanings, though the research ultimately did not support such interpretations. One difficulty that surfaced in the work of geneticists in the 1940s and early 1950s, for example, was that units of recombination and mutation appeared to be mapping *within* a unit responsible for a phenotypic characteristic.[28]

The interesting feature of the Watson-Crick discovery of DNA's tertiary structure was that it offered Seymour Benzer a means to *unify these prima facie disparate gene concepts*. Benzer utilized a number of mutants of the bacteriophage T4 to construct a genetic map at a very high degree of resolution, and on the basis of this work observed:

> The classical "gene," which served at once as the unit of genetic recombination, of mutation, and of function, is no longer adequate. These units require separate definition. (1956, 116)[29]

In a section of his discussion on the "relation of genetic length to molecular length," he wrote:

> We would like to relate the genetic map, an abstract construction representing the results of recombination experiments, to a material structure. The most promising candidate in a T4 particle is its DNA component, which appears to carry its hereditary information. [Reference to Hershey and Chase 1952.] DNA also has a linear geometry. [Reference to Watson and Crick 1953c.] The problem then is to derive a relation between genetic map distance (a

probability measurement) and molecular distance. In order to have a unit of molecular distance which is invariant to change in molecular configuration, the interval between the two points along the (paired) DNA structure will be expressed in nucleotide (pair) units, which are more meaningful for our purposes than, say, angstrom units. (1956, 128–129)

Benzer introduced three concepts in terms of which to designate the gene, the recon, the muton, and the cistron. He noted that there were at that time (in 1955 or 1956) difficulties on both the genetic and the molecular sides due to insufficient knowledge, but he felt that he could offer a "rough estimate" of the size of the three genetic units on the basis of his work with T4 and the Watson-Crick structure. He proposed that "the size of the recon [the unit of recombination] would be limited to no more than two nucleotide pairs," that the muton [the unit of mutation] was "no more than five" nucleotide pairs, and that the cistron or unit of function "turns out to be a very sophisticated structure" probably about one hundred times larger than the muton (1956, 130).

Benzer's proposals have by and large been universally accepted. His term "cistron" is used widely, and though the *terms* "recon" and "muton" have not enjoyed the same acceptance, the *concepts* for which they stand have become entrenched in the biomedical sciences. Thus, rather than causing a rejection of the classical notions, the molecular biological advances permitted more precise connections *among* the classical notions as well as a relation of them to the underlying biochemistry.

Further work on conceptual clarification of the gene notion continues, as is evidenced by comments in Keeton's (1980) edition of his textbook. Keeton remarks:

Though defined essentially as the unit of recombination, the gene in classical genetics was also regarded as the unit of mutation and the unit of function, i.e., as the smallest unit whose alteration by mutation would change the phenotype and as the smallest unit of control over the phenotype. This concept of the gene was satisfyingly unified. But from what is now known of the structure of genetic material and its function it is clear that the units of recombination, mutation, and function are not identical. (1980, 656)

Keeton also notes that most geneticists accept a *biochemical definition of the gene*, which he characterizes as the "one gene–one polypeptide principle," adding that this involves regarding "the gene as equivalent to the cistron" (1980, 657). At the same time that there is near universal acceptance of this definition of the gene, however, Keeton observes that geneticists "often find it inapplicable to work on higher plants or animals," essentially because not much is yet known about the DNA of these higher organisms. Thus from a working point of view, geneticists still continue to use the Morganian recombination definition. This, however, does not introduce any dissonance into the relation between classical and molecular genetics, as Kitcher seems to think, but rather indicates the still incomplete nature of the disciplines.

In an important additional comment Keeton explicitly addresses the point that Kitcher stressed with respect to the nontranscription of some portions of DNA. It is worth quoting his two paragraphs on this issue:

> Although our discussion of the biochemical gene has focused on the function of determining a polypeptide chain, it must not be overlooked that some functional units of DNA, instead of determining polypeptide chains, act as templates for transfer RNA or ribosomal RNA. The functional definition of the gene is usually taken to include such units; thus it would perhaps be more accurate to say that the gene is the length of DNA that codes for one functional product. In addition, some parts of the DNA molecule serve exclusively in the control of genetic transcription [such as the operator]. These are usually called *regions* rather than genes. [my emphasis]
>
> Besides the DNA in genes and control regions, there is much DNA of unknown function. Some of this nongenic DNA occurs between adjacent genes, but there are also other large regions of apparently nongenic DNA in chromosomes, especially near the centromeres. In some cases, as much as one fifth of all the chromosomal DNA may be nongenic. (1980, 657)

On my reading of both Benzer's work and the above comments and suggestions by Keeton, what molecular genetics has done is to produce a deeper unity among large portions of classical and molecular genetics. The definitions of the gene and other "bridge principles" are quite complex, but it is patently not the case that such principles are not of any interest to biologists; it is also highly likely that a complex but rich set of "bridge principles" will continue to be sought and found by those biologists. I also see no reason why such carefully formulated and robust bridge principles should not yield generalizations which support counterfactuals (see Kitcher 1984, 345). I accordingly believe that (R2) has *not* been shown to be false.

Are the Connections "Many-Many" in the Rosenberg Sense? In addition to Kitcher's and Hull's questioning of the possibility of defining the relationship between classical and molecular genetics, a somewhat different variant of Hull's many-many problem with respect to the connectability of these two fields has recently been raised by Rosenberg (1985). His orientation might best be characterized as one of "boggled skepticism" (P.S. Churchland 1986, 315–316).

Rosenberg's Argument. Rosenberg claims:

> Molecular considerations explain the composition, expression, and transmission of the Mendelian gene. The behavior of the Mendelian gene explains the distribution and transmission of Mendelian phenotypic traits revealed in breeding experiments. But the identity of Mendelian genes is ultimately a function of these same breeding experiments. Mendelian genes are *identified* by identifying their effects: the phenotypes observationally identified in the breeding experiments. So, if molecular theory is to give the biochemical identity of Mendelian genes, and explain the assortment and segregation, it will have to be linked *first* to the Mendelian phenotypic traits; otherwise it will not link up with and explain the character of Mendelian genes. But there is no *manageable* correlation or connection between molecular genes and Mendelian phenotypes. So there is no prospect of manageable correlation between Mendelian genes and molecular ones. The explanatory order is from molecules to genes to phenotypes. But the order of identification is from molecules to phenotypes and back to genes. So to meet the reductive requirement of connectability between terms, the concepts of the three levels must be linked in the order of molecules to phenotypes to genes, not in the explanatory order of molecules to genes to pheno-

types. And this, as we shall see, is too complex an order of concepts to be of systematic, theoretical use. (1985, 97)

Rosenberg refers to problems similar to those that have concerned Hull (as described above), and indicates that the overwhelming complexity of biosynthetic pathways will defeat any attempt at formulating a concise or even manageable set of relations between classical and molecular genetics. He concludes, like Hull, that "the relation between the molecular gene and the Mendelian phenotype is not a one-to-one relation, or a one-to-many relation, or even a many-to-one relation. It is a many-to-many relation" (1985, 105). Rosenberg asserts that, consequently, "there cannot be actual derivation or deduction of some regularity about the transmission and distribution of phenotypes, say their segregation and independent assortment, from any complete statement of molecular genetics" (1985, 106). He qualifies, however, on the force of this conclusion, adding "the 'cannot' is not a logical one; it has to do with limitations on our powers to express and manipulate symbols: The molecular premises needed to effect the deduction will be huge in number and will contain clauses of staggering complexity and length" (1985, 106).

The situation as Rosenberg describes it seems to me to be unduly pessimistic. *Part* of Rosenberg's problem is, I think, his view that a reduction has to be completely explicit in all its detail. However, geneticists can (and typically do) proceed by collapsing much of this detail into packages to be drawn on as needed. Thus the elaborate machinery of transcription, splicing, and translation (protein synthesis on the ribosomes) lies in the background, assumed and from time to time cited in discussions and papers, but only as needed to make a specific point or where the behavior of the machinery is in some respect(s) anomalous or exceptional. This means of proceeding by a kind of "information hiding" has significant analogies with the practice of object-oriented programming (OOP) mentioned in chapters 2 and 3. More importantly, the research programs of geneticists constitute counterexamples to Rosenberg's thesis. Classical techniques are being used *together* with molecular techniques to identify the DNA sequences of genes and the protein(s) which they make (or fail to make). A few words about these research programs and their techniques will make the point clearer.

Classical and Molecular Mapping Techniques. Classical techniques of locating genes on chromosomes are based on a determination of how often two traits are inherited together. Because of crossing-over (recombination) in meiosis, the genes causing the traits can be separated. Geneticists can construct a map of the likelihoods of proximity of the genes based on the frequencies of observed traits in a breeding population. In the early history of genetics, Morgan and his coworker Sutton constructed such maps for *Drosophila* and found that there were four independent linkage groups; these were identical to the four chromosomes of the organism. For the human, detailed linkage-analysis gene mapping required gathering information on many individuals from large families, since a great amount of data on the association of traits was needed.

In the 1970s, new molecular techniques were developed that have enabled alternative approaches to gene mapping. These new techniques are usually collectively referred to as recombinant DNA technology. One of these advances was the discovery of a series of enzymes in procaryotes that recognized specific six-nucleotide sequences of DNA and cut the strands at those recognized sites. These enzymes are known as "restriction enzymes" because they acted *against* or "restricted" foreign DNA. More than a hundred of these enzymes have been discovered; each is quite specific for a different nucleotide sequence. Their advent led to the further discovery that humans (and other eucaryotic organisms) have fairly extensive variations in their DNA, termed "polymorphisms," at which the restriction enzymes can act. These polymorphisms constituted a new series of inheritable genetic "markers." This (usually benign) variation is detectable by the restriction enzymes because variant individuals have their DNA fragmented differently by the enzymes. DNA can be obtained easily (from white blood cells, for example) and subjected to this type of analysis to yield a "restriction fragment length polymorphism (RFLP—pronounced "riflip") map." Medical geneticists can do linkage analyses looking for a close association between an RFLP marker and a harmful gene, and then utilize the RFLP to distinguish healthy individuals (or fetuses) from those that have inherited the defective gene. Such a test has been developed for Duchenne muscular dystrophy and has led to the births of at least 16 healthy male infants who probably would not otherwise have been carried to term by their mothers, who were known carriers of this serious X-linked disorder (Nichols 1987, 49).

The use of RFLP mapping has enabled researchers to take several further steps toward obtaining full sequence maps of or-

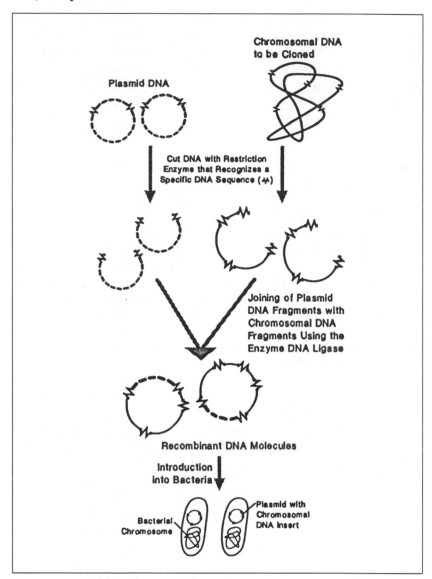

Figure 9.1 DNA cloning in plasmids. Source: Office of Technology Assessment, 1988.

ganisms' genomes. A recent report from the U.S. Office of Technology Assessment (OTA) notes that "as physical markers that can be followed genetically, RFLPs are the key to linking the genetic and physical maps of the human genome" (1988, 30). The restriction fragments can be separated by placing them onto a gel and applying an electrostatic field across the gel. They can then be physically joined to other DNA molecules (cloning vectors) to constitute an independent, circularized piece of DNA (a plasmid or "minichromosome")[30] and inserted into an organism such as *E. coli*, where they can be replicated many times over (see figure 9.1) as *cloned* fragments. Watson et al. write of this methodology as applied to the common fruit fly *Drosophila*:

> Study of individual pieces of cellular DNA only became possible with the advent of recombinant DNA procedures. These allow the separation of even very similar-size DNA pieces by individually inserting them into cloning vectors. All the restriction fragments from genomes even as large as *Drosophila* can be inserted in only some 40,000 different *E. coli* plasmids. The subsequent multiplication of these individual vectors (known as a "gene library") can generate all the pure DNA ever needed for exhaustive molecular characterization. (Watson et al. 1987, 273)

These fragments can be analyzed and the sequence of the nucleotides determined. Two powerful techniques are commonly used for this, one due to Maxam and Gilbert (1977) and the other developed by Sanger et al. (1977). The details can be found in any basic molecular genetics text; a summary of the process for the Maxam and Gilbert variant is given in figure 9.2. The sequencing proceeds by generating radioactively labelled subchains (from the DNA chain chosen) of different lengths. When these subchains are separated by gel electrophoresis, the DNA sequence can be easily read directly off an X-ray film left in contact with the migrating radioactive subchains in the gel, which expose the film at points of contact. These techniques are more easily applied to simple genomes than to complex genomes such as that of the human. Even for *E. coli*, however, enormous labor is required to generate a physical map and to sequence all the DNA. Watson et al. (1987) estimate that *E. coli* has a DNA sequence of 4×10^6 base pairs and between 2,000 and 5,000 functional genes.

The Relation between Genetic and Physical Maps. The notion of a "physical" map was introduced briefly at several points in the above discussion. It will be useful to say a bit more about the differ-

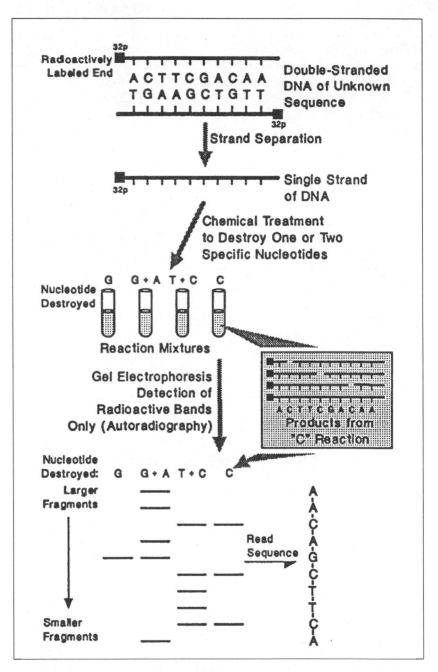

Figure 9.2   DNA sequencing by the Maxam and Gilbert method. Details of the process are given in the text. Source: Office of Technology Assessment, 1988.

ent types of physical maps that can be constructed and also about their relation to the "genetic" map.

A genetic map is essentially one obtained by linkage analysis of recombination frequencies. The techniques and elementary mathematical formulae utilized in such an analysis were reviewed by Watson et al. (1987, 15-17). These authors also note that there are very good (but not exact) correlations between such genetic maps and sequences determined by high resolution molecular techniques with a simple organism such as the bacterial virus phage λ (1987, 234-237).

Physical maps of genomes may be placed on a rough continuum of resolutions, from the low resolution of banding patterns visible on chromosomes through a light microscope to the highest resolution, of the specific nucleotide sequence of the DNA. The former type of mapping has resulted in the identification of about 1,000 landmarks (visible bands) in the human (OTA 1988, 30). Another form of relatively low resolution physical maps can be obtained from the use of complementary DNA sequences (cDNA) used as probes to identify various expressed genes on chromosomes. These cDNA maps have determined the chromosomal location of about 1,200 of the 50,000–100,000 human genes. Of higher resolution are maps made by cutting up the entire genome with restriction enzymes and "contiguously" ordering the resultant DNA sequences as they originally were in the chromosomes. This type of map is known as a *contig* map. The philosophical point to be stressed in connection with the existence of these various mapping methodologies is that there is a fairly *smooth* transition as one moves from lower to higher resolutions, and not the re-sorting and reclassification that such philosophers as Hull, Rosenberg, and Fodor (to be discussed below) would seem to have expected.

This point about smoothness can be illustrated by citing a recent study of a rare form of human color blindness known as "blue cone monochromacy." Individuals who have this X-linked disorder "display little or no color discrimination at either high or low light levels" (Nathans et al. 1989) and were suspected of having mutant red ($R^+ \rightarrow R^-$) and green ($G^+ \rightarrow G^-$) pigment genes. Nathans and his coinvestigators studied 12 blue cone monochromat families and characterized the pedigrees for the affected males and the normals. These researchers were able to generate restriction maps comparing cloned color-normal and mutant

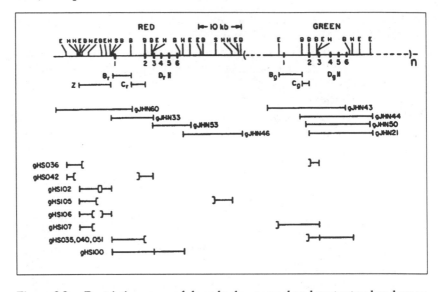

Figure 9.3   Restriction maps of cloned color-normal and mutant red and green pigment genes. (Top) Restriction map of normal genomic DNA. B, Bam HI; E, Eco RI; H, Hind III; N, Not I; S, Sal I. Numbers 1 to 6 mark red and green pigment gene exons. The number of green pigment genes varies among color-normals as indicated by subscript n. Restriction fragments shown below the genes refer to DNA blot hybridization bands [provided in another figure — not shown here]. Center, genomic phage clones from color-normal DNA are labeled gJHN. (Bottom) Genomic phage clones from X-linked incomplete achromats. Deleted sequences are indicated by brackets. . . . Two or more independent recombinants were isolated and analyzed for each mutant. Deletion breakpoints were defined by restriction mapping to a resolution of several hundred base pairs. Figure and legend from Nathans et al. (1989), p. 834, copyright © 1989 by the AAAS. With permission of author and publisher.

(disordered) red and green pigment genes and also to determine the specific nucleotide sequence of these lengths of the DNA of the affected individuals, revealing various deletions in the genes (see figure 9.3).

Nathans et al. (1989) also provide a "working model" to "explain G-R- phenotype of upstream deletions" (see Nathans 1989, fig. 8B). The appeal to a "working model" indicates that the details of the causal mechanism of gene expression are not yet fully confirmed.

This gap in our knowledge indicates where the problem of reductive explanations is more appropriately localized. The problems are *not* in the *many-many* complexities that have disturbed Hull and boggled Rosenberg, but rather are of the type discussed above in chapter 7: incomplete aspects of the causal sequences at the molecular level. Such gaps in our knowledge are expected to be remedied over time as powerful molecular techniques become applied to such problems. Watson et al. (1987) described the necessity of using recombinant DNA techniques in a brief quotation above. They have underscored this in connection with the approach to determining physiological "function":

> Effective experimentation on the structure and functioning of the eucaryotic genome is only possible using recombinant DNA techniques. To understand how eucaryotic genes work, we must first isolate them in pure form through gene-cloning procedures and then reintroduce them into cells where their expression can be studied. . . .
>
> . . . By using [these currently available techniques in the study of the eukaryotic yeast genome], any desired normal or mutant gene can be retrieved and its structure subsequently worked out. Integrative recombination now allows any yeast gene to be replaced with its [naturally existing or artifically synthesized] mutated derivitive and so provides a powerful way to probe the physiological role of genes whose function is not known. (Watson et al. 1987, 616–617)

This methodology seems to me to be a potent molecular realization of Claude Bernard's method of comparative experimentation discussed in chapter 4. The research program of contemporary molecular genetics thus seems to uphold the characterization of Rosenberg's views as pessimism that is not supported by current achievements.

By the same token, however, an overly optimistic interpretation of the simplicity of unravelling genetics is not warranted either. Particularly where genetic traits are the resultant of multiple genes in interaction, it will be difficult to articulate the reduction relations in any simple fashion. Watson et al. (1987, 277) discuss the extent to which analyzing DNA sequence information is already dependent on powerful computers and sophisticated software. I suspect that computer-assisted analysis of genetics may well provide for the reduction that Rosenberg finds so implausible, and in lieu of which he seems to favor a "supervenience" approach — see p. 461).

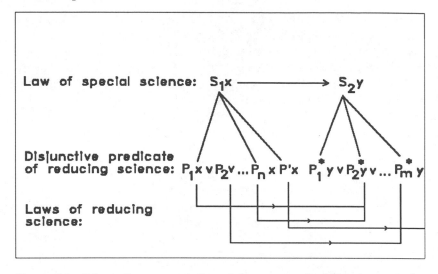

Figure 9.4   Schematic representation of the proposed relation between the reduced and reducing science on a revised account of the unity of science. If any S_1 events are of the type P', they will be exceptions to the law $S_1x \rightarrow S_2y$. From Fodor, 1975, p. 20, with permission.

Is Reduction in Biology and Medicine "Token-Token?"

Fodor and Kimbrough on "Token-Token" Reduction. I mentioned earlier (p. 437) that Hull's criticisms of reduction in the biomedical sciences bore some analogy to arguments by Jerry Fodor on the relation between psychology and the natural sciences, primarily neurophysiology. Fodor has suggested:

> The problem all along has been that there is an open empirical possibility that what corresponds to the kind predicates of a reduced science may be a heterogeneous and unsystematic disjunction of predicates in the reducing science. (1975, 20)

To put it another way,

> the predicates appearing in the antecedent and consequent will, by hypothesis, not be kind predicates. Rather, what we will have is something that looks [like figure 9.4]. That is, the antecedent and consequent of the reduced law will each be connected with a disjunction of predicates in the reducing science. (1975, 20)

Fodor illustrates this connection (which Kimbrough terms "to-ken-token reduction") by the diagram presented in figure 9.4. In this relation "the antecedent and consequent of the reduced law will each be connected with a disjunction of predicates in the reducing science (of the form)$P_1x \lor P_2x \lor \ldots \lor P_nx \to P_1{}^*y \lor \ldots \lor P_ny$" (1975, 21). This relation, though true, Fodor argues, cannot plausibly be considered a law because it mixes natural kinds in peculiar ways. It is a kind of token-to-token reduction at best.

Steven Kimbrough has argued that Fodor's token-token type of reduction is what we find in the relationship between genetics and molecular biology. Kimbrough's tack is to consider the relation between the traditional gene concept and the concepts introduced by the DNA sequence of the promoter and operator regions in the *lac* operon. He finds it difficult to offer a general characterization of the gene at any reasonably general level which does not admit of exceptions. For example, he asserts that if something is DNA we cannot infer that it is a gene, though he does not give any example of DNA which is not a gene. He also maintains that specification of the transcription or translation mechanisms of protein synthesis will not clarify what is a gene, since the promoter gene is not transcribed but (a part of) the operator gene is transcribed. Kimbrough proposes that what one finds in this case is not a Nagelian "type-type" reduction but rather a token-token reduction:

> Our problem can be solved by distinguishing yet another kind of reduction. Following Fodor . . . again, I shall call this kind of reduction token-token reduction. Where token-token reduction occurs, *individuals* described in the language of one science are identified with *individuals* described in the language of another science. This is a weak sort of reduction. (1978, 403; my emphasis)

Rosenberg and Supervenience. In his 1978, Rosenberg proposed a related thesis using Davidson's (1980 [1970]) and Kim's (1978) notion of supervenience. Rosenberg's aim was "to provide a new statement of the relation of Mendelian predicates to molecular ones in order to provide for the commensurability and potential reducibility of Mendelian to molecular genetics" (1985, 368). Rosenberg's paper appeared prior to Kimbrough's, and he did not use the Fodor token-token terminology but rather attempted to provide a means of responding to Hull's concerns about reduction discussed earlier.

In his more recent book, Rosenberg (1985) elaborated on this notion of supervenience, but the concept as he presents it in his 1985 is essentially equivalent to his earlier characterization.[31]

Supervenience is a notion that was introduced by Davidson, who argued against the *reducibility* of the mental to the physical but in favor of the *dependence* of the mental on the physical. In Kim's precise analysis of the concept, this emergentist use is disavowed and establishing supervenience appears to be equivalent to determining a correlation between two parallel sets of predicates that cannot be explicitly represented because of the complexity of the mappings. Rosenberg characterized a supervenient relation of Mendelian and molecular predicates in the following terms:

> Call the set of all Mendelian predicates M, and the set of all properties constructable from M, M*. Call the parallel sets of predicates of molecular genetics, L and L*. The set of Mendelian predicates, M, is supervenient on the set of molecular predicates L if and only if any two items that both have the same properties in the set L* also have the same properties in M*. Thus, on the assumption if an item exemplifies a certain set of Mendelian properties, then there is a set of molecular properties and relations that it also exemplified, and if any other item also exemplified the same set of molecular properties and relations, it manifests exactly the same Mendelian properties as well. (1978, 382)

In the light of the foregoing discussions about reduction in genetics, however, it is unclear what the notion of supervenience adds. If supervenience is associated with an emergentist thesis it has interesting implications, but, as noted, it is not. On the other hand, if it is not, it appears weaker than the synthetic identity thesis interaction of connectability assumptions defended above. Supervenience may guarantee a token-to-token predicate mapping relation between reduced and reducing theories, but this seems trivial. Supervenience does not exclude more interesting stronger classifications of token predicates, but neither does it guarantee them. Hull himself was pessimistic about the utility of the notion and wrote in response to Rosenberg's earlier views:

> Supervenience is clearly a well-defined relation but as Rosenberg is aware it is much weaker than the traditional conception of theory reduction. In fact all that has been

salvaged is ontological reduction. . . . Supervenience does not seem to capture our intuitions about the actual relation between Mendelian genetics and molecular biology. (1981, 135)

More recently Kim summarized a number of investigations into the notion of supervenience, including his own reanalysis of the concept, and identified a major problem with supervenience:

The main difficulty has been this: if a relation is weak enough to be nonreductive, it tends to be too weak to serve as a dependence relation; conversely when a relation is strong enough to give us dependence, it tends to be too strong—strong enough to imply reducibility. (1989, 40)

Kim concludes that nonreductive materialism, of which supervenience is one variant, "is not a stable position." He adds that "there are pressures of various sorts that push it either in the direction of outright eliminitivism or in the direction of an explicit form of dualism" (1989, 47). Earlier in his essay he also suggests that the "physicalist has only two genuine options, eliminitivism and reductionism" (1989, 32). I submit that Kim's searching analysis of supervenience in the realm of the mental has parallels for the relation of classical genetics to molecular genetics. As Hull suggested in the quotation above, supervenience is a weak and uninteresting relation. It is at best a preliminary surrogate for a reductionistic relation. I think that the existence of reductionistic relations of the sort described in my discussion of the fit between Mendelian and molecular genetics demonstrates the viability of a reductionist position and renders the need to appeal to a supervenience relation unnecessary.

Though there is some truth in Fodor's speculations and in Kimbrough's contentions, and perhaps in Rosenberg's supervenience in areas other than genetics,[32] I believe they are overstated in connection with reduction in the biomedical sciences generally and particularly in the area of genetics. First, it should be noted that, in genetics, it is not specific individuals demarcated in space and time that are identified; rather, the *lac p* and *o* genes present in many individual bacteria are identified with DNA sequences presumed to be repeated in many (a potentially infinite number of) instances. The sequence for *E.coli lac p* and *o* is given in Figure 9.5, and this diagram, if linguistically represented, would be a paradigm instance of an entity-reduction function.

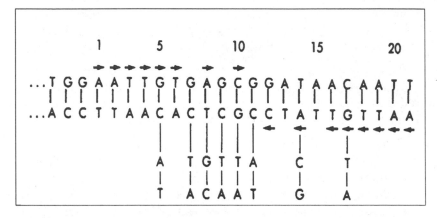

Figure 9.5   The *lac* operator sequence, showing its relation to the starting point for transcription of *lac* mRNA (nucleotide 1). Base-pair changes that lead to poor binding of the *lac* repressor are shown below their wild-type equivalents. The horizontal arrows designate bases having identical counterparts located symmetricaly in the other half of the operator. The center of symmetry is at nucleotide 11. Legend and figure adapted from *Molecular Biology of the Gene*, Vol. I, Fourth Edition, by Watson et al. (Menlo Park, CA: Benjamin/Cummings Publishing Company), p. 471.

Thus we do not have the kind of presumed variation associated with the thought and neurophysiology of a single individual that Fodor draws on, where true nonrepeatability may be more likely. Accordingly, there is a question whether Fodor's suggestion can be legitimately extended to biology, as Kimbrough suggests.

This prima facie dissimilarity between reduction in the mental realm and in the biological sciences is further supported by the preservation of the generalizations in biology as one moves to levels of increased resolution.[33] Contrary to Hull's earlier speculations concerning the probable dismantling and restructing of genetics because of reductions, the pictures one obtains of the *lac* DNA region through careful traditional genetic techniques and through modern chemical sequencing are *not* at variance with each other — recall the references made earlier to empirically correlated genetic and physical maps (p. 455). Most generalizations at the higher level are confirmed at the more specific level. Exceptions to genetic generalizations and paradoxical relations of dominance (as found in the "Pajama" experiment in the development of the operon theory, to be discussed on p. 485) become explained at the DNA-protein synthesis level. The few modifications required at the level of the reduced theory represent the shift from T_2 to T_2^* discussed as part of the general model introduced earlier in the chapter.

In spite of these considerations, there is an element of truth in Kimbrough's concerns. Reduction in genetics and, I suspect, much of biology and medicine appears to be more specific; it does not yield the broad generalizations and identities one finds in physics. This, I think, is due in part to the systems one studies in biology, and also to the kinds of theories one finds at what I have termed in chapter 3 the "middle range." Let me clarify this situation vis-à-vis reduction by a brief digression into an example from physics, in order to demonstrate the essential deep-structure parity between reduction in the physical sciences and in biology and medicine.

Consider how one explains, in terms of an underlying mechanical or quantum mechanical theory, the behavior of middle range objects we encounter in everyday life, simple machines such as inclined planes, car jacks, hydraulic elevators, and so on. By using Newtonian mechanics plus initial and boundary conditions, we can adequately explain all of the above. The types of initial conditions vary quite extensively. Our systems of classification are also not terribly sharp—for example, is a wedge which is used for a door stop an inclined plane or not?

The same problems afflict biology, though their source is different. If we began from classes of physical mechanisms and *then* developed fundamental mechanics we would encounter the kinds of problems Kimbrough and Hull discuss. The biochemical universals of the genetic code and protein synthesis are sufficient when the appropriate number and types of initial conditions are specified to allow derivation of the *lac* system in all of its forms, including mutant types. However, what is of great interest in this is the fact that biomedical scientists can formulate theories which do not require this type of knowledge. At the "middle range" level, such scientists employ a range of (often) overlapping polytypic models which are universals of narrow scope. But though these have impact for theory construction, their use does not significantly affect the abstract problem of reduction beyond complicating the type and number of initial conditions.

The answer, then, to the leading question of this section, "is reduction in the biomedical sciences 'token-token'?" is at most weakly affirmative, and with these important qualifications: (1)

this kind of reduction does not entail the dissociation of concepts and generalizations Fodor indicates occurs in other areas of to-ken-token reduction; (2) this form of token-token reduction also occurs in physics when one attempts to "reduce" classes of middle-range objects; (3) a less misleading gloss of "token-token" in these contexts would be to construe the term "token" as a "restricted type" in accordance with the view of theories developed in chapters 3 and 5.

Problems Posed by Construing Connectability Assumptions as Synthetic Identities.

Do Identities Capture Reductional Asymmetry? To this point I have been treating the identity interpretation of reduction functions as uncontroversial, though the specificity (type or token connections) and the character (many-one, one-many, etc.) have been critically examined. In several articles, and in his 1977 monograph, Robert Causey has provided several arguments for a deeper account of this identity interpretation. His account was subsequently criticized by Enç, who proposed a rather different account of predicate relations in reduced and reducing theories. I believe, to an extent, that both philosophers are correct but that they are characterizing different components of a dynamic reduction process. Let me first briefly sketch their positions and then defend the views. The Causey and Enç analyses are complementary if not taken too strictly.

Causey's focus is on microreductions in which, for example, a micro-level theory such as the kinetic theory of gases reduces a thermodynamic characterization of gas behavior. One of Causey's major themes is that, in a reduction, predicates of the nonsortal or nonentity type (which he terms "attributes") are to be construed as constituting synthetic or contingent identities. He argues it is only via this identity interpretation that scientists obtain explanations and not (mere) correlations, which would only suffice for (mere) derivation of the reduced theory from the reducing theory.

Causey attempts to specify "special nonsyntactical conditions," which, taken together with derivability, are severally necessary and jointly sufficient for reduction. Restricting reductions to contexts of nonmodal and nonpropositional attributes, Causey proposes what he contends is a necessary condition for contingent attribute identities:

Let 'A', 'B' be attribute-predicates, and let D_1, D_2 be derivations such that D_2 is obtainable from D_1 by uniform substitution of 'B' for 'A', and such that D_1 is obtainable from D_2 by uniform substitution of 'A' for 'B'. Then: If A and B are identical, then D_1 and D_2 are explanatorily equivalent. (1972, 419)

The notion of explanatory equivalence is characterized by Causey as follows:

For any two derivations D_1, D_2, . . . ,D_1, D_2 are explanatorially equivalent if D_1 and D_2 either represent the same explanation or none.

Enç reviews Causey's account, contending that the symmetry involved in it is incorrect, misleading, and vacuous. For Enç, there is an important directionality involved in reductions, and he locates this directionality in what he terms a "generative relation." This relation is causal. Enç puts his thesis as follows:

I can now state my thesis more succinctly: Suppose a heterogeneous reduction of T_2 into T_1 is attempted. Then T_2 will contain attribute-predicates (call them 'φ_i' that do not occur in T_1, and there will be sentences of T_2 of the type, "x is φ," where 'x' designates an individual of the domain T_2. T_1, on the other hand, will contain predicates (call them ψ_i) that are expected to be connected via the bridge laws to the predicates of T_2, and there will be statements of T_1 of the type, "y is ψ_i." where 'y' designates the same individual as 'x'. My thesis is that the reduction will be successful only if the fact that y is ψ_k is shown in T_1 to be generatively related to the fact that x is φ_k. (1976, 295)

Enç illustrates his view by referring to a case history that he admits is the "overworked example of the reduction of classical thermodynamics to the kinetic theory of gases." For Enç such expressions as

(P) Pressure of a gas is the average rate of change per unit area and time of the linear momentum of the gas molecules

and

(T) Temperature of a gas is the mean (translational) kinetic energy of the gas molecules are bridge laws or connectability assumptions that exemplify the generative relation and embody explanatory asymmetry (1976, 296). For example, he states that one "cannot explain why the rate of change of momentum of the molecule is such and such by the fact that the gas exerts such and such a pressure on them all" (1976, 296).

Enç is correct in stressing the asymmetry in reductions, though I believe he has misanalyzed it by thinking of it *only* in terms of a causal relation. In my view, causal connections can be invoked in reductions either (1) as (exploded) correspondence rules in replacements or (2) as parts of the reducing theory in cases of reduced theory preservation, as in the earlier discussion of the double arrow in genetics examples. Still, synthetic identities are required for preserved theories. Enc's arguments have prima facie plausibility because he has illustrated his thesis using partially homogeneous reductions. Thus, since the terms "momentum" and "pressure" occur in a mechanical theory of small objects, it is a straightforward procedure to relate (enthymematically) the term "pressure" that occurs in phenomenological thermodynamics to the average force ($= \Delta mv/\Delta t$) produced by rebounding molecules per unit area. However, this begs the question whether the concept of pressure$_{kinetic}$ is synthetically identical with pressure$_{thermodynamic}$: the enthymematic synthetic identity premise should be made explicit. Enç suppresses the requisite identity because it does not appear necessary in this type of reduction. I suspect we have a situation here that is analogous to the earlier case of genetic dominance, where both causal and identity claims were required for full-scale reductions. Recall that these causal sequences, however, are highly detailed microlevel sequences that are part of the reducing *theory* but not necessarily part of the connectability assumptions.

The weakness of Enç's position can be seen in his second example. He views the reduction of the temperature concept as "more interesting and illuminating." Without going into the details of the kinetic theory, let me note that, for Enç, "the relation [between kinetic energy and temperature] is generative because kinetic theory shows how the motion of the molecules, which is an essential component of the concept of mean kinetic energy of the molecules, causes the energy of the gas, which, in turn, is an essential component of the concept of temperature" (1976, 300). But such a notion of cause is purely formal inasmuch as **v**, a measure of the motion of the molecules, appears in the kinetic energy expression, $1/2\ mv^2$, and does not display the efficient causal type of asymmetry claimed. The situation would, I suspect, be similar in the case of the reduction of the concept of entropy.

The kind of asymmetry that is inherent in reductions depends, in my view, on three factors. First, the reducing theory is usually more general, that is, of greater scope than the reduced theory. (Cf. Hooker's view on this point in his 1981, 211.) Second, the reducing theory is usually a theory of the parts of some whole, and the part-whole relation is a source of asymmetry. (These factors can also be coupled with my view of correspondence rules as telescoped causal sequences.) Finally, the reducing theory can be a causal theory and it can account for some causal consequence, such as the molecules rebounding from the wall of the container under pressure in Enç's above example. However, the pressure is not the "effect" of the causal sequence(s) as described by the theory; the individual impulses of the molecules over an area are the "effects," which are *synthetically identical* to the pressure.

What Does Identity Mean, and How Are Synthetic Identities Established? A number of philosophers have concerned themselves with the notion of *identity*, and it would take us far beyond the scope of this book to undertake a comprehensive review and analysis of all that has been written on the concept. Nonetheless, because of the importance of synthetic identities in reduction, a brief account of some of the main modern positions, and of difficulties with them, is desirable. I begin with a short review of contemporary notions of identity and of the ways in which identities may be established in reductions. In the following section, I discuss the provocative thesis of Kripke and Putnam that such synthetic identities as are found in reductions are *necessarily true in all possible worlds*.

In his 1967 monograph *Identity and Spatial Temporal Continuity*, David Wiggins reviewed the notion of personal identity. Wiggins suggested that one key to analyzing identity was to consider his version of Leibniz's law, which asserts, assuming some sortal or individuative covering concept, say f, that if two entities a and b are identical, then for all predicates φ, φ is true of a if and only if it is also true of b, or symbolically:

$$(a =_{df} b) \supset (\varphi) (\varphi a \equiv \varphi b).$$

This is termed by Kalish and Montague (1960, 223) Leibniz's "principle of the indiscernibility of identicals." One could also consider the converse of Leibniz's law, namely, that for all properties φ, if *every* property which s has is also possessed by *b*, then *a* is identical with *b*, or symbolically:

$$(\varphi) [(\varphi a \equiv \varphi b) \supset (a = b)].$$

This is equivalent to the famous (or infamous) principle of identity of indiscernibles. This principle, in point of fact, is one way by which identity can be introduced into and defined in a logical calculus.

Wiggins argued that though Leibniz's law and its contraposition could be used to indicate *necessary* conditions of *identity* and *sufficient* conditions of *difference*, together they would not suffice for determining identity; in addition, he held, persistence of identicals through time and space under the aforementioned sortal covering concept (*f*) would be required. (Wiggins expressed some uneasiness about the proper explication of identity in reductions, suggesting that one should not think "that any one explanation of (the) reductive 'is' (is) possible," since the proper explanation "depends on the reduction" (1967, 26).) The use of Leibniz's law in reductions has also been considered by Wimsatt (1976b), who has suggested that we use Leibniz's law as a "rigorous detector" of the failure or incompleteness of reductions. This is an interesting proposal and I shall return to it later in this section.

In his 1981, Hooker outlined an explication of predicate identity that is a generalization of Putnam's (1970) views on property identity. Hooker's explication is also congruent with Causey's proposal quoted on p. 467 and with suggestions made by Kim and Achinstein (though Hooker also disagrees with certain features of the latter two accounts). Hooker proposes, on a "rough" epistemic criterion of contingent property identity, that:

> The designata of two predicates, P, Q say, are to be accepted as contingently identical if and only if (P and Q are not logically equivalent and) (i) the extension of P is identical to that of Q, and (ii) there is a homomorphism between the abstract determinate/determinable structure in which P is embedded and that in which Q is embedded,

and (iii) there is a homomorphism between the nomic roles of P and Q, all as specified by theory. Provided we add the qualification that only ultimately clarified, true sciences are involved, this is the criterion of contingent property identity. (1981, 219)

This appears to be a prima facie reasonable suggestion, though it should be noted immediately that the theories and sciences which enter into such a criterion are to be "ultimately clarified" and that this condition is rarely if ever satisfied. I pointed out earlier that we usually deal with continuously *evolving* theories, and that part of the evolutionary pressures which change theories are putative reduction relationships. Thus Hooker's criterion requires that we come to some final, stable equilibrium, where a stable identity exists between some reducing T_1^{n*} and a reduced T_2^{m*}, where n amd m have ceased to change. (Here I use the notation T_1^{2*} for T_1's successor and likewise for T_2. This is similar to chapter 6's notation for an extended theory, the only alteration being the * representing correction due to reduction rather than some other reason.) I shall have more to say about this in section 9.5.

Though Hooker's criteria for property identity are reasonable ones, they are not additions to the conditions for reduction in the general reduction-replacement model. In point of fact, if the conditions of the model are met, Hooker's criteria follow. (An alternative way of construing this relation would be to see Hooker's criteria as an alternative way of providing conditions of adequacy for a reduction.)

Hooker's condition (i) follows from the extensional interpretation of predicates given earlier, and condition (ii) follows from the existence of a reduction function for predicates and functions. A homomorphism is defined as a mapping φ from $/A/$ to $/B/$ under the assumptions that "for all nonlogical symbols f and p and all $a_1, \ldots, a_n$ in $/A/$

$$\varphi(f_A(a_1, \ldots, a_n)) = f_B(\varphi(a_1), \ldots, \varphi(a_n))$$

and

$$p_A(a_1, \ldots, a_n) \rightarrow p_B(\varphi(a_1, \ldots, \varphi(a_n)).$$

(See Shoenfield 1967, 94.)

The mapping φ can be construed as a many-one reduction function from the reducing theories' domain $/A/$ into the reduced theories' domain /B/. These two conditions "preserve the structure." (The separate application of φ to functions, in addition to predicates, can be absorbed into the predicate expression since an n-ary function can be defined as an (n + 1)-ary predicate with a premise requiring a unique value for the function as the n + 1 place of the predicate.) But if such a (homomorphic) reduction function exists, then it guarantees the satisfaction of Hooker's condition (ii), which is a verbal statement of the above conditions.

It is a bit more difficult to show how Hooker's condition (iii) follows from the general reduction-replacement model, but this is because of what I see as some conflation of current science (or science as it is actually) with Putnam's idealized "clarified science." For Hooker,

> the notion that . . . clinches contingent property identity is sameness of nomological role. For what Putnam's schema suggests, or rather the ideas which back it suggest, is that in a clarified science there will be a unique set of fundamental properties governed by an unambiguous set of fundamental laws, for then if all complex properties are constructable, all laws can be derived from fundamental laws. Correspondingly, every distinct complex property is uniquely associated with certain roles in a certain class of laws and, conversely, from identity of nomological role (hence of law class), identity of construction, and so identity of a property will follow. (1981, 218)

Such a clarified science will not follow from the general reduction-replacement model, but any criterion which appeals to a to-be clarified science seems fairly useless as a criterion to apply to current or any real science. And if we relax condition (iii), as Hooker seems wont to do (see his 1981), then a weaker analogue of condition (iii) will follow from the already derived conditions (i) and (ii), if we supplement them with the generalization of Nagel's condition of derivability, that the "corrected" laws of the reduced theory are derivable from the "corrected" reducing theory, supplemented with appropriate reduction functions. This argument assumes that the "nomic roles" of predicates are determined by the laws of the theory in which they appear, which seems to be a reasonable assumption. The analogue of Hooker's

(iii) is a weaker condition, since we are dealing at best with a temporally stable identity and not with clarified science.

Several caveats must be added to this discussion concerning predicate identity. First, some type of restriction must be introduced on either the entities or the predicates that are identified. Most writers follow Quine and exclude modal predicates (such as having beliefs, desires, etc.; see Hooker 1981), but some, following Frege, do not, preferring to qualify on the objects rather than the properties (see Wiggins 1980). Second, we are discussing evolving science and not an ultimately stable science ("clarified science") or even only a temporarily stable science. Attention must be paid to the interesting process of predicate modification that occurs as $T_2 \rightarrow T_2^*$ under the stress of an attempted reduction to T_1, since it illustrates important features of dynamic theory structure, as were discussed in chapter 5. Accordingly, we may in many cases of actual science have to be content with "close analogues" or "very similar properties" rather than identical properties.

The dynamic nature of science must also be invoked when we consider how predicate and entity identities are established. It is impossible, in an ultimate sense, to separate predicate reduction and entity reduction, as was pointed out in note 21, since all identities are ultimately entity (or colligations of entity) identities. However, the connections must be so established that there is an isomorphism or homomorphism of extensions and structures, such that the entities identified in the reduced and reducing theories must *behave* identically (that is, must have the same or identical properties, subject to the modal restrictions cited). To repeat the version of Leibniz's law noted above,

$$(a = b) \supset (\varphi) (\varphi a \equiv \varphi b).$$

That is, if a is identical to b, then if a has a property, b must have that property, and vice versa.

We obtain access to identities in terms of their properties, some of which are observable *consequences* of the entity's properties and some of which are more "directly" associated with them (see the discussion in chapter 4, p. 136 ff.). In establishing entity identities, we make use of properties that are, for the state of science, empirically applicable to the entities to be identified. Accordingly, for establishing $gene_1 = DNA_1$, for example, we need to show that the presence or absence of a gene is associated with the presence or absence of a DNA sequence. Since genes duplicate in mitosis we need to be able to say that DNA similarly duplicates, and since genes mutate we also require an identity between substances that affect DNA and substances that are mutagens. This is akin to implementing methodologically the contrapositive form of Leibniz's law or the principle of the identity of indescernibles:

$$(\varphi)\ (\varphi a \equiv \varphi b) \supset (a = b).$$

Such a scientific review of properties that establishes entity identification is not an easy task, since the reduced (and probably the reducing) theory will need to change to accommodate the strict identification. Thus a provisional $gene_1 = DNA_1$ reduction function may require that contexually different DNAs be introduced; that is, within the vocabulary of the reducing theory we may need to define subtypes of DNA — say, whether DNA is transcribed and translated or not. For example, only one strand of the double helix of DNA is transcribed and translated, and in many eukaryotic organisms much of the DNA is silent, representing intervening sequences of as-yet-unknown function(s). Thus not all DNA is identifiable with Mendelian $genes_1$, though the converse may be true. Furthermore, as noted above, Benzer (1956) argued that the traditional Mendelian definition of a gene as a coextensive unit of mutation, recombination, and function needed further dissection and correction if it is to accord with our knowledge of how heredity modifications occur at the level of DNA. These difficulties make reduction functions *complex*, but they do not, contra earlier comments of Hull, Kitcher, and Rosenberg, make it either impossible or impractical. There is, then, a progressive shifting and mutual accommodation of T_1, T_2, and the reduction functions as a reduction occurs. The nomic connections cited in Hooker's condition (iii) vary as this shifting and accommodation occur.

There are, in addition, limits to such accommodations, though they are difficult to specify. Essentially, the limits on either theory appear to be the same as were developed in chapter 5 in regard to theory individuation, that is, high-level central properties and assumptions of either theory cannot be eliminated or denied lest the theory be replaced rather than altered (though the replaced theory's domain may be "reduced"). In point of historical fact, this failure of a reduction due to essential theory change occurred in physics when an Einsteinian interpretation of Maxwellian electrodynamics precluded any coherent mechanical aether reduction of Maxwell's theory (see Schaffner 1972).

Are Identities in Reductions Necessary A Posteriori Truths? The last issue under the general heading of the synthetic identity interpretation of connectability assumptions or reduction functions I want to consider involves the epistemic and metaphysical interpretation of these assertions. Comparatively recently a theory of such identities was developed by Kripke, Donnellan, and Putnam. The theory has some plausibility in connection with its interpretation of identity statements involving well defined individuals, such as when one identifies the two names of a planet, such as, for example, Hesperus = Phosphorus, the two names for Venus in its guises as the evening star and the morning star respectively. This theory of identities, however, has been extended to more general examples involving mass terms such as "heat = molecular agitation" by Kripke, and "water = H_2O" by Putnam, where its conclusions are less certain and more controversial. Since these latter types of examples are the kind of identities involved in reductions, and because the Kripke-Putnam theory is a bold, even startling, account of the logical, epistemological, and metaphysical nature of these identities, a brief summary of their views is desirable. Any searching analysis is beyond the scope of this book, but the interested reader can consult Schwartz's anthology, which includes reprints of Kripke's and Putnam's original papers as well as critical commentaries on this view of reference.[34]

One of the most provocative claims of this Kripke-Putnam theory is the thesis that synthetic identities of the type found in reductions are not contingent but are rather *necessary* truths. They are, however, not known a priori but are discovered. Thus they represent a class of *necessary a posteriori* truths.

In a sense the claim is not that novel. Ramsey argued that identities in the sense of x = y were tautologies (1931, 51–53). In her 1947, Ruth Barcan-Marcus *proved* in an axiomatic treatment of modal logic that if two objects are identical they are necessarily identical. The proof follows from Leibniz's law introduced above if one of the properties P is allowed to range over such a modal property as "is necessarily identical with a." Substitution of that property in the expression for Leibniz's law followed by several simple steps yields the theorem:

$$(a = b) \supset \Box\,(a = b)$$

where $\Box$ is read, as usual, "it is necessary that." (However, recall that following Quine I adopted a restriction on the range of predicates in Leibniz's law above to *exclude* modal predicates, such as having beliefs, desires, and the like. Such a position is, however, controversial and is, of course, denied in the Barcan-Marcus argument.)

Kripke's and Putnam's contribution was at least partially to provide a series of arguments for a theory of reference, which informally undergirded the interpretation of this formal theorem. For Kripke there is an important distinction between those terms that name or designate the same objects in all possible worlds, and those terms that do not. The former are characterized as "rigid designators," and it follows that, if rigidly designating terms flank an identity sign, then that identity is true in all possible worlds, which is another way of characterizing necessity. The identities can come to be discovered, however, via their *accidental* designators; for example, "cause of heat sensations" is an accidental designator whereas "heat" and "molecular motion" are rigid designators. This allows a proponent of Kripke's view to answer Causey's (1977, 97) concern that Krip-kean identities seem to require necessarily true identities of the type that we do not appear to find in scientific reductions (but see Causey 1977, 96–97 and 104 n. 4 for further qualifications).

The proper way to understand rigid designators, especially as applied to general mass terms like "water," is not very clear. Putnam has argued in the light of this theory of rigid designators that "if there is a hidden structure (like H_2O for water) then generally it determines what it is to be a member of a natural kind not only in the actual world but in all possible worlds." Barcan-Marcus and others have seen that this type of view leads to essentialism. She writes:

> What . . . [a rigid designator] seems to designate is an essential property; a property which if something has it, it has necessarily, whatever world it is in. (1947, 138)

This interpretation is consistent with Putnam's claim that if we were to discover a substance phenomenologically identical to water but chemically different (made of XYZ and not H_2O) it would not be water. Water, he argues, is necessarily identical with H_2O in all possible worlds.

The argument is sound, given the premises, but its victory is Pyrrhic. By defining rigid designators as true in all possible worlds and by attributing essential substructural properties to substances, the theory begs the interesting questions: (1) Are there any rigid designators? and (2) Are they the kind that are represented by "water = H_2O" [or, for our purposes, "gene = DNA"]? I submit that, as regards interesting problems in reduction, the answer to both of these questions is "no." Let me indicate my reasons.

The methodology of verifying reductions is to begin from a well characterized theory and then to attempt to discover and construct entity and predicate (attribute) identities. The reduced theory will possess evidential support in its own terms, and what scientists seek is some existing support and confirmable realization in another domain of those terms which permit identity claims. The theory can in principle be realized in a number of ways. In another world an entity that was the heredity determiner and that segregated, mutated, or combined in accord with the Mendel-Morgan theory of genetics would be termed a "gene." For those who would follow Putnam and doubt this, consider that in a number of viruses, such as the tobacco mosaic virus and the HIV-1 or AIDS virus, RNA and not DNA carries the heredity information. The RNA in such organisms represents the "genes" of those organisms according to standard scientific usage. I, accordingly, do not find the arguments of the Kripke-Putnam analysis of identities either compelling or very helpful in elucidating the nature of those identities that function in reductions. Others' intuitions may differ.

9.4.3 *Derivability Problems*

In this comparatively brief section I want to address the question whether reduction involves derivation. In this connection I shall consider Kitcher's objections to what he conceives of as yet a third key assumption made by any Nagelian model of reduction. I shall also in this section consider the problems of approximation and of strong analogy, which arise in connection with conditions (3) and (4) of the general reduction-replacement model of theory reduction, outlined on p. 429. Some of the distinctions and structures of what I termed an extended theory in chapter 5 will prove useful here.

Kitcher on Derivational Reduction

Let us first begin by noting that Kitcher has argued that Nagelian models of reduction (applied to genetics) are committed to the following thesis, which he terms (R3):[35]

> (R3) A derivation of general principles about the transmission of genes from principles of molecular biology would explain why the laws of gene transmission hold (to the extent that they do). (1984, 339)

Kitcher maintains that this (R3) thesis is *false*. He elaborates his criticism of (R3) by stating that, even if he were to grant the truth of the earlier theses (R1) and (R2), "exhibiting derivations of the transmission laws [of classical genetics] from principles of molecular biology and bridge principles would not explain the laws, and, therefore, would not fulfill the major goal of reduction" (1984, 347).

His argument seems to go as follows. Providing a molecular mechanism for the "laws" of classical genetics, such as the law of independent assortment, would not add anything to the cytological narrative of homologous chromosomal pairing and post-metaphase meiotic segregation. A molecular account would in point of fact destroy the simplicity and unity afforded by the cytological perspective. The cytological explanation is both superior to a molecular explanation and is in a methodological sense sui generis, since rather different molecular realizations are possible, but these would not add (or subtract) from the cytological level explanation of Mendel's law.[36] Appealing to specific molecular level realizations would, however, subtract from the explanation because explaining meiosis involves appealing to "PS-processes" (for pairing-separating). These PS-processes, when analyzed *at the molecular level*, are not natural kinds (Kitcher 1984a, 349).

It appears to me that there are several mistakes in this argument. First, I see no reason for giving a special priority to the cytological level as regards explanation. Just as we saw before that molecular discoveries have resulted in clarification and unification of the gene concept, it seems eminently plausible to me that additional explanatory unification and power will be forthcoming from a molecular explanation. Evidence for this can be seen if we examine various failures, or perhaps better, limitations of Mendel's theory (or laws). Recombination and crossing over are *not* well understood at the cytological level. Spindle formation, segregation, and segregation failure, which results in the tragic nondisjunctions producing Down's syndrome, are at best described, but not explained, at the cytological level. Current research programs in *molecular* genetics are directed at these topics (see Watson et al. 1987, in chapter 11, "Recombination at the Molecular Level," and the review of the production of haploid yeast cells [583–585]).

Second, I believe that Kitcher's argument concerning PS processes is either too strong or too weak. It is too strong if taken at face value because it eliminates *any* biological entities as being natural kinds. Kitcher writes that:

> PS-processes are heterogeneous from the molecular point of view. There are no constraints on the molecular structure of the entities which are paired or on the ways in which fundamental forces combine to pair them and to separate them . . . I claim, therefore, that PS-processes are realized in a motley of molecular ways. (1984a, 349–350)

But surely we can envisage different biological bases other than the cellular type we are familiar with that would constitute realizations of cytological generalizations, and clearly genes or the heredity determiners could be different from what they are in this world. Such possibilities have in fact, as we noted in chapter 3, led J. J. C. Smart to argue that there are *no* biological laws, a view which has an element of truth but which requires a good bit of further analysis and correction. If this claim is correct, then Kitcher's argument is too strong because it removes the entities of cytology and genetics from the domain of natural kinds, which either is a startling conclusion that needs additional argument, or, I would maintain, constitutes a counterargument to Kitcher's view. If we do not wish to take such a strong interpretation of Kitcher's notion, then it seems to me that there are constraints at the molecular level that lead to every bit as compelling an argument for natural kinds at the molecular level as at the cytological and/or genetic levels. An examination of such molecular processes as genetic coding and protein synthesis disclose just how limited a set of options are followed by quite diverse organisms. Natural selection exercises powerful constraints on replicating populations, and chemical features such as bonding constraints introduce additional limitations as regards the flexibility Kitcher envisages at that level.[37]

A rather separate criticism of Kitcher's critique is that his objection to explanation *by derivation* misses the mark. His cytological account could as easily be framed within a deductive pattern as within the framework of a molecular explanation. Thus it is misleading to construe, as he himself seems to do, his argument as directed against explanation by derivation. The argument rather is against an explanation at any level deeper than the cytological level, and this, I have suggested in the previous paragraph, is not supportable.

Finally, I have several general objections to the use of early twentieth-century cytological theory to argue against the Nagel and Nagelian models of reduction. First, it could be claimed that cytological theory represents one of the earlier reductions of Mendelian genetics. I suspect it is at most a *partial* reduction, but the history of the interactions between genetics and cytology does suggest that both theories were mutually corrective at different points in time, and that the cytology was functioning in certain explanatory capacities.[38] Thus to use cytology as a vantage point from which to criticize the reduction model seems to beg the question, unless it can be shown that the genetics-cytology relation cannot be captured by a Nagelian reduction. Mendel's second law seems to be a limiting case for genes on independent chromosomes, but the same idea can be put in the language of genetics by speaking of independent "linkage groups." Much of the work by Sutton and Morgan in the early twentieth century was directed at working out the relations between genetics and cytology, and my reading of the history does not indicate that all the illumination by any means came from cytology.[39]

Kitcher's account, then, seems to me not to offer any serious, telling objections to the classical account of reduction. His (R1) thesis, that there are laws that need to be invoked in biological reductions but that are not available, as I argued earlier is based on an overly strict interpretation of the nature of biological theory structure, which, when appropriately relaxed along the lines suggested in this book, permits a reasonably close analogue to the classical approach to reduction to go through. His view of the (R2) thesis, that bridge laws are required but not findable, is false, as I have also argued (that is, R2 is true), though for quite complex reasons. Kitcher's (R3), it seems to me, is also defensible against his objections, along the lines just sketched. Finally, it should be pointed out that, as regards the *logic* involved in explanation, Kitcher's own model (see chapter 6, p. 312) subscribes to a derivational approach, though one supplemented with a unification criterion. As I shall indicate shortly (see p. 492ff.), appealing to a deductive relation in order to achieve deductive systematicity is both powerful and innocuous, when interpreted in the correct manner.

The Problem of Analogy in Reduction

In addition to the criticisms of the derivational approach per se, criticisms have also been raised in regard to the introduction of the conditions of correction and of strong analogy that appear in the GRR model. Recall, for example, Hull (1974, 42–44, as quoted above on p. 438), who is concerned that a "reduction" may actually be a "replacement." In one sense this type of objection has already been met by broadening the GRR model to encompass the continuum of reduction-replacement relations. In another sense the issues (1) are not peculiar to reduction — they affect scientific change in its most general aspects — and (2) do not affect the logical core of reduction. I can best argue for these two points by presenting of an extended historical example. This example serves the function of illustrating how an earlier reducing theory (the generalized induction theory) is *replaced* by a successor reducing theory (the operon theory) that explains enzyme induction. The example will also indicate how the operon theory in its first form becomes progressively modified as it attempts to explain additional experiments associated with enzyme induction, these successive forms displaying strong analogies with each other as the operon theory is itself reduced to a detailed molecular account. Some of the latter story has already been told in chapter 4, where the work of Gilbert and Muller-Hill was discussed, so it need not be repeated in detail here.

The Historical Background to the Operon Theory. Consider the early development of the *lac* operon theory of genetic regulation, which in its more definitive later forms has been discussed at several different points in this book. Though, as will be noted in a later section, reduction was not the aim of Jacob and Monod's work, significant progress toward a complete chemical explanation of enzyme induction has been a consequence of their research. For example, in a previous section (p. 464) I described the sequencing of the operator and promoter genes in the *lac* region.

In the development of the operon theory, Monod, working with Melvin Cohn, initially began from a very different theory involving an instructive type of hypothesis. This early theory was known as the generalized induction theory (GIT). Stated all too briefly to provide a sense of the complex issues that were invoked as its experimental basis, the essence of the GIT is as follows:

1. A unitary hypothesis concerning enzyme-forming systems was asserted, that the fundamental production mechanisms of both constitutive and induced enzymes are identical.

2. The difference between induced and constitutive enzyme production (the latter type is continuously being produced, while the production of the former can be turned on and off) was accounted for by supposing that induction is really universal but that the induction mechanism is masked or hidden in the cases of constitutive enzyme production because a "natural" internal or endogenous inducer is continuously inducing production of those enzymes.

Explicitly rejected in Cohn and Monod's generalized induction theory was an alternative to an endogenous inducer hypothesis which would still have allowed the assertion of a unitary hypothesis. This rejected alternative was termed the "secondary induction hypothesis"; it asserted that "induction is only a secondary and contingent phenomenon which does not directly impinge on the mechanism of enzyme synthesis" (1953, 134). The secondary induction hypothesis was rejected because it tacitly implied that *the enzyme exists before induction* (1953, 134), or at least reducible as discussed earlier. (I say "reducible" here rather than simply explainable since the operon theory is now a biochemical theory and the experimental domain of the generalized induction theory was genetics.) Such information had to be available since enzymes are extremely "specific," or individually distinct. The remarkable, complementary "lock-and-key" structural relationship of inducer and induced enzyme seemed to require that the inducer play some important role in molding the active or catalytic site of the enzyme. To put it somewhat metaphorically, it seemed extremely implausible to Cohn and Monod that a "lock" could have been designed without some active informational role being played by the "key," much in the way antigens were believed to "instruct" antibody formation via the antigen-antibody complex. I shall term this belief the "inducer-template hypothesis"; such a template hypothesis is essentially equivalent to what has been termed, in our discussions of immunology in earlier chapters, an "instructive" hypothesis. From the point of view of this type of hypothesis, structural information can pass from the small molecule (the inducer) into a protein (the induced enzyme). Though Cohn and Monod accepted the "one gene–one enzyme" hypothesis of Beadle and Tatum, they were at that time, and for good reasons, reluctant to accept the truth, only much later established, that genes completely determine the structure, especially the three-dimensional "tertiary structure," of the enzyme.

The "Pajama" Experiment. In the mid-1950s, F. Jacob, working with E. Wollman, clarified the mechanisms of chromosomal transfer from "male" to "female" *E. coli* cells. Thus a most important genetic tool became available for analyzing the interaction of the i, z, and y genes in the *lac* region of the *E. coli* genome. An experiment to study these interactions was planned in early 1957, and the specific mutants to be used were selected for in Jacob's laboratory. With the assistance of A. Pardee, who visited the Pasteur Institute during 1957–58 while on a sabbatical year, Jacob and Monod conjugated straints of *E. coli* that were variously inducible and constitutive for the production of β-galactosidase and permease. The investigations are collectively referred to as the "Pa-ja-mo" or sometimes the "Pajama" experiment (after the names of three investigators). I wish to focus on two types of crosses or matings that were carried out (the technical details of the experiments will not concern us here).

The result of the cross of bacteria of genotypes:

$$z^- i^- \times z^+ i^+ \text{ (I)}$$

which fed $z^- i^-$ genes into the cytoplasm of a "female" of the $z^+ i^+$ strain of *E. coli*, producing partially diploid or merozygotic "progeny" with genotype $z^- i^-/z^+ i^+$, was that *no* enzyme synthesis was detected either immediately or even after several hours. On the other hand, the cross

$$z^+ i^+ \times z^- i^- \text{ (II)},$$

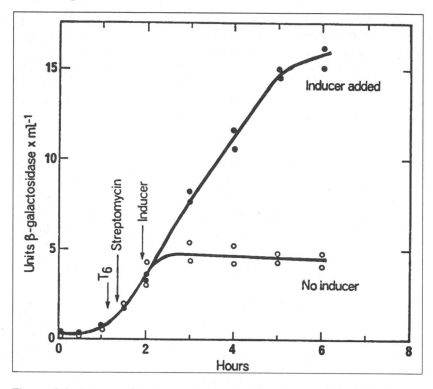

Figure 9.6   Enzyme kinetic graph representing the results of the Pajama experiment, Cross II (see text). (The arrows indicating when the T6 bacteriophage and streptomycin were added are not of concern to us.) The graphs clearly show the commencement of β-galactosidase synthesis very soon after the entrance of the z^+ gene and also the conversion of the merozygotes from the constitutive form to the inducible form after about two hours. (From Pardee, Jacob, and Monod, 1959, with permission.)

in which the z^+i^+ genes enter the z^-i^- cytoplasmic environment, resulted in the synthesis of β-galatosidase at a normal rate beginning about 3-4 minutes after the predicted penetration of the z^+ gene. After about two hours, however, synthesis ceased, but it was found to be restartable by the addition of an external inducer (the induction kinetics are shown in figure 9.6). In other words, the phenotype of the merozygotes resulting from a cross of type II changed from constitutive to inducible. The absolute contrast of the immediate results of crosses I and II indicated that the i-z interaction took place through the cytoplasm. This also seemed to be supported by the two-hour delay in the change from constitutivity to inducibility. A cross not specifically cited here showed that no cytoplasmic substances are transferred during conjugation, in agreement with results obtained several years before by Jacob and Wollman, so the genes must have been the cause of the change. It is clear then, using traditional genetic language, that inducibility is "dominant" over constitutivity, though the dominance is slowly expressed. According to the generalized induction theory, constitutivity should have been dominant over inducibility, since this theory understood constitutive enzyme production to be governed by a natural internal inducer that should have directed the synthesis of β-galactosidase (see hypothesis 2 of the GIT above). The reversal of this expected result by the Pajama experiment seemed to suggest another interpretation of the control of enzyme synthesis. In the preliminary three-page announcement of their results in the 28 May 1958 numbers of *Comptes Rendus*, Pardee, Jacob and Monod wrote:

> It had appeared reasonable up to the present to suppose that constitutive mutants of a given system synthesized an endogenous inducer absent in the case of the inducible type. The results described here suggest a hypothesis which is exactly opposite. The facts are explained if one supposes that the *i* gene determines (through the mediation of an enzyme) the synthesis, not of an inducer, but of a "repressor" which [diffusing throughout the cytoplasm] *blocks* synthesis of the β-galactosidase, and which the exogenous inducers remove [déplacent] restoring the synthesis. The *i⁻* allele present in the case of the constitutives being inactive, the repressor is not formed, the galactosidase is synthesized, the exogenous inducer is without effect. (1958, 3127)

The generalized induction theory was thus in effect overthrown by the Pajama experiments,[40] and a more selection-oriented, negative-control, repressor-based theory proposed. It was this theory which developed into the operon theory (see pp. 76–82, figure 3.1, and Technical Discussion 2).

As work proceeded on the operon theory various changes in that theory occurred. In its very early (1959) stages, the inducibility gene, *i*, was incorrectly mapped between the *z* and *y* genes and there was no operator gene. In the 1960–61 form of the theory, the operator and associated structural genes were introduced and the gene order was corrected, but initially the repressor was conjectured to be a species of RNA or an RNA-protein complex and not a pure protein, as it later was recognized to be. In 1965 the importance of the promoter locus was discovered. As recounted in chapter 4, in 1966 the molecular nature of the repressor was elucidated by Gilbert and Müller-Hill, and, in the years since, the operon theory, initially an interlevel theory as characterized in chapter 3, has itself become reduced to an almost completely molecular theory (see Watson et al. 1987, 475–480 for details of the specific DNA sequences in the *lac* control region). A relationship of strong analogy exists between these successive forms of the operon theory, to be distinguished from the *replacement* relation holding between the GIT and the operon theory of 1960–61.

Lessons of the "Pajama" Experiment. Two points should now be clear: (1) the generalized induction theory was *replaced,* though its experimental domain is (later) explained by the operon theory, and (2) there is no *single,* timeless operon theory—rather, there is a changing extended theory, time-slices of which bear similarity and analogical relations among themselves. We can, I think, use the terminology developed in chapter 5 and to be elaborated further in connection with reduction below to elucidate, at least partially, the differences between these theories. When central γ-level assumptions change, such as the general instructive thesis involved in the generalized induction theory, the theory is replaced. However, when (1) peripheral assumptions change (such as the belief that the operon messenger RNA was broken down into separate RNA molecules for each gene z, y, a) or (2) central σ-level assumptions (that introduction of a promotor was necessary) or δ-level assumptions (that the repressor was RNA rather than protein) change, we have change *within* the extended theory. This is the case *as long as there is central* γ-level continuity (continuity of belief in the existence of negative control interactions, i.e., control is by repression, at the level of transcription between induction gene product, the repressor, and the operator. (I should add that even when the theory is replaced, its *experimental domain* may be reducible, as discussed earlier. I say "reducible" here rather than simply explainable since the experimental domain of the operon theory is now biochemistry and the experimental domain of the generalized induction theory was genetics.)

This suggests that the kind of reduction exemplified by the operon theory — and this example is a paradigm of the reduction of biology to physics and chemistry — has both informal and formal features. We should be willing to say that T_1, say, biochemistry, reduces T_2, say, regulatory genetics, if there are versions (time slices) of T_1 and T_2 in the extended sense that satisfy the connectability and derivability conditions precisely. The successive relations within the extended theories, however, are only amenable to characterization by similarity measures. Whether these *diachronic* relations can be made formally precise and quantified is an interesting question vis-à-vis the issue of theory individuation and theory discrimination, but this question is not peculiar to the problem of reduction and it need not be resolved in order to set out a clear model of theory reduction.

9.5 Multiple Levels, Causes, and the Possibility of an Alternative Causal/Mechanical Model of Reduction

9.5.1 *Multiple Levels of Analysis in Reduction*

I shall begin this discussion by recalling again that biological theories are typically interlevel. This is the case, I believe, with respect to both the level of aggregation and the level of generality. In the present chapter we were reminded of the first sense by Mendel's first paper — in his suggestion that a cytological basis for his "factors" could explain his law of independent assortment. Here we dealt only with what I have referred to in a previous chapter as the γ and the σ levels, or in one interpretation, the most general level in a theory and its cytological realization.[41] Mendel was not familiar with the primitive biochemistry of his day, but almost from the beginning of the rediscovery of genetics in 1900 various biologists began to develop biochemical or molecular speculations about genetics. For example, Beadle and Tatum note in one of their early papers:

> The possibility that genes may act through the mediation of enzymes has been suggested by several authors. See Troland, L. T., *Amer. Nat.*, *51*, 321–350 (1917); Wright, S., *Genetics*, *12*, 530–569 (1927); and Haldane, J.B.S., in *Perspectives in Biochemistry*, Cambridge Univ. Press, pp. 1–10 (1937) for discussion and references. (1941, 506, n. 1)

Similarly, Muller in his writings in the 1920s, long before anything resembling "molecular genetics" was developed, wrote:

> The chemical composition of the genes, and the formulae of their reactions, remain as yet quite unknown. We do know for example, that in certain cases a given pair of genes will determine the existence of a particular enzyme (concerned in pigment production) . . . [and other examples are available]. Each of these effects, which we call a "character" of the organism, is the product of a highly complex, intricate, and delicately balanced system of reactions, caused by the interaction of countless genes. (1922, 87)

The point of these quotations is to support the thesis that, even in the heyday of recombination-based genetics, geneticists were concerned with more than the cell-and-organelle basis of their discipline. Both experimentally warranted and speculative δ-level, or biochemical, realizations of genetics were to be found in the genetics literature.[42] These molecular realizations are primitive in comparison to those of the present day and are usually quite at variance with a nucleic acid basis for the genes, since virtually all biologists prior to about 1950 believed that the gene would be found to be a proteinaceous entity.[43] Nevertheless, the existence of what I shall call a full (if impoverished) set of theory realization levels suggests that the later reduction of classical genetics to molecular genetics is likely to be more complex than a simple *two-level* schema that some interpretations of the standard model of reduction would seem to indicate. Exactly how to elaborate still further on the above-described general reduction-replacement (GRR) model is the issue to which I now turn my attention.

In order to apply an analogue of the standard reduction model to theories which are interlevel both in aggregation and in generality, the notion of partial reduction and the concept of reduction as replacement must be kept in mind. The historical record in many other disciplines in addition to genetics suggests that reductions will preserve a number of earlier scientific achievements, though some components will be modified and others will be rejected in the light of newer knowledge. Usually, but not always, what have often been referred to as "empirical generalizations" have the greatest stability across both reductions and scientific revolutions (even more so than specific data observations, I would argue). These generalizations may figure in defining a scientific theory, though per se they usually lack sufficient explanatory and unificatory power to be characterized as constitutimg a theory. Mendel's laws are only a prima facie exception, for his theory of genetics involves (as has been argued earlier and supported by quotation from his 1865 paper) several theoretical elements pertaining to cytology in addition to his more directly warranted empirical claims.

A scientific theory that is a candidate for reduction, then, will typically have a set of assumptions that intertwine several levels of both aggregation and generality. Some of the more "theoretical" assumptions may be preserved in a reduction, sometimes with slight modifications. Often many of the empirical underpinnings of a previously successful theory will be retained, though even here those elements may be partially reclassified and reattributed to different disciplines. It is difficult to propose any *universal* requirements for such reductions since they represent science in flux, often during periods of intense activity and deepening insight. Nevertheless, it would appear that one should expect γ-level assumptions that are close to direct empirical verification to be retained. Preservability is likely to decrease as one examines a reduced theory's δ-level assumptions, since here one is obtaining, via the reducing theory, what is usually characterized as a *new mechanism* to explain some heretofore puzzling phenomena. Thus there is likely to be sharp contrast between the older δ-level mechanisms and those of the new reducing theory. Such is by no means invariably the case, however, and it can occur that the new reducing theory is seen as a significant amplification of older, speculative δ-level hypotheses, as for example Beadle and Tatum's advances on Muller's and others' proposals concerning gene activity, previously discussed.

The complexities introduced by the interlevel nature of biomedical theories do not argue against the reduction-replacement model introduced earlier, though they do underscore the difficulties with achieving a simple and syntactically precise formal characterization of the relation. It may be that the nature of these partial and analogical relations can best be comprehended in specific examples of the type examined in the previous section, pending the development of some stronger forms of knowledge representation discussed in chapter 3, such as OOP techniques.

9.5.2 *Might a Fully Causal/Mechanical Approach of Reduction Be Possible?*

Bracketing for a moment this further complexity of reductions suggested by the typically interlevel character of the involved theories, there are several important points to *re*emphasize about the above lengthy account of reduction and of reduction in genetics specifically. In this section, my discussion will strongly re-echo the account given in chapter 6 of *explanation* (in neurobiology). This should be expected because of the close relation between explanation and reduction. Here, however, the focus will be on genetics and in the context of the relation of one scientific domain to another.

First, I must agree with Wimsatt (1976a, 1976b) and Kitcher (1984) that we do not have anything *quite* like the "laws" we find so prevalent in physics explanations. This point was introduced in connection with explanation in neuroscience in chapter 7, but it has broader application with implications for reduction. There are generalizations of a sort (of varying degrees of generality) that we could extract from molecular explanations of genetics, though they are usually left implicit, typically having been introduced in other (perhaps earlier and more didactic) contexts.[44] Further, these generalizations are typically borrowed from a very wide-ranging set of models (protein synthesis models, biochemical models, etc.). Recall that the set in biology is so broad it led Morowitz's (1985) committee to invoke the notion of still another sense of a "many-many" in biology: a many-many modeling in the form of a complex "matrix" (see Morowitz (1985). But even when such generalizations, narrow or broad, are made explicit, they need to be supplemented with the details of specific "hook-up" connections in the system in order to constitute an explanation.[45] These are not quite like the "initial conditions" of traditional philosophy of science because they are an integral part of the reducing mechanism, for instance, that the gene sequence in the *lac* system is *i-p-o-z-y-a* and that the repressor binds to the DNA operator sequence ACCTTAACACT (Watson et al. 1987, 476–480). Some of the generalizations that we can glean from such molecular mechanisms may have quite a narrow scope and typically need to be changed to *analogous* generalizations (or mechanisms) as one changes organism or behavior, for instance to RNA as the material basis of the gene for TMV or the AIDS virus (HIV-1), or to the different eukaryotic gene regulation principles as one moves away from prokaryotes.

What we appear to have in most of our "reduction" examples are rather intricate *systems* describable using both broad and narrow *causal generalizations* that are typically not framed in purely biochemical terminology but that are characteristically *interlevel* and *interfield*. As noted earlier, this is a feature importantly stressed by Darden and Maull in their 1977, and in chapters 3 and 5 and the subsection immediately above I reemphasized this interlevel feature of typical biological theories and also suggested that such theories often explain by providing a temporal sequence as part of their models. As an explanation of a phenomenon like dominance or enzyme induction is given in molecular terms, one maps parts of the phenomenon into a molecular vocabulary, sometimes by utilizing synthetic identities, sometimes by exhibiting an entity previously characterized in molecular terms as a causal consequence of a reducing mechanism. Enzyme induction becomes not just the phenomenon as Monod encountered it in his early research but is *reinterpreted as* a causal consequence of derepressed protein synthesis. Thus something *like* Nagel's condition of connectability is found, but it is laden with new causal freight.

Is reduction as characterized above, in terms of the examples given, also in accord with reduction by derivation from a theory, as in the GRR model? Again, I think the answer is generally yes, but with some important caveats. We do not have, as I have argued above, a very general set of sentences (the "laws") that can serve as a small set of premises from which we can deduce the conclusion. Rather, what we have is *a set of causal sentences of varying degrees of generality,* many of them quite specific to the system in question, and many left implicit. It may be that in some distant future all of these causal sentences of narrow scope, such as "the *i* gene determines . . . the synthesis of . . . a 'repressor' which blocks synthesis of the β-galactosidase, and which the exogenous inducers remove" (Pardee, Jacob, and Monod 1959, 3127), will be explainable by general laws of protein chemistry, but such is not the case at present. In part this failure of unilevel explanation is a consequence of our inability to infer the three-dimensional structure of a protein such as the repressor from a complete knowledge of the sequence of amino acids which make up this tetrameric (four-segmented) protein. Fundamental and very general principles will have to await a more developed science than we will have for some time. Thus the reductans, the explaining generalizations in such an account, will be a *complex web* of interlevel causal generalizations of varying scope, and will typically be expressed in terms of an idealized system of the types discussed, complicated by all of the intertwined γ-, σ-, and δ-level features, along with some textual elaboration on the nature of the causal sequence leading through the system.

Reduction in the biomedical sciences, then, is a kind of *partial model reduction with largely implicit generalizations*, often of narrow scope, licensing temporal sequences of causal propagations of events through the model. It is not unilevel reduction, to, say, biochemistry, but it is characteristically what is termed a *molecular biological explanation*.[46] The model effecting the "reduction" is typically interlevel, mixing different levels of aggregation from cell to organ and back to molecule, and the reducing model may be further integrated into another model, as the later operon model is integrated into positive control circuitry (see chapter 3). The model or models also may not be robust across one or another organism; there may well be a narrow domain of application, in contrast to what we typically encounter in physical theories (we saw this in chapter 3 with respect to other modes of gene regulation).

In spite of all of these qualifications, however, there is no reason that the *logic* of the relation between the reductans and the reductandum cannot be *cast* in deductive form. Typically this is not done because it requires more formalization than it is worth, but some fairly complex engineering circuits, such as the full adder introduced in chapter 6 (figure 6.7 and textbox), can effectively be represented in the first-order predicate calculus and useful deductions made from the premises, which in the adder example numbered around thirty.

The picture of reduction that emerges from any detailed study of molecular biology as it is practiced is thus not an elegant one. There are, in the above characterization, indications that reduction may perhaps be better conceived of, as Wimsatt (1976b) has urged, more along causal/mechanical lines. I think there is some truth in this suggestion, but it only captures one dimension of the relationships that exist between reduced and reducing domains. The relation between the GRR approach and the causal/mechanical approach is the subject of the next section.

9.5.3 *The Relation between the Causal/Mechanical Account of Reduction and the GRR Model and Two Versions of the GRR Model — Simple and Complex*

In subsection 9.5.2 immediately above the discussion is strongly focused on the causal characterization of reduction. At several points, however, I addressed the relations of that account to Nagel's conditions of connectability and derivability, which continue to figure prominently in the GRR model introduced earlier in this chapter. In the present subsection, I want to consider those relations more systematically.

It appears to me that the GRR account, which might be termed, following Salmon, a more "epistemic" approach to reduction, may *best* capture the relations that exist in a "clarified" science where a unilevel reductans (and a unilevel reductandum at a different level of aggregation) has been fully developed. We might term this a *simple interpretation* of the GRR model; it allows us to construe the model as comprising a *set of conditions* that must be met if a *complete* reduction is to have been judged as accomplished. Under this interpretation, the GRR model falls into what might be termed the justificatory or evaluative sphere. The requirements of connectability and derivability are seen in this light to be both reasonable and benign: connectability *must* be established if two languages are to be related, and derivability is just the implementation of a well-understood, truth-preserving mode of inference — one that carries impeccable credentials.

This *simple interpretation* of the GRR model does not, however, without elaboration and interpretation of its tenets along the lines proposed in subsection 9.5.2, adequately capture the heavy reliance of scientific explanation on causal mechanisms of the type that Wimsatt and Hull (and in a sense Enç) have stressed. This is particularly true if the causal mechanisms are *interlevel,* in accord with the position advanced in chapters 3, 5, and 6. In terms of active scientific investigation and of the language in scientific research reports (and textbooks), a causal/mechanical analysis *seems* much more suitable. In point of fact it is just this approach that I favored in chapter 6 for explanation, though there I was also willing to incorporate aspects of unificatory or syntactic approaches to explanation.

Along similar lines, it is thus tempting to think of the causal reduction analysis presented above (in terms of interlevel causal generalizations that become progressively better characterized at complex δ-levels of aggregation and specificity) as perhaps *another sense* of reduction, analogous with Carnap's probability$_1$ and probability$_2$ and especially with Salmon's explanation$_1$ and explanation$_2$. On such a view, there would be a reduction$_{grr}$ and a reduction$_{cm}$, representing the epistemic "*general reduction-replacement model*" at one extreme and for the ontic "*causal mechanism*" at the other, perhaps with some overlapping (mixed) analyses likely between these two extreme types.

Though tempting, I think this view would be mistaken without keeping in mind four additional clarificatory comments. First, recall that an appeal to "mechanisms" also requires appeals to the "*laws* of working" that are implemented in the mechanisms and which provide part of the analysis and grounding of the "causal" aspect of the causal/mechanical approach. Second, if we appeal to *any* general notion of a theory (i.e., to a semantic or a syntactic analysis) it would seem that we would have to deal with "generalizations" and with connecting the generalizations' entities and predicates, as in the GRR model. For example, if we consider the semantic conception of a scientific theory as elaborated in chapters 3 and 5 as it is involved in reductions,[47] such "theories" are set-theoretic (or other language) predicates which are essentially constituted by component generalizations.[48] Thus if we were to think about attempting to characterize a "causal/mechanical" approach to reduction with the aid of a semantic construal of theories, we would *still* require recourse to traditional generalizations. Third, appeals to the semantic (or syntactic) notion of theories still require that entity (the η's) and predicate (the Φ's) terms be used (in addition to the *generalizations*—the Σ's) to characterize the theories which we consider. Thus some form of connectability assumptions relating terms such as "gene" and "DNA sequence" will be required to effect a reduction. Fourth and finally, in those cases in which we wish to verify the *reasoning* supporting some *causal consequence* of a reducing theory (whether it be a general result or a particular one), we can do no better than utilize the principles of *deductive* reasoning, other forms of logic and reasoning being significantly more suspect.[49]

It seems to me, however, that we can effect a "rapprochment" of sorts between the two CM and the GRR senses of reduction, or, if we cannot, we can at least identify the source of certain confusions that are prevalent in the reduction literature. To disentangle several potentially conflatable distinctions, let us consider parsing the approaches to reduction in a way that explicitly exhibits the spectrum of reductions from partial or interlevel to unilevel along one dimension and the CM-GRR distinction along another orthogonal dimension. (See table 9.2.) This analysis is based on the fact that reductions in science frequently have two aspects: (1) ongoing advances that occur in *piecemeal* ways, for instance, as some features of a model are further elaborated at the molecular level or perhaps a new "mechanism" is added to the model, and (2) assessments of the explanatory fit between two theories (viewed here as a collection of models) or even between two *branches* of science. Under aspect (1), as scientists further develop reducing theories in a domain, they frequently elaborate various parts of the theories, both by (a) modifying a δ-level assumption or proposing a δ-level assumption that accounts for (part of) a σ-level process and by (b) describing these new assumptions in *causal* terms. Thus the result of such advances are typically complex interlevel connections that appeal, in part, to causal processes. (Part-whole or constituent relationships may also be appealed to in such situations.) These various theoretical developments and attendant connections — bushy and weblike though they may be — frequently have the ability to "explain" at least partially some features of a higher level domain, for example a phenomenon such as sensitization in *Aplysia* or self-tolerance in vertebrate immunology.

This task of formulation is typically done by scientists, and reflects the *ontic* dimension.[50] This ongoing process will establish connections at several different levels, and prior to arriving at something like a unilevel theory in a clarified science many complex and reticulate connections can be expected. Describing this process (Box 1) is much easier to do in CM language, which is tolerant of gappy and patchy causal connections (see chapter 6); the GRR approach in such a situation highlights the gappiness and thus *seems* to fail or at least does not appear to be the most felicitous approach under such circumstances.

These reticulate relations, however, do not count *against* a reduction; they can be thought of as part of the process leading *toward* a "simplified" unilevel reduction. On the other hand, *if* a science has progressed (stultified?) to the point where it is reasonably well clarified and complete, and can be formulated in a unilevel ontology in terms of a relatively small number of generalizations of wide scope, the GRR approach is most natural. In addition, the GRR approach explicitly *tests* for the adequacy of a reduction in a straightforward and transparent manner (see next paragraph). The traditional question of reduction, then, is a question of the adequacy of the explanatory relationship viewed in a more *global* or gross sense, which appeals (usually) to preexisting disciplines or fields (or theories). Working out this type of relation is typically done by the philosopher or by a scientist interested in reviewing very broad questions of domain relation. Such a relation(s) is much more systematic than the ontic dimension referred to in the previous paragraph.

TABLE 9.2 CM AND GRR APPROACHES IN DIFFERENT STATES OF COMPLETIONS OF REDUCTIONS

State of Completion\ Approach	CM	GRR
Partial/patchy/ fragmentary/ interlevel	Box 1 – CM approach usually employed; interlevel causal language is more natural than GRR connections.	Box 2 – Complex GRR Model: the connections are bushy and complex when presented formally, but GRR does identify points of identity, as well as the generalizations operative in mechanisms.
Clarified science/ unilevel at both levels of aggregation	Box 3 – Either approach could be used here, but where theories are collections of prototypes, the bias toward axiomatization or explicit generalization built into the GRR approach will make it less simple than CM.	Box 4 – Simple GRR Model: best match between Nagelian reduction and scientific practice.

In connection with this global question, the various features of the GRR model can be appealed to as providing the *logical* conditions that must be satisfied, but usually satisfied in a post hoc evaluative manner. Thus one looks for (1) synthetic identities, which introduce basic ontological economies, and (2) derivability of the corrected reduced science (with the help of causal generalizations in the reducing science), which insures that security of relation that only truth-preserving, nonampliative inference can provide. A representation of intertheoretic relations using the GRR model thus is a kind of "executive summary" of much scientific work that has gone on to establish interdisciplinary connections; such analysis also typically falls into the justificatory arena of the philosophy of science. The GRR model is thus useful in providing us with a kind of systematic summary and regulatory ideal, but it should not in general be confused with the *process* of establishing reductions in the ongoing elaboration of the complex web of connections that typically unite reduced and reducing theories.

I believe that the failure to keep these aspects of reductions distinct has led to confusion about the adequacy of the GRR model, for example, by Wimsatt in his 1976b. Patchy CM reduction (Box 1 in table 9.2) is akin to what Mayr (1982) has termed explanatory reduction, a notion that has been further elaborated by Sarkar (1989, 1991). Box 4 represents the more traditional notion of intertheoretic reduction. Box 2 suggests that a more complex form of the GRR approach than we would find under the conditions in Box 4 will have value, particularly in such cases as described in the discussion above of the connectability issue in Benzer's analysis of the gene concept, and also in the response to Rosenberg's concerns about the relation between Mendelian and molecular mapping. Similar discussions on the issue of *derivability* have taken place, though primarily in the physical sciences.[51] Thus, though the GRR model can be conceived of as a summary and a regulatory ideal, it *can* also accommodate two interlevel theories that have patchy relations. This would not be the *simple interpretation* of the GRR model discussed in the earlier parts of this chapter, but there is no reason in principle why a theory which was *interlevel but primarily cellular* could not be explained by a theory which was *interlevel but primarily molecular*. Insofar as the explanation was adequate, this type of theory would be akin to a type of homogeneous but now interlevel reduction discussed by Nagel in his 1961.[52] Perhaps it might be termed a "complex homogeneous" reduction. The GRR model could accommodate this form of reduction, but its reduction functions would reflect the *mixed* interlevel character of the theories. Such a *complex interpretation* of the GRR model (Box 2) may be more realistic than the simple interpretation (Box 4) discussed earlier, where unilevel theories functioned as reductans and reductandum.

Certain general methodological principles are likely to govern the implementation of this complex GRR model. For example, using the terminology developed in chapter 5, it seems likely that:

(1) $T_2^{(*)}$'s central γ-level hypotheses will be preserved unless the relation falls on the replacement side of the reduction/replacement continuum.

(2) $T_2^{(*)}$'s σ-level hypotheses will either be replaced or amplified.

(3) $T_2^{(*)}$'s δ-level hypotheses will either be replaced or amplified.

A good example that shows just how this works in practice can be seen in connection with the development of the clonal selection theory developed in chapter 5. Current theories of antibody diversity generation and of T-lymphocyte stimulation (see Watson et al. 1987, chap. 23) suggest that these types of methodological developments are continuing to take place in those fields studying the molecular biology of the immune response.

Scientists presenting a reasonably complete reduction typically would use the approach represented by Box 3 in their writings, and those cases would be philosophically interpretable using the Box 4 approach. Something close to Box 3 can be found in optics or electromagnetic theory textbooks, but we are a long way from seeing a unilevel theory in most of biology and medicine.

The GRR model, particularly in its *simple* (Box 4) interpretation, is also an appropriate framework in terms of which deeper logical questions, such as predicate analysis, the nature and means of establishing synthetic identities, and the metaphysical implications of such identities, can be pursued, though it will also have some value under Box 2 conditions as well, where partial or incomplete identities can be framed and the scope of the explaining generalizations can be made explicit. In either Box 2 or 4 conditions, the GRR framework forces an actual ongoing reduction into a "rational reconstructive" mode.

Accordingly, I believe that the GRR model, in spite of its syntactic (epistemic?) flavor, and though it may prima facie appear to be intuitively less in accord with the strong causal flavor of the examples of middle-range theories (whether used in explanatory or reduction contexts) presented in this book, is a useful and defensible account of reduction. Though the causal/mechanical alternative is a valuable approach representing an important aspect of reductions, it is not the whole story by any means. As argued above, it seems to me that deeper analysis of what a causal/mechanical alternative involves leads us back to many of those assumptions which constitute the GRR model.

In two recent publications, Kitcher (1989) and Culp and Kitcher (1989) have elaborated further on the views presented in Kitcher's 1984a essay, where he proposed that we might better replace the notion of reduction with the idea of an "explanatory extension." An explanatory extension was characterized as follows: "a theory T' provides an *explanatory extension* of a theory T just in case there is some problem-solving pattern of T one of whose schematic premises can be generated as the conclusion of a problem-solving pattern of T'" (1984a, 365).[53] In his (1989) Kitcher again affirms this recommendation stating that "the outmoded concept of reduction, which is tied to an inadequate account of scientific theories, should be replaced with the notion of an explanatory extension, and disputes about the virtues of reductionism reformulated accordingly" (1989, 448). Similarly, Culp and Kitcher write "the intertheoretic relationships that philosophers have often tried to describe in terms of reduction are best reconceived in terms of the embedding of the problem-solving schemata of one field of science in those of another" (Culp and Kitcher 1989, 479). I think these suggestions are valuable and correct if they are meant to amplify the concept of reduction to accommodate both the CM approach and the complex interpretations of the GRR account described above, but insofar as they recommend a full replacement of anything like the GRR model, I believe this is shortsighted. I have indicated above what I take to be the strengths and limitations of the simple (and complex) forms of the GRR model, and these do not need to be repeated in any detail in reply to Kitcher's (and Culp's) suggestions. It should be noted, however, that the accounts recommended in the present chapter have resources that are not present in the Kitcherean alternative. First, Kitcher's account is causally limited; for him causation is only derivative from unificatory strong theories, and this, it seems to me, ignores a fundamental feature of biological and medical explanations, as developed in chapter 6 and employed in the discussion of reduction above. Second, Kitcher's analysis eschews the important searches for connectability that find a natural interpretation in both forms of the GRR model. I do think that the "embedding" metaphor captures, in only slightly different language, the features of extended interlevel theories that have been elaborated in this book, and thus view that aspect of Kitcher's suggestions as congruent with the proposals presented here. Kitcher does not as yet seem to be sensitive to the need to conceive of theories as families of overlapping prototypical models, however, but I do not see this perspective as necessarily inconsistent with his (and Culp's) approach. The GRR account in particular forces us to think carefully about the scope of the generalizations found in such overlapping models. Finally, both of us agree with the importance of deductive connections, though I construe this as more closely connected with causal processes than does Kitcher.

In summary then, I think that the account of reduction presented above is not at serious variance with Kitcher's positive proposals, provided it be kept in mind that there are more approaches to reduction (e.g., Boxes 2 and 4) in science than explanatory extension or embedding, which I interpret as falling essentially into Box 1 of table 9.2. This may be as far as we can take the discussion of models of reduction at the present time. Such a view of the GRR and the CM analyses as has been sketched provides some parallel to the views of the philosophy of science community on scientific explanation as characterized by Salmon (1989) and discussed in chapter 6, and it may well be that, as further progress is made on the issue of scientific explanation, additional advances can also be made on the topic of reduction. In the remaining sections of this chapter, I shall reexamine the issues of emergence and also touch on the notion of reduction as a research program, while drawing on a number of the features of the GRR model as it has been further developed in the context of rebuttals to its critics.

9.6 Arguments against In-Principle Emergentism

In section 2 of this chapter I reviewed some biologists' and philosophers' arguments in favor of various types of in-principle emergentism. Now that we have examined what I have taken to be the core sense of reduction as exemplified by the general re- duction-replacement model, as well as some criticisms directed against it, we are in a good position to reconsider the cogency of the emergentists' views. The most basic issues arise out of the prospects of satisfying the connectability condition and the derivability condition. These must be met even if some (or even all) biological theories are to be "replaced," since the experimen- tal/observational realm of biology must be explained by the re- ducing theory (or theories) drawn from the physicochemical sciences.

In connection with this point it would be wise to stress, as Nagel has done previously, that it is not that properties are de- rived from properties, but rather that derivations are formulated in the context of suitable observational reports, generalizations, and theories. Thus the concern of someone like Grobstein's (see his 1965 and 1969) about the pragmatically emergent property of the tertiary structure of enzymes needs to be expressed in terms of a *theory* of enzyme kinetics and molecular folding, including a description of the molecular structure and physicochemical forces (say, covalent sulfhydryl bonds and various forms of weak forces such as van der Waals and hydrogen bond interactions). Research on this specific front is proceeding under those as- sumptions and from this physicochemical approach,[54] and to date no mysterious features have been discovered which would indicate that biological entities such as enzymatic-active sites could *not* be identified with *complex structures of chemical entities*. A similar thesis holds for Weiss's arguments concerning higher- level structures and controls, as was indicated in the previous chapter, but there are some logical distinctions that need to be made in connection with such arguments to which I will return in a moment.

9.6.1 *Polanyi Reconsidered*

In the last paragraph I emphasized the phrase "complex struc- tures of chemical entities," since the theories of the irreducibility of structure (and system) is another recurrent theme of the emer- gentist position. As noted in some of the quotations earlier in this chapter, organization above the simple molecular level is a major feature of living organisms. Weiss and especially Polanyi in this chapter discerned in this organization and hierarchical arrange-

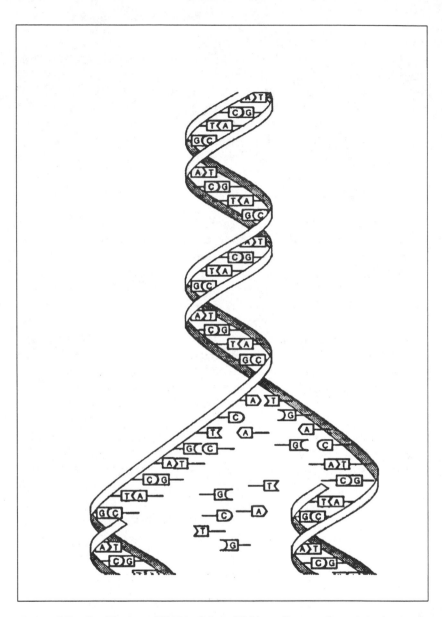

Figure 9.7 Replication of DNA. When DNA replicates, the original strands unwind and serve as templates for the building of new, complementary strands. The daughter molecules are exact copies of the parent, each daughter having one of the parent strands. Source: Legend and figure from Office of Technology Assessment, 1988. Readers shoul be aware of the fact that this graphic represents a very simplified version of the multienzymatic replication process for DNA.

ment a significant source of the irreducibility of biology to physics and chemistry. From the perspective of the general reduction-replacement model, an account of these complex structures must be provided on the basis of the fundamental entities of physics and chemistry. As Polanyi notes, however, in connection with the sequences of bases in the DNA molecule, the sequence is "extraneous to the chemical forces at work in the DNA molecule." (1968, 1309) This is correct, however, only if Polanyi means the specific nucleotide sequence in the DNA daughter strand *taken independently of the sequence information in the parent strand.* In point of fact, the sequence of the daughter strand is a consequence of that DNA strand's parent sequence, the synthesis governed by complementary Watson-Crick pairing of thymine (T) with adenine (A) and cytosine (C) with guanine (G) in semiconservative replication. (See figure 9.7 for an illustration as to how this occurs in very oversimplified outline form).[55]

This reply to Polanyi, however, simply moves the problem one step back—to the organization inherent in the *parent molecule.* The reply also does not yet adequately address Weiss's arguments cited earlier, since DNA replication does not occur in isolation; in point of fact replication takes place in the cell with a number of specific and complex enzymes, presynthesized molecules T, A, G, and C, and cellular energy sources being only a few of the necessary coconditions for DNA replication. Accordingly, in order to account for DNA structure in physical and simple chemical terms one will have to explain the *origin* of the cell in chemical terms as well as the DNA sequence order.

9.6.2 *Structural versus Ultimate Reductionism*

At this point it will be useful to distinguish two types of reduction in addition to those characterized thus far. Even if it is not possible to account for the origin of the structure from simple chemical molecules, say in terms of self-assembly,[56] a weaker form of reductionism may hold. In this weaker form the chemical structure would be taken as a given element in the initial conditions of an explanans. These initial conditions would be contained in the connectability assumptions or reduction functions of the generalized reduction-replacement model. If this chemical structural information (in conjunction with available theories in physics and chemistry, such as the principles of hydrogen bonding, ionic binding forces, principles of chemical diffusion, energy thermodynamics, and enzyme kinetics) is sufficient to entail deductively all sentences describing biological laws and processes, then this weaker form of reductionism, which we can call *structural reductionism*, will succeed. (How this form of reduction might conceivably *fail* will be discussed below in connection with Elsasser's views.)

There is, however, another, stronger form of reductionism which we can call *ultimate reductionism* in contrast with the weaker structural reductionism. (This distinction parallels comments on the distinction between *proximate* [physiological] causes and *ultimate* [evolutionary] causes [Mayr 1982, 67].) This strong form of reductionism requires a *historical* account expressed in purely physicochemical terms and theories which would explain the *origins* of those structures assumed in the weaker form of reductionism. It is here that one would have to appeal to a theory of chemical evolution (Schaffner 1969b). This approach was briefly introduced in my discussion of Oparin's emergentist argument, and his objections to conceiving of chemical evolution as support for ultimate reductionism must be addressed.

Oparin's argument concerned the fact that only a very few chemical processes and chemical structures out of many chemically possible ones have been implemented in living systems. These were the result of natural selection and constituted specific biological adaptations. Oparin, however, does not give any arguments why purely chemical replication processes with differential rates of reproduction and different efficiencies of replicating in varying environments cannot account for the selection of these few processes and entities. In point of fact, Oparin's pioneering research and all subsequent inquiries into the origins of life proceed from this ultimate reductionistic premise. It would take us beyond the scope of this book to rehearse this research, but a perusal of texts such as Orgel's *The Origins of Life*, the discussion of the origin of life in Watson et al. (1987, chapter 28), or Morowitz's recent monograph (1992), will confirm this. Accordingly, it is the opinion of this author that Oparin implicitly presents the solution to the ultimate reductionist's problem of how to account for structure. This type of solution is a somewhat Pyrrhic victory, however, since it is very highly unlikely that even in special laboratories scientists will be able to replicate exactly the sequence of processes which occurred billions of years ago. In addition, even if such a sequence was by chance replicated, it does not seem

possible, short of developing time-travel, that we could ever verify that it was that type of sequence which occurred on this
earth — chemical evolution does not leave a (simple) fossil trail.[57]

To all intents and purposes, then, we are left with the
weaker form of structural reductionism. I believe that this is a
defensible reductionist position and that it vitiates in principle
emergentist theses. The position is, however, potentially still vul-
nerable from one direction which could rescue a Polanyi-type of
emergentism. I also believe that such a structural reductionism is
not terribly interesting if it is interpreted as a research program
and that my defense of it could easily be misconstrued methodologically. Let me first address the question of a rescued Polanyi emergentism and then, in the subsequent section, turn to
the relation between structural reductionism and research programs in contemporary biology.

There are at least two further ways in which a thesis of structural reductionism could be legitimately criticized: if it could be
shown either that the structures were in principle unknowable
(failure of the connectability condition) or, if knowable, that the
explananda of biological laws and processes could not be derived (failure of the derivability condition).

9.6.3 *Bohr, Elsasser, and Generalized Quantum Complementarity*

Both of these tacks have been taken by several distinguished
physicists and developed more recently by two medical scholars.
Niels Bohr, the founder of the Copenhagen interpretation of
quantum mechanics, suggested in 1933 in his essay "Light and
Life" that the principle of complementarity, so important in
quantum physics, might have an important generalization in biology. Bohr introduced his notion of generalized complementarity in the following manner:

> It must be kept in mind, however, that the conditions
> holding for biological and physical researches are not
> directly comparable, since the necessity of keeping the
> object of investigation alive imposes a restriction on the
> former, which finds no counterpart in the latter. Thus, we
> should doubtless kill an animal if we tried to carry the
> investigation of its organs so far that we could describe the
> role played by single atoms in vital functions. In every
> experiment on living organisms, there must remain an

uncertainty as regards the physical conditions to which they are subjected, and the idea suggests itself that the minimal freedom we must allow the organism in this respect is just large enough to permit it, so to say, to hide its ultimate secrets from us. On this view, the very existence of life must be considered as an elementary fact just as in atomic physics the existence of the quantum of action has to be taken as a basic fact that cannot be derived from ordinary mechanical physics. Indeed, the essential non-analyzability of atomic stability in mechanical terms presents a close analogy to the impossibility of a physical or chemical explanation of the peculiar functions characteristic of life. (1987 [1933], 9)

As we have seen, however, the techniques of contemporary molecular biology have been able to outflank this problem and the connectability condition has been satisfied in a number of areas. Specific, detailed structures at the chemical level have been determined. DNA replication is (typically) extraordinarily conservative (mutation rates normally are on the order of 1 nucleotide in 10,000,000) and one can, using such organisms as *E. coli*, assume identity of structure in a large (if narrow) class of organisms. The discovery of (nearly) universal biochemical processes (see chapter 3) at certain levels is further evidence against Bohr's early speculations.

Arguments against the *derivability* of biological laws and processes have generally focused on quantum physics. These arguments, principally due to the work of W. M. Elsasser (1958, 1966), but interestingly developed and exemplified in biological organisms by J. P. Isaacs and J. C. Lamb (1969), have two rather different aims. First, arguments are elaborated to show that quantum mechanics cannot be used to predict the trajectories of all physical particles which constitute organisms. Second, a type of emergence is defended in which there is some nomic regularity, but these regularities are *only permitted, not entailed* by quantum mechanics. Their possible source is never indicated. (From one point of view these arguments are irrelevant to the issue of reductionism, since they are directed against the reducibility of biology by quantum physics and not the reduction of biology by the chemistry of large and complex molecules. In most discussions of the autonomy of biology, the issue is the reducibility of biology to a combination of physics and chemistry, not to physics per se. Curiously, the antireductionistic proponents do not seem to be very interested in the in-principle emergence of chemistry.)

The replies that can be made to proponents of such quantum mechanics–based emergentism, however, arise not only from the fact that they may have missed the main point at issue. Some other objections to these emergentist theses are, in my view, much more serious, for it appears that (1) at least one chemical premise of the argument is false, (2) the specificity and detail of what one wants to derive is misconstrued, (3) quantum mechanics not only is in point of fact applicable to such molecules as DNA and its replication process but has been applied to them with reasonable results, and (4) not one instance of an emergent law licensed by such arguments has yet been offered. It would take us too far afield to examine the arguments of Elsasser (or of Isaacs and Lamb) in detail, and the reader must be referred elsewhere (see Kauffman 1974). It should be pointed out, however, in support of the first three points made, that the biological individuality of test organisms is not so extensive that what Elsasser terms his "principle of finite classes" can function as a defensible premise in his arguments.

Elsasser introduces the principle of finite classes by suggesting that, in contrast with atomic physics, where we can obtain atoms and molecules in the same composition and set of quantum states as often as needed to conduct experiments, "we may quite simply run out of specimens of an organism during the process of selection before we reach a point of adequate homogenization" (1966, 36). (Elsasser's arguments were put forth before the advent of cloning technology.) From an assumed irreducible homogeneity and a rather vague speculation that multiple feedback loops in metabolism will cascade errors, delocalizing them, Elsasser conjectures that extraordinary imprecise predictions would result.

But it is unclear that the biochemists and molecular biologists, for the same reasons that were utilized in objecting to Bohr, cannot obtain homogeneous classes. These classes are in point of fact sufficient, not to compute future quantum mechanical states of the organism, but rather to trace biosynthetic pathways with well-defined inputs and outputs, to systematize these as generalizations (e.g., in a theory of protein synthesis and the genetic code), and to predict within the limits of available current theory what modifications in DNA sequence will produce a new genetic product.[58]

Though quantum mechanics is not very useful as yet in its applications to large molecules, there have been some attempts to apply it to this domain.[59] The practical difficulties of solving the Schroedinger equation in complex systems are extraordinary and for specific, complex time-dependent systems may be insuperable. However, for some time-independent systems, good results that are in agreement with experiments can be obtained.[60] I conclude, then, that quantum mechanics will not serve as an appropriate basis for the type of indeterminism or generalized complementarity which might vitiate the structural form of reductionism and support an in principle emergentism.

9.7 The Peripherality of Reductionism as a Research Program and the Need for Research Methodologies of the Middle Range

The essence of the general reduction-replacement model outlined above as applied to the relation between biology and physicochemistry is to explicate all biological entities and relations in terms of physicochemical entities and relations. This would represent the type of structural reductionism discussed in the preceding section. A reductionist *research program* that takes its orientation from such a model will aim at discovering the exact molecular sequences and arrangements of biological entities and will attempt to explain biological processes in terms of physical and chemical sequences of events. As examples of what the methodology practiced will involve, I might mention amino acid and nucleotide sequencing of biological molecules, X-ray crystallographic analysis of the three-dimensional structure of relevant proteins and other chemical species, and the working out of the chemical diffusion processes and quantum mechanical bindings of biological molecules in the appropriate, chemically characterized environment.

The thrust of a strictly reductionist research program is toward obtaining the complete chemical characterization of the chemical side of the reduction functions and toward strengthening the physical and chemical theories that appear as the reducing theories so that the biological processes can be completely accounted for by those theories. From such a perspective, a gene is satisfactorily characterized if and only if it is replaceable by a particular DNA (or RNA) sequence, and a biological generalization or theory is adequately understood only when all the entities appearing in the generalization or theory are completely specifiable in chemical terms and the generalization is derivable from theories of known physical and chemical interactions, such as chemical binding theories, diffusion theory, chemical equations, and chemical thermodynamics.

9.7.1 *The Peripherality of Reductionism Thesis*

There are very few interesting aspects of biology in which the chemical analysis has proceeded far enough so that *complete* reduction functions are specifiable for *all* the relevant entities in a problem area.[61] Furthermore, an examination of major advances in molecular biology and molecular genetics indicates that such detail is not of primary interest to molecular biologists, and that rarely will they orient their research in such a way as to attempt to provide such extensive detail.[62] The apparent exceptions are interesting ones, since I believe they take place in a research context which supports the general point. This view is what I have previously termed the thesis of the "peripherality of reductionism" in molecular biology (see my 1974b).

To put the peripherality thesis in another more positive way, I believe that most molecular biologists who are at the frontiers of "molecular" research plan their research in such a way as to attempt to uncover interesting biochemical generalizations, but that such generalizations are not physicochemically complete in the sense that they do not as yet fulfill the conditions of the reduction model presented in this paper, and that many of these molecular biologists are interested in providing physicochemical details only in order to choose among competing, physicochemically incomplete alternative theories. This thesis will make more sense and carry added credibility when illustrated by some examples from molecular biology.[63] I will first briefly consider some of the implications which the Watson-Crick model of DNA had for molecular biology, after which I shall *re*consider the extraordinary, conceptually rich discovery of the Jacob-Monod operon theory of genetic regulation.

9.7.2 *Watson-Crick Replication and the Peripherality Thesis*

It is clear that the Watson-Crick model of DNA, with its two intertwining right-handed helices displaying sugar phosphate backbones and a central, irregularly varying sequence of purine and pyrimidine bases, represents a major accomplishment and a significant advance in the reduction of biology to physics and chemistry. The helices are held together by weak hydrogen bonds, which are explicable by quantum mechanics, and the purines and pyrimidines—the nucleotide bases—are fully and completely characterizable in terms of physics and chemistry. How then, it might be asked, do the implications of the Watson-Crick structure support a thesis of the peripherality of reductionism in the development of molecular genetics?

The Watson-Crick model, I submit, had the major impact it did on the development of molecular genetics because (1) it was easy to see, to quote Watson and Crick, "that (the model) immediately suggests a mechanism for its self-duplication" and (2) it was not difficult to envision how the sequence of nucleotide bases could be "the code which carries the genetical information" (1953, 737 and 934). Now, it must be stressed that the mechanism by which self-duplication or replication (as well as transcription) occurs is still not *completely* explicable in physico-chemical terms. Various models have been proposed over a long period of time, but the source of the uncoiling energy, the exact mechanism of complementary pairing and the enzyme(s) involved remain unclear. (For example, the Kornberg polymerase, which had earlier seemed responsible for replication, was subsequently discovered to be a DNA repair enzyme.) Watson et al., in their recent (1987) account of DNA duplication, write in confirmation of the long process of understanding DNA replication:

> The replication of even the simplest DNA molecule is a complicated multi-step process, involving many more enzymes than was initially anticipated following the discovery of the first DNA polymerizing enzyme. Fortunately it *now seems likely* that all the key enzymatic steps involved in the replication of . . . DNA have been described and that the general picture of DNA replication presented here will not be seriously modified. (1987, 282; my emphasis)

The account of self-duplication was, accordingly, physicochemically incomplete, and is still so if all the specific details are wanted. Nevertheless, the Watson-Crick model has had a most important influence in suggesting experiments and clarifying the revisions of genetics, necessitated by the fine structure analyses of the gene. The Watson-Crick model is also a fundamental background assumption of an elaborate theory of protein synthesis that constitutes one of the most powerful theories of molecular biology. One point I would like to make on the basis of this example is that *physicochemically incomplete* theories that significantly *aid* in the reduction of classical biology, in this case classical genetics, can still play a most important role in conditioning the development of molecular biology. A second and related point is that, though highly specific problems associated with the uncoiling, replication, and transcription of the double helix are legitimate research topics, most molecular biologists found that this type of problem could be left until later while the more interesting issues of protein synthesis, genetic control, and the working out of the genetic code were explored. A physicochemically complete identification and explanation is not to be taken as a sine qua non for developing theories utilizing the "molecular" discovery.

In this very brief discussion of the Watson-Crick model I have not treated the rationale behind specific research strategy. The Watson-Crick example is intended primarily to make the peripherality thesis plausible by showing that important and interesting generalizations, which are quintessentially "molecular," are nonetheless physicochemically incomplete. I would now like to relate another example, which I believe offers a more specific argument for the irrelevance of reduction at certain crucial stages in the development of a molecular biological theory.

9.7.3 The Operon Theory Revisited – Again

Early in this chapter I reviewed the historical background of the development of the Jacob-Monod operon theory, which was discussed in its current form in some detail in chapters 3 and 4. Recall the key experiment leading to the operon theory was the "Pajama" experiment. In 1960, several similar experiments with additional constitutive and inducible mutants clarified the nature of the genetic interactions.

In their 1961 paper, Jacob and Monod proposed that repressor-making genes be termed "regulator genes" to distinguish them from the more ordinary "structural genes." In that paper they also proposed that a specific target or site of action of the repressor had to exist, and they considered as alternative possibilities whether the target was associated with each gene controlled by the regulator gene or whether there was one target, the present-day operator, which controlled several genes adjacent to it. The alternative hypotheses predicated the existence of different types of mutants that could be selected for in the laboratory and examined for their capacities to synthesize the various enzymes associated with the structural genes. Data were gathered in 1960 and the operator (or operon) hypothesis came to be corroborated over the alternatives. In their research, Jacob's knowledge of the phage λ system and lysogeny offered many insights because of its fundamental analogies with the *lac* system.

Let us step back from this rapid overview of the development of the operon theory and note some features relevant to our concerns. First recall that the chemical nature of the repressor was not known at this time. In 1961, in fact, it was thought possibly to be a species of RNA. Second, it should be noted that the interactions of the constituent parts of the theory are not described in terms of DNA, RNA polymerase, and the like, but rather in terms of a modified classical genetics. Jacob and Monod did not, in their research program, aim initially at providing chemical characterizations of the entities with which they worked, even though methods for at least beginning such characterizations were available. Such chemical analyses were extremely tedious and probably would not have provided any information about the interactions of the genes and their expression for a very long period of time.[64] Accordingly, we can conclude that we have before us a paradigmatic example of theory construction in an area that is usually termed molecular biology or molecular genetics but that found many of the methods that would yield physicochemical characterizations of its elements irrelevant to its development. The short-term aim of Jacob and Monod was not to reduce genetics to physics and chemistry; it was to determine the principle governing the causal interactions of the entities responsible for enzyme induction and repression and for phage synthesis and latency. These principles and causally relevant entities are both "biological" and "chemical"; Jacob and Monod did not work at the strictly chemical level but at levels "intertwining" the biological and chemical. This research methodology is a kind of parallel to the thesis developed in chapter 3, that biology and medicine are importantly populated by theories of the "middle range"; it represents a "methodology of the middle range." The distinctions of the γ-, σ-, δ-levels introduced in chapter 5 and again applied to reduction in this chapter also serve to highlight another dimension of such theories and their methodology.

It can be added, nonetheless, that the operon theory has brought us closer to the day when the genetic interactions will be completely understood in terms of the chemistry of the theory's constituent parts. As discussed earlier, in 1966 and 1967 Gilbert and Müller-Hill and Ptashne isolated repressors and chemically characterized these as proteins. Since then, studies have continued on the chemical nature of the repressor: it has been sequenced and its tertiary and quaternary structures are now well understood.[65] Further studies on the binding constants and manner of binding have also been made (see Miller and Reznikoff 1978). It is clear that determining more about the repressor and its mode of action helps fulfill the aim of the reduction model sketched earlier. This, however, does not mean that, at all stages of its development, molecular biology functioned with such an intention. If one conceives of molecular biology in this way, one's perception of its history and research methodology is likely to be rather distorted.

9.8   Suggestion for a Bayesian Explication of the Peripherality Thesis

One possible way of explicating and at the same time providing a degree of rigor for this peripherality thesis is to use a form of Bayesian decision theory. As noted in chapter 5, this theory is not a descriptive theory about how people reason and behave, and this qualification would naturally include molecular biologists. Rather, the theory is a normative or prescriptive account of behavior that is based on subjective probability and ordered preferences, or "utilities" of anticipated outcomes. It is thus a kind of "rational reconstruction" of behavior. Bayesian theory might find useful application in the context of explication of the peripherality thesis in the following ways.

(1) Bayesian theory involves specifying rewards and penalties or costs of taking particular actions; in our case, this could be the propounding of different types of molecular genetic theories. The rewards and penalties are different depending on which state of nature is actually realized, that is, which propounded theory is "true." The alternative theories must be assigned initial or prior probabilities, and these could be dependent on various

background theories and experiments as well as certain methodological and pragmatic criteria (see chapter 5).

(2) Bayesian theory also allows one to represent explicitly the costs of alternative samplings or of obtaining additional information about the situation one is investigating. Such samplings are equivalent to experiments, and it is possible in various interesting cases to determine if such costs are worth the added information in terms of increases in expected utilities. This would be reflected in our examples as the consideration of alternative types of experiments with different specified costs or penalties imputed to the experiments. The value of doing the experiments can be evaluated prior to performing them if all possibilities of outcomes can be envisaged and if the different outcomes can be so connected with the alternative theories being considered that the experimental outcomes alter the prior probabilities in a calculable manner.

(3) Bayes's theorem, discussed in chapter 5, permits an explicit calculation of the redistribution or alteration of the probability of alternative theories, if the prior probabilities of the theories are known and if one can make reasonable estimates of the likelihood of obtaining the specific alternative outcomes of those experiments given the "truth" of the alternative theories. (In the Pajama experiments considered earlier, an instance of such an estimate would involve an educated guess at the probability of discovering the possible experiment outcome that i^- was dominant over i^+, first on the basis of an early instructive internal-inducer model and, second, on the assumption of the truth of the repressor model.)

(4) Bayesian theory also allows the possibility of using what is termed a "normal form of analysis," which (a) "puts less stringent demands on the numerical codification of . . . [an investigator's] judgment," and (b) often allows and provides a rationale for the isolation of a limited class of potentially good strategies of experimentation and action and for the choice of a best strategy from among them.[66]

The cost of performing the extensive sequencing of x-ray crystallographic analysis, for example, which would be required to obtain completely specified reduction functions, could be estimated to be quite high. Further, the information that such studies would produce would probably not be much in excess of the information provided by more "biological" experiments, such as those involving bacterial conjugation, as regards the choice between the various models of genetic regulation discussed above. These various parameters seem to be specifiable in Bayesian terms, and it is thus suggested that the Bayesian approach might provide a rigorous explication and rationale for the peripherality thesis.

These Bayesian suggestions are somewhat speculative but are congruent with the Bayesian orientation of chapter 5. I also think that some of Wimsatt's (1980) views concerning reductionistic and nonreductionistic research strategies find a natural interpretation in terms of the Bayesian framework.

It is important to understand that, in proposing a peripherality thesis concerning reductionistic research programs, I am talking about (1) a rather precise model of reduction, and (2) short-term methodologies. These points can be misunderstood, as they have been by Fuerst in his generally illuminating 1980. Fuerst takes a number of rather general comments by prominent molecular biologists concerning long-term methodologies as evidence against my thesis. However, he has not looked at what those biologists do in their work and in their research papers, the substance of which would support my thesis. Second, he and, unfortunately, a number of biologists as well, often confuse the *applicability of physicochemical methods to biological entities* with a *reduction of those entities*. Most of the comments concerning methodology cited by Fuerst do not make such a distinction.

9.9 Conclusion

In this chapter I have examined several senses of reduction and sketched a general model for reduction (or, better, reduction-replacement). I have also considered a number of objections to that model and attempted to provide answers which I think are both reasonable and anchored in the actual accomplishments of the biomedical sciences. It remains to draw together a number of strands from this and previous chapters, especially those on historicity and teleology, since they may seem most at variance with the theses developed in this chapter.

The viewpoint, which I believe serves as a constant, unifying theme, is one of logical pragmatism. Such a viewpoint takes both the practices and the results of the sciences seriously, as not to be analyzed away with neat logical distinctions but rather to be explicated in all their complexity and richness with the aid of both historical and philosophical tools. Major tools of this perspective are elementary logical analysis and simple formalization, as well as the probability calculus with a Bayesian interpretation.

The use of heuristic techniques (such as generational constraints, gappy generalizations, and teleological and functional language), the importance of taking organization quite seriously, and the crucial utility of theorizing proceeding on many different and interacting levels are seen as facets of this logical pragmatism. The prima facie tension that I have defended between (1) the utility of providing a clear and, I think, persuasive quasi-formal model and (2) a thesis of the peripherality of reductionism, together with a defense of the aforementioned value of interlevel, overlapping, polytypic theoretical models, is an attempt to make sense of significant scientific achievements without forcing them into a preconceived philosophical version of the procrustean bed.

CHAPTER TEN

Conclusion and Research Issues for the Future

10.1 Introduction

THIS BOOK HAS BEEN an examination of philosophical issues in the areas of biology and medicine and their intersection—sometimes referred to as the "biomedical sciences." In contrast to traditional and also recent work in the philosophy of biology, in the work I have attempted to draw on examples and sciences that have hitherto not been looked at closely, stressing immunology in particular, but also examining relevant work in bacterial and human genetics, the neurosciences, and internal medicine. One of my themes was that much recent work in the philosophy of science in such areas as scientific discovery, theory structure, scientific progress, and the logics of confirmation and explanation illuminates the nature of biological and medical science, and that many of the tools of the more empirically minded philosophers of science could be applied together with insights drawn from more "historical" schools of philosophy of science.

10.2 Discovery, Evaluation, and the Experimental Testing of Hypotheses and Theories

I began this book with a partially historical analysis of philosophers' work on scientific discovery and argued that the logic of scientific discovery needed to be parsed in ways that were somewhat different from the pioneering work of Hanson. My thesis there was that, as has been recognized in recent work in psychology and artificial intelligence, we needed a logic of generation, and in addition, a logic of preliminary evaluation, both of which fall into what the traditional analysis saw as the context of discovery. I maintained that rational accounts of what occurs in the sciences in such discovery contexts could be developed, and I provided several examples from immunology, in particular looking at Jerne's selective theory and Burnet's clonal selection theory as detailed cases in point. The latter example was revisited in chapter 5, where more specific details of a logic of preliminary evaluation were developed and applied to Burnet's further elaboration of the clonal selection theory. In spite of the advances in this area of the logic of scientific discovery, however, I believe that philosophical analyses, and their sister subjects' approaches to this topic, are still in the preliminary stages of being able to provide us with a detailed and robust account of scientific innovation and creativity. In recent years philosophers have become reinterested in the topic and the recent work of Thagard (1989), Darden (1991), and Bechtel and Richardson (1992) illustrates the ways in which philosophical research in this area is being influenced by approaches borrowed from the cognitive sciences. A recent international symposium on the subject of "Creativity and Discovery in the Biomedical Sciences" (Holmes et al. 1991), which involved seven Nobel Laureates and philosophers of science, among others, confirms this reawakened interest.

One of the theses developed in chapter 2 was that, even in the preliminary stages of gestation of a new hypothesis or theory, the new idea is "evaluated." In this volume such evaluation was presented as having a number of aspects. Traditionally, a new hypothesis or theory was thought to be judged primarily in terms of how it measured up to laboratory tests. Chapter 4 of this book ("The Logic and Methodology of Empirical Testing in Biology and Medicine") discussed how hypotheses and theories make contact with the empirical world. This discussion reanalyzed the logical empiricists' concept of a "correspondence rule" and indicated with the help of an important experiment in immunology how empirical control over theories is provided. There I also developed a position I termed "generalized empiricism," which I view as much more flexible than "logical empiricism" and which tolerates (indeed requires) metaphysics at certain points (see also chapter 6 and my account of causation on this issue). My approach was then embedded in a discussion of Mill's methods and Claude Bernard's criticism of them. The importance of Mill's "method of difference," and how it relates to Bernard's "method of comparative experimentation" and to the little-analyzed "deductive method" of Mill, were pursued and then illustrated using a key set of experiments from recent molecular biology: the isolation and characterization of the "re-pressor" of the *lac* operon. This analysis also permitted me to dis-cuss the issue of "direct evidence," considered with respect to physics by Shapere (1982) and Galison (1987). I view the ap-proach developed here as resonating with similar recent work on the importance of experiments in science, conducted mainly in the philosophy and recent history of physics, by such authors as Hacking (1982), Galison (1987), and Franklin (1986, 1989).

Though chapter 4 represented a beginning discussion of the ways that experimental or empirical findings related to theory, a fuller account required both an analysis of more general "evalu-ation" in science and attention to the structure of scientific theo-ries in both their synchronic and their diachronic, or historical, dimensions.

10.3 Evaluation and Theory Structure

The second of these questions, the nature of scientific theories in biology and medicine and how best to represent them, was dis-cussed in chapter 3 ("Theories and Laws in Biology and Medi-cine"), and I returned to it again in chapter 5 ("Local and Global Evaluation: A Bayesian Approach"); it also formed an important part of the discussion in chapter 9 (on "Reduction").

Chapter 3 proposed that many of the theories we encounter in the biomedical sciences have a structure different from the standard type that we find in physics. More specifically, I argued that in the medically related biological sciences such as molecu-lar genetics, immunology, physiology, embryology, and the neurosciences, we find "theories of the middle range," midway in a sense between the universal mechanisms of biochemistry and the universal generalizations of neo-Darwinian evolution and typically also involving what might be termed "middle-sized" levels of aggregation—organelles, cells, and cell net-works. I reexamined the problem of "generalizations" in biology and medicine, looking at Smart's rather negative response to the question as to whether there are any "laws" in biology and car-rying the issue forward touching on contributions to this discus-sion by Ruse (1973), Wimsatt (1976b), Beatty (1981), Kitcher (1984), Rosenberg (1985), the U.S. National Academy of Sciences (Morowitz 1985), Lloyd (1988), van der Steen and Kamminga (1991), and again by Beatty (1992). I presented an account of sev-eral senses of "universal" within the framework of theories of the middle range and argued that this analysis provided a solution to at least important parts of this debate. I also suggested that the semantic approach to scientific theories, which has attracted considerable interest on the part of problems raised by philosophers of biology in the 1980s, is a natural context in which to give added structure to these theories of the middle range and generalized the set-theoretic characterization from previous accounts (such as Lloyd's 1988 and Thompson's 1989). In addition, I responded to some criticisms posed by Suppe in his recent (1989) book. Finally, I addressed a set of suggestions recently made by Beatty (1992) and suggested that their important views can be better expressed in terms of the account developed in chapter 3.

In chapter 5 I argued that the concept of a "theory of the middle range" had to be still further generalized to take into account its changes throughout time in order to represent the manner in which theories are actually evaluated. This generalized notion of a theory I called a "temporally extended theory." I discussed this notion, described some of its features, and tried to show how it raises and provides at least the beginnings of answers to interesting questions about the largely ignored subject of theory individuation. Along the way, I also criticized the relativistic theses of Kuhn and Feyerabend, as well as the "constructivist program" of Latour and Woolgar (1979) and Knorr-Cetina (1981, 1983) for misunderstanding and mislocating the nature of experimental control of models and theories in biology, though I did not deny the important role that "social knowledge" plays in scientific experiments.

My extension of theory structure took place within a lengthy argument for the appropriateness of a Bayesian "framework" within which we can locate many of the notions involved in theory comparison and evaluation in a natural way. Because of its importance, I briefly characterized the "received" classical or frequentist view of statistical hypothesis testing, so widespread in both the basic biological and the clinical sciences, and then went on to develop and defend a Bayesian position. I suggested that this Bayesian position can accommodate (in a translated and reconceptualized way) traditional statistical testing, and it can also be used as a general framework within which to develop a more "global" notion of intertheoretic comparison and evaluation. In this chapter I also indicated how other important evaluational concepts, such as simplicity, the freedom from ad hoc hypotheses, and the effect of the theoretical context, can be brought together within this Bayesian framework. I applied these ideas to a quite detailed historical example drawn from immunology: the competition between the instructive theory and the clonal selection theory of the immune response in the years 1957–67. At various places in this chapter I sketched what I believe are the strengths and weaknesses of the Bayesian approach in contrast with other approaches that might be taken to theory evaluation, including Glymour's (1980) bootstrapping approach. The position that I developed in chapter 5 might be termed a type of critical Bayesianism. Like Savage, I believe that whatever form the foundations of statistics may ultimately take, it is reasonably certain it will be different from contemporary views. I noted that Savage himself wrote toward the end of his career that: "Whatever we may look for in a theory of statistics, it seems prudent to take the position that the quest is for a better one, not for the perfect one" (1977, 7). It is a recurring thesis of this book that the Bayesian approach is currently the best and most general foundation from which to search for such a theory. Readers might find it of interest that when I attempted to rewrite the lengthy historical example developed in this chapter for a special issue of the journal *Theoretical Medicine* (see Schaffner 1992) free of the Bayesian gloss that I give to it in this book, much of the story about theory competition was not tellable. Thus in this 1992 essay I was forced to reintroduce parts of the Bayesian framework that is developed much more extensively in this book. Some will view this reliance on Bayesianism as a failure of my imagination; I see that failed attempt as underscoring the power and naturalness of the Bayesian framework.

10.4 Explanation and Reduction in Biology and Medicine

In chapter 6 ("Explanation in Biology and Medicine"), I began to develop what became a lengthy account of scientific explanation with applications to the neurosciences, molecular genetics, Mendelian genetics, and population genetics. This chapter is a watershed chapter: it uses the earlier material on theory structure and the generalization of the semantic approach to scientific theories as well as the Bayesian framework and develops a six-component model of explanation. The central notion involves an appeal to (possibly probabilistic) causal model systems that instantiate interlevel generalizations of varying scope: some are narrow generalizations and some have broad domains of applicability. I related the assumptions in this model to traditional writings on scientific explanation by philosophers of science. My preferred analysis of causation developed some of Mackie's (1974) insights within a broader framework, drawing on work by Collingwood and Hart and Honoré. The account involves an important "metaphysical" component to causation, but it also relies on the natural history of that concept in human thought as well as on ways in which individual humans come to learn and apply notions of causation.

I view the emphasis on causation in explanation developed in this chapter as both fundamental and preliminary. There has in recent years been an increased interest in causation, and the articulation of a complex analysis that takes the subject forward in ways I find congenial and fruitful can be found in the recent book by Cartwright (1989) and also in the more formal recent work by Spirtes, Glymour, and Scheines (1993). More details on how I might extend the views developed in this book in these directions can be found in my (1993) essay.

This account of explanation developed in chapter 6 was then further elaborated in the context of some issues in scientific explanation that are more specific to the biological and medical sciences. In chapter 7 I reexamined an old debate about historical explanation, tried to present it in a new light, and argued that, though the explanations provided by evolutionary theory are indeed "explanations," they are quite weak and conjectural ones. I supported this claim by using a detailed example—the sickle cell trait and sickle cell disease research of Allison and Livingstone. I tried to show just how many empirically *un*substantiated assumptions need to be made in order to construct even the strongest examples of "historical explanation in biology and medicine." I related the view developed in this chapter to Brandon's recent (1990) approach to ideally complete adaptation explanations, from which, though I view it as largely correct, I take a different lesson. I think that the view developed in this chapter raises questions about the generally accepted view in biology, medicine, and philosophy of biology, which holds that evolutionary theory can provide us with appropriate explanatory paradigms.

In chapter 8 I examined the role of "functional" statements and "teleological" explanations in biology and medicine. My main thesis there was that the most common interpretation of functional statements (and their "explanatory" force) is licensed by a "vulgar" understanding of evolution that lacks *scientific* support. I maintained, however, that such functional language *is* heuristically important; it is also in my view irreducible to efficient causal language. I developed this thesis through a comprehensive review of what I termed intentional, cybernetic, evolutionary, and anthropomorphic accounts of function and teleology, discussing the important contributions of Nagel, Ruse, Brandon, Hempel, Wimsatt, and Wright. I also furnished a "translation schema" for functional language which explicitly provides for the irreducibility of such locutions to efficient causal language. I suggested that discovery of "the function" of the thymus comported well with my analysis, and provided a historical account of this discovery.

In chapter 9 I briefly reviewed some of the claims that have been made by biologists working in a number of different subfields about the nonreducible character of biology and then turned to an in-depth, partially historical analysis of intertheoretic reduction. I considered the problem of the connectability of different levels of analysis (such as "gene" and "DNA"), and the appropriateness of thinking of reduction along deductive versus causal lines. The subject was pursued with extended attention to the relation between Mendelian and molecular genetics, and the important critiques of Hull, Wimsatt, Fodor, the Churchlands, Rosenberg, and Kitcher, as well as their positive views about reduction, were discussed.

I concluded that a fairly complex model that I termed the general reduction-replacement model (GRR) was the most plausible, but that it had two subforms. If one was examining the relation between "unilevel" theories, the GRR model had a fairly straightforward, simple application that was close to the traditional Nagelian model of reduction. On the other hand, if the theories to be related were only partially reducible (and this would typically be the case where the "theories" fit the characterizations of theories of the middle range developed in chapters 3 and 5), the GRR model was hard to apply and a more "causal" account was more natural, though the model would generate important insights even in this more complex case. I also compared these two subforms of the GRR model with some of the recent proposals by Kitcher to replace talk of reduction by talk about explanatory extensions and embeddings. It seems to me that additional work is needed at this interface between traditional reduction discourse and "explanatory extension" terminology, and that clarification of these relations may assist us also in understanding deep issues associated with scientific discovery and scientific advances in a number of the biomedical sciences. That, however, is material for future research. The chapter concluded with attention to an application of Bayesianism to reductionistically oriented research, which I term the "peripherality thesis."

As I stated at the conclusion of the preceding chapter, I believe the viewpoint that unifies the themes in this very long book might best be termed "logical pragmatism." This position takes both the practices and the results of the sciences seriously, as not to be analyzed away with neat logical distinctions, but rather to be explicated in all their complexity and richness with the aid of both historical and philosophical tools. Important tools of this perspective are elementary logical analysis and simple formalization, as well as the probability calculus. Bayesianism, taken critically, appears to me at this point in the development of inductive logic and statistics to be a natural, normative component of this approach. The use of incomplete and heuristic techniques and language such as generational constraints and the open-textured language of gappy generalizations, and teleological and functional expressions, the importance of taking organization seriously, and the crucial utility of theorizing proceeding on many different and interacting levels, are viewed in these pages as representing facets of this logical pragmatism.

As I have mentioned several times, I suspect that some will object that the recurrent Bayesian theme is a somewhat Procrustean constraint. I think differently and have tried to show that taken critically at this point in time, it is the most plausible candidate for both accommodating the results of mathematical statistics and serving as a heuristic tool to sharpen the issues for more global concerns.

In the above chapters I have reviewed examples from genetics, immunology, internal medicine, the neurosciences, and evolutionary theory. I believe these range over representative areas of inquiry in biology and medicine. The approach has been both historical and philosophical, and, appropriately enough, only the test of time and further critical philosophical scrutiny will determine its ultimate worth.

Notes

Chapter One

1. The term "theories of the middle range" is originally due to R.K. Merton; see his (1968).

Chapter Two

1. Also see H. Reichenbach 1938, 7 and 382. For a defense of Reichenbach's distinction in the light of more recent developments in the philosophy of science, see W. C. Salmon's (1970).

2. This simile comparing antigens and antibodies to keys and locks is, I believe, a variant of Paul Ehrlich's original simile which likened toxins and antibodies to keys and locks. Arthur Silverstein has pointed out to me (personal communication) that Ehrlich borrowed the simile (with acknowledgment) from Emil Fischer's description of enzyme-substrate interactions.

3. Instructive theories in immunology were also paralleled by instructive theories in genetics. See chapter 9 below for a discussion of the "Generalized Induction Theory" and also my 1974a for a discussion and references.

4. Thus I take exception to Laudan's (1980) views that methods of generation *as such* must have special epistemic force. On this view also see McLaughlin (1982), Laudan (1983), and Nickles (1985).

5. For a series of detailed papers describing DENDRAL see Lindsay, Buchanan, Feigenbaum, and Lederberg (1980).

6. The most accessible source for a description of INTERNIST-1 is Miller, Pople, and Myers' (1982) essay. CADUCEUS is described in Pople's (1982) article and the path toward CADUCEUS is discussed in Pople (1985) and Schaffner (1985). QMR (Quick Medical Reference) is the subject of Miller, Masarie, and Myers's (1986) and also Miller et al.'s (1986) essays.

7. An independent but similar phase of scientific inquiry has been considered by L. Laudan and A. Grünbaum, who have termed such a phase in the analysis of budding research traditions a "logic of pursuit" or a "context of pursuit." For detailed comments on the latter see Laudan's (1977, esp. 108–114).

8. See the essays cited in note 6.

9. This case is taken from the unpublished essay by Pople, Myers, and Miller (1974). For a more complex published case see Myers (1985) which demonstrates similar stages.

10. See note 9 for source of this case.

11. Exactly how much "separation" there must be between competing disease candidates to warrant a concluding diagnosis has been the subject of extensive discussion among the developers of the program. A rough rule of thumb is that the separation be equivalent to slightly more than the value given a pathognomonic manifestation taken by itself as described above. Exactly how such a separation is computed is discussed in my (1985, 17–18).

12. See the 1967 proceedings of the Cold Spring Harbor meeting on "Antibodies," with opening remarks by Burnet and concluding comments by Jerne in *Cold Spring Harbor Laboratory of Quantitative Biology* 32 (1967).

13. See for example Watson et al. (1987, Vol. 2, 838).

14. In the present discussion, I focus primarily on Burnet's work to illustrate certain salient features of scientific discovery. There is a more complex story to tell including Talmage's (1957) near simultaneous discovery of clonal selection and Lederberg's (1956) anticipatory near discovery of a selective theory of antibody response. Lederberg's account of his work in his (1988) suggests that what I describe below as analogical reasoning and what I refer to in chapter 5 as "theoretical context sufficiency" constraints on the acceptability of scientific theories were factors impelling him toward and the same time away from an early discovery of clonal selection. These more complex issues will be discussed in my forthcoming paper "The Discovery of the Clonal Selection Theory."

15. The quotations and general account of Burnet's discovery of the clonal selection theory follow his autobiography's account in his *Changing Patterns* (1968, see esp. chap. 15). (Very recently a new biography of Burnet was published (see Sexton 1992) but I have not been able to use it to inform this book.) I have had to question only one minor point concerning that account on the basis of an examination of the primary literature: see below, p. 42, and especially Burnet's (1957a). A parallel account which adds essentially only one further point of information can be found in Burnet's opening remarks at the 1967 conference, cited in note 12 above. The additional point is a reference to work by Mackay and Gajdusek (published in 1958) noting that a case of Waldenstrom's macro-globulenemia had an extremely high titer in Gajdusek's AICF test. This also, Burnet remarks in that (1967, 2) address, impressed "the cellular aspect of immunity on me."

16. CAM is an abbreviation for the chorioallantoic membrane, that delicate sheath found clinging to the inside of a chick's eggshell.

17. Burnet's 1957 formulation of the Clonal Selection Theory is as follows: "The plasma γ-globins comprise a wide variety of individually patterned molecules and probably several types of physically distinct structures. Amongst them are molecules with reactive sites which can correspond probably with varying degrees of precision to all, or virtually all, the antigenic determinants that occur in biological material

other than that characteristic of the body itself. Each type of pattern is a specific product of a clone of mesenchymal cells and it is the essence of the hypothesis that each cell automatically has available on its surface representative reactive sites equivalent to those of the globulin they produce. For the sake of ease of exposition these cells will be referred to as lymphocytes, it being understood that other mesenchymal types may also be involved. Under appropriate conditions, cells of most clones can either liberate soluble antibody or give rise to descendant cells which can.

"It is assumed that when an antigen enters the blood or tissue fluids it will attach to the surface of any lymphocyte carrying reactive sites which correspond to one of its antigenic determinants. The capacity of a circulating lymphocyte to pass to tissue sites and there to initiate proliferation is now relatively well established (cf. Gowens 1957; Simonsen 1957). It is postulated that when antigen-natural antibody contact takes place on the surface of a lymphocyte the cell is activated to settle in an appropriate tissue, spleen, lymph node, or local inflammatory accumulation, and there undergo proliferation to produce a variety of descendants. In this way preferential proliferation will be initiated of all those clones whose reactive sites correspond to the antigenic determinants on the antigen used. The descendants will include plasmacytoid forms capable of active liberation of soluble antibody and lymphocytes which fulfill the same functions as the parental forms. The net result will be a change in the composition of the globulin molecule population to give an excess of molecules capable of reacting with the antigen, in other words the serum will now take on the qualities of specific antibody. The increase in the number of circulating lymphocytes of the clones concerned will also ensure that the response to a subsequent entry of the same antigen will be extensive and rapid, i.e. a secondary type immunological response will occur.

"Such a point of view is basically an attempt to apply the concept of population genetics to the clones of mesenchymal cell within the body." (F. M. Burnet 1957b, 68)

18. For a discussion of the "self-marker" hypothesis and difficulties with it, see F. M. Burnet, (1959, 51–56).

19. See F. M. Burnet (1968, 91–92) for an account of his early work with the chorioallantoic membrane.

20. See Simonsen (1962).

21. See Burnet (1957a).

22. The term "mechanism" will be encountered frequently in this book. In particular, in chapter 6 I will be proposing an extension of Salmon's approach to explanation as the most suitable general analysis of the notion of "scientific explanation." In the present chapter "hypothesis" and "mechanism" are largely used interchangeably. Wimsatt favors the use of "mechanism" (see his 1976b; also in personal conversation) in distinction with any reliance on "generalizations" in explanation (and reduction). In chapter 6 I shall explore the notion of

mechanism in more depth and indicate the extent to which it is importantly dependant on the notions of "generalization" and "scientific law."

23. The notion of a "blackboard" has had a significant influence on the development of a number of AI programs. Nii in her (1986, 47) notes that the first implemented "blackboard system," HEARSAY-II, was the result of Simon's suggestion to Erman and Reddy. Nii (1986) reviews both the background to such systems as well as a number of different blackboard implementations. Also see Engelmore and Morgan's (1989) recent book.

24. High level "selective" types of theories often seem to play important roles in scientific discovery. See my (1974) account of such a theory's influence on Lederberg's approach to the problem of enzyme induction; also see Darden and Cain's (1989) essay on selection type theories.

25. The "short paper" is Burnet's (1957b). The quotations that follow are all from this paper.

26. This also seems to be Nickles' (1985, 190) position. In support he cites Buchanan (1985, 95), who in turn cites my earlier (1974) views, which while stronger than ones I favor at present, provide evidence in support of such constraints.

27. I cite "accessory informational structures" in the present sentence intending to refer to domains and disciplinary matrices. It is of interest to note, however, that another somewhat more formal apparatus heavily influenced by cognitive science and AI considerations has been advanced by Holland, Holyoak, Nisbett, and Thagard (1986). Their analysis construes scientific theories as "mental models," and relies extensively on default hierarchies and production system notions. I will offer some comments on this approach in chapter 3 below where I discuss different approaches to analyzing scientific "theories." I will also briefly comment on this group's use of analogy further below.

28. These terms will be analyzed in later chapters. See chapter 5 for a discussion of research programs and positive heuristic, and chapter 6 for views on explanation sketches and gappy causal generalizations. The role of analogy in discovery is discussed later in the present chapter.

29. Recently, Simon working with Kulkarni extended the production system approach to scientific discovery in a high-fidelity simulation of Sir Hans Kreb's discovery of the urea cycle based on information obtained from Holmes's (1981) and from Krebs himself. This computer program, named KEKADA, is considerably more complex than was BACON, is implemented in the computer language OPS5 and contains a number of classes of heuristics such as "problem choosers," "strategy choosers," "experiment proposers," and the like that generate and guide the discovery of new scientific knowledge in the biochemical area. A detailed description of KEKADA is contained in a recent essay by Kulkarni and Simon (1988) and in Kulkarni's dissertation (1989).

30. For details see Langley et al. (1987, 9–10 and 69–70).

31. In a later discussion of this example, velocities rather than accelerations are measured (cf. Langley et al. 1987, 155–156).

32. See further below, however, for a suggestion I make that perhaps analogical reasoning is too difficult to capture in any traditional computational perspective, and that perhaps an "object-oriented" programming mode of knowledge representation may be a better way to represent (and also bypass) this feature of scientific discovery (and knowledge representation). Also, see my suggestion (p. 62 below) that a "connectionist" or neural net approach may help.

33. In addition to Winston's work, which includes his later (1984) and (1986) extensions, there are a number of other recent papers on the use of analogies in AI implementations such as Burstein (1986), Carbonell (1986), Darden and Rada (1986), and Forbus and Gentner (1986) which also provide promising directions for further development along these lines. Also see the two recent anthologies in this area by Helman (ed.) (1988) and Prieditis (ed.) (1988). (I thank Lindley Darden for these anthology references.)

34. Karp notes that this component is similar to Forbus' Qualitative Process Theory — see Forbus (1984).

35. I will discuss "object-oriented" knowledge representation in chapter 3 below.

36. OOP techniques do not eliminate the need for the modeler (the programmer) to deal with the problem of encoding similarity (analogy). The designer (programmer) of a system that models biological objects must decide what objects are similar, and must arrange them in a (possibly tangled) hierarchy with necessary *exceptions* built into override slots that captures the identity and difference that constitutes the similarity (analogies). The point here (and in chapter 3) is that OOP techniques provide a powerful means of representation, not that they do away with the difficult problems of such representation.

37. Quite recently Darden (1991) presented a highly detailed analysis of the strategies of theory change in Mendelian-Morganian genetics, and Bechtel and Richardson (1992) explored an account of scientific discovery based on the psychological heuristics of decomposition and localization. Darden's various strategies are suggestive and work well in her areas of application, but would need to be extended to be applied in the more highly detailed areas. (For example, the use of analogy in classical genetics is likely to be quite different when applied to immunology or to molecular genetics, where there are special background constraints operative due to cellular interactions and special biochemical information.) Bechtel and Richardson's analysis is also suggestive, but their focus on only two psychological heuristics is somewhat limiting. They do sketch the outlines of a more speculative account of scientific development, including further constraints (in addition to the two psychological heuristics cited), but they themselves admit that the analysis is quite preliminary. Both contributions do sup-

port the importance of the discovery and preliminary evaluational phases of scientific inquiry and thus complement the current chapter in valuable ways.

Chapter Three

1. As noted earlier, the expression "theories of the middle range" is originally due to R. K. Merton; see his 1968.

2. See Ruse (1975) for a useful critique of Woodger's program.

3. The issue is a bit more complex, and Ruse wants, after Hempel and Oppenheim, to distinguish between "fundamental" and "derivative" laws, but the main point still stands (see Ruse 1973, 29).

4. For other useful criticisms of Smart see Munson (1975), Rosenberg's comments on Smart's views in his 1985 (chapter 2, esp. 24–25), as well as van der Steen and Kamminga (1991) and Beatty (1992).

5. Beckner's reference here is to Arber 1954, 46.

6. Interestingly, Thompson's recent (1989) assessment of the Ruse and Beckner (and others') positions on this point also supports Beckner (Thompson 1989, 3–4 and 14).

7. I should add here in passing that I think Hull has overlooked an important sense of systematization caught by the term "deductive statistical." The population genetics of infinite populations falls in this area. For the distinction between deductive nomological, deductive statistical, and inductive statistical, see Hempel (1965, 335–93). Also see the discussion of Wright's model in section 4.5.2.

8. I first made this type of observation in my 1980a and, in spite of the extensive amount of work in philosophy of biology in the past ten years, I think that this point continues to be valid. Even those texts that deal with theories outside the evolutionary domain, such as Rosenberg's, discuss theory structure primarily within the context of evolutionary theory. The burgeoning work in the neurobiological area, paradigmatically represented by Patricia Churchland's 1986 book, offers many examples of neurobiological theories, but does not address the issue of theory structure.

9. See Judson's 1979 (chapter 6) and Whitehouse's 1973 (chapters 12 and 14) for a history and extensive references, and also Olby (1974, 427–32) for more details on Watson and Crick's (1953a, 1953b) and Gamow's (1954) contributions.

10. See my 1974a for a detailed description of the development of the operon theory.

11. CRP stands for "cyclic AMP receptor protein" in Strickberger's notation; he notes that CRP is also referred to as CAP (catabolite activator protein), which I believe is actually the more standard term.

12. Actually, the arabinose C protein is *both* an activator and a repressor and, moreover, acts as a repressor in two different ways. See Watson et al. (1987, 483–485).

13. Darden and Maull (1977) use "interfield" terminology, which I believe is actually the derivative notion, in the sense that the need to employ different "fields" follows from the fact that biological theories (as collections of models) are intertheoretic.

14. See figure 9.5 in chapter 9 and also Watson et al. (1987, 471) for the *lac* operator sequence. Also to be noted are the existence of various base-pair changes that are given as part of "the" sequence.

15. Though Burnet favored somatic mutation as his preferred mechanism of antibody diversity, later work by molecular immunologists indicated that somatic *rearrangement* of the immunoglobulin genes contributed more diversity than did mutation, though the latter phenomenon also occurs (Watson et al. 1987, 853–867).

16. A reader familiar with immunology might raise the interesting question of whether the subject matter of this subsection is best termed a "theory." In the current immunological literature, what I refer to as the two-component theory is not characterized as such, perhaps because the system has been so well confirmed. In the early stages the theory was referred to as the disassociation "hypothesis" or "concept," and as it became further clarified other "hypotheses," such as the synergism hypothesis, were added. Accordingly, I believe we are justified in using the term "theory" to describe this entity. For early references see Cooper, Peterson, and Good (1965) and Peterson, Cooper, and Good (1965).

17. See Arnason, Jankovic, and Waksman (1962). I qualify the "independence" here because of the reference to Archer and Pierce (1961) in the former.

18. For an in-depth discussion of Wright's work and influence see Provine (1986).

19. For an elementary treatment see Mettler and Gregg (1969, 47–49).

20. The discussion of the solution of equation (1) essentially follows Jacquard (1974).

21. See Merton's influential essay "On Sociological Theories of the Middle Range," originally published in 1949 reprinted in the enlarged edition of his *Social Theory and Social Structure* (1968). Also, see Stinchcomb (1975) for an interesting critique of Merton's claim that he was really opposed to general theory.

22. As noted earlier, I first advanced this thesis in my 1980a, and, as also noted, arguing independently and largely from evolutionary considerations, Rosenberg proposed a similar view in his 1985 (219–225).

23. See Munson (1975), who disputes Lederberg's (1960) suggestion that extraterrestrial organisms "may have alternative solutions," say, to genetic coding.

24. Though simple population genetics is formulated at the single-locus genetic level of aggregation, it must be remembered that the unit is actually the gene pool of the population, one of the largest units of aggregation. Whether population genetics might not be required to

construe the unit of selection in higher-level terms is an interesting question discussed by Lewontin (1974, chapter 6) and by G. C. Williams (1966).

25. The term "typical" here has several not necessarily exclusive senses covering not only "most frequent" but also "most important" (in describing central features of biological mechanisms). See the discussion of "prototypicality" in relation to Rosch's research in section 7.1, illustrating the complex character of these notions.

26. I have speculated on the extent to which my suggestion that we need to find efficient means of representing biological variation is analogous to Mayr's long-held thesis that "population thinking" is mandatory in biology. Mayr writes: "Population thinkers stress the uniqueness of everything in the organic world. . . . There is no 'typical' individual, and mean values are abstractions. Much of what in the past has been designated in biology as 'classes' are populations consisting of unique individuals" (1982, 46). I think my view, in a sense may be an extension *to mechanisms* of what Mayr recommends with respect to individuals. In another sense, however, I see the need to use "typical" individuals (and mechanisms) as "prototypes" to capture the biomedical world in our conceptual net. (Even the term "mechanism" needs further analysis, however, as is done in chapters 6 and 9.)

27. Suppe's important essays on the semantic conception have very recently been gathered together and supplemented with additional materials in his 1989.

28. The point has also sometimes been overlooked. In Holland et al. (1986, 327) we find a *contrast* between the semantic approach and a "mental models" approach, which is similar to the frame-based proposal developed below. I view this contrast as a category mistake, since the semantic approach is appropriately contrasted with the syntactic approach but not with various linguistic implementations.

29. But see Worral's (1984) views on this.

30. Suppe in his 1989, (4 and 84) characterizes his approach as "relational" and distinct from the set-theoretic and state space approaches, though it seems to me that it is sufficiently close to the state space approach as used that it is appropriate to consider it a variant of that implementation.

31. The question whether "levels" per se are sufficient to demarcate interacting entities in any useful way in such an analysis might be raised here. Bechtel (1986, 9) suggests that Shaperean domains (Shapere 1974, 1977) might be invoked to help clarify any ambiguities, and perhaps Toulmin's notion of a discipline as well. The need for additional characterization is also noted by Bechtel (1986, 44–46) in connection with Darden and Maull's (1977) "interfield" theories. As I see it, if we are dealing with the extended interlevel theories of the type described in chapters 3 and 5, the theories themselves are likely to provide sufficient constraints to pick out the types of entities and their permissible interactions. We can, if necessary, also refer to Shaperean

domains (introduced in chapter 2), and we can even, to discriminate further, introduce Kauffmanian "perspectives," as Wimsatt has done in the article discussed earlier. I doubt the context will require this finer discrimination be made explicit, except in special cases.

32. Also compare Rosenberg, who writes, commenting on respiration and the type of detail at the level of the Krebs cycle, that:

> The chemical reactions are of course universal, and the molecular mechanisms whereby the enzymes catalyze steps in the glucolysis and oxidative phosphorylation are perfectly universal. But the complete details of any particular mechanism—its particular steps, chemical conditions, reaction rates, the primary structure of its catalyzing enzymes—will *differ, sometimes only slightly, sometimes greatly, from species to species.* There will be important *similarities,* large enough in number and *close enough* in structure to make empirical generalizations worthwhile, even though we know they have *exceptions* that cannot be reduced or eliminated in a systematic way. (1985, 221; my emphasis.)

Rosenberg concludes from such a situation that biology is (largely) a series of "case studies." In my 1980a and further below, I propose an alternative view.

33. The concept of polytypy has been criticized by Hull (1964) and by Suppe (1974a), a fact which suggests, if they are correct, that the "smearing out" feature or variation in the generalizations holding for individuals in a species will be increased in evolutionary theory.

34. See Beatty's (1981) example and also Balzer and Dawes's 1986 on genetics and molecular biology.

35. For example, compare Winston and Horn's second (1984) and third (1989) editions. The recent addition of OOP capabilities to version 5.5 (and later versions) of Turbo Pascal will increase the utilization and visibility of OOP methods, as will the widely available OOP programs needed to develop WINDOWS programming tools.

36. Holland et al. (1986, 12) argue that the frame concept is quite inflexible as a tool for knowledge representation and develop their alternative "mental model" approach in their book. I would agree with them if they intend only the very simplest form of a "frame" as warranting the name, but this does not appear to me to be in accord with standard usage. As will be shown below, frames are quite versatile and are easily extended to incorporate rules. The OOP approach discussed later utilizing objects is intended to bundle together data and procedures (rules). Thus I think that the sense I am giving to "frame" has all of the capabilities that Holland et al. ascribe to their mental models.

37. For examples of more complex frames for the gene concept, see Darden (1991, chap. 11) and Overton, Koile, and Pastor (1990).

38. There are different programming environments as well as language standards that can be utilized to implement these ideas. Karp, as noted in chapter 2 and below, uses KEE; others feel that for maximum

portability the Common LISP Object System (CLOS) may be best. For an excellent introduction to CLOS, see Winston and Horn (1989, chap. 14).

39. I say "ultimately" because this program is still in its comparatively early stages of its development. Karp indicates (personal communication) that currently HYPGENE (that is, in the current experiment) conjectures change to the SKB only, though in a more developed version one will want to alter the CKB and PKB as well.

40. I have stated that elaboration "usually" occurs at a lower level. Lindley Darden (personal communication) suggested that this ampliative development might occur at a "higher" level, a point with which I agree (see, e.g., my discussion of testing various molecular mechanisms of repressor-operator interactions at the genetic level in the development of the operon theory, in Schaffner 1974a, 126).

41. The amplification might, however, be *recast* into a *deductive* formulation if the theories and models drawn on in the elaboration and testing are conceived of as *added premises*, as in analogy with Duhem's auxiliary theories. Such an approach would be in accord with my earlier comments on the untrustworthiness of nonmonotonic logic in knowledge representation. It still might be wise to stress, though, (1) the complex extent to which this premise-adding occurs along both horizontal and vertical dimensions of connectivity among biological theories ("reticularity"), and (2) the "overlapping" or smearedness of many of the "auxiliary" theories in their own right. In the biomedical sciences one does not usually borrow one or two clearly articulated laws (as in the use of auxiliary theories or laws in physics, such as when Newton's second law is borrowed and used in solving an electrodynamical problem). In biomedicine, a more individualized set of complex conditions is selected from a robust set of overlapping models as part of the downward elaboration.

42. This point is a major theme to be developed in chapters 5 and 9 in terms of levels of generality (and aggregation) at what I term the γ, σ, and δ levels.

43. A subtle qualification is required in Hull's (1974) case, inasmuch as his view is quite a bit weaker than, say, Ruse (1970, 1973), Simon (1971), and Munson (1975). Also Rosenberg's view (1985, 219) that, with the exceptions of general molecular biology and evolutionary theory, biology is a series of case study–oriented research programs does not comport with this prevailing tendency. As noted above, some very recent discussions, such as van der Steen and Kamminga's (1990) and Beatty (1992), go in a different direction and one that I interpret as more in accord with the theses presented in this chapter.

44. This second point is based on what I think is an incorrect analogy with electronics and is easily answered, though the answer is, in my view, largely irrelevant to my thesis. In fact, there are important principles of, for example, electrical engineering, such as Ohm's law and "Kirchoff's laws." These latter laws are used in electronic circuit analy-

sis and can be formulated (following Sommerfeld 1964, 135) as: $\Sigma I_n = 0$ and $\Sigma I_n R_n + \Sigma V_{nm} =$ loop emf, where I_n are the currents into (+) and out of (–) branch point, R_n are the resistances, V_{nm} is the electromotive force between points n and m, and emf is the electromotive force. These laws are enormously useful in explanations and predictions in electrical theory; they are also understood to be as universal as Newton's laws of motion.

45. The distinction appears in my 1980a, however.

46. The terms "essential" and "historical" are intended to make explicit concepts that have perhaps been implicit in philosophical discussions of biology (see, e.g., Hull 1974, 71–72).

47. See Nagel (1961, 49–73) for the example and a discussion of counterfactuals and scientific laws.

48. The extent to which the scope of these generalizations varies will be considered in chapter 6 (and also again in chapter 9). I should add here also that I am unconvinced by the thesis advanced in Beatty (1992) that there will be a *continuity* of differing degrees of contingency. As suggested above, I believe this view conflates the *scope*-related and *causal* senses of generalization in biology.

49. Though I think the sentiment expressed by Simpson serves as a useful corrective here, and one that is congruent to the theme of the present chapter, the thesis can, unless qualified, lead to conclusions with which I would disagree, such as the primacy of the social sciences (Hull, personal communication; see also Simon 1971).

50. Suppe does not believe that fuzzy set extensions to the basic semantic conception are needed to incorporate interlevel theories with overlapping models — see his recent 1989 (266–277). In this appendix I introduce the fuzzy-set approach as one means of applying the state space variant to the middle-range theories discussed in the present chapter. Note that the extensions making use of the frame approach and OOP programming techniques do not necessarily subscribe to fuzzy-set principles, so to this extent Suppe is correct. Whether *no* extensions to his analysis are required to accommodate the types of theories and models I discuss above, as he argues in his recent book, is less clear to me and will have to be addressed in later work.

Chapter Four

1. The sense I give to "simplicity" and the role it plays will be discussed in chapter 5.

2. Another excellent example of how antecedent theoretical meaning is created can be found in Darden's account of the role of the "thread" and "beads on a string" analogies used by Morgan and his group for reasoning about chromosomes. Darden (1991, chap. 10) analyzes the role of this analogy using Boyd's (1979) "theory-constituent metaphor" approach, though it seems to me that what the analogy is doing is be-

ing drawn on to create the "antecedent theoretical meaning" of certain components of the then still partially "theoretical" chromosomes.

3. Recall the discussion about the two senses of "universal generalizations" in chapter 3, p. 121. This will be the case for almost all hypotheses. One could conjecture a situation in which a scientist would hypothesize the existence of a specific entity, such as a "black hole," but this would typically be handled as an "initial condition," as discussed below.

4. I leave aside the subtleties of the logical form of the premises, as well as the asymmetry between confirmation and falsification which Sir Karl Popper (1959 [1934]) has emphasized so much. These issues are discussed in almost any elementary philosophy of science text, such as, for example, Hempel's (1965).

5. Burnet (1968, 207) and Lederberg (1988).

6. See, for example, Burch and Burwell (1965, 253), who characterize the theory as: "The clonal selection theory of Burnet (1957; 1959; 1961; 1965) and Lederberg (1959)."

7. Nossal and Lederberg (1958).

8. Arthur Silverstein (personal communication) has commented on the reasoning I set out below, suggesting that what is confirmed by the Nossal-Lederberg experiment is a weaker statement than Premise 1, namely only that "not *all* antibody-forming cells can form *all* antibodies." Dr. Silverstein also adds that "one cell—one antibody" was not critical to the clonal selection theory. I discuss the latter point in chapter 5, but it would seem that there was a silent simplicity assumption at work in the Nossal-Lederberg reasoning that led them to focus their attention on the stronger hypothesis, which is also confirmed but not so clearly as the weaker hypothesis.

9. The account of confirmation just sketched is presented in syntactic terms, an approach that is both more traditional and, I think, more natural. (Recall that in chapter 3 I argued that the semantic and syntactic approaches to theories were "equivalent," but that heuristically one might be more natural, in the sense of easier to work with, than the other in different contexts.) However, it should be noted that a semantic approach to testing can and has been presented by Suppe (1974b, 1989) and Giere (1979, 1984), a brief sketch of which, in light of the discussion of the previous chapter, might be useful. (Thompson's 1989 monograph on the semantic approach to theories does not discuss in any detail the empirical testing dimension of this approach. Lloyd, in her 1988, chapter 8, explores a semantic conception of confirmation of evolutionary models and theories. Her work relies to some extent on P. Suppes's 1962 but differs from it.)

To use the semantic terminology of chapter 3, what the Nossal-Lederberg experiment involves is a "phenomenal system," namely the adult Wistar rat lymph cells immunized with the two types of *Salmonella* antigens. The deduction sketched above is equivalent to the construction of an abstract biological system that has certain idealized features representing those of the actual phenomenal system. This theory-induced biological system is but one of many models (*potentially* an infinite number) which satisfy by definition the conditions of the theory.

Testing, from the perspective of the semantic conception of theories, has two aspects. For *confirmation*, one shows that the truth condition "the set of theory-induced . . . [biological systems] for [theory] T is identical with the class of causally possible . . . [phenomenal] systems holds" (Suppe 1974b, 80). For *falsification*, one demonstrates that this condition and a second truth condition do *not* hold. This second (violated) truth condition states that "the possible values of parameters $p_1 \ldots p_n$ allowed by T are attributes [that] particulars in the phenomenal systems in . . . [the intended scope of the theory T] do possess, or else idealizations of these" (Suppe 1974b, 80).

Since we can show identity between the theory-induced systems and the phenomenal systems only partially, both with respect to (1) the limited number of systems tested and (2) the comparability of only the observational aspects (or those aspects calculable from observations), we obtain only "relative confirmation of T" (Suppe 1974b, 83). This account is only a bare-bones sketch of the semantic approach to theory testing; see Suppe (1974b; 1989, chapters 3 and 4) and van Fraassen (1970) for more details. Omitted from my present discussion is an account of the appropriate ceteris paribus conditions, a theory of experimental design, and a theory of the data, all of which are required in a full-scale analysis according to Suppe (1989, 135). Analogues of these notions appear in my syntactic account of the Nossal-Lederberg experiment presented earlier.

10. For some other conditions imposed on sentences that are "observation" sentences see Carnap (1956).

11. It should be noted that Shapere, in some of his later writings, such as his 1984 (342–351), does not commit himself to any sharp theoretical-observational distinction. The existence of a sharp and temporally stable distinction is also not required in the account I present in this chapter (and book).

12. Billingham and Silvers (1971, 9).

13. The Duhemian thesis and problems with it are discussed in chapter 5. Also see Grünbaum (1960) and Laudan (1965) on further refinements of the Duhemian thesis.

14. We shall see shortly that what I have outlined as the method of testing above — of deriving consequences from hypotheses — is one that is most criticized by Mill. The extent to which the criticism is justified and the extent to which it is misguided will be discussed in section 6.4.

15. See Mill (1973 [1843], 283) and also the excellent discussion by Cohen and Nagel (1934, 249–265).

16. See Nagel's comment on this claim, however, in his 1961 (366–369) .

17. Support for this rather sweeping assertion is discussed in chapter 6, where I also cite the views of Mackie (1974) on this point.

18. In chapter 9, p. 459, I shall discuss some very recent methods of synthesizing modified genes and reinserting them into an organism's genome, an approach that appears to be another modern variant of comparative experimentation.

19. This experimental approach can easily be extended to lower level entities such as genes or nucleotide sequences. See Gilbert and Müller-Hill's experiments discussed on p. 161, and also the powerful new molecular techniques described in chapter 9, p. 459.

20. Cohen in the foreword to Bernard's 1957 [1865], 1-2.

21. As noted earlier, similar conclusions were reported independently and almost simultaneously from R. A. Good's laboratory by Good, Dalmasso, Archer, Peirce, Martinez, and Papermaster (1962); see chapter 3.

22. See Murphy (1974, 234-236) for a discussion of "parastasis."

23. This bears an analogy to Mackie's INUS condition discussed in chapter 6.

24. I say strong support but not "certain proof," as Mill seems to have thought. The replacement of the Newtonian theory of gravitation by Einsteinian general relativity both confirms this and also supports my view about the "relativity" of direct evidence to be developed below.

25. Though not correct in prokaryotes, this is the case (among other forms of regulation) in the more complex forms of regulation found in eukaryotes.

26. In Stent's (1964) scheme, the regulator genes coded not for a repressor protein that bound the operator but rather for enzymes such as transfer RNA-specific nucleases, which would destroy one or another species of a certain type of transfer RNA responsible for translation. The operator genes—what are mapped *genetically* as the operator genes—would in this view code for corresponding species of what Ames and Hartman (1963) had termed "modulating" transfer RNA. Since the genetic code was thought to be (and is) degenerate, more than one transfer RNA codon for each amino acid could exist, and with one codon conceived of as a major and another as a minor representation, these differences could be taken as signals to cease or to begin translation of the associated proteins.

27. See Gilbert and Müller-Hill (1966, 1967).

28. I discuss additional aspects of Glymour's account and also his criticisms of a Bayesian analysis in chapter 5. For a number of critiques of Glymour's theory as well as defenses and discussion, see Earman (1983).

Chapter Five

1. Further below, however, I will raise a problem with the "more subjective" character of likelihood expressions for deterministic theories.

2. The term "deterministic" is placed in quotes here because frequently the variation found in biological systems will be handled by statistical methods, rather than through reclassification of the data into finer subgroups in order to achieve generalizability and data reduction, even though the underlying processes are thought not to be probabilistic or stochastic ones.

3. I should add that either deterministic or probabilistic hypotheses may be *causal* hypotheses, and in chapter 7 I shall discuss how this is possible in the context of an analysis of probabilistic causality. For a discussion as to how Bayesian theory can be used to confirm causal hypotheses see Howson and Urbach (1989, 250-253).

4. Though most commentators on this issue have thought "probability" was relevant, Popper (1959) seems to disagree. Whether he can do so without being impaled on the horns of Salmon's 1968 (especially 28) artfully crafted dilemma I find doubtful.

5. Though the recent book by Howson and Urbach (1989) became available too late to inform the writing of this chapter, I have incorporated as many references to their pro-Bayesian views as is feasible.

6. See their papers in Kyburg and Smokler (1980).

7. See, for example, the arguments by Putnam (1963), Hesse (1974), Shimony (1970), Dorling (1979), and Teller (1976).

8. Also see Teller (1976) and Hesse (1974, 120 n. 1).

9. The term is Herbert Simon's; see his 1957, (204-206) and chapters 14 and 15.

10. These terms are defined later in this chapter.

11. Also see Hacking's rejection of the Fisherian simple hypothesis test without alternatives in his 1965, (82-83) as well as Howson and Urbach on Fisher's approach, (1989, chaps. 5 and 6).

12. A cursory examination of almost any biomedical journal, particularly in the more clinical areas, will confirm the strong hold that the Neyman-Pearson approach exerts on contemporary science.

13. See Seidenfeld (1979) and also Howson and Urbach (1989, chap. 7) for support for this view.

14. This primary hypothesis (H_0) is often called the "null" hypothesis. The term "null" arises because in the discipline of statistical *medical* testing, an investigator often wishes to compare two treatments, say A and B, and a hypothesis asserting there is no, or zero, or *null* difference between treatments is called the "null hypothesis."

15. This alternative hypothesis is "fanciful" but primarily so in the context of well-entrenched Mendelian and post-Mendelian theories of

inheritance; it is introduced here because the numbers proposed allow for easy calculations on the part of the reader. The hypothesis is, however, not so "fanciful" as it may prima facie seem. Lindley Darden notes (personal communication) "that there might be a sex difference that affects dominance wouldn't be such a fanciful hypothesis in the early 20th century," and in support of this view cites some Darwinian calculations that predict 11% recessives (Darden 1976, 160). Bill Wimsatt (personal communication) has drawn my attention to Morgan's (1919) speculations concerning the possibilities of specifically maternal effects on genes (see especially Morgan 1919, chapter 18). Joshua Lederberg (personal communication) views the difficulty of proposing *plausible* alternative hypotheses to the 3 : 1 Mendelian prediction to be a result of our very strong current confidence in the Mendelian hypothesis. He also notes that the *statistical discrimination* between the Mendelian hypothesis and the fanciful alternative is swamped by the entrenched character of the Mendelian hypothesis and its integration into a broad context of other biological theories. This point of Lederberg's finds a natural interpretation in the role of "theoretical context sufficiency" and the importance of Bayesian experimental evidence convergence discussed later in the present chapter.

16. The situation is a bit more complicated, since the needed sample size will also be a function of the difference between the two hypotheses being tested, sometimes referred to as Δ.

17. These advances follow on the earlier foundational work of Ramsey (1931) and DeFinetti (1937); also see the anthology by Kyburg and Smokler (1980).

18. See Neyman (1957), for example.

19. See, for example, Vickers (1965), Hacking (1967), Shimony (1970), and Hesse (1974, 113–114), but also see Armendt (1980) for a contrasting position.

20. This follows since by the probability calculus $P(E \mid E) = 1$.

21. The parameter α is given by a rather complex expression, $(1/2) \log (q/p)/((1 - q)/(1 - p))$, and can be any real number. Here p is the probability of an event at time t and q is the probability of that event at a later time t' (see Field 1978, 364).

22. There is a nice unification of conditionalization and Jeffrey's rule in Williams's (1980) generalization.

23. For example, a q or α expression would then appear in the odds form for comparing hypotheses (see below). For Jeffrey's later thoughts on the debate he initiated, see his 1983, (181–183).

24. An alternative suggestion is favored by Levi (1967) and adopted by Howson and Urbach (1989, 287–288), namely to be able to assign to some data, which has probability 1 in one context, a probability of less than 1 in another. Though we may be forced to limit conditionalization to local contexts, and thus have to adopt a somewhat "patchy"

Bayesian epistemology (see further discussion below), I feel this move should be resisted to the extent possible.

25. Also see Hesse (1974, 136–137) and Salmon (1967, 119) for a similar thesis. Salmon's account is quite complex; see n. 26.

26. I also once thought this simple argument worked; see my 1974 (71). It should be noted that Pap's general thesis can be captured in the Bayesian framework by other means. Salmon (1967, 119) provides a more complex expansion of the denominator in Bayes's theorem and interprets parts of that expression so as to incorporate the (larger) effect of surprising evidence. Howson and Urbach (1989, 86) also rewrite Bayes's theorem so as to make explicit a contrast between H and ¬H to make a similar point, and further below I argue that the odds form of Bayes's theorem permits us to do the same.

27. This raises the problem of the as-yet-undiscussed "catchall" hypothesis considered further below.

28. See p. 179 for a description of the way in which the odds form might help bypass this problem of old evidence, but also see the following note and the discussion of "old evidence" later in this chapter.

29. I say "preliminarily" because the old evidence problem is highly likely to require some form of a "counterfactual" treatment, as discussed below. The problem of old evidence (where the old evidence has a probability = 1, i.e., p(e) = 1) will affect the odds formulation (with a background knowledge term) treatment of novelty, as well as Howson and Urbach's (1989, 86) explication of the force of novel evidence. In the latter, a reformulation of Bayes's theorem is given as:

$$\frac{P(h \mid e)}{P(h)} = \frac{P(e \mid h)}{P(e)} = \ldots$$

and the second expression in this equation will not do its work on old evidence if p(e) = 1.

30. See Garber (1983) and Howson and Urbach (1989, 270–275).

31. See Earman's detailed discussion of the old evidence problem in chapter 5 of his recent book on Bayesianism as well as Technical Discussion 8 below. There is a consensus among those of a Bayesian persuasion, but it is not shared by those who believe other approaches to inductive logic may be necessary. See Chiara's 1987, which raises additional problems regarding old evidence in the Bayesian approach, as well as van Fraassen's 1988, which questions the reliability of any counterfactual approach to the old evidence problem.

32. Also see Good's (1977) discussion of "dynamic probability."

33. Glymour proposes that old evidence is confirming if P(h | e & b & (h ⇒ e)) > P(h | b & e), where b represents the background beliefs (1980, 92).

34. I thank John Earman for this reference. Earman has pursued this issue of convergence in considerable depth in his 1992 (especially in chaps. 6 and 9), and is very skeptical of the force of convergence argu-

ments for nonstatistical theoretical hypotheses. For local evaluations of the type developed in appendix 2, however, these concerns do not seem warranted. For the extension of Bayesianism to the types of comparative theoretical evaluations presented in the later sections of this chapter, additional investigation of the conditions of convergence are almost certainly going to be required.

35. I must add a caveat about my use of a "Bayesian" approach to hypothesis testing. Even in Savage's early work it was noted that "hypothesis testing" has an odd flavor for Bayesians since it singles out the situation in non-Bayesian ways (see Edwards, Lindman, and Savage 1963, 214). Nonetheless there have been explicitly "Bayesian" treatments of hypothesis testing. Kadane (personal communication) and Kadane and Dickey (1980), however, maintain that the entire approach is misconceived, and that all that one should do in hypothesis testing contexts is examine the ways in which our prior and posterior distributions change. This is a fairly radical view, and I shall not follow it at this point, but it will be reconsidered further below after I have had a chance to introduce an extended example in terms of which to raise the question more specifically.

36. This appears to be the way favored by Edwards, Lindman, and Savage, though there is no Bayesian approach in anything like a consensus sense for "hypothesis testing" (see the previous footnote). For the purposes of comparison with the classical tradition of hypothesis testing, however, this use of the odds form for comparing "prior" and "posterior" distributions seems a reasonable one. For additional support for this approach see Barnett (1982, 192–196), but also compare his discussion (202–204) to be commented on below.

37. This is not, of course, to say that the Bayesian approach cannot be embedded in a decision-theoretic context; in point of fact, that is one of its most natural extensions. See Edwards, Lindman, and Savage (1963).

38. Several alternative Bayesian approaches to representing something like Neyman-Pearson hypothesis testing have been proposed; see appendix 2 for an example and references to the literature.

39. In a book of this type, not all of the issues raised by a Bayesian approach to science can be considered. For other salient issues, see Hesse (1974) and Howson and Urbach (1989), both of which are very general defenses of a Bayesian-oriented philosophy of science. For a "mixed review" of Bayesianism, see Earman's 1992.

40. For a statistically oriented set of further readings in this area see Lindley's 1965, Rosenkrantz's 1977, and Howson and Urbach's 1989.

41. Here I shall summarize those elements that are most germane to the issues raised by "local evaluation"; in chapter 6 those points more closely related to "global evaluation" as well as deterministic theories will be considered.

42. The Lindley-Savage argument can be stated formally, following Giere's exposition, as a theorem:

Theorem. Being indifferent between two tests t = (α , β) and t' = (α', β') is equivalent to holding H and K with prior probabilities in the ratio

$$P(H)/P(K) = - U_{II}/U_I \text{ slope } (t, t')$$

where U_I and U_{II} represent the utilities (or disutilities) of making a Type I or Type II error respectively.

Proof. Assume that indifference between t and t' implies that the expected value of the two tests is the same.

$EU(t) = P(H) \times \alpha \times U_I + P(K) \times \beta \times U_{II}$.

$EU(t') = P(H) \times \alpha' \times U_I + P(K) \times \beta ' \times U_{II}$.

Setting these equal yields the desired result. (Giere 1977, 49)

43. See the note on Birnbaum in Giere (1977, 69 n. 29).

44. Some time ago Harold Jeffreys (1961) and E. T. Jaynes (1968), and, more recently, R. Rosenkrantz (1977) attempted to specify objective prior probabilities, and they argued that maximum entropy priors supplemented with indifference procedures generate objective priors. Subjective or personalist Bayesians such as Savage did not agree. Savage, in a posthumous article commenting on Jeffrey's and Jaynes's position, which he termed "necessarian," wrote that "we personalists feel that necessarians claim to get something for nothing, and this seems particularly conspicuous in necessarian statistics" (1977, 13). More forceful criticisms against Jaynes's views were developed in Friedman and Shimony (1970) and in Shimony (1970) arguing that Jaynes's priors were inconsistent with the principles of probability theory. Also Efron (1978) argued that an analysis of "Stein's phenomenon" indicates that classical analyses yield better results for estimating a multiparameter data vector than objective Bayesian approaches. Seidenfeld (1980) criticized Rosenkrantz's (1977) explication and extension of Jaynes's necessarian approach as inconsistent with Bayesian conditionalization. (But also see Rosenkrantz's (1980) reply to Seidenfeld.) Finally, Howson and Urbach (1989, 288–290) argue that Jaynes's objective priors neither exist nor do Bayesians need them.

45. See, for example, Freedman and Spiegelhalter (1983).

46. See Edwards, Lindman, and Savage (1963), and also Lindley (1965a, 1965b), Barnett (1982, chapter 6), Kadane and Dickey (1980), and Howson and Urbach (1989, chapter 10).

47. See Jeffrey (1975, 155–156).

48. See Teller 1975, as well as Miller's (1976) critique of Popper on verisimilitude and Laudan's (1973) criticism of Peircean views.

49. For an example of the diverse theses that different realists have held (and antirealists denied) see Leplin (1984, 1–2).

50. See Laudan (1973) and Sellars (1977).

51. See Nagel's discussion in his 1961 (129–152) and also Fine's (1984, 98), in which Fine develops a notion of a "natural ontological attitude" (NOA) which is "neither realist nor antirealist."

52. I use the notion of a Kantian type of intuition here, in the sense that Kant believed particular scientific truths, such as that space was Euclidean, were synthetic a priori and given as "certain" forms of our knowledge.

53. I do admit that form of hypothetical truth and falsity needed for truth functional logic, however. See Fine (1984) for a similar incorporation of truth into an antirealist approach.

54. See the discussion earlier in this chapter of this sense of acceptance.

55. See Feyerabend's discussion of his early conversations with Kuhn in his 1970 (197–198).

56. I spend time in refuting the Feyerabend and Kuhn positions described not so much because I feel I need to convince philosophers of science (even Kuhn evidently relaxed his strong position about incommensurability in his 1970 postscript) but because what is written in *The Structure of Scientific Revolutions* has become so entrenched in the scientific (and the sociological) culture over the past 25 or so years. As an example, see Latour and Woolgar's 1986 (275–276).

57. See p. 137, chapter 4, and also my 1970 for an earlier argument on this issue.

58. I put aside for the moment the radical thesis of historical discontinuity that the paradigm notion seems to entail.

59. See the festschrift for Robert K. Merton edited by L. Coser (1975) for examples such as the essays by J. Cole and H. Zuckerman and by S. Cole. The former two authors write "Kuhn's model of revolutionary change has been especially influential in studies of scientific specialties."

60. Lakatos (personal communication).

61. See chapter 2, p. 52.

62. Thus what are seen as "central" in this sense will depend on how a theory is axiomatized. Maxwell, in his account of his electromagnetic theory, used the *vector potential* as a fundamental notion, whereas Hertz (and Heaviside), axiomatizing the "same" theory, did not (see Schaffner 1972, chapters 5 and 6).

63. See Jacob and Monod (1961, 352).

64. The subjective element could be objectified with the aid of a "theory of generality," but this is best left for the future.

65. See chapter 3, p. 106 for a discussion of the formalism needed.

66. See above, p. 204.

67. See Kordig (1980) on Laudan for a similar point; also see Hempel (1970).

68. I am not strongly committed to only these three factors for global theory evaluation. In my 1974a (376), I also proposed a principle of the unity of fundamental biological processes, though I now think that the scope of such a principle is quite narrow and that the principle might better be formulated as one that gives weight to closely analogous precedent mechanisms or narrow generalizations. Other writers have suggested still additional criteria for theory assessment, among them Newton-Smith (1981) and Darden (1991, chap. 15).

69. See Laudan (1977, 109-114) for a discussion of the logic of pursuit.

70. I think that this might amount to something like a Glymorean computation — see p. 166 above.

71. What we could term a "direct" test by analogy with the term "direct evidence" developed in chapter 4 could be introduced here via an odds form of Bayes's theorem.

72. This complicates the dynamics because b contains other T's, but does not qualitatively change the dynamics.

73. Shimony, for example, disagrees with this suggestion (personal communication) and proposes reconditionalization, somewhat akin to Levi's suggestion (1967).

74. Often τ^1 will be preservable and some component of κ modifiable (though not central γ-level assumptions), but this will not affect the general argument.

75. This point was raised by Adolf Grünbaum on the basis of my 1974b (personal communication).

76. Perhaps the frame or OOP approach might be applied to such an issue. To the best of my knowledge, this critically important problem of theory individuation has received little attention in the philosophy of science.

77. This hypothesis does not specify the *number* of types; it embodies the sequence hypothesis. Hypothesis σ_7 limits this type number to one (probably) or two (possibly). I thank Dr. Arthur Silverstein for bringing the distinction between hypotheses 5 and 7 to my attention.

78. Dr. Silverstein (personal communication) suggests that this hypothesis may reflect an expansion of the original clonal selection theory.

79. For example, δ_5 is probably derivable from the central dogma of protein synthesis, taken together with the other hypotheses.

80. For a good introductory account of these theories see Burnet (1959, chapter 4) and also Talmage's earlier (1957) review.

81. Silverstein in his recent (1989) history of immunology also cites Topley's (1930) work. Also see Silverstein's interesting report of a personal communication with Haurowitz (Silverstein 1989, 84–85 n. 39).

82. See Haurowitz (1965) for an excellent review of the instructive theory vis-à-vis the CST.

83. Landsteiner's work is summarized in his classic monograph (1945) *The Specificity of Serological Reactions*.

84. Haurowitz (1965, 32–33).

85. The resolution of the problem with the Simonsen phenomenon is somewhat murky, a situation confirmed by Arthur Silverstein (personal communication).

86. See section 15 below for additional comments on the normative character of Bayesian inference and the extent to which scientists may be Bayesians.

87. Determining how to combine different individuals' probabilistic judgments into a summary assessment is a complex undertaking and though some progress has been made in this area there is as yet no consensus on how to model consensus. See Genest and Zidek (1986). (I thank Jay Kadane for this reference.)

88. See my 1970 and also Hesse (1974, chapter 10) for a general discussion of simplicity in connection with comparative theory evaluation. Readers should also note Howson and Urbach's (1989, 290–292) suggestion that simplicity is such a difficult notion to analyze that perhaps one should not do anything other than allow it to function in various individuals' priors.

89. See Glymour (1980, 78–79) and also the discussions in Hesse (1974, 226–228) and Howson and Urbach (1989, 292).

90. Shimony (personal communication, but also see his 1970) suggests that, when b changes, we should not use Bayesian conditionalization but should rather start over again. This has similarities to Levi's (1967) and Howson and Urbach 's (1989) suggestions but leaves the kinematics ill-defined.

91. I suspect that extensive indeterminancy would be the consequence of attempting to compare the probabilities of two different theories on the basis of two different backgrounds.

92. See Part I above for a discussion of this principle.

93. See the discussion in Edwards, Lindman, and Savage (1963, 199–201).

94. See Bayarri, DeGroot, and Kadane (1988).

95. Box and Tiao discuss the measurement of a physical constant and provide a standardized likelihood function represented by a "normal curve." Shimony (personal communication) also seems to favor something like this approach.

96. See his comment (1977, pp. 15–16) that Bayesians, by recognizing subjectivity, are more objective, in the sense of more constrained, than those who are typically characterized as "objectivist."

97. See Salmon (1967, 117) for this suggestion, and also the comment by Howson and Urbach (1989, 81).

98. I say "analogue" since, if we accept Shimony's "tempering" suggestion, we do not obtain a 0 probability.

99. The account here follows my 1974a. For a more recent Bayesian account of ad hocness see Howson and Urbach (1989, 110).

100. Grünbaum (personal communication) and Laudan (personal communication and also 1977, 235).

101. Redhead wished to translate the analysis I offered back into Zahar's (1973) approach. Redhead writes:

> Schaffner proceeds to discover ad hocness as a property of an hypothesis as a constituent part of a theory, but in order to keep the argument as simple as possible we shall follow Zahar in considering the ad hocness of theories. (1978, 356)

This move on Redhead's part is contrary to a necessary distinction in my analysis, since h has near 0 prior probability but the remainder of the theory does not. Amalgamating the hypothesis with the theory blocks the analysis I gave in my (1974a) article. It also leads Redhead into making the mistake of attributing to me a use of Zahar's ad hoc$_3$. A more serious confusion is Redhead's attempt to provide a different Bayesian explication of Zahar's ad hoc$_2$. Redhead develops some symbolism which it is not necessary to discuss here, for what Redhead takes ad hoc$_2$ to be seems to me *so far* from what scientists and methodologists mean by ad hoc that in any sense the analysis is foundationally faulty. Redhead writes:

> We can now explain that if a theory is *ad hoc$_2$* with respect to the experiment e then = 1, i.e., the explanation of e by T in no way depends on the truth or falsehood of T, both of which eventualities lead with certainty to the result e. This is just what a scientist means when he says that T was an *ad hoc* explanation of e, namely T was devised for the express purpose of explaining e, so the explanation of e is guaranteed independently of whether T is true or false (1978, 357)

This, however, is not an explication of *ad hoc;* it is rather an explication of *the irrelevance of T (and ~T) to e,* and e is guaranteed on this account by b.

102. Haurowitz (1978).

103. See figure 5.1 above and accompanying text.

104. This example is based on Hoel (1976, 188–190).

105. If there is no evidence that a specific distribution is involved, statisticians often use what is termed a "nonparametric" test. See Silvey (1970, chapter 9), for a discussion and examples, and also Lehmann (1959) for details of optimal properties of nonparametric procedures.

106. Following Hoel (1976) I use the circumflexed $\hat{p}$ to represent the proportion of the n entities with the property in question.

107. For examples of other distributions, see Lindley (1965b).

108. There are other ways that this subject of statistical hypothesis testing might have been approached. See Kadane and Dickey (1980), as

mentioned in n. 35, and also see Howson and Urbach's discussion of Bayesian statistical hypothesis testing (1989, chapter 10).

109. This is a fairly simple example, and others that are more complex do not allow as direct a comparison between classical and Bayesian approaches. See Barnett (1982, 202–203) for indications that simple translations between the approaches may break down in two-sided tests.

Chapter Six

1 *Webster's Ninth New Collegiate Dictionary* (Springfield, Mass.: Merriam-Webster, 1983), 293.

2. Though I tend to use the interrogative "why" in examples 1, 2, 3,and 4, it may be that "why" is interestingly best reserved for more evolutionary questions and answers and that "how" would be more suitable. I discuss this issue in chapter 8.

3. See Jacob and Monod (1961). To be complete, I should add the proviso "in the absence of glucose in the environment."

4. Kandel and Schwartz (1985, 819).

5. Strickberger (1976, 206).

6. Jacquard (1974, 410).

7. Miller (1961).

8. For a superb, immensely detailed overview of the historical developments in scientific explanation see Salmon (1989).

9. Hempel (1965) and Nagel (1961).

10. Nagel, in developing his account, of D-N explanation (1961, 33–37) to apply it to scientific laws, does not detect any serious problems with the extension. Hempel and Oppenheim, in their original (1948) account, were concerned with special problems that such an extension posed, and elaborated on their reservations in what Salmon (1989) terms their "notorious" note 33 (Hempel 1965, 273). Salmon indicates Hempel never adequately addressed this problem in any of his subsequent writings.

11. See Hempel (1965, 365).

12. I use more standard notation than did Salmon in his 1970.

13. Curiously, van Fraassen dropped the emphasis on Aristotle between 1977 and 1980 but did retain in his (1980) many of the criticisms of the traditional Hempelian models of explanation. See p. 313.

14. See Brody (1972).

15. These asymmetries are the asymmetries between prediction and explanation or deduction and explanation discussed earlier.

16. Some of these asymmetries that concern van Fraassen, such as Scriven's paresis and the barometer examples, are the classic counterexamples for scientific explanation cited earlier in our discussion of Hempel's D-N model. Van Fraassen subsequently (in his 1980) pro-

vided a somewhat different, though still largely *causal*, resolution of these counterexamples, and I shall discuss van Fraassen's (1980) account further below.

17. For Bromberger's flagpole example see his 1961. For a more easily accessible description see Salmon (1971, 71–76). It should be noted that much of the literature on scientific explanation over the past 40 years has been concerned with what might be termed classic counterexamples to the Hempelian model of deductive nomological explanation. Bromberger's example attempts to show that predicting the height of a flagpole from the length of its shadow does not amount to an explanation of the height, contra Hempel's model. Scriven produced several counterexamples, only one of which I will describe here, namely his paresis example. Paresis, a form of paralysis found in some patients with tertiary syphilis, is explained by citing that the patient had syphilis, even though only very few patients with syphilis ever develop paresis. This amounts to an explanation even though the prediction would have been the reverse (i.e., given primary syphilis, one should not predict that the afflicted individual would develop paresis). For Hempel's discussion of the paresis example see his 1965, (369–370). For a recent introduction to the role of these examples in the history of explanation, see those pages referenced in the index of Kitcher and Salmon's 1989 under the terms "flagpole" and "paresis."

18. I have resisted using the phrase "the Salmon watershed essay."

19. A good introduction to *Aplysia* can be found in Kuffler, Nichols, and Martin (1984, chapter 18) and also in Kandel (1979). More advanced details are given in Kandel and Schwartz (1985, chapter 62) and in other articles from Kandel's laboratory cited below.

20. Habituation is the decrease in sensitivity to a stimulus as it is repeated over time, sensitization is defined immediately below, and classical and operant conditioning in these contexts have their usual meaning. See Kandel and Schwartz (1985, chapter 62) for an extended discussion of these terms as applied to *Aplysia*.

21. Recent work by Frost, Clark, and Kandel (1988) indicates there are at least four sites of circuit modification involved in short-term sensitization in *Aplysia*. These further complexities will be discussed further below.

22. This is a generalizable point and is not based only on the present example; it has been argued for by Wimsatt (1976b) and Kitcher (1984), primarily in the context of reduction. I will pursue the issue again in my discussion of reduction in chapter 9, where I explicitly consider Kitcher's views about the paucity of "laws" in biology.

23. The significance of the C-kinase mechanism for learning in *Aplysia* is the source of some controversy in the field. For an alternative to the approach of Kandel's group, see Alkon's (1989) account.

24. See my 1987 for an account of some of the deliberations of Morowitz's committee and also Morowitz (1985).

25. *Because* of this interlevel character of biological models, it is natural to find inter*field* theories (see Darden and Maull 1977) employed widely in biology.

26. I should add that there is not simply *one* causal sequence being described but a rather complex *set* of parallel sequences.

27. This "reinterpretation" has implications for the analysis of intertheoretic reduction models and will be readdressed in chapter 9.

28. From Kandel et al. (1987, 120–121).

29. The causal sequence mixing various levels of aggregation can be fully causally deterministic even though not all the details of the underlying molecular mechanisms are known.

30. I will return to this issue again both further below and also in chapter 9 and indicate what I mean by "first approximation" in those contexts.

31. One means of representing efficiently the varying scope of the generalizations encountered in the *Aplysia* example discussed above may be to utilize some tools developed in artificial intelligence and computer programming that I discussed in chapters 2 and 3. What has been termed an "object-oriented" style of programming with a complex "inheritance" structure may well be a natural way to represent these types of conceptual structures. I have recently begun to explore a simulation of short-term sensitization using Common Lisp with its Common Lisp Object System (CLOS), and the preliminary results are theoretically promising.

32. Though the full adder described here uses the first-order predicate calculus for its knowledge representation, the same circuit could have been represented in either frames or in an object-oriented program approach (OOP), as discussed in chapters 2 and 3. For a treatment of the full adder using a frame system with inheritance that its authors say is "more object-oriented," see Fulton and Pepe's (1990) article on model-based reasoning.

33. The following was initially motivated by Searle's (1985, 1987) causal view of the mind-brain problem, but it applies as well to some hierarchically oriented embryological and evolutionary theorists, to be discussed in chapter 9 below.

34. The prime example of such an exception can be found in theoretical population genetics, where a small number of abstract principles can be conjoined to constitute an axiomatized theory and important theorems proved on their basis. See for an example Jacquard (1974) and also the discussion in chapters 3 and 8.

35. I believe that even a cursory reading of standard textbooks and research papers in biochemistry, microbiology, and physiology will support the claim that most explanations that are provided are of the causal/mechanical type. This fact, however, raises the philosophical problem, acknowledged by Salmon and stressed by such unificationists as Kitcher (1989 and in personal communications), that we lack any

consensus on characterizing causality and causal interactions. Much of Salmon's 1984 (especially chapters 5–7) attempts to respond to this hoary conundrum first raised by Hume by developing some of the logical empiricist Reichenbach's views in new directions. In section 6.7 below I shall offer yet another alternative, couched more in the pragmatic tradition.

36. See Coulson, Feltovich, and Spiro (1989).

37. See my discussion about the two senses of generality in chapter 3, p. 121.

38. In section 8, I will generalize the properties to include probabilistically causal influences.

39. In his search for consensus and rapprochement, Salmon also finds a way to integrate the "pragmatic" tradition of van Fraassen and Achinstein; I shall reconsider Salmon's comments on these writers further below in section 6.9.

40. The example involves explaining the direction of motion of a helium-filled balloon in an accelerating airliner (see Salmon 1989, 183); the balloon paradoxically moves *forward*.

41. My sense is that when biomedical scientists find laws of coexistence they view these as provisional surrogates for deeper causal explanations.

42. I will also add, after reviewing some of van Fraassen's (1980) suggestions about the pragmatic character of scientific explanations, what I will term a "doubly comparative" component to the causal explanation account that I have developed to this point.

43. In some comments on an earlier account of the above model of explanation (and reduction), Philip Kitcher also cautioned me (in correspondence) that the analysis I favored would require an explication of causation that would permit me to respond to Hume's criticism— see section 6.1.

44. Others have stressed this contrast as well. Lewis (1973) notes that "Hume defined causation twice over." Earman in his (1986) sees the first two definitions as the basis of empiricist accounts of laws of nature and the conditional definition as "the inspiration of the non-Humean necessitarian analyses" (1986, 82).

45. See Brand (1976) for a representative collection of these diverse approaches; for more on the various conditional analyses, see Sosa (1975).

46. This expression will permit probabilistic causation as I shall explain further below.

47. The notion of "causal priority" is defined and discussed on p. 299.

48. See p. 300 for a discussion of the relation of conditionals to their epistemological warrant.

49. See chapter 4, p. 151.

50. It should also be noted that interpreting causation as involving a judgment of "necessity in the circumstances" still permits stochastic and probabilistic causal sequences. Mackie notes that "Saying that A is likely to cause B does not put likelihood into the causing itself: it could (though it does not) mean that A is likely to necessitate B, and I think it does mean that A is likely to be, in some particular case, necessary in the circumstances for B" (1974, 50).

51. It will not be possible to review Mackie's argument for this conclusion, which can be found in his 1974, (40–43), in any great detail in this book. Suffice it to say that Mackie is attempting to clarify our intuitions whether "necessity in the circumstances" or "sufficiency in the circumstances" in some strong sense is the better explicandum for our notion of "causation." To this end Mackie has us imagine three chocolate bar dispensing machines, which he terms K, L, and M. These machines operate through the insertion of a shilling into a coin slot, and they have glass fronts so one can see the mechanism that accepts the shilling and dispenses the chocolate bar. K is a deterministic machine and under normal circumstances insertion of the coin into this machine is both necessary and sufficient to release the chocolate. (The machine *can* fail to work, but we can detect the reason for the failure.) Both L and M are indeterministic machines, but of different sorts. L requires a shilling, but it may fail to dispense a chocolate bar. It acts like a slot machine. M on the other hand will typically produce a chocolate bar if a shilling is inserted, but occasionally it will produce a bar without the need for a coin (analogous to a slot machine that, when you walk by it, pays out a jackpot!). Mackie argues that, in M's case, since even if we put in a coin we cannot know whether it was necessary, we would not want to say that putting in the coin caused the chocolate bar to be dispensed, whereas we would want to say that insertion of the coin in L's case caused the chocolate bar to appear (though it might not have).

52. For additional comments relating "necessity in the circumstances" to probabilistic causality, see n. 50.

53. See Mackie (1974, 262) for his interpretation of when a causal account is "explanatory."

54. These "gaps" can exist at the same level; they can be gaps in our adequately complete knowledge of some causes or gaps in "lower" level knowledge regarding the mechanisms underlying some phenomenon well understood at a grosser level. Kandel's treatment of sensitization above illustrates this second sense of "gappy."

55. In some cases a feedback system will result in a decrease ($\downarrow$) rather than an increase ($\uparrow$) in a factor in such a causal chain. This type of notation is frequently used by biomedical scientists in discussion and in seminars, though I have seen it used in print only infrequently. See, however, Schaffner (1986) for examples and references to some published cases.

56. This is an issue to which I shall return under point (3) below; see especially note 60.

57. This is a view that Collingwood and also Hart and Honoré (1985) maintain—though Mackie disagrees (1974, 120–126).

58. It seems to me, however, on the basis of the arguments developed in chapter 4, that it is preferable to cite Mill's method of difference in the weaker sense found in Claude Bernard's method of comparative experimentation, as providing the empirical support for causal sequences.

59. For a critique of Salmon's views on causation see Sober (1987).

60. See Collingwood's discussion on this point in his 1940 (chapter 31). Collingwood's argument for continuity in both temporal and spatial senses arose in the context of his seeking to distinguish the modern scientific conception of causation—his sense III above—from his other two senses. He wrote:

> Cause in sense III is simultaneous with effect.
>
> Similarly, it is coincident with its effect in space. The cause of an explosion is where the explosion is. For suppose x causes y, and suppose that x is in position p_1 and y in position p_2, the distance from p_1 to p_2 being δ. If 'cause' is used in sense II, δ may be any distance, so long as it is bridged by a series of events which are *conditiones sine quibus non* of x causing y. But if 'cause' is used in sense III, δ must = 0. For if it did not, p_2 would be any position on the surface of a sphere whose center was p_1 and whose radius would = δ; so the relation between p_1 and p_2 would be a one-many relation. But the relation between x and y, where x causes y in sense III, is a one-one relation [because in sense III, a cause "leads to its effect by itself, or 'unconditionally'; in other words the relation between cause and effect is a one-one relation" (1940, 313)]. Therefore, where δ does not = 0, x cannot cause y in sense III. (1940, 315)

61. Mackie does not go so far as to say we also observe *laws* directly, but he does indicate that such laws are reached by the framing and testing of hypotheses and that as such they are no less objective. See his 1974 (230).

62. My (1991) discusses these complexities and criticizes Giere's views. It should be noted here that counterfactuality is needed if what has been termed Simpson's paradox is to be avoided. See Cartwright (1979) on this problem.

63. The measure of effectiveness introduced here is essentially identical to what the epidemiologists have termed a "measure of effect" for "attributable risk." Giere does not comment on this notion, but see Fletcher, Fletcher, and Wagner (1982, 101).

64. See Salmon (1989) for an extensive discussion of the relation of some of these notions to scientific explanations, as well as Salmon (1980), Cartwright (1979), Skyrms (1980), Otte (1981), Eels and Sober (1983), and Sober (1984, chapter 7). Also see my 1987 and 1990a.

65. See chapter 5.

66. I have in mind here the account I gave of the case of the competition between various versions of the instructive theory and the clonal selection theory in chapter 5.

67. Van Fraassen does cite Aristotelian doctrines, such as the four cause theory, which he views, however, as overly simplified (1980, 131).

68. There are some similarities between van Fraassen's (1980) erotetic theory of explanation and Achinstein's illocutionary approach (1983), but there are also a number of significant differences. For clarifying comments about their interrelations, as well as both views' relation to the causal/mechanical approach, see Salmon (1989, section 4.4).

69. There are some revealing similarities between these comparative aspects of van Fraassen's (1980) theory of explanation and Skyrms's account of explanation independently developed in his (1980, 140–142). See my (1983, 95–97) for comments on Skyrms's desiderata for scientific explanations.

70. Van Fraassen is concerned that screening off, for example, may eliminate some specific useful information in an answer. Such information, though useful, nonetheless may generate a posterior probability of the topic, given on an alternative screening off answer, that is less than a more general vague answer. See van Fraassen (1980, 150–151) for details.

71. See Salmon (1971, 71-76) for a discussion of this example, and also see van Fraassen's interesting adaptation of the problem in his story "The Tower and the Shadow" (1980, 132–134).

72. Strickberger (1976, 206).

73. The explanation here involves the aa genotype hiding any color potentially generated by the B locus — see Strickberger (1976, 204–206).

74. Salmon would probably say that this appeal to "inductive support" is a relic of the epistemic approach to explanation and is not required in an "ontic" analysis. It seems to me, however, that we need to make explicit the nature of the connections holding between explanans and explanandum, and simply telling a story (exhibiting causal factors) without attention to the ties that bind the story together leads to an incomplete analysis of explanation.

Chapter Seven

1. Many of these arguments are old disputes in the philosophy of biology, and some philosophers of biology may view the issues as long settled. See M. Williams (1981, 385–386) for this view. Some biologists writing in a philosophical vein, such as Mayr (1982), just quoted, disagree with Williams's view, and think that these matters are of critical importance in understanding the differences between the biological and the physical sciences. I view the arguments to be reviewed in section 7.2 as very useful background to introduce the question of the

types and strengths of historical explanations in biology. As I shall try to show in section 7.4, a number of philosophical distinctions, introduced by such philosophers as Woodger, Gallie, Goudge, and Beckner, can help us comprehend better the strengths and weaknesses of explanations in contemporary embryology and evolutionary theory.

2. See Watson et al. (1987, chapter 10) for an account of DNA replication. This process has become an extremely complex story in comparison with the simple, semiconservative replication hypothesis proposed by Watson and Crick in their 1953b.

3. For a recent analysis of these "just so" stories see Lennox (1991).

4. For a different position on the ability of adequate explanations to simplify and abstract from detailed situations, see Horan (1988, 1989); but compare her views with Cartwright (1983).

5. For additional comments relating "necessity in the circumstances" to probabilistic causality, see n. 50 in chapter 6.

6. Compare Mackie (1974, 262) for his interpretation of when a causal account is "explanatory."

7. Compare Beckner on this point with Cartwright (1983), who sees such *false* assumptions as being pervasive in the physical sciences; for a criticism of Cartwright (and thus also of Beckner) on this point in the biological sciences, see Horan (1988).

8. The percentage given here is taken from Jacquard (1974, 410). More recent data suggests the percentage is higher, perhaps 8–10% (Forget 1982). The exact numbers are not critical given the thesis developed below.

9. See Rosenberg (1985, 73–83), who discusses this example in extenso under the rubric of "A Triumph of Reductionism."

10. Williams's axiomatization is extensively critiqued by Sober (1984c), who argues that in some respects it is too weak and in others it is too strong.

11. The issue of whether population genetics should be conceived of as a "core" component of evolutionary theory is part of a larger issue as to what the theory *is*. Burian (1988) agrees with Depew and Weber's (1988) suggestion that neo-Darwinism be conceived of more as a *treaty* than a theory. Recent scholarship in evolutionary theory, such as was reviewed by Burian (1988), encompasses a very diverse set of approaches to the foundational aspects of the field.

12. These selective values are sometimes described by the term "relative adaptive value" or even identified with "fitness"; see, for example, Sober (1984b, 40) or the table on p. 344. The issue of the proper meaning of "fitness" is one that has (strenuously) exercised philosophers of biology. A consensus of sorts seems to have emerged that construes the notion along the lines proposed by Brandon (1978) and Mills and Beatty (1979) and further developed by Brandon (1982); also see Sober (1984b, 1984c) and Rosenberg (1985, chapter 6). Burian (1984) suggests that there are three different aspects to the notion. These discussions,

interesting both in their own right and in connection with the question of the circularity of Darwinian (and neo-Darwinian) evolutionary theory, do not have a direct impact on the points covered in the present chapter, and thus I shall not be discussing the notion further. "Fitness" has also generated appeals to "supervenience" to account for its diverse implementations. The notion of "supervenience" will be discussed in chapter 9.

13. Here I follow a syntactic approach, which suffices here and which I think is clearer than a semantic approach for the purposes of this chapter. These assumptions could, however, be conjoined so as to constitute the basis for an analogue to a "set-theoretic predicate" semantic approach. See Beatty (1981) and Thompson (1989, chapter 5). I am not persuaded by Thompson's claim (1989, 96) that the semantic approach facilitates the "interaction" of the theories of natural selection and population genetics better than does a syntactic approach, since the axiomatization and derivation discussed above seems to perform that function quite well. Also see the critique by Sloep and van der Steen (1987) and the replies of Beatty (1987), Lloyd (1987), and Thompson (1987) on the utility of the semantic approach in the evolutionary domain.

14. I have already outlined Jacquard's strategy, though perhaps overly briefly, in chapter 3.

15. Also compare Kitcher's account of the sickle cell case in his 1985 (46–47).

16. Forget indicates the disease is very variable with a mean lifespan of approximately 40 years, though a significant number of infants expire within the first three years because of overwhelming sepsis and/or acute splenic sequestration crises (in which, for unknown reasons, large amounts of blood pool in the liver and spleen producing circulatory collapse). (1982, 891).

17. Also see Horan (1988) for a discussion of some of the differences between physicists' and biologists' controls.

18. See the discussion of van Fraassen's (and Skyrms's) approach to explanation in chapter 6, which involved evaluative components.

19. Recall the discussion about the ability of the SR model to account for explanations of low weight. Sober (1984b, 142) also seems to accept this application of the Jeffrey-Salmon view (as distinguished from the early Hempelian view) to evolutionary explanations.

20. On this score it is instructive to compare Cartwright's (1983) comments about the laws of physics; but also see Horan (1988) for a criticism of Cartwright in the biological sciences.

21.There are several useful anthologies which reprint some of the major papers and also capture the nature of the interaction among these various issues. See Brandon and Burian 1984, and Sober 1984a, as well as Depew and Weber 1985. Also several monographs touch on these issues, such as Sober 1984b, Eldredge 1985, and Lloyd 1988.

Chapter Eight

1. The stellar and chemical evolution referred to here are taken in the senses of evolution of the stars from hydrogen atoms and the evolution of the chemical elements.

2. Further below I will return to a rather different type of approach which also appears to ascribe animistic aspects to nature when I discuss Rosenberg's (1985) "intentionality" argument.

3. "Neutral" here is taken in the sense that the account would apply *both* to intentional and to non-intentional systems.

4. The term is based on the Greek word for governor: kubernetes.

5. Page references here are to the version reprinted in Canfield 1966.

6. The notion of "causal priority" is defined and discussed on p. 299 above.

7. Ruse's most recent observations about function and teleology can be found in his introductory handbook on the philosophy of biology (1988, chapter 5). Also see his (1986) essay for additional comments on function and teleology.

8. See chapter 7, p. 355 for a discussion of Brandon's ecological explanation.

9. I ignore migration here because I do not believe it affects this argument.

10. Not all philosophers of biology would agree with this view. In particular James Lennox (personal communication) believes that Lewontin's suggestion leaves out the important focus that should be retained on *selective* features, and my reading of Brandon, who writes that "whatever the importance of natural selection relative to other evolutionary mechanisms [such as drift or pleiotropy], only natural selection can lead to adaptations" (1990, 175).

11. See Crow and Kimura (1970, chapter 5). Also see Kitcher's comments on this issue (1985, chapter 7).

12. In n. 34, I recount the highly idealized parable from Simon about the watchmakers Tempus and Hora, which shows how a part-whole relation is likely to be established by natural selection.

13. Compare Kitcher's views in chapter 7 of his 1985, which argues against the adaptationist program and an optimality thesis, though it does not stress the implications of his arguments for purposive views of evolutionary theory.

14. Moore's arguments that "good" cannot be defined naturalistically have led to a large critical literature, primarily in philosophical ethics. For a criticism of Moore, as well as linkage to Hume's problem of the *is-ought* distinction, see Bernard Williams's insightful 1985, chapter 7.

15. For a discussion of "synthetic identities" see chapter 9, p. 466.

16. I think this hope for at least a *neo*-Aristotelian picture of the world is what motivates some of Lennox's recent (1992) analyses of teleology. Lennox usefully distinguishes between two types of teleology, an extrinsic Platonic type and an "internal" Aristotelian form. Using these distinctions, the position I defend in the present chapter can perhaps be stated as one that sees the Aristotelian form as depending on a covert Platonic type which has important heuristic advantages.

17. See Williams (1985, especially chapters 3, 7, and 8) and also Mackie (1977).

18. Page references are to the version reprinted in Sober (1984a).

19. Wimsatt (personal communication) indicates that he is "bothered" by the "cloner" example given above and suggests that it plays the role of a "Deus ex machina" permitting me to postulate no complexity of the reproduced entities, and therefore no genotype-phenotype distinction. If such complexity were incorporated, he further suggests, the conclusions I draw would not follow.

But it seems to me that the needed complexity could be added and that it would not affect my conclusions. In place of the cloner, substitute for the "ball bearings" small, "simple" unicellular creatures that look like ball bearings. Provide them with a nucleic acid-based genome that can produce the *a*, *b*, and *c* surface roughness phenotypes, which perhaps originated through simple mutations. Also provide them with a reproductive mechanism that is sensitive to surface contact and has temporal limitations, such that the *a* type of cells do not spend a sufficient amount of time in contact with the surface to permit their nucleic acid unwinding and replication occurring before they are "in the air" again, and thus they do not replicate. Keep this system sufficiently simple that we can characterize the replication and genotype → phenotype causal chains in full detail. Then I submit that we have incorporated the requested Wimsattian complexity but have not altered the force of the argument.

20. This expression could be made more complex so as to postulate that health, survival, or (and) reproductive fitness is (are) a G state(s) and that the "purpose" of various systems is to contribute to that (those) state(s).

21. I provide a detailed example of how this is done on p. 385.

22. "Creationists," for example, are not likely to hold this view.

23. See Watson et al. (1987, 834), who describe "The *need* [of the immune system] to constantly monitor the entire body for invading substances." Also compare Lewin's description of bacteria in his introductory remarks about the operon mechanism, where he writes: "Bacteria *need* to be able to respond swiftly to changes in their environment" (1985, 221; my emphases).

24. See Campbell (1974).

25. Following Gould and Vrba (1982), this would be a stage *after* feathers had been coopted into assisting flight.

26. The force of Cummins's argument may depend on his theory of functional ascription, though I will argue further below that his account is flawed and begs the question at a critical point.

27. Three Mile Island is the location of a near meltdown of a nuclear power plant. Excess radiation is believed to have been released into the atmosphere in this area.

28. Wimsatt (personal communication) would argue for a weaker "satisficing" interpretation, though I do not think that replacing "optimality" by "satisficing" makes any difference here. My colleague James Lennox (personal communication), however, disagrees.

29. Such strengthening could be accomplished by satisfying Brandon's five conditions for "ideally complete adaptation explanations"; see chapter 7.

30. In some higher animals, ends-in-view based on memories and primitive imagination may well come into play.

31. We do this, as Braithwaite pointed out in his 1953, when we attribute a goal to a homing torpedo as it corrects its trajectory in pursuit of a target's evasive behavior.

32. Such an argument may be made in the case of some higher animals or even in the case of certain very advanced (and not yet built) artificial intelligences.

33. I should qualify this point. Identification of a general end or an appropriate quantity that was "maximized" would do the trick here, but that is not the *only* way that evolution could be made to support an account of functional analysis. More specific types of goals, if defensible, would also suffice. I owe this point to James Lennox.

34. Herbert Simon has developed a little parable to explain the evolution of complex systems in which part/whole relationships develop. The sketch is a kind of "genetic argument" of the sort analyzed in chapter 7, but of an intentionally very general sort rather than one of the more specific types of sequences I have instanced in the previous chapter.

Simon suggests we consider what would happen to two watchmakers who bear the appropriate names of Tempus and Hora. The two watchmakers had different working methods: Hora built his watches out of subassemblies, each containing 10 parts, 10 of which could be put together to form a larger subassembly. Ten of those larger units would then in turn be linked to form the 1000-part watch. Tempus, on the other hand, constructed a similarly complex 1000-part timepiece in sequence, *without* subassemblies. Both watch makers were continually interrupted by telephone calls, with the result that Tempus had to begin his assembly *anew* each time, whereas Hora could rebuild from pre-asssembled components.

Simon outlined a rough probabilistic account of the effect of interruptions on Tempus's and Hora's tasks. If the probability that an interruption will occur before an assembly (or subassembly) is completed is p, the probability that Tempus will complete his task is $(1 - p)^{1000}$, whereas Hora's is $(1 - p)^{10}$. (The exponents in the expressions are, of course, the numbers of parts which must be assembled in sequence.) Simon points out that if p is 0.01, or "one chance in one hundred that either watchmaker will be interrupted while adding any one part to an assembly [or subassembly], then a straightforward calculation shows that it will take Tempus on the average of about four thousand times as long to assemble a watch as Hora" (Simon 1981, 201). (Details of the numerical argument can be found in Simon (1981, 202).)

Simon suggests that the parable can be applied to biological evolution:

> The time required for the evolution of a complex form from simple elements depends critically on the numbers and distribution of potential intermediate stable forms. In particular, if there exists a hierarachy of potential stable "subassemblies," with about the same span, s, at each level of the hierarchy, then the time required for a subassembly can be expected to be about the same at each level—that is, proportional to $1/(1 - p)^s$. The time required for the assembly of a system of n elements will be proportional to $\log_s n$, that is, to the number of levels in the system. One would say—with more illustrative than literal intent—that the time required for the evolution of multicelled organisms from single-celled organisms might be of the same order of magnitude as the time required for the evolution of single-celled organisms from macromolecules. The same arugment could be applied to the evolution of proteins from amino acids, of molecules from atoms, of atoms from elementary particles. (1981, 202–203)

Simon is aware that this is a very oversimplified scheme, but it seems to me to show the role that evolutionary theory and generalized genetic accounts can play in rationalizing explanations in a variety of domains in biology and medicine.

35. I have in mind here such expressions as the "*task* for these enzymes" emphasized by Rosenberg in his quotation from Stryer's textbook; see p. 401 for Rosenberg's full quotation. I should add here that Rosenberg's account of teleology *in biology*, which follows to some extent Cummins's views, is *not* perceived by Rosenberg as involving intentionality.

36. Case I: The *teleological* sense of function:

DFT: $'F_t (B(i), S, E, P, T) = C' =_{df}$.

(i) B(i) is a *proper subsystem* of S or B(i) and S are elements in a closed functional loop, and according to the causal laws of T under conditions (B(i), S, E', E):

(ii) *Ceteris paribus*, B(i) does C in E' with frequency or probability, $q \ (0 < q \leq 1)$.

(iii) *Ceteris paribus,* that C is done by B(i) in E' with frequency or probability q promotes the attainment of P by S in E with frequency or probability r (0 <r ≤1), where P is a *simple, primary* purpose, and E is identical with or a temporal successor of E. (1972, 41)

Case 2: The *evaluative* sense of function:

$$DFE: 'F_e (B(i), S, E, P, T) = C' = {}_{df}.$$

(i) Same as (i) of DFT

(ii) Same as (ii) of DFT

(iii) *Ceteris paribus,* that C is done by B(*i*) in E' with frequency or probability q promotes the meeting of P by S in E with frequency or probability r (0< r ≤ 1), where P is a logically simple criterion of an evaluative standard, and E is identical with or a temporal successor of E'. (Wimsatt 1972, 42)

The E and E' are distinguished to take into account the possibility that a process performed at an earlier time in environment E' may have later functional consequences in environment E. Specifically this augmentation is introduced to take into account the example of the discovery of the immunological function of the thymus gland. The *ceteris paribus* clause introduces some vagueness into the analysis, and Wimsatt attempts to defend the necessity of its incorporation and its legitimacy. I will not be able to comment on this issue and must refer the reader to Wimsatt's article (1972, 51–55).

37. Cummins discusses the classic counterexample of the heart's effect of pumping blood versus it's effect of producing heart sounds in his (1975, 404), but the difference to him is based on sounding right versus sounding wrong.

38. Rosenberg accepts Cummins's account (1985, 58 and 68). Rosenberg appears to be able to outflank the criticism I developed above only by introducing a notion of "the body's needs" (1985, 58). But this strategy begs the question, in my view, by introducing an unanalyzed concept of "needs" that picks out those capacities that are biologically significant. For reasons introduced in the section on Nagel's account, I also do not think that appeals to "directively organized systems" will help resolve this problem (see Rosenberg 1985, 52–59).

39. It also appears to me that the quotation from Harvey which Rosenberg uses to support his (and Cummins's) analysis (see his 1985, 47) makes better sense in Harvey's milieu on the divine designer (or Aristotelian final cause grounds) and in the present day on evolutionary grounds.

40. It is unfortunate that the difficulty of the problem is also compounded by the two rather different senses of the word "intentional" that are involved here: intentional in the sense of "intend" versus intentional in the sense of "aboutness."

41. As I have suggested in chapter 7 and again in the present chapter, I doubt that this can be done.

42. Also compare Rosenberg (1985) for somewhat similar but, I think, much stronger views.

Chapter Nine

1. From time to time vitalist or vitalist-like theses surface in contemporary biology. For one such example see Sheldrake (1981). (I add the caveat "essentially" in urging this distinction since defenders of in-principle emergentism would strongly object to being labeled vitalists, and would deny the existence of special vital forces. Whether in-principle emergentism makes sense in the absence of such an ontological claim is, I think, a debatable one.)

2. Also see Mayr (1982, 863 n.9).

3. Also see analyses of this notion by Nagel (1961, 380–397) and by Wimsatt (1985).

4. In Simpson's account, historical explanations are added in addition to these two types of explanation.

5. Mayr (1982) has usefully distinguished reduction into three forms: (1) constitutive, (2) explanatory, and (3) theory reduction. He takes a strong unilevel interpretation of the latter, one that I do not take in my analysis of theory/model reduction further below. S. Sakar has developed Mayr's notion of "explanatory" reduction in very fruitful ways in his 1989.

6. Nagel's example of some of these are the Newtonian axioms of mechanics in the kinetic theory of gases (1961, 347).

7. Darden (personal communication) has suggested that the Kemeny-Oppenheim model might best be conceived of as "eliminative" since it does not require the retention of the reduced theory's ontology.

8. Philosophers since Nagel (1947) have characterized as "reductions" even those theories which seem to be on the same "level." Nagel's term for this type of reduction is "homogeneous" reduction (1961, 339). Also compare Feyerabend (1962) on Aristotle, the impetus theorists, Galileo, and Newton in the area of mechanics. Nickles (1973) suggests we treat homogeneous and heterogeneous forms of reduction quite differently, but this does not seem right to me; see my 1976 (624–628) for counterarguments. I will later consider a generalization of this notion to "complex homogeneous" reductions.

9. The features of the general reduction model as of 1967 were stated as follows (some of the vocabulary is technical to permit logical precision):

GENERAL REDUCTION MODEL
T_1 — the reducing theory
T_2 — the original reduced theory
T_2^* — the "corrected" reduced theory

Reduction occurs if and only if: (1) All primitive terms $q_1 \ldots q_n$ appearing in the *corrected* secondary theory T_2^* appear in the primary theory T_1 (in the case of homogeneous reductions) or are associated with one or more of T_1's terms, such that (a) it is possible to set up a one-to-one correspondence representing synthetic identity between individuals or groups of individuals of T_1 and T_2^* or between individuals of one theory and a subclass of groups of the other, in such a way that a reduction function can be specified whose values exhaust the universe of T_2^* for arguments in the universe of T_1; (b) all the primitive predicates of T_2^* are effectively associated with an open sentence of T_1 in n free variables such that F^n_i is fulfilled by an n-tuple of values of the reduction function always and only when the open sentence is fulfilled by the corresponding n-tuple of arguments . . . ; (c) all reduction functions cited in (a) and (b) be specifiable, have empirical support, and in general be interpretable as expressing referential identity. (2) Given fulfillment of condition (1), that T_2^* be derivable from T_1 when T_1 is conjoined with the reduction functions mentioned above. (3) T_2^* corrects T_2 in the sense of providing more accurate experimentally verifiable predictions than T_2 in almost all cases, and should also indicate why T_2 was incorrect (e.g., crucial variable ignored), and why it worked as well as it did. (4) T_2 should be explicable by T_1 in the non-formal sense that T_1 yields a deductive consequence (when supplemented by reduction functions) T_2^* which bears a close similarity to T_2, and produces numerical predictions which are "very close" to T_2's. Finally (5) the relations between T2 and T2* should be one of strong analogy—that is (in current jargon) they possess a large "positive analogy." (Schaffner 1967, 144)

10. Paul Churchland's position seems closest to the general reduction-replacement model I proposed in my 1977, which is elaborated further below.

11. See chapters 3 and 5 above for a discussion of the usefulness of the semantic approach to scientific theory.

12. I will occasionally use the terms "reductans" and "reductandum" for "reducing theory/model" and "reduced theory/ model" respectively.

13. Watson et al. (1987, 8–11) use both "law" and "principle" as terms to describe independent segregation and independent assortment.

14. Olby reissued his 1966 monograph in a second edition in 1985. Also see Darden (1991, chapter 11), who shows that Mendel's two laws were not clearly conceptually separated until anomalies with independent assortment forced that distinction early in this century.

15. See the papers in Voeller (1968) as well as the account of Darden (1990).

16. Quotes from Hull (1974) above and in the following paragraphs are taken from pages 39–44 of his book.

17. Compare Strickberger (1976, 1985), who has a chapter (11) on the notion in his textbook, but uses that chapter to introduce a number of

topics only weakly related to "dominance." Also compare Watson et al. (1987), who introduce the notion in their discussion of Mendel's laws and then effectively outflank the need for the notion in the remainder of a very large book. Also see n. 19.

18. David Hull, in comments at an informal symposium on reduction held in Chicago in 1973, argued that a cellular environment should also be specified since changes in that environment can affect dominance. I view this point as correct, but I also think that it can be handled as part of normally understood ceteris paribus conditions.

19. Muller's original article suggesting his analysis of dominant and recessive genes into amorph, hypomorph, and hypermorph classes appears in his 1932 (213). A more recent account of this quantitative theory of dominance can be found in Wagner and Mitchell's 1964.

20. This lack of a complete account, as I see it, is a problem for Balzer and Dawe (1986), who contend they provide an axiomatic and quite formal treatment of the reduction of classical genetics by molecular genetics. Kitcher, in his 1984, argues against the need (or possibility in terms of "natural kinds") of such a complete account, but, I think, incorrectly. See my discussion of Kitcher and his (R3) thesis further below.

21. The synthetic identity interpretation of entity reduction functions and the extensional construal of n-ary predicates as ordered n-tuples of entities suggests that, from a logical (syntactic) point of view, ultimately all reduction functions connect reduced entities with reducing entities. This point was noted as a footnote in the textbox introducing the formal conditions of the GRR model earlier.

22. From a syntactical point of view this seems correct and reasonable. Wimsatt (1976b) questions whether this is the best way to conceive of reduction. It seems to me that it offers clarity, but that it may need to be supplemented with a more causal/mechanical view to be complete; see section 9.5.3.

23. The terminology is not often used now, but Strickberger (1985, chapter 11) and Wagner and Mitchell (1964, 394–401) cover gene interactions and biochemical explanations of them. The term "epistasis" does not appear in Watson et al.'s (1987) lengthy index, presumably because so many other genetic (DNA, etc.) interactions have been found to exist that this one is not viewed as very salient.

24. See my 1974a for an analysis of Jacob and Monod's reasoning.

25. Kitcher actually uses the weaker biconditional "≡" rather than the stronger "=."

26. Kitcher does note that some genes are made of RNA but sees this as an added complication supporting his own argument.

27. Paraphrased from Kitcher (1984, 343–346).

28. The first indication that recombination and mutation might be occurring within a functional genetic unit seems to have been noted by

C. P. Oliver in his 1940. Corwin and Jenkins suggest that "Oliver's paper was received with great surprise and skepticism" (1976, 113).

29. Page references are to the version of Benzer's 1956 reprinted in Corwin and Jenkins' 1976.

30. Other "cloning vectors" including phage λ, cosmids, and "yeast artificial chromosomes" are also used (OTA 1988, 36).

31. Pedagogically useful in Rosenberg's account is his introduction of the notion in terms of an example using "clocks" and all devices which have time-keeping properties (1985, 114–115). Rosenberg also introduces an argument intended to show that the type of ontological reduction he defends under the rubric of "supervenience" will not permit any indeterministic emergent properties (see his 1985, 116).

32. I suspect that supervenience may have more utility in connection with definitions of "fitness," to which Rosenberg also applies the notion (see his 1985, 164–166).

33. I say "prima facie dissimilarity" since some philosophers, notably Paul and Patricia Churchland (1986), have argued the contrary. Also see Kim's 1989 (38) where he argues that species-specific biconditional laws may "breathe new life into psychophysical reductionism."

34. See Schwartz (1977).

35. Recall that (R1) and (R2) were introduced and criticized above.

36. Paraphrased from Kitcher (1984, 347–350).

37. A good introductory but elegant account of the types of constraints which may have been operative on chemically evolving systems can be found in Eigen et al. 1982. In his discussion of physicochemical forces, Kitcher appears to be thinking of those forces as they function in strictly physicochemical and nonbiological systems, and this may be the source of his error. The confusion between two forms of reductionism, what I call below structural reductionism, which I think is defensible, and ultimate reductionism, which is a fantasy, is rather common in the philosophy of biology.

38. A good introduction to the complexities of the relations between genetics and cytology can be found in the collection of extracts from the papers of that time edited by Voeller (1968) and also in Darden's (1991) forthcoming book.

39. See the papers in Voeller (1968) and also Darden (1990, chapter 10). Darden indicates that in many ways genetics led the cytology.

40. Also referred to as "the Pa-ja-mo experiment," but called "pajama" not only for the names of the experimenters but also because it was a "mating" experiment (Monod, personal comunication).

41. But see n. 42 as a reminder that these levels are primarily ones of generality rather than aggregation.

42. A good example of the distinction between a low level of generality (what I refer to as a δ-level) and a low level of aggregation (which is often de facto a molecular or chemical level) can be found in

Bateson's early speculations that genes were like Larmorean singularities in an aether field. Here we have an example of a nonmolecular δ-level hypothesis. See Coleman's 1970 for a discussion of Bateson's ideas, and Schaffner (1972) for more information about Larmor's aether.

43. See Olby (1973) for a good discussion of these views.

44. Thus a molecular geneticist will *assume* extensive knowledge on the part of her readers of DNA, RNA, etc.

45. I added the term "hook-up" here to distinguish these connections within a system from reduction functions or "bridge laws" that are connections (of a different sort) between reduced and reducing systems.

46. It may seem paradoxical that molecular biological explanations are not unilevel reductions, but the empirical evidence for this view is overwhelming. Bill Bechtel (personal communication) has argued that thus we are not capturing "reduction" by admitting interlevel features. I would admit that we are not capturing a *unilevel* reduction, but the account given suggests that the higher-level theory is itself not unilevel, and the examples suggest that what occurs is that we move closer to a biochemical explanation but do not typically achieve it in any full sense (with very few exceptions, and those primarily in very simple biochemistry). I elaborate on this issue in more detail below.

47. We could accept the Suppes-Adams approach as described above for reduction, though this would have to be supplemented by a syntactic requirement of connectability that was more than isomorphism (or, more generally, homomorphism) and also a semantic requirement to interpret the connectability assumptions as synthetic identities (for entities).

48. See Suppes (1957, 294–298) for such a predicate, containing Newton's second and third laws of motion as axioms P7, P5, and P6.

49. For probabilistic consequences we would have to use some form of inductive logic, where particular cases were concerned. Other forms of logic, e.g., nonmonotonic logics, are notoriously suspect (see Ginsberg 1987).

50. Further below I will relate this approach to Kitcher's proposal that we replace a discussion of traditional reduction with an analysis that focuses on explanatory extensions and embedding.

51. Good examples are Maxwell's concern about the derivability of Snell's laws (see Schaffner 1972, chapter 5) and Poincaré's troubles over the recurrence theorem in connection with mechanics and thermodynamics (Brush 1966, introduction and papers 5 and 6).

52. See n. 8 for a discussion of Nagel's "homogeneous reduction." For Nagel, the distinction was introduced to allow for "reduction" even when one did not go to a new level of aggregation but only to a new level of generality. At the time, Nagel thought the meanings of the terms would not change as one moved, say, from Galilean motions to

Newtonian motions (this was pre-Kuhn and pre-Feyerabend). As discussed in chapter 5, I do not see meaning variance as a serious issue, but the reader should be aware that Nagel is assuming stable theoretical meaning in his classical account.

53. See my discussion of Kitcher in chapter 6, p. 312, for a discussion of his notion of a problem-solving pattern, and also generally his 1989 essay.

54. See Chothia (1985) and, more generally, Watson et al. (1987, chapter 5). Our appreciation of the complexity of the protein-folding process recently increased considerably with the discovery of so-called molecular chaperones, whose function is to assist the proper folding of proteins in vivo. See the recent review of Langer et al. (1992) for a discussion of chaperone-mediated protein folding.

55. Compare this historically important but very oversimplified, diagrammatic account of base pairing with Watson et al's (1987) very complex and still not fully understood account, as quoted on p. 510.

56. Many processes in biology are understood to involve self-assembly, from the construction of the quaternary structure of the hemoglobin molecule to that of collagen and of viral and phage particles. See Watson et al. (1987, 159–160).

57. This does not mean that there are no chances for experimental determinations of chemical fossils. Watson et al. (1987, chapter 28) suggest means of conjecturing such fossils.

58. See the references cited in n. 54 on the prospects of determining tertiary structure from primary structure.

59. For a recent discussion of quantum-mechanical effects on enzymology, see Cha, Murray, and Klinman (1989) on hydrogen tunneling.

60. If semi-empirical results are permitted, the problem may not be so insuperable. Calculations from first principles (or what are termed "a priori" calculations) present severe computational problems.

61. I would include biochemistry in this since most of the important biochemical processes involve enzymes and thus tertiary structures.

62. Not that such detail is unimportant in providing the ultimate explanation of biology in terms of biochemistry. The examples to be cited below will, I think, indicate the complex dimensions of the "peripherality thesis."

63. Since I first put forth this thesis in my 1974b, there have been two interesting types of developments relevant to it. The major movement in molecular biology has been toward more detailed characterization of the entities at the molecular level, but there is a realization that "sequence" is not all that is important (on this also see my 1989). Also of interest was Wimsatt's (1976b) expansion of the peripherality thesis toward a "functional" model of reduction.

64. In this respect, this type of research is akin to the kind of research in which the human genome project is engaged. The monotonous and boring nature of detailed genetic mapping work has led to concerns

about the speed with which this major scientific enterprise can be completed. A recent article, "Creation of Linkage Map Falters, Posing Delay for Genome Project" *The Scientist* 4, [Jan 1990]: 1 and 10–12), notes that: "The reasons why genome mapping has stumbled point to the pitfalls of big science. Some scientists have rebelled at the numbingly repetitive nature of the work, while others who had actually embarked on large scale mapping projects have redirected their research at the first sign of a possibly interesting disease gene" (4: 10). The article also chronicles social pressures: "Adds NIH Panel member Philip Sharp, a cancer researcher at the Massachusetts Institute of Technology, 'young people have to do something interesting within five to seven years [of receiving their degree]. If they don't, they'll get bored, they won't get promoted or get tenure, and they won't get grants.'" (4: 12).

65. See Watson et al. (1987, 146) for indications that the *lac* repressor has a standard modular construction.

66. See Raiffa's 1968.

Bibliography

American Association for Artificial Intelligence. 1986. *Proceedings AAAI-86: Fifth National Conference on Artificial Intelligence.* 2 vols. Los Altos, Calif.: Morgan Kaufmann.

Achinstein, P. 1968. *Concepts of Science.* Baltimore: Johns Hopkins Press.

_____. 1970. "Inference to Scientific Laws." In *Historical and Philosophical Perspectives of Science,* ed. R. Stuewer, 87–104. Minnesota Studies in the Philosophy of Science, vol. 5, Minneapolis: University of Minnesota Press.

_____. 1971. *Law and Explanation.* Oxford: Oxford University Press.

_____. 1983. *The Nature of Explanation.* New York: Oxford University Press.

_____. 1987. "Scientific Discovery and Maxwell's Kinetic Theory." *Philosophy of Science* 54:409–434.

Aczél, J. 1966. *Lectures on Functional Equations and Their Applications.* New York: Academic Press.

Ada, G., and Nossal, G. 1987. "The Clonal Selection Theory," *Scientific American* 257 (August): 62–68.

Adams, E. 1959. "The Foundations of Rigid Body Mechanics and the Derivation of Its Laws from Those of Particle Mechanics." In *The Axiomatic Method,* ed. L. Henkin, P. Suppes, and A. Tarski. Amsterdam: North-Holland.

Alexander, J. 1931. "Some Intracellular Aspects of Life and Disease." *Protoplasma* 14:296–356.

Alkon, D. 1989. "Memory Storage and Neural Systems." *Scientific American* 261 (July): 42–50

Allison, A. 1955. "Aspects of Polymorphism in Man." *Population Genetics: The Nature and Causes of Genetic Variability in Populations.* Cold Spring Harbor Symposia on Quantitative Biology, vol. 20, 239–255. Cold Spring Harbor, N.Y.: The Biological Laboratory.

_____. 1964. "Polymorphism and Natural Selection in Human Populations." *Human Genetics.* Cold Spring Harbor Symposia on Quantitative Biology, vol. 29, 137–150.

Ames, B., and Hartman, P. 1963. "The Histidine Operon." *Synthesis and Structure of Macromolecules.* Cold Spring Harbor Symposia on Quantitative Biology, vol. 28, 349–356.

Anderson, J. 1938. "The Problem of Causality." *Australasian Journal of Psychology and Philosophy* 14:127–142.

Anscombe, E. 1971. *Causality and Determination*. London: Cambridge University Press.

Arber, A. 1954. *The Mind and the Eye*. Cambridge: Cambridge University Press.

Archer, O., and Pierce, J. C. 1961. "The Role of the Thymus in Development of the Immune Response." *Federation Proceedings* 20:26.

Armendt, B. 1980. "Is There a Dutch Book Argument for Probability Kinematics?" *Philosophy of Science* 47:583–588.

Arnason, B. G.; Jankovic, B. D.; and Waksman, B. H. 1962. "Effect of Thymectomy on 'Delayed' Hypersensitive Reactions." *Nature* 194:99–100.

Arnold, A., and Fistrup, K. 1982. "The Theory of Evolution by Natural Selection: A Hierarchical Expansion." *Paleobiology* 8:113–129.

Asquith, P., and Giere, R., eds. 1980 and 1981. *PSA–1980: Proceedings of the 1980 Biennial Meeting of the Philosophy of Science Association*. 2 vols. East Lansing, Mich.: Philosophy of Science Association.

Attardi, G.; Cohn, M.; Horibata, K.; and Lennox, E. 1959. "On The Analysis of Antibody Synthesis at the Cellular Level." *Bacteriological Reviews* 23:213–223

———. 1964. "Antibody Formation by Rabbit Lymph Node Cells: I, II, and III." *Journal of Immunology* 92:335–345, 346–355, 356–371.

Ayala, F. J. 1968. "Biology as an Autonomous Science." *American Scientist* 56:207–221.

———. 1970. "Teleological Explanations in Evolutionary Biology." *Philosophy of Science* 37:1–15.

Bacon, F. 1960 [1620]. *The New Organon*. Indianapolis, Ind.: Bobbs–Merrill.

Balzer, W., and Dawe, C. M. 1986. "Structure and Comparison of Genetic Theories: Part 1, Classical Genetics; Part 2, The Reduction of Character–Factor Genetics to Molecular Genetics." *British Journal for the Philosophy of Science* 37:55–69, 177–191.

Barcan[–Marcus], R. 1947. "The Identity of Individuals in a Strict Functional Calculus of the Second Order." *Journal of Symbolic Logic* 12:12–15.

Barnett, V. 1982. *Comparative Statistical Inference*. 2d ed. Chichester: Wiley.

Barrett, J. 1988. *Textbook of Immunology*. 5th ed. St. Louis: Mosby.

Bayarri, M.; DeGroot, M.; and Kadane, J. 1988. "What Is the Likelihood Function?" In *Statistical Decision Theory and Related Topics IV*, vol. 1, ed. S. Gupta and J. Berger, 3–16. New York: Springer-Verlag.

Beadle, G., and Tatum, E. 1941. "Genetic Control of Biochemical Reactions in *Neurospora*." *Proceedings of the National Academy of Sciences USA* 27:499–506.

Beatty, J. 1981. "What's Wrong with the Received View of Evolutionary Theory?" In Asquith and Giere, 397–439.

_____. 1987. "On Behalf of the Semantic View." *Biology and Philosophy* 2:17–23.

_____. 1992. "The Evolutionary Contingency Thesis and Its Role as a Unifying Principle in Philosophy of Biology." (draft manuscript.)

Bechtel, W. 1986a. "The Nature of Scientific Integration." In *Integrating Scientific Disciplines*, ed. W. Bechtel, 3–52. Dordrecht: Martinus Nijhoff.

_____. 1986b. "Teleological Functional Analyses and the Hierarchical Organization of Nature." In ed. Rescher, 1986, 26–48.

Bechtel, W., and Richardson, R. 1992. *Discovering Complexity: Decomposition and Localization as Strategies in Scientific Research*. Princeton: Princeton University Press.

Beckner, M. 1959. *The Biological Way of Thought*. New York: Columbia University Press.

_____. 1969. "Function and Teleology." *Journal of the History of Biology* 2:151–164.

Beckwith, J., and Zipser, D. eds. 1970. *The Lactose Operon*. Cold Spring Harbor, N.Y.: Cold Spring Harbor Laboratory of Quantitative Biology.

Benzer, S. 1956. "The Elementary Units of Heredity." In *A Symposium on the Chemical Basis of Heredity*, ed. W. D. McElroy and B. Glass, 70–93. Baltimore: Johns Hopkins University Press.

Bernard, C. 1957 [1865]. *An Introduction to the Study of Experimental Medicine*. Trans. H. C. Green. New York: Dover.

Bernardo, J. 1980. "A Bayesian Analysis of Classical Hypothesis Testing." In Bernardo et al. 1980.

Bernardo, J.; DeGroot, M.; Lindley, D.; and Smith, A. 1980. *Bayesian Statistics: Proceedings of the First International Meeting Held in Valencia, Spain, May 28 to June 2, 1979*. Valencia, Spain: Valencia University Press.

Beth, E. 1949. "Towards an Up-to-Date Philosophy of the Natural Sciences." *Methods* 1 (no. 2): 178–85.

Bibel, D. J. 1988. *Milestones in Immunology: A Historical Exploration*. Madison, Wis.: Science Tech Publishers.

Billingham R., and Silvers, W. 1971. *The Immunobiology of Transplantation*. Englewood Cliffs, N.J.: Prentice-Hall.

Blackburn, R., ed. 1966. *Interrelations: The Biological and Physical Sciences*. Chicago: Scott, Foresman.

Blum, R. L. 1982. "Discovery and Representation of Causal Relationships from a Large Time–Oriented Clinical Data Base." Ph.D. diss., Stanford University.

Bock, W. 1979. "A Synthetic Explanation of Macroevolutionary Change — A Reductionist Approach." *Bulletin Carnegie Museum of Natural History* 13:20–69.

Bohr, N. 1987 [1933]. "Light and Life." In *Essays 1932–1957 on Atomic Physics and Human Knowledge*, by N. Bohr, 3–12. Woodbridge, Conn.: Ox Bow Press. Essay originally appeared in *Nature* 131:421–423.

Box, G., and Tiao, G. 1973. *Bayesian Inference in Statistical Analysis*. Reading, Mass.: Addison-Wesley.

Boyd, R. 1979. "Metaphor and Theory Change: What Is 'Metaphor' a Metaphor for?" In *Metaphor and Thought*, ed. A. Otorny, 356–408. Cambridge: Cambridge University Press.

Brachman, R. 1985. "'I Lied about the Trees' or Defaults and Definitions in Knowledge Representation." *AI Magazine* 6 (no. 3): 80–93.

Brand, M., ed. 1976. *The Nature of Causation*. Urbana, Ill.: University of Illinois Press.

Brandon, R. 1978. "Adaptation and Evolutionary Theory." *Studies in History and Philosophy of Science* 9:181–206.

———. 1981. "Biological Teleology: Questions and Explanations." *Studies in History and Philosophy of Science* 12:91–105.

———. 1982. "The Levels of Selection." In *PSA–1982*, vol. 1, ed. P. Asquith and T. Nickles, 315–324. East Lansing, Mich.: Philosophy of Science Association.

———. 1990. *Adaptation and Environment*. Princeton: Princeton University Press.

Brandon, R., and Burian, R. eds. 1984. *Genes, Organisms, Populations: Controversies over the Units of Selection*. Cambridge, Mass.: MIT Press.

Breinl, F., and Haurowitz, F. 1930. "Chemische Unterschungen des Praezipitates aus Haemoglobin und Antihaemoglobin–Serum und Bemerkungen über die Natur der Antikörper." *Zeitschrift Physiologie Chemie* 192:45–57.

Britten, R. J., and Davidson, E. H. 1969. "Gene Regulation for Higher Cells: A Theory." *Science* 165:349–57.

Brody, B. 1972. "Towards an Aristotelian Theory of Scientific Explanation." *Philosophy of Science* 39:20–31.

Bromberger, S. 1961. "The Concept of Explanation." Ph.D. diss. Harvard University.

Brush, S. G. 1966. *Kinetic Theory I and II*. Oxford: Pergamon Press.

Buchanan, B. 1985. "Step Toward Mechanizing Discovery." In *Logic of Discovery and Diagnosis in Medicine*, ed. K. F. Schaffner, 94–114. Berkeley: University of California Press.

Buckley, C.; Whitney, P.; and Tanford, C. 1963. "The Unfolding and Renaturation of a Specific Univalent Antibody Fragment." *Proceedings of the National Academy of Sciences USA* 50:827–834.

Burian, R. 1988. "Challenges to the Evolutionary Synthesis." *Evolutionary Biology* 23:247–269.

Burian, R. 1989. "The Influence of the Evolutionary Paradigm." In *Evolutionary Biology at the Crossroads*, ed. M. Hecht, 149–166. New York: Queens College Press.

Burch, P., and Burwell, R. 1965. "Self and Not-Self: A Clonal Induction Approach to Immunology." *Quarterly Review of Biology* 40: 252–279.

Burnet, F.M. 1957a. "Cancer—A Biological Approach." *British Medical Journal* 1:779–786, 841–847.

_____. 1957b. "A Modification of Jerne's Theory of Antibody Production Using the Concept of Clonal Selection." *The Australian Journal of Science* 20:67–69.

_____. 1959. *The Clonal Selection Theory of Acquired Immunity*. Nashville, Tenn.: Vanderbilt University Press.

_____. 1962. *The Integrity of the Body*. Cambridge: Harvard University Press.

_____. 1963. "Theories of Immunity." In *Conceptual Advances in Immunology and Oncology*, 7–21. Symposium on Fundamental Cancer Research, M. D. Anderson Hospital and Tumor Institute, Houston, Texas, 1962. New York: Harper and Row.

_____. 1964. "A Darwinian Approach to Immunity" *Nature* 203:451–454.

_____. 1967. "The Impact of Ideas on Immunology." In *Antibodies*. Cold Spring Harbor Symposia on Quantitative Biology, vol. 32, 1–8. Cold Spring Harbor, N.Y.: Cold Spring Harbor Laboratory of Quantitative Biology.

_____. 1968. *Changing Patterns*. Melbourne: William Heinemann.

Burnet, F. M., and Fenner, F. 1949. *The Production of Antibodies*. London: Macmillan.

Burstein, M. H. 1986. "Concept Formation by Incremental Analogical Reasoning and Debugging." In Michalski, Carbonell, and Mitchell, 1986, 351–369.

Campbell, N. 1920. *Physics: The Elements*. Cambridge: Cambridge University Press.

Canfield, J. 1964. "Teleological Explanation in Biology." *British Journal for the Philosophy of Science* 14:285–295.

_____, ed. 1966. *Purpose in Nature*. Englewood Cliffs, N.J.: Prentice-Hall.

Carbonell, J. 1986. "Derivational Analogy." In Michalski, Carbonell, and Mitchell, 1986, 371–392.

Carnap, R. 1950. *Logical Foundations of Probability*. Chicago: University of Chicago Press.

_____. 1956. "The Methodological Character of Theoretical Concepts." in *The Foundations of Science and the Concepts of Psychology and Psychoanalysis,* ed. H. Feigl and M. Scriven, 38–76. Minnesota Studies in the Philosophy of Science, vol. 1. Minneapolis: University of Minnesota Press.

Cartwright, N. 1979. "Causal Laws and Effective Strategies." *Nous* 13:419–437

_____. 1983. *How the Laws of Physics Lie.* New York: Oxford University Press.

_____. 1989. *Nature's Capacities and Their Measurement.* New York: Oxford University Press.

Causey, R. 1972. "Attribute–Identities in Microreductions." *Journal of Philosophy* 69:407–422.

_____. 1977. *Unity of Science.* Dordrecht: Reidel.

Cha, Y.; Murray, C.; and Klinman, J. 1989. "Hydrogen Tunneling in Enzyme Reactions." *Science* 243:1325–1330.

Charniak, E., and McDermott, D. 1985. *An Introduction to Artificial Intelligence.* Reading, Mass.: Addison–Wesley.

Chihara, C. 1987. "Some Problems for Bayesian Confirmation Theory." *British Journal for the Philosophy of Science* 38:551–560.

Chothia, C. 1984. "Principles That Determine the Structure of Proteins." *Annual Review of Biochemistry* 53:537–572.

Churchland, P. M. 1979. *Scientific Realism and the Plasticity of Mind.* Cambridge: Cambridge University Press.

_____. 1981. "Eliminative Materialism and the Propositional Attitudes." *Journal of Philosophy* 78:67–90.

_____. 1984. *Matter and Consciousness: A Contemporary Introduction to the Philosophy of Mind.* Cambridge, Mass.: MIT Press.

Churchland, P. M., and Hooker, C., eds. 1985. *Images of Science.* Chicago: University of Chicago Press.

Churchland, P. S. 1986. *Neurophilosophy.* Cambridge: MIT Press.

_____. 1988. "The Significance of Neuroscience for Philosophy." *Trends in Neurosciences* 11:304–306.

Claman, H. N.; Chaperon, E. A.; and Triplett, R. F. 1966. "Immunocompetence of Transferred Thymus–Marrow Cell Combinations." *Journal of Immunology* 97:828–32.

Cohen, B. 1982. "Understanding Natural Kinds." Ph.D. diss. Stanford University.

Cohen, B., and Murphy, G. L. 1984. "Models of Concepts." *Cognitive Science* 8:27–58.

Cohen, M., and Nagel, E. 1934. *An Introduction to Logic and the Scientific Method.* London: Routledge and Kegan Paul.

Cohen, R. S.; Hooker, C.; Michalos, A.; and van Evra, J., eds. 1976. *PSA–1974: Proceedings of the 1974 Biennial Meeting Philosophy of Science Association.* Dordrecht: Reidel.

Cole, J., and Zuckerman, H. 1975. "The Emergence of a Scientific Specialty: The Self-Exemplifying Case of the Sociology of Science." In Coser, 1975, 139–174.

Cole, S. 1975. "The Growth of Scientific Knowledge: Theories of Deviance as a Case Study." In Coser, 1975, 175–220.

Coleman, W. 1970. "Bateson and Chromosomes: Conservative Thought in Science." *Centaurus* 15:228–314.

Collingwood, R. G. 1940. *An Essay on Metaphysics.* Oxford: Clarendon Press.

Cooper, M. D.; Peterson, R. D. A.; and Good, R. A. 1965. "Delineation of the Thymic and Bursal Lymphoid Systems in the Chicken." *Nature* 205:143–46.

Corwin, H., and Jenkins, J. 1976. *Conceptual Foundations of Genetics.* Boston: Houghton Mifflin.

Coser, L., ed. 1975. *The Idea of Social Structure: Papers in Honor of Robert K. Merton.* New York: Harcourt Brace Jovanovich.

Coulson, R.; Feltovich, P.; and Spiro, R. 1989. "Foundations of a Misunderstanding of the Ultrastructural Basis of Myocardial Failure: A Reciprocation Network of Oversimplifications." *Journal of Medicine and Philosophy* 14:109–146.

Cox, R. 1946. "Probability, Frequency, and Reasonable Expectation." *American Journal of Physics* 14:1–13.

———. 1961. *The Algebra of Probable Inference.* Baltimore: Johns Hopkins Press.

Crick, F. H. C. 1958. "On Protein Synthesis: Biological Replication of Macromolecules." *Symposium of the Society of Experimental Biology* 12:138–163.

Crick, F. H. C.; Barnett, L.; Brenner, S.; and Watts–Tobin, R. J. 1961. "General Nature of the Genetic Code for Proteins." *Nature* 192:1227–32.

Crown, J. F., and Kimura, M. 1970. *An Introduction to Population Genetics Theory.* New York: Harper and Row.

Culp, S., and Kitcher, P. 1989. "Theory Structure and Theory Change in Contemporary Molecular Biology." *British Journal for the Philosophy of Science* 40:459–483.

Cummins, R. 1975. "Functional Analysis." *Journal of Philosophy* 72:741–765.

Damuth, J., and Heisler, L. 1988. "Alternative Formulations of Multilevel Selection." *Biology and Philosophy* 3:407–430.

Darden, L. 1991. *Theory Change in Science: Strategies from Mendelian Genetics.* New York: Oxford University Press.

Darden, L., and Cain, J. A. 1989. "Selection Type Theories." *Philosophy of Science* 56:106–129.

Darden, L., and Maull, N. 1977. "Interfield Theories." *Philosophy of Science* 44:43–64.

Darden, L., and Rada, R. 1986. "Hypothesis Formation via Interrelations." In ed. A. Prieditis, 109–127. Rutgers, N.J.: Rutgers University Computer Science Department.

Davidson, D. 1980 [1970]. "Mental Events." In *Essays on Actions and Events*, D. Davidson, 207–225. Oxford: Oxford University Press. Essay first published in 1970.

Davidson, D.; Suppes, P.; and Siegle, S. 1957. *Decision Making: An Experimental Approach*. Stanford, Calif.: Stanford University Press.

Dawkins, R. 1976. *The Selfish Gene*. Oxford: Oxford University Press.

DeFinetti, B. 1937. "La prévision; ses lois logiques, ses sources subjectives." *Annales de l'Institut Henri Poincaré* 7:1–68. Reprinted in English translation in Kyburg and Smokler, 1980, 97–158.

de Kleer, J. 1979. "Causal and Teleological Reasoning in Circuit Recognition." *Report TR–529*. Cambridge, Mass.: Massachusetts Institute of Technology Artificial Intelligence Laboratory.

Delbruck, M. 1947. "A Physicist Looks at Biology." *Transactions of the American Academy of Arts and Sciences* 38:173–190. Reprinted in Blackburn, 1966, 117–129.

Depew, D., and Weber, B. 1988. "Consequences of Nonequilibrium Thermodynamics for the Darwinian Tradition." In *Entropy, Information, and Evolution: Perspectives on Physical and Biological Evolution*, ed. B. Weber, D. Depew, and J. Smith, 317–342. Cambridge: MIT Press.

Depew, D., and Weber, B. eds. 1985. *Evolution at the Crossroads: The New Biology and the New Philosophy of Science*. Cambridge: MIT Press.

Descartes, R. 1960 [1701]. "Rules for the Direction of the Mind." In *Philosophical Essays*, by R. Descartes. Trans. L. J. Lafleur. Indianapolis: Bobbs-Merrill.

Dobzhansky, T. 1955. "A Review of Some Fundamental Concepts and Problems of Population Genetics." *Population Genetics: The Nature and Causes of Genetic Variability in Populations*. Cold Spring Harbor Symposia on Quantitative Biology, vol. 20, 1–15.

_____. 1970. *Genetics of the Evolutionary Process*. New York: Columbia University Press.

Dobzhansky, T.; Ayala, F. J. S.; Stebbins, G. L.; and Valentine, J. W. 1977. *Evolution*. San Francisco: W. H. Freeman.

Domotor, Z. 1980. "Probability Kinematics and the Representation of Belief Change." *Philosophy of Science* 47:384–403.

Donnellan, K. 1966. "Reference and Definite Descriptions." *Philosophical Review* 75:281–304.

Doolittle, W., and Sapienza, C. 1980. "Selfish Genes, the Phenotype Paradigm, and Genome Evolution." *Nature* 284:601–603.

Dorland's Illustrated Medical Dictionary 1981. 26th ed. Philadelphia: W. B. Saunders.

Dorling, J. 1979. "Bayesian Personalism, the Methodology of Research Programmes, and Duhem's Problem." *Studies in History and Philosophy of Science* 10:177–187.

Dounce, A. L. 1952. "Duplicating Mechanism for Peptide Chain and Nucleic Acid." *Enzymologia* 15:251–258.

Dray, W. 1957. *Laws and Explanation in History*. Oxford: Oxford University Press.

Driesch, H. 1908. *The Science and Philosophy of the Organism*. London: A. C. Black.

Duhem, P. 1914. *Aim and Structure of Physical Theory*. 2d ed. Trans. P. P. Wiener. New York: Atheneum.

Dupre, J., ed. 1987. *The Latest on the Best: Essays on Evolution and Optimality*. Cambridge: MIT Press.

Earman, J. 1986. *A Primer on Determinism*. Dordrecht: Kluwer.

———. 1992. *Bayes or Bust? A Critical Examination of Bayesian Inference*. Cambridge: MIT Press.

———. 1983. *Testing Scientific Theories*. Minnesota Studies in the Philosophy of Science, vol. 10. Minneapolis: University of Minnesota Press.

Eberle, R.; Kaplan, D.; and Montague, R. 1961. "Hempel and Oppenheim on Explanation." *Philosophy of Science* 28:305–318.

Edwards, W.; Lindman, H.; and Savage, L. 1963. "Bayesian Statistical Inference for Psychological Research." *Psychological Review* 70:193–214.

Eells, E. 1985. "Problems of Old Evidence." *Pacific Philosophical Quarterly* 66:283–302.

Eells, E. and Sober, E. 1983. "Probabilistic Causality and the Question of Transitivity." *Philosophy of Science* 50:35–57.

Efron, B., and Morris, C. 1977. "Stein's Paradox in Statistics." *Scientific American* 236 (May): 119–127.

Eigen, M.; Gardiner W.; Schuster, P.; Winkler–Oswatitsch, R. 1982. "The Origin of Genetic Information." In Smith, J. M., 1982, 10–33.

Einstein, A. 1949. "Autobiographical Notes." In *Albert Einstein: Philosopher-Scientist*, ed. P. A. Schilpp, 1–95. La Salle, Ill.: Open Court.

Eldredge, N. 1985. *Unfinished Synthesis: Biological Hierarchies and Modern Evolutionary Thought*. New York: Oxford University Press.

Eldredge, N., and Gould, S. 1972. "Punctuated Equilibria: An Alternative to Phyletic Gradualism." In ed. T. Schopf, *Models in Paleobiology*. San Francisco: Freeman, Cooper. Pp. 82–115.

Elsasser, W. 1958. *The Physical Foundation of Biology*. London: Pergamon.

578 \ Bibliography

_____. 1966. *Atom and Organism*. Princeton: Princeton University Press.

Enç, B. 1976. "Identity Statements and Microreductions." *Journal of Philosophy* 73: 285–306.

_____. 1979. "Function Attributions and Functional Explanation." *Philosophy of Science* 46:343–365.

Engelmore, R. and Morgan, A. eds.. 1989. *Blackboard Systems*. Reading, Mass.: Addison-Wesley.

Etherington, D., and Reiter R. 1983. "On Inheritance Hierarchies with Exceptions." In *AAAI–83: The National Conference on Artificial Intelligence*, 3d National Conference on Artificial Intelligence, Washington, D.C., 104–108. Los Altos, Calif.: Kaufmann.

Fahlman, S. 1979. *NETL: A System for Representing and Using Real World Knowledge*. Cambridge: MIT Press.

Feigenbaum, E. A.; Buchanan, B. G.; and Lederberg, J. 1971. "On Generality and Problem Solving: A Case Study Using the DENDRAL Program." *Machine Intelligence* 6:165–190.

Feyerabend, P. K. 1962. "Explanation, Reduction, and Empiricism." In *Minnesota Studies in the Philosophy of Science*, edited by H. Feigl and G. Maxwell. Vol. 3. Minneapolis: University of Minnesota Press, 28–97.

_____. 1970. "Consolations for the Specialist." In Lakatos and Musgrave 1970, 197–230.

Field, H. 1975. "Theory Change and the Indeterminancy of Reference." *Journal of Philosophy* 70:462–481.

_____. 1978. "A Note on Jeffrey Conditionalization." *Philosophy of Science* 45: 361–367.

Fikes, R., and Kehler, T. 1985. "The Role of Frame–Based Representation in Reasoning." *Communications of the ACM* 28 (no. 9): 904–920.

Fine, A. 1984. "The Natural Ontological Attitude." In Leplin 1984, 83–107.

Fine, A., and Earman, J. 1977. "Against Indeterminacy." *Journal of Philosophy* 74:535–538.

Fine, A., and Machamer, P. eds. 1986 and 1987 *PSA–1986: Proceedings of the 1986 Biennial Meeting Philosophy Science Association*. 2 vols. East Lansing, Mich.: Philosophy of Science Association.

Fisher, R. A. 1970. *Statistical Methods for Research Workers*. 14th ed., rev. and enl. New York: Hafner.

Fletcher, R. H.; Fletcher, S. W.; and Wagner, E. H. 1982. *Clinical Epidemiology – The Essentials*. Baltimore: Williams and Wilkins.

Fodor, J. 1975. *The Language of Thought*. New York: Crowell.

Forbus, K. D., and Gentner, D. 1986. "Learning Physical Domains: Toward a Theoretical Framework." In Michalski, Carbonell, and Mitchell, 1986, 311–348.

Forget, B. 1982. "Sickle-Cell Anemia and Associated Hemoglobinopathies." In *Cecil Textbook of Medicine*. 16th ed., ed. J. Wyngaarden and L. Smith, 887–893. Philadelphia: Saunders.

Fox, S. 1965. "A Theory of Macromolecular and Cellular Origins." *Nature* 205:328–331.

Frankfurt, H., and Poole, B. 1965. "Functional Analyses in Biology." *British Journal for the Philosophy of Science* 17:69–72.

Franklin, A. 1986. *The Neglect of Experiment*. Cambridge: Cambridge University Press.

Freedman, D., and Spiegelhalter, D. 1983. "The Assessment of Subjective Opinion and Its Use in Relation to Stopping Rules for Clinical Trials." *The Statistician* 32:153–160.

Friedland, P., and Kedes, L. 1985. "Discovering the Secrets of DNA." *Computer*, 18 (Nov.): 49–69.

Friedman, M. 1974. "Explanation and Scientific Understanding." *Journal of Philosophy* 71:5–19.

Frost, W. N.; Clark, G. A.; and Kandel, E. R. 1988. "Parallel Processing of Short-Term Memory for Sensitization in *Aplysia*." *Journal of Neurobiology* 19:297–334.

Fudenberg, H. H.; Good, R. A.; Hitzig, W.; Kunkel, H. G.; Roit, I. M.; Rosen, F. S.; Rowe, D. S.; Seligmann, M.; and Soothill, J. R. 1970. "Classification of the Primary Immune Deficiencies: WHO Recommendation." *New England Journal of Medicine* 283:656–57.

Fuhrmann, G. 1991. "Note on the Integration of Prototype Theory and Fuzzy–Set Theory." *Synthese* 86:1–27.

Fulton, S., and Pepe, C. 1990. "An Introduction to Model–Based Reasoning." *AI Expert* 5 (no. 1): 48–55.

Fuerst, J. A. 1982. "The Role of Reductionism in the Development of Molecular Biology: Peripheral or Central?" *Social Studies of Science* 12:241–278.

Gaifman, H., and Snir, M. 1982. "Probabilities over Rich Languages, Testing, and Randomness." *Journal of Symbolic Logic* 47:495–548.

Galison, P. 1987. *How Experiments End*. Chicago: University of Chicago Press.

Gallie, W. 1955. "Explanations in History and the Genetic Sciences." *Mind* 64:160–180.

Gamow, G. 1954. "Possible Relations between Deoxyribonucleic Acid and Protein Structures." *Nature* 173:318.

Garber, D. 1980. "Field and Jeffrey Conditionalization." *Philosophy of Science* 47:142–145.

———. 1983. "Old Evidence and Logical Omniscience in Bayesian Confirmation Theory." In Earman, 1983, 99–131.

Genesereth, M., and Nilsson, N. 1987. *Logical Foundations of Artificial Intelligence*. Los Altos, Calif.: Morgan Kaufmann.

Genest, C., and Zidek, J. 1986. "Combining Probability Distributions: A Critique and an Annotated Bibliography." *Statistical Science* 1 (no. 1): 114–148.

Ghiselin, M. 1966. "On Psychologism in the Logic of Taxanomic Controversies." *Systematic Zoology* 15:207–215.

———. 1974. "A Radical Solution to the Species Problem." *Systematic Zoology* 23:536–544.

Giere, R. 1975. "The Epistemological Roots of Scientific Knowledge." In *Induction, Probability, and Confirmation Theory,* ed. G. Maxwell and R. Anderson, 212–261. Minnesota Studies in the Philosophy of Science, vol. 6. Minneapolis: University of Minnesota Press.

———. 1976. "Empirical Probability, Objective Statistical Methods, and Scientific Inquiry." In Harper and Hooker, 1976, vol. 2, 63–101.

———. 1977. "Testing Versus Information Models of Statistical Inference." In ed. *Logic, Laws and Life,* ed. R. Colodny, 19–70. University of Pittsburgh Series in the Philosophy of Science, vol. 6. Pittsburgh: University of Pittsburgh Press.

———. 1980. "Causal Systems and Statistical Hypotheses." In *Applications of Inductive Logic,* ed. L. Cohen and M. Hesse, 251–270. Oxford: Oxford University Press.

———. 1984a. *Understanding Scientific Reasoning.* 2d ed. New York: Holt, Reinhart and Winston.

———. 1984b. "Causal Models with Frequency Dependence." *Journal of Philosophy* 81:384–391.

———. 1988. *Explaining Science: A Cognitive Approach.* Chicago: University of Chicago Press.

Gilbert, W., and Maxam, A. 1973. "The Nucleotide Sequence of the *lac* Operator." *Proceedings of the National Academy of Sciences USA* 70:3581–3584.

Gilbert, W., and Müller–Hill, B. 1966. "Isolation of the *Lac* Repressor." *Proceedings of the National Academy of Sciences USA* 56:1891–1898.

———. 1967. "The *Lac* Operator is DNA." *Proceedings of the National Academy of Sciences USA* 58:2415–2421.

———. 1970. "The Lactose Repressor." In *The Lactose Operon,* ed. J. R. Beckwith and D. Zipser, 93–109. Cold Spring Harbor, N. Y.: Cold Spring Harbor Laboratory.

Ginsberg, M. 1987. *Readings in Nonmotonic Reasoning.* Los Altos, Calif.: Morgan Kaufmann.

Glick, B. 1964. "The Bursa of Fabricius and the Development of Immunologic Competence." In Good and Gabrielsen, 1964, 343–358.

Glick, B.; Chang, T. S.; and Japp, R. G. 1956. "The Bursa of Fabricius and Antibody Production." *Poultry Science* 35:224–34.

Glymour, C. 1975. "Relevant Evidence." *Journal of Philosophy* 72:403–426.

_____. 1980. *Theory and Evidence*. Princeton: Princeton University Press.

Goldschmidt, R. 1940. *The Material Basis of Evolution*. New Haven: Yale University Press.

Good, I. J. 1950. *Probability and the Weighing of Evidence*. London: C. Griffin.

_____. 1961 and 1962. "A Causal Calculus." Parts 1, 2. *British Journal for the Philosophy of Science* 11:305–318; 12:43–51.

_____. 1977. "Dynamic Probability, Computer Chess, and the Measurement of Knowledge." In *Machine Intelligence*, vol. 8, ed. E. Elcock and D. Michie, 139–150. New York: Wylie.

Good, R. A. 1971. "Disorders of the Immune System." In Good and Fisher, 1971, 3–16.

Good, R. A., and Fisher, D. W., eds. 1971. *Immunobiology*. Stamford, Conn.: Sinauer Associates, Inc.

Good, R. A., and Gabrielsen, A. B. eds. 1964. *The Thymus in Immunobiology*. New York: Harper and Row.

Good, R. A.; Martinez, C.; and Gabrielsen, A. E. 1964. "Clinical Considerations of the Thymus in Immunobiology." In Good and Gabrielsen, 1964, 3–47.

Goudge, T. 1961. *The Ascent of Life*. Toronto: University of Toronto Press.

Gould, S. 1980. "Is a New and General Theory of Evolution Emerging?" *Paleobiology* 6:119–130.

_____. 1982. "Darwinism and the Expansion of Evolutionary Theory." *Science* 216:380–387.

_____. 1989. *Wonderful Life*. New York: W. W. Norton.

Gould, S. and Eldredge, N. 1977. "Punctuated Equilibria: The Tempo and Mode of Evolution Reconsidered." *Paleobiology* 3:115–151.

Gould, S., and Lewontin, R. C. 1978. "The Spandrels of San Marco and the Panglossian Paradigm: A Critique of the Adaptationist Programme." *Proceedings of the Royal Society of London* 205:581–598. Reprinted in Sober, 1984a, 252–270.

Gould, S., and Vrba, E. 1982. "Exaptation— A Missing Term in the Science of Form." *Paleobiology* 8:4–15.

Grene, M. 1978. "Individuals and Their Kinds: Aristotelian Foundations of Biology." In *Organism, Medicine, and Metaphysics*, ed. S. Spicker, 121–136. Dordrecht, Reidel.

Griesemer, J., and Wade, M. 1988. "Laboratory Models, Causal Explanation, and Group Selection." *Biology and Philosophy* 3:67–96.

Grobstein, C. 1965. *The Strategy of Life*. San Francisco: W. H. Freeman & Co.

_____. 1969. "Organizational Levels and Explanation." *Journal of the History of Biology* 2:199–221.

582 \ Bibliography

Grünbaum, A. 1960. "The Duhemian Argument." *Philosophy of Science* 11:75–87.

Hacking, I. 1965. *Logic of Statistical Inference.* Cambridge: Cambridge University Press.

_____. 1967. "Slightly More Realistic Personal Probability." *Philosophy of Science* 34:311–325.

_____. 1980. "Panel Discussion: The Rational Explanation of Historical Discoveries." In Nickles, 1980b, 24–25.

_____. 1983. *Representing and Intervening.* Cambridge: Cambridge University Press.

Hanks, S., and McDermott, D. 1986. "Default Reasoning, Nonmonotonic Logics, and the Frame Problem." In *American Association for Artificial Intelligence*, vol. 1, 1986, 328–333. Los Altos: Morgan Kaufmann.

Hanson, N. R. 1958. *Patterns of Discovery.* Cambridge: Cambridge University Press.

_____. 1961. "Is There a Logic of Scientific Discovery?" In *Current Issues in the Philosophy of Science*, ed. H. Feigl and G. Maxwell, 21–42. New York: Holt, Rinehart and Winston.

_____. 1963. "Retroductive Inference." In *Philosophy of Science: The Delaware Seminar*, ed. B. Baumrin, 21–37. New York: Wiley.

_____. 1967. "An Anatomy of Discovery." *Journal of Philosophy* 64:321–352.

Harman, G. H. 1965. "The Inference to the Best Explanation." *Philosophical Review* 74:88–95.

_____. 1968. "Enumerative Induction as Inference to the Best Explanation." *Journal of Philosophy* 65:529–533.

Harper, W., and Hooker, C. eds. 1976. *Foundations of Probability Theory, Statistical Inference, and Statistical Theories of Science.* 3 vols. Dordrecht: Reidel.

Hart, H. L. A., and Honoré, A. M. 1985. *Causation in the Law.* 2d ed. Oxford: Oxford University Press.

Haurowitz, F. 1963. "The Template Theory of Antibody Formation." In *Conceptual Advances in Immunology and Oncology*, 22–36. New York: Harper and Row. Paper originally presented at Symposium on Fundamental Cancer Research, M. D. Anderson Hospital and Tumor Institute, Houston, Texas, 1962.

_____. 1965. "Antibody Formation." *Physiological Reviews* 45:1–47.

_____. 1967. "Evolution of Selective and Instructive Theories of Antibody Formation." *Antibodies.* Cold Spring Harbor Laboratory Symposium on Quantitative Biology, vol. 32, 559–568.

_____. 1978. "The Foundations of Immunology." In *Basic and Clinical Immunology.* 2d ed., ed. H. Fudenberg, 1–9. Los Altos: Lange.

Helman, D. 1988. *Analogical Reasoning.* Dordrecht: Reidel.

Hempel, C. G. 1965. *Aspects of Scientific Explanation*. New York: Free Press.

_____. 1966. *Philosophy of Natural Science*. Englewood Cliffs, N.J.: Prentice-Hall.

_____. 1969. "Reduction: Ontological and Linguistic Facets." In *Philosophy, Science and Method*, ed. S. Morgenbesser, P. Suppes, and M. White, 179–199. New York: St. Martins.

Hempel, C. G., and Oppenheim, P. 1948. "Studies in the Logic of Explanation." *Philosophy of Science* 15:135–175. Reprinted with a postscript in Hempel, 1965, 245–295.

Herbert, W. J., and Wilkinson, P. C. 1971. *A Dictionary of Immunology*. Oxford: Blackwell.

Hershey, A., and Chase, M. 1952. "Independent Functions of Viral Protein and Nucleic Acid in Growth of Bacteriophage." *Journal of General Physiology* 36:39–56.

Hesse, M. B. 1966. *Models and Analogies in Science*. Notre Dame, Ind.: Notre Dame Press.

_____. 1974. *The Structure of Scientific Inference*. Berkeley: University of California Press.

Hillis, D. M., and Moritz, C., eds. 1990. *Molecular Systematics*. Sunderland, Mass.: Sinauer.

Hoel, P. 1971. *Introduction to Mathematical Statistics*. 4th ed. New York: Wiley.

_____. 1976. *Elementary Statistics*. 4th ed. New York: Wiley.

Hofstadter, A. 1941. "Objective Teleology." *Journal of Philosophy* 38: 29–39.

Holland, J. H.; Holyoak, K. J.; Nisbett, R. E.; and Thagard, P. R. 1986. *Induction: Processes of Inference, Learning, and Discovery*. Cambridge, Mass.: MIT Press.

Holland, P. W. H. 1991. "Cloning and Evolutionary Analysis of msh-like Homeobox Genes from Mouse, Zebrafish, and Ascidian." *Gene* 98:253–257.

Holloway, C. A. 1979. *Decision Making under Uncertainty: Models and Choices*. Englewood Cliffs, N.J.: Prentice-Hall.

Holmes, F. L. 1980. "Hans Krebs and the Discovery of the Ornithine Cycle." *Federation Proceedings* 39:216–225.

Holmes, F. L., et al. 1991. *Creativity and Discovery in the Biomedical Sciences*. Paper presented at a symposium organized by F. L. Holmes and J. Lederberg, sponsored by the Royal Society of Medicine Foundation, London and New York. Manuscript.

Hood, L., and Talmage, D. 1970. "Mechanisms of Antibody Diversity: Germ Line Basis for Variability." *Science* 168:325–334.

Hooker, C. 1981. "Towards a General Theory of Reduction. Part I: Historical and Scientific Setting. Part II: Identity in Reduction. Part III: Cross–Categorical Reduction." *Dialogue* 20: 38–59, 201–236, 496–529.

Horan, B. 1988. "Theoretical Models, Biological Complexity, and the Semantic View of Theories." In *PSA–1988: Proceedings of the 1988 Biennial Meeting Philosophy of Science Association.* vol. 2, ed. A. Fine and J. Leplin, 265–277. East Lansing, Mich.: Philosophy of Science Association.

_____. 1989. "Functional Explanations in Sociobiology." *Biology and Philosophy* 4:131–158.

_____. 1992. "What Price Optimality?" *Biology and Philosophy* 7:89–109.

Howson, C., and Urbach, P. 1989. *Scientific Reasoning: The Bayesian Approach.* La Salle, Ill.: Open Court.

Hull, D. 1964. "The Logic of Phylogenetic Taxonomy." Ph.D. diss., Indiana University.

_____. 1973. *Darwin and His Critics.* Cambridge: Harvard University Press.

_____. 1974. *Philosophy of Biological Science.* Englewood Cliffs, N.J.: Prentice-Hall.

_____. 1976a. "Informal Aspects of Theory Reduction." In Cohen, et al., 1976, 653–670. Dordrecht: Reidel.

_____. 1976b. "Are Species Really Individuals?" *Systematic Zoology* 25:174–191.

_____. 1978. "A Matter of Individuality." *Philosophy of Science* 45:335–360.

_____. 1980. "Individuality and Selection." *Annual Review of Ecology and Systematics* 11:311–332.

_____. 1981. "Reduction and Genetics." *Journal of Medicine and Philosophy* 6:125–143.

_____. 1988. *Science as a Process: An Evolutionary Account of the Social and Conceptual Development of Science.* Chicago: University of Chicago Press.

Hume, D. 1927 [1777]. *Enquiries.* Ed. L. Selby–Bigge. Oxford: Oxford University Press.

Isaacs, J., and Lamb, J. 1969. *Complementarity in Biology.* Baltimore: Johns Hopkins Press.

Jacob, F. 1966. "Genetics of the Bacterial Cell." *Science* 152:1470–1478.

Jacob, F., and Monod, J. 1961. "Genetic Regulatory Mechanisms in the Synthesis of Proteins." *Journal of Molecular Biology* 3:318.

Jacquard, A. 1974. *The Genetic Structure of Populations.* New York: Springer-Verlag.

Jaynes, E. T. 1968. "Prior Probabilities." *IEEE Transactions in Systems Science and Cybernetics,* 4:227–241.

Jeffrey, R. 1965. *The Logic of Decision*. Chicago: University of Chicago Press.

_____. 1975. "Replies." *Synthese* 30:149–157.

_____. 1983a. *The Logic of Decision*. 2d ed. Chicago: University of Chicago Press.

_____. 1983b. "Bayesianism with a Human Face." In Earman, 1983, 133–156.

Jeffreys, H. 1961. *Theory of Probability*. 3d ed. Oxford: Clarendon Press.

Jeffreys, H., and Wrinch, D. 1921. "On Certain Fundamental Principles of Scientific Inquiry." *Philosophical Magazine* 42:269–298.

Jerne, N. K. 1955. "The Natural–Selection Theory of Antibody Formation." *Proceedings of the National Academy of Sciences USA* 41:849–57.

_____. 1967. "Waiting for the End." In *Antibodies*. Cold Spring Harbor Symposia on Quantitative Biology, vol. 32; 591–603. Cold Spring Harbor, N.Y.: Cold Spring Harbor Laboratory of Quantitative Biology.

_____. 1969. "The Natural Selection Theory of Antibody Formation: Ten Years Later." In *Phage and The Origins of Molecular Biology*, ed. M. Delbruck and J. Cairns, 301–313. Cold Spring Harbor, N.Y.: Cold Spring Harbor Laboratory of Quantitative Biology.

Jerne, N. K., and Nordin, A. 1963. "Plaque Formation in Agar by Single Antibody–Producing Cells." *Science* 140:405.

Judson, H. F. 1979. *The Eighth Day of Creation*. New York: Simon and Schuster.

Kadane, J., and Dickey, J. 1980. "Bayesian Decision Theory and the Simplification of Models." In *Evaluation of Econometric Models*, ed. J. Kimenta, 245–268. New York: Academic Press.

Kalish, D., and Montague, R. 1964. *Logic*. New York: Harcourt, Brace and World.

Kandel, E. 1987. "Preface." In *Molecular Neurobiology in Neurology and Psychiatry*, ed. E. Kandel, vii–ix. New York: Raven Press.

Kandel, E., and Schwartz, J., eds. 1985. *Principles of Neural Science*. 2d ed. New York: Elsevier.

Kandel, E.; Castellucci, V.; Goelet, P.; and Schacher, S. 1987. In *Molecular Neurobiology in Neurology and Psychiatry*, ed. E. Kandel, 111–132. New York: Raven Press.

Karp, P. D. 1989a. "Hypothesis Formation as Design." In *Computational Models of Scientific Discovery and Theory Formation*, ed. J. Schrager and P. Langley, 275–317.

_____. 1989b. "Hypothesis Formation and Qualitative Reasoning in Molecular Biology." Ph. D. diss., Calif.: Stanford University.

Karr, C. 1991. "Applying Genetics to Fuzzy Logic." *AI Expert* 6(3): 38–43.

Karush, F. 1958. "Structural and Energetic Aspects of Antibody–Hapten Interactions." In *Serological and Biochemical Comparisons of Proteins*, ed. W. H. Cole, 40–55. Rutgers, N.J.: Rutgers University Press.

Kauffman, S. A. 1974. "Elsasser, Generalized Complementarity, and Finite Classes: A Critique of His Antireductionism." in *PSA–1972*, ed. K. F. Schaffner and R. S. Cohen, 57–65. Dordrecht: Reidel.

Keene, S. 1989. *Object-Oriented Programming in COMMON LISP*. Reading, Mass.: Addison–Wesley.

Keeton, W. T. 1980. *Biological Science*. 3d ed. New York: W. W. Norton.

Kemeny, J., and Oppenheim, P. 1956. "On Reduction." *Philosophical Studies* 7:6–17.

Keosian, J. 1968. *The Origin of Life*. 2d ed. New York: Reinhold.

Kim, J. 1978. "Supervenience and Nomological Incommensurables." *American Philosophical Quarterly* 15:149–156.

_____. 1989. "The Myth of Nonreductive Materialism." *Proceedings and Addresses of the American Philosophical Association* 63 (no. 3): 31–47.

Kimbrough, S. O. 1979. "On the Reduction of Genetics to Molecular Biology." *Philosophy of Science* 46:389–406.

Kimura, M., and Ohta, T. 1971. *Theoretical Aspects of Population Genetics*. Princeton, N.J.: Princeton University Press.

Kitcher, P. 1976. "Explanation, Conjunction, and Unification." *Journal of Philosophy* 73:207–213.

_____. 1981. "Explanatory Unification." *Philosophy of Science* 48:507–531.

_____. 1983. *The Nature of Mathematical Knowledge*. New York: Oxford University Press.

_____. 1984a. "1953 and All That. A Tale of Two Sciences." *Philosophical Review* 93:335–373.

_____. 1984b. "Species." *Philosophy of Science* 51:308–333.

_____. 1985. *Vaulting Ambition: Sociobiology and the Quest for Human Nature*. Cambridge: MIT Press.

_____. 1987. "Why Not the Best?" In Dupre, 1987, 77–102.

_____. 1989. "Explanatory Unification and the Causal Structure of the World." In *Scientific Explanation*, ed. P. Kitcher and S. Salmon, 410–505. Minneapolis: University of Minnesota Press.

Kitcher, P., and Salmon, W. 1987. "Van Fraassen on Explanation." *Journal of Philosophy* 84:315–330.

Knorr-Cetina, K. 1981. *The Manufacture of Knowledge*. Oxford: Pergamon Press.

Kordig, K. 1978. "Discovery and Justification." *Philosophy of Science* 45:110–117.

Koshland, M., and Engelberger, F. 1963. "Differences in the Amino Acid Composition of Two Purified Antibodies from the Same Rabbit." *Proceedings of the National Academy of Science* 50:61–68.

Kripke, S. 1971. "Identity and Necessity." In *Identity and Individuation*, ed. M. Munitz, 135–164. New York: New York University Press.

Kuffler, S.; Nichols, J.; and Martin, A. 1984. *From Neuron to Brain*. 2d ed. Sunderland, Mass.: Sinauer Associates.

Kuhn, T. S. 1970. *The Structure of Scientific Revolutions*. 2d ed. Chicago: University of Chicago Press.

_____. 1977. "Objectivity, Value Judgments, and Theory Choice." In *The Essential Tension*, by T. S. Kuhn, 320–339. Chicago: University of Chicago Press.

Kulkarni, D. 1989. "The Processes of Scientific Discovery: The Strategy of Experimentation." Ph.D. diss., Carnegie-Mellon University.

Kulkarni, D., and Simon, H. A. 1988. "The Processes of Scientific Discovery: The Strategy of Experimentation." *Cognitive Science* 12:139–175.

Kyburg, H. 1974. *The Logical Foundations of Statistical Inference*. Dordrecht: Reidel.

Kyburg, H., and Harper, W. 1968. "Reply to Levi." *British Journal for the Philosophy of Science* 19:247–258.

Kyburg, H., and Smokler, E., eds. 1980. *Studies in Subjective Probability*. Huntington, N.Y.: Krieger.

Lakatos, I. 1970. "Falsification and the Methodology of Scientific Research Programmes." In Lakatos and Musgrave, 1970, 91–196.

Lakatos, I., and Musgrave, A., eds. 1970. *Criticism and the Growth of Knowledge*. Cambridge: Cambridge University Press.

Landsteiner, K. 1945. *The Specificity of Serological Reactions*. 2d ed. Springfield, Ill.: C. C. Thomas.

Langer, T.; Lui, C.; Echols, H.; Flanagan, J.; Hayer, M.; and Hartl, F. 1992. "Successive Action of KnaK, DnaJ, and GroEL Along the Pathway of Chaperone-Mediated Protein Folding." *Nature* 356:683–689.

Langley, P.; Simon, H. A.; Bradshaw, G. L.; and Zytkow, J. M. 1987. *Scientific Discovery: Computational Explorations of the Creative Process*. Cambridge: MIT Press.

Langman, J. 1981. *Medical Embryology*. 4th ed. Baltimore: Williams and Wilkins.

Latour, B., and Woolgar, S. 1986. *Laboratory Life: The Construction of Scientific Facts*. 2d ed. Princeton: Princeton University Press.

Laudan, L. 1965. "Grünbaum on the Duhemian Argument." *Philosophy of Science* 32:295–299.

_____. 1973. "C. S. Peirce and the Trivialization of the Self-Corrective Thesis." In *Foundations of Scientific Method in the 19th Century*, ed. R. Giere and S. Westfall, 275–306. Bloomington, Ind.: Indiana University Press.

_____. 1977. *Progress and Its Problems*. Berkeley: University of California Press.

_____. 1980. "Why Was the Logic of Discovery Abandoned?" In Nickles, 1980a, 173–183.

_____. 1981. "A Confutation of Convergent Realism." *Philosophy of Science* 489–49.

_____. 1983. "Invention and Justification." [reply to McLaughlin] *Philosophy of Science* 50:320–322.

Lederberg, J. 1956. "Comments on Gene-Enzyme Relationship." In *Enzymes: Units of Biological Structure and Function*, ed. Gaebler, O. H., 161. New York: Academic Press.

_____. 1959. "Genes and Antibodies." *Science* 129:1649–1653.

_____. 1960. "Exobiology: Approaches to Life beyond Earth." *Science* 132:393–400.

_____. 1988. "Ontogeny of the Clonal Selection Theory of Antibody Formation: Reflections on Darwin and Ehrlich." In *Molecular Basis of the Immune Response*, ed. C. A. Bona. *Annals of the New York Academy of Sciences* 546:175–187.

Lehmann, E. 1959. *Testing Statistical Hypotheses*. New York: Wiley.

Lehninger, A. 1975. *Biochemistry*. 2d ed. New York: Worth.

Lenat, D. 1977. "Automated Theory Formation in Mathematics." *Proceedings of the Fifth International Joint Conference on Artificial Intelligence*, 833–842. Cambridge, Mass.:

Lennox, J. 1991. "Darwinian Thought Experiments: A Function for Just-So Stories." *In Thought Experiments in Science and Philosophy*, ed. T. Horowitz and G. Massey, 175–195. Savage, Md.: Roman and Littlefield.

_____. 1992. "Teleology." In *Keywords in Evolutionary Biology*, ed. E. Lloyd and E. Fox–Keller, 324–333. Cambridge, Mass.: Harvard University Press.

Leplin, J, ed. 1984. *Scientific Realism*. Berkeley: University of California Press.

Levene, H.; Pavlovsky, O.; and Dobzhansky, T. 1954. "Interaction in the Adaptive Values in Polymorphic Experimental Populations of *Drosophila pseudoobscura*." *Evolution* 8:335–349.

Levins, R. 1966. "Strategy of Model Building in Population Biology." *American Scientist* 54:421–31.

_____. 1968. *Evolution in Changing Environments*. Princeton, N. J.: Princeton University Press.

Levi, I. 1967. *Gambling with Truth*. New York: Knopf.

_____. 1967. "Probability Kinematics." *British Journal for the Philosophy of Science* 18:197–209.

_____. 1980. *The Enterprise of Knowledge*. Cambridge: MIT Press.

Levins, R. 1968. *Evolution in Changing Environments: Some Theoretical Explorations*. Princeton: Princeton University Press.

Levitan, M., and Montague, A. 1977. *Textbook of Human Genetics*. 2d ed. New York: Oxford University Press.

Lewin, B. 1985. *Genes*. 2d ed. New York: John Wiley.

_____. 1990. *Genes IV*. New York: Oxford University Press.

Lewis, D. 1973. "Causation." *Journal of Philosophy* 70:556–557.

Lewontin, R. C. 1965. "Selection in and out of Populations." In *Ideas in Modern Biology*, ed. J. Moore, 299–311. New York: Natural History Press.

_____. 1969. "The Bases of Conflict in Biological Explanation." *Journal of the History of Biology* 2:35–45.

_____. 1970. "The Units of Selection." *Annual Review of Ecology and Systematics* 1:1–18.

_____. 1974. *The Genetic Basis of Evolutionary Change*. New York: Columbia University Press.

_____. 1977. "Fitness, Survival, and Optimality." In *Analysis of Ecological Systems*, ed. D. J. Horn, G. R. Stairs, and R. D. Mitchell, Columbus, Ohio: Ohio State University Press.

Li, C. C. 1961. *Human Genetics: Principles and Methods*. New York: McGraw-Hill.

Lindley, D. 1965a. *Introduction to Probability and Statistics from a Bayesian Viewpoint*. vol. 1. *Probability*. Cambridge: Cambridge University Press.

_____. 1965b. *Introduction to Probability and Statistics from a Bayesian Viewpoint*. vol. 2. *Inference*. Cambridge: Cambridge University Press.

Lindsay, R. K.; Buchanan, B. G.; Feigenbaum, E. A.; and Lederberg, J. 1980. *Applications of Artificial Intelligence for Organic Chemistry: The DENDRAL Project*. New York: McGraw-Hill.

Livingstone, F. 1967. *Abnormal Hemoglobins in Human Populations*. Chicago: Aldine.

Lloyd, E. 1984. "A Semantic Approach to the Structure of Population Genetics." *Philosophy of Science* 51:242–264.

_____. 1986. "Evaluation of Evidence in Group Selection Debates." In Fine and Machamer, 1986 and 1987, vol. 1, 483–493.

_____. 1987. "Response to Sloep and van der Steen." *Biology and Philosophy* 2:23–26.

_____. 1988. *The Structure and Confirmation of Evolutionary Theory*. Westport, Conn.: Greenwood Press.

Loeb, J. 1964 [1912]. *The Mechanistic Conception of Life*. Ed. Donald Fleming. Cambridge: Harvard University Press.

Mäkelä, O. 1967. "The Specificity of Antibodies Produced by Single Cells." In *Antibodies*. Cold Spring Harbor Symposia on Quantitative Biology, vol. 32, 423–430.

Mackie, J. 1974. *The Cement of the Universe*. Oxford: Oxford University Press.

_____. 1977. *Inventing Right and Wrong*. New York: Penguin.

Martin, A.; Naylor, G.; and Plaumbi, S. 1992. "Rates of Mitochondrial DNA Evolution in Sharks Are Slow Compared with Mammals." *Nature* 357:153–155.

Marx, J. 1992. "Homeobox Genes Go Evolutionary." *Science* 255:399–401.

Masterman, M. 1970. "The Nature of a Paradigm." In Lakatos and Musgrave, 1970, 59–89.

Maull, N. L. 1977. "Unifying Science without Reduction." *Studies in History and Philosophy of Science* 8 (no. 2): 143–71.

Maxam, A., and Gilbert, W. 1977. "A New Method for Sequencing DNA." *Proceedings of the National Academy of Sciences USA* 74:560–564.

Mayo, D. 1986. "Understanding Frequency-Dependent Causation." *Philosophical Studies* 49:109–124.

Mayr, E. 1963. *Animal Species and Evolution*. Cambridge: Harvard University Press.

_____. 1982. *The Growth of Biological Thought*. Cambridge: Harvard University Press.

_____. 1985. "How Biology Differs from the Physical Sciences." In Depew and Weber, 1985, 43–63.

_____. 1988. *Toward A New Philosophy of Biology*. Cambridge: Harvard University Press.

McDermott, D., and Doyle, J. 1980. "Nonmonotonic Logics." *Artificial Intelligence* 13:41–72.

McGee, V. E. 1971. *Principles of Statistics: Traditional and Bayesian*. New York: Appleton-Century-Crofts.

McLaughlin, R. 1982. "Invention and Induction: Laudan, Simon, and the Logic of Scientific Discovery." *Philosophy of Science* 49:198–211.

McMillan, C., and P. Smolensky 1988. "Analyzing a Connectionist Model as a System of Soft Rules." In *Proceedings of the Tenth Annual Conference of the Cognitive Science Society*. Montreal, 62–68.

Mendel, G. 1966 [1865]. "Experiments on Plant Hybrids." In *The Origin of Genetics: A Mendel Sourcebook*, ed. C. Stern and E. Sherwood. San Francisco: Freeman.

Merton, R. K. 1968. "On Sociological Theories of the Middle Range." In *Social Theory and Social Structure*. New York: Free Press.

Merz, J. T. 1904–1912. *A History of European Scientific Thought in the Nineteenth Century*. Reprint. New York: Dover, 1965.

Mettler, L., and Gregg, T. G. 1969. *Population Genetics and Evolution*. Englewood Cliffs, N.J.: Prentice–Hall, Inc.

Michalski, R.S.; Carbonell, J.G.; and Mitchell, T. M. eds. 1986. *Machine Learning*. vol. 2. Los Altos, Calif.: Morgan Kaufmann.

Michotte, A. 1963. *The Perception of Causality*. New York: Basic Books.

Mill, J. S. 1959 [1843]. *A System of Logic*. London: Longmans, Green and Co.

Miller, D. 1976. "Verisimilitude Redeflated." *British Journal for the Philosophy of Science* 27:363–372.

Miller, R., and Masarie, F. E. 1986. "The INTERNIST – 1/Quick Medical Reference Project: Status Report." *Western Journal of Medicine* 145: 816–822.

Miller, R. A.; Pople, H. E., Jr.; and Myers, J. D. 1982. "INTERNIST-1: An Experimental Computer–Based Diagnostic Consultant for General Internal Medicine." *New England Journal of Medicine* 307:468–476.

Miller, J., and Reznikoff, W. eds. 1978. *The Operon*. Cold Spring Harbor, N.Y.: Cold Spring Harbor Laboratory of Quantitative Biology.

Miller, J. F. A. P. 1961. "Immunological Function of the Thymus." *Lancet* 2 (September 30): 748–749.

_____. 1962. "Effect of Neonatal Thymectomy on the Immunological Responsiveness of the Mouse." *Proceedings of the Royal Society of Edinburgh B* 156:415

_____. 1971. "The Immunological Role of the Thymus." In *Immunological Diseases*. 2d ed. Ed. M. Samter. Boston: Little, Brown and Co.

Miller, J. F. A. P.; Doak, S. M. A.; and Cross, A. M. 1963. "Role of the Thymus in Recovery of the Immune Mechanism in the Irradiated Adult Mouse." *Proceedings of the Society for Experimental Biology and Medicine* 112:785–792.

Miller, S. J. 1953. "A Production of Amino Acids under Possible Primitive Earth Conditions." *Science* 117:528–529.

Minsky, M. 1975. "A Framework for Representing Knowledge." In *The Psychology of Computer Vision*, ed. P. Winston, 211–277. New York: McGraw-Hill.

Mishler, B., and Brandon, R. 1987. "Individuality, Pluralism, and the Phylogenetic Species Concept." *Biology and Philosophy* 2:397–414.

Monod, J. 1966. "From Enzymatic Adaptation to Allosteric Transitions." *Science* 154:475–483.

Montefiore, A. 1956. "Professor Gallie on 'Necessary and Sufficient Conditions.'" *Mind* 65:534–541.

Morowitz, H. 1985. *Models for Biomedical Research: A New Perspective*. Washington, D.C.: National Academy of Sciences Press.

Mudd, S. 1932. "A Hypothetical Mechanism of Antibody Formation." *Journal of Immunology* 23:423–427.

Muller, H. J. 1976 [1922]. "Variation Due to Change in the Individual Gene." *American Naturalist* 56:32–50. Reprinted in Corwin and Jenkins, 1976, 86–94.

Muller, H. J. 1932. "Further Studies on the Nature and Causes of Gene Mutations." *Proceedings of the 6th International Congress of Genetics* 1. Ithaca, N.Y., 213–255.

Mueller, A. P.; Wolfe, H. R.; and Meyer, R. K. 1960. "Precipitin Production in Chickens." *Journal of Immunology* 85:172–179.

Munson, R. 1971. "Biological Adaptation." *Philosophy of Science* 38:200–215.

_____. 1975. "Is Biology a Provincial Science?" *Philosophy of Science* 42:428–447.

Murphy, E. 1974. *Logic of Medicine.* Baltimore: Johns Hopkins Press.

Murtha, M.; Leckman, J.; and Ruddle, F. 1991. "Detection of Homeobox Genes in Development and Evolution." *Proceedings of the National Academy of Sciences USA* 88:10711–10715.

Nagel, E. 1949. "The Meaning of Reduction in the Natural Sciences." In *Science and Civilization,* ed. R. Stauffer, 97–135. Madison, Wis.: University of Wisconsin Press.

_____. 1961. *The Structure of Science.* New York: Harcourt, Brace and Co.

Nathans, J.; Davenport, C. M.; and Maumenee, I. H. 1989. "Molecular Genetics of Human Blue Cone Monochromacy." *Science* 245:831–838.

Newell, A.; Shaw, J.; and Simon, H. 1962. "The Processes of Creative Thinking." In *Contemporary Approaches to Creative Thinking,* ed. H. Gruger, G. Terrell, and M. Wertheimer, 63–119. New York: Atherton Press.

Newton-Smith, W. 1981. *The Rationality of Science.* Boston: Routledge and Kegan Paul.

Neyman, J. 1957. "'Inductive Behavior' as a Basic Concept of Philosophy of Science." *Review of the International Statistical Institute* 25:7–22.

Nickles, T. 1977. "Heuristics and Justification in Scientific Research: Comments on Shapere." In *The Structure of Scientific Theories,* ed. F. Suppe, 571–589. 2d ed. Urbana, Ill.: University of Illinois Press.

_____, ed. 1980a. *Scientific Discovery, Logic, and Rationality.* Dordrecht: Reidel.

_____, ed. 1980b. *Scientific Discovery: Case Studies.* Dordrecht: Reidel.

_____. 1985. "Beyond Divorce: Current Status of the Discovery Debate." *Philosophy of Science* 52:177–206.

Nii, H. P. 1986. "Blackboard Systems: Part 1: The Blackboard Model of Problem Solving and the Evolution of Blackboard Architectures; Part 2: Blackboard Application Systems, Blackboard Systems from a Knowledge Engineering Perspective." *The AI Magazine* 7: 38–53, 82–106.

Niiniluoto, I. 1983. "Novel Facts and Bayesianism." *British Journal for the Philosophy of Science* 34:375–379.

Nirenberg, M. W., and Matthaei, J. H. 1961. "The Dependence of Cell-Free Protein Synthesis in *E. coli* upon Naturally Occurring or Synthetic Polyribonucleotides." *Proceedings of the National Academy of Sciences USA* 47:1588–1602.

Nossal, G. 1967. "Discussion Comment" [on Mäkelä 1967]. In *Antibodies*. Cold Spring Harbor Symposia on Quantitative Biology, vol. 32, 430.

———. 1978. *Antibodies and Immunity*. 2d ed. New York: Basic Books.

Nossal, G., and Lederberg, J. 1958. "Antibody Production by Single Cells." *Nature* 181:1419–1420.

Nossal, G., and Mäkelä, O. 1962. "Elaboration of Antibodies by Single Cells." *Annual Review of Microbiology* 16:53–74.

Nowell, P. C. 1960. "Phytohemagglutinin: An Initiator of Mitosis in Culture of Normal Human Leukocytes." *Cancer Research* 20:462–466.

Office of Technology Assessment. 1988. *Mapping Our Genes: Genome Projects: How Big, How Fast?* Washington, D.C.: Government Printing Office.

Olby, R. C. 1966. *Origins of Mendelism*. Chicago: University of Chicago Press.

———. 1974. *The Path to the Double Helix*. London: Macmillan Co.

Oliver, C. P. 1940. "A Reversion to Wild-Type Associated with Crossing Over in *Drosophila melanogaster*." *Proceedings of the National Academy of Sciences USA* 26:452–454.

Oparin, A. I. 1962. *Life, its Nature, Origin, and Development*. Trans. Ann Synge. Edinburgh: Oliver and Boyd.

Orgel, L. 1973. *The Origins of Life*. New York: Wiley.

Orgel, L., and Crick, F. H. C. 1980. "Selfish DNA: The Ultimate Parasite." *Nature* 284: 604–607.

Osherson, D., and Smith, E. 1981. "On the Adequacy of Prototype Theory as a Theory of Concepts." *Cognition* 9:35–58.

Oster, G. F., and Wilson, E. O. 1978. *Caste and Ecology in the Social Insects*. Princeton: Princeton University Press.

Otte, R. 1981. "A Critique of Suppes' Theory of Probabilistic Causality." *Synthese* 48:167–181.

Overton, G.; Koile, K.; and Pastor, J. 1990. "GeneSys: A Knowledge Management System for Molecular Biology." In *Computers and DNA*, ed. G. Bell and T. Marr, 213–239. Redwood City, Calif.: Addison-Wesley.

Pardee, A.; Jacob, F.; and Monod, J. 1958. "Sur l'expression et le rôle des allèles inducible et constitutif dans la synthèse del la β–galactosidase chez de zygotes d'*Escherichia coli*." *Comptes Rendus Academie des Sciences, Paris* 246:3125–3127.

Pardee, A.; Jacob, F.; and Monod, J. 1959. "The Genetic Control and Cytoplasmic Expression in the Synthesis of β–galactosidase of *E. coli*." *Journal of Molecular Biology* 1:165.

Pauling, L. 1940. "A Theory of the Structure and Process of Formation of Antibodies." *Journal of the American Chemical Society* 62:2643–2657.

Pearmain, G.; Lycette, R.; and Fitzgerald, P. 1963. "Tuberculin–Induced Mitosis in Peripheral Blood Leucocytes." *Lancet* 1:637–638.

Perry, R. B. 1921. "Purpose." *Journal of Philosophy* 18:85–105.

Peterson, R. D. A.; Cooper, M. D.; and Good, R. A. 1965. "The Pathogenesis of Immunologic Deficiency Diseases." *American Journal of Medicine* 38:579–604.

Pittendriegh, C. S. 1958. "Adaptation, Natural Selection, and Behavior." In Behavior and Evolution, ed. A. Roe and G. G. Simpson, 390–416. New Haven: Yale University Press.

Platt, J. R. 1964. "Strong Inference." *Science* 146:347–353.

Polanyi, M. 1962. *Personal Knowledge*. Rev. ed. Chicago: University of Chicago Press.

———. 1969. "Life's Irreducible Structure." *Science* 160:1308–1312.

Pople, H. E., Jr. 1977. "The Formation of Composite Hypotheses in Diagnostic Problem Solving: An Exercise in Synthetic Reasoning." *Advance Papers of the Fifth International Joint Conference on Artificial Intelligence*. Cambridge: Artificial Intelligence Laboratory.

Pople, H. E., Jr.; Myers, J. D.; and Miller, R. A. 1974. "The DIALOG Model of Diagnostic Logic and Its Use in Internal Medicine." Mimeo.

Pople, H. E., Jr.; Myers, J. D.; and Miller, R. A. 1975. "DIALOG: A Model of Diagnostic Logic for Internal Medicine." *Advance Papers of the Fourth International Joint Conference on Artificial Intelligence*, Vol. 2 Cambridge: Artificial Intelligence Laboratory, 848–855.

Popper, K. 1957. "The Aim of Science." *Ratio* 1:24–35.

———. 1959 [1934]. *The Logic of Scientific Discovery*. New York: Free Press.

———. 1962. *Conjectures and Refutations*. New York: Basic Books.

Pratt, J. 1976. "A Discussion of the Question: For What Use are Tests of Hypotheses and Tests of Significance." *Commun. Statist.-Theor. Meth.*, A5: 779–787.

Price, G. 1970. "Selection and Covariance." *Nature* 227:520–521.

———. 1972. "Extension of Covariance Selection Mathematics." *Annals of Human Genetics* 35:485–490.

Prieditis, A., ed. 1988. *Analogica*. Los Altos, Calif.: Morgan Kaufmann.

Provine, W. 1986. *Sewall Wright and Evolutionary Biology*. Chicago: University of Chicago Press.

Ptashne, M. 1967. "Isolation of the λ Phage Repressor." *Proceedings of the National Academy of Sciences USA* 56:306–313.

Putnam, H. 1961. "What Theories Are Not." In *Logic, Methodology and Philosophy of Science*, ed. A. Tarski, 240–251. Stanford, Calif.: Stanford University Press.

_____. 1963. "'Degree of Confirmation' and Inductive Logic." In *The Philosophy of Rudolph Carnap*, ed. P. Schilpp, 761–784. La Salle, Ill.: Open Court.

_____. 1973. "Meaning and Reference." *Journal of Philosophy* 70:699–711.

_____. 1975. "The Meaning of 'Meaning.'" In *Language, Mind, and Knowledge*, ed. K. Gunderson. Minnesota Studies in the Philosophy of Science, vol. 7, 131–193. Minneapolis: University of Minnesota Press.

_____. 1975–76. "What Is Realism?" *Proceedings of the Aristotelian Society*: 177–194.

_____. 1978. *Meaning and the Moral Sciences*. London: Routledge and Kegan Paul.

_____. 1988. *Representation and Reality*. Cambridge: MIT Press.

Quine, W. V. 1951. "Two Dogmas of Empiricism." *Philosophical Review* 60:20–43.

_____. 1960. *Word and Object*. New York: Wylie.

_____. 1964. "Ontological Reduction and the World of Numbers." *Journal of Philosophy* 61:209–216.

Race, R. R., and Sanger, R. 1954. *Blood Groups in Man*. 2d ed. Oxford: Basil Blackwell.

Raiffa, H. 1968. *Decision Analysis*. Reading, Mass.: Addison-Wesley.

Railton, P. 1980. *Explaining Explanation*. Ph.D. diss., Princeton University.

Ramsey, F. 1931. *The Foundations of Mathematics and Other Logical Essays*. London: Routledge and Kegan Paul.

_____. 1931. "Truth and Probability." In *The Foundations of Mathematics and Other Logical Essays*, ed. F. Ramsey, 156–198. Reprinted in Kyburg and Smokler, 1980.

Redhead, M. 1978. "Ad Hocness and the Appraisal of Theories" *British Journal for the Philosophy of Science* 29:355–361.

Reichenbach, H. 1938. *Experience and Prediction*. Chicago: University of Chicago Press.

_____. 1949. *The Theory of Probability*. Berkeley: University of California Press.

_____. 1956. *The Direction of Time*. Berkeley: University of California Press.

_____. 1958. *The Rise of Scientific Philosophy*. Berkeley: University of California Press.

Renwick, J. 1971. "The Mapping of the Human Chromosome." *Annual Review of Genetics* 5:81–120.

Rescher, N., ed. 1986. *Current Issues in Teleology*. Lanham, Md.: University Press of America.

Richerson, P., and Boyd, R. 1987. "Simple Models of Complex Phenomena: The Case of Cultural Evolution." In ed. J. Dupré, 1987, 27–52. Cambridge: MIT Press.

Robinson, J. A. 1962. "Hume's Two Definitions of Cause." *Philosophical Quarterly* 12:162–171.

Romer, A. 1941. *Man and the Vertebrates*. Chicago: University of Chicago Press.

Rosch, E. 1976. "Classification of Real-World Objects: Origins and Representations in Cognition. In *Thinking: Readings in Cognitive Science*, ed. P. N. Johnsen–Laird and P. C. Wason, 212–222. Cambridge: Cambridge University Press.

Rosch, E., and Mervis, C. 1975. "Family Resemblances: Studies in the Internal Structure of Categories." *Cognitive Psychology* 7:573–605.

Rosenberg, A. 1978. "Supervenience of Biological Concepts." *Philosophy of Science* 45:368–386.

_____. 1985. *The Structure of Biological Science*. Cambridge: University of Cambridge Press.

Rosenbleuth, A.; Wiener, N.; and Bigelow, J. 1943. "Behavior, Purpose, and Teleology." *Philosophy of Science* 10:18-24.

Rosenkrantz, R. 1977. *Inference, Method and Decision*. Dordrecht: Reidel.

Ruse, M. 1970. "Are There Laws in Biology?" *Australasian Journal of Philosophy* 48:234–46.

_____. 1971. "Function Statements in Biology." *Philosophy of Science* 38:87–95.

_____. 1972. "Biological Adaptation." *Philosophy of Science* 39:525–528.

_____. 1973. *Philosophy of Biology*. London: Hutchinson.

_____.1975. "Woodger on Genetics: A Critical Evaluation." *Acta Biotheoretica* 24:1–13.

_____. 1976. "Reduction in Genetics." in Cohen, et al., 1976, 653–670.

_____. 1977. "Is Biology Different from Physics?" In *Logic, Laws and Life*, ed. R. Colodny, 89–127. University of Pittsburgh Series in the Philosophy of Science, vol. 6. Pittsburgh: University of Pittsburgh Press.

_____. 1986. "Teleology and the Biological Sciences." In Rescher, 1986, 56–64.

_____. 1988. *Philosophy of Biology Today*. Albany: State University of New York Press.

Russell, B. 1948. *Human Knowledge, Its Scope and Limits*. New York: Simon and Schuster.

Salmon, W. C. 1967. *The Foundations of Scientific Inference*. Pittsburgh: University of Pittsburgh Press.

____. 1968. "The Justification of Inductive Rules of Inference." In *The Problem of Inductive Logic*, ed. I. Lakatos, 24–43. Amsterdam: North-Holland.

____. 1970. "Bayes's Theorem and the History of Science." In *Historical and Philosophical Perspectives of Science*, ed. R. Stuewer, 68–86. Minnesota Studies in the Philosophy of Science, vol. V. Minneapolis: University of Minnesota Press.

____. 1971. *Statistical Explanation and Statistical Relevance*. Pittsburgh: University of Pittsburgh Press.

____. 1980. "Probabilistic Causality." *Pacific Philosophical Quarterly* 61: 50–74.

____. 1984. *Scientific Explanation and the Causal Structure of the World*. Princeton: Princeton University Press.

____. 1989. "Four Decades of Scientific Explanation." In Kitcher and Salmon, 1989, 3–219.

____. 1990. "Rationality and Objectivity in Science, or Tom Kuhn Meets Tom Bayes." In *Scientific Theories*, ed. C. W. Savage, 175–204. Minnesota Studies in the Philosophy of Science, vol 14. Minneapolis: University of Minnesota Press.

____. 1992. "Scientific Explanation." In *Introduction to the Philosophy of Science*, ed. M. Salmon, 7–41. Englewood Cliffs, N.J.: Prentice-Hall.

Sanger, F.; Nicklen, S.; and Coulson, A. R. 1977. "DNA Sequencing with Chain-Terminating Inhibitors." *Proceedings of the National Academy of Sciences USA* 74:5463–5467.

Sarkar, S. 1989. "Reductionism and Molecular Biology: A Reappraisal." Ph.D. diss., University of Chicago.

____. 1992. "Models of Reduction and Categories of Reductionism." *Synthese* 91:167–194.

Savage, L. 1954. *The Foundations of Statistical Inference*. New York: Wylie.

____. 1962. *The Foundations of Statistical Inference: A Symposium*. London: Methuen.

____. 1977. "The Shifting Foundations of Statistics." In *Logic, Laws, and Life*, ed. R. Colodny, 3–18. University of Pittsburgh Series in the Philosophy of Science, v. 6. Pittsburgh: University of Pittsburgh Press.

Schaffner, K. 1967. "Approaches to Reduction." *Philosophy of Science* 34:137–147.

____. 1969a. "Correspondence Rules." *Philosophy of Science* 36:280–290.

____. 1969b. "The Watson-Crick Model and Reductionism." *British Journal for the Philosophy of Science* 20:235–248.

____. 1970. "Outlines of a Logic of Comparative Theory Evaluation with Special Attention to Pre- and Post-Relativistic Electrodynamics." In *Historical and Philosophical Perspectives of Science*, ed. R.

598 \ Bibliography

Stuewer, 311–364. Minnesota Studies in the Philosophy of Science, vol. 5, Minneapolis: University of Minnesota Press.

_____. 1972. *Nineteenth-Century Aether Theories.* Oxford: Pergamon Press.

_____. 1974a. Logic of Discovery and Justification in Regulatory Genetics." *Studies in the History and Philosophy of Science* 4:349–385.

_____. 1974b. "Einstein versus Lorentz: Research Programmes and the Logic of Comparative Theory Evaluation." *British Journal for the Philosophy of Science* 25:45–78.

_____. 1974c. "The Peripherality of Reductionism in the Development of Molecular Biology." *Journal of the History of Biology* 7:111–139.

_____. 1976. "Reduction in the Biomedical Sciences: Problems and Prospects." In Cohen et al., 1976, 613–632.

_____. 1977. "Reduction, Reductionism, Values and Progress in the Biomedical Sciences." In *Logic, Laws and Life,* ed. R. Colodny, 143–171. *University of Pittsburgh Series in the Philosophy of Science,* vol. 6. Pittsburgh: University of Pittsburgh Press.

_____. 1980a. "Theory Structure in the Biomedical Sciences." *The Journal of Medicine and Philosophy,* 5:57–97.

_____. 1980b. "Discovery in the Biomedical Sciences: Logic or Irrational Intuition?" In *Scientific Discovery: Case Studies,* ed. T. Nickles, 171–205. Dordrecht: Reidel.

_____. 1982. "Biomedical Knowledge: Progress and Priorities." In *Seventh Interdisciplinary Symposium on Philosophy and Medicine,* ed. H. T. Engelhardt, W. Bondeson, and S. S. Spicker, 131–151. Dordrecht: Reidel.

_____. 1983. "Explanation and Causation in the Biomedical Sciences." In *Mind and Medicine,* ed. L. Laudan, 79–124. Berkeley: University of California Press.

_____. 1985. "Introduction." In *Logic of Discovery and Diagnosis in Medicine,* ed. K. F. Schaffner, 1–32. Berkeley: University of California Press.

_____. 1986. "Exemplar Reasoning about Biological Models and Diseases: a Relation between the Philosophy of Medicine and Philosophy of Science." *Journal of Medicine and Philosophy* 11:63–80.

_____. 1987. "Computerized Implementation of Biomedical Theory Structures: An Artificial Intelligence Approach." in Fine and Machamer, 1986 and 1987, 17–32.

_____. 1991. "Causing Harm: Epidemiological and Physiological Concepts of Causation." In *Acceptable Evidence: Science and Values in Hazard Management,* ed. D. G. Mayo and R. Hollander, 204–217. Oxford: Oxford University Press.

_____. 1992a. "The Discovery of the Clonal Selection Theory." Paper presented at Hershey Conference on Conceptual Change in Medicine, April 1990.

____. 1992b."Theory Change in Immunology: The Clonal Selection Theory, Part I: Theory Change and Scientific Progress; Part II: The Clonal Selection Theory" *Theoretical Medicine* 13 (no. 2): 191–216

____. 1993. "Clinical Trials and Causation: Bayesian Perspectives."*Statistics in Medicine*, in press.

Scheffler, I. 1967. *Science and Subjectivity*. Indianapolis: Bobbs-Merrill.

Schiller, F. C. S. 1917. "Scientific Discovery and Logical Proof." In *Studies in the History and the Methods of the Sciences*, vol. 1, ed. C. Singer, 235–289. Oxford: Clarendon Press.

Schwartz, S. 1977. *Naming, Necessity, and Natural Kinds*. Ithaca: Cornell University Press.

Scriven, M. 1959. "Explanation and Prediction in Evolutionary Theory." *Science* 130:477–482.

Searle, J. 1985. *Minds, Brains, and Science*. Cambridge: Harvard University Press.

____. 1987. "Minds and Brains without Programs." in *Mindwaves: Thoughts on Intelligence, Identity, and Consciousness*, ed. C. Blakemore and S. Greenfield, 206–233. Oxford: Blackwells.

Seidenfeld, T. 1979. *Philosophical Problems of Statistical Inference*. Dordrecht: Reidel.

____. 1979. "Why I Am Not an Objective Bayesian; Some Reflections Prompted by Rosenkrantz." *Theory and Decision* 11:413–440.

Sellars, W. 1977. "Is Scientific Realism Tenable." In PSA–1976: *Proceedings of the 1976 Biennial Meeting Philosophy of Science Association*, vol. 2, ed. F. Suppe and P. Asquith, 307–334. East Lansing, Mich.: Philosophy of Science Association.

Sessions, S.; Gardiner, D.; and Bryant, S. 1989. "Compatible Limb Patterning Mechanisms in Urodeles and Anurans." *Developmental Biology* 131:294–301.

Shapere, D. 1964. "The Structure of Scientific Revolutions." *Philosophical Review* 73:393–394.

____. 1974. "Scientific Theories and Their Domains." In Suppe, 1977, 518–565.

____. 1982. "The Concept of Observation in Science and Philosophy." *Philosophy of Science* 49:485–525.

____. 1984. *Reasons and the Search for Knowledge*. Dordrecht: Reidel.

Sheldrake, R. 1981. *A New Science of Life: The Hypothesis of Formative Causation*. Los Angeles: J.P. Tarcher. Distributed by Houghton Mifflin.

Shimony, A. 1970. "Scientific Inference." In *The Nature and Function of Scientific Theories*, ed. R. Colodny, 79–172. Pittsburgh: University of Pittsburgh Press.

Shoenfeld, R. 1967. *Mathematical Logic*. Reading, Mass.: Addison-Wesley.

600 \ Bibliography

Silverstein, A. M. 1989. *A History of Immunology*. San Diego: Academic Press.

Silvey, S. 1970. *Statistical Inference*. Baltimore: Penguin.

Simon, H. 1957. *Models of Man*. New York: Wiley.

_____. 1962. "The Architecture of Complexity." *Proceedings of the American Philosophical Society* 106:467–482.

_____. 1977. *Models of Discovery*. Dordrecht: Reidel.

_____. 1981. *The Sciences of the Artificial*. Enlarged ed. Cambridge: M.I.T. Press.

Simon, H.; Langley, P.; and Bradshaw, G. 1981. "Scientific Discovery as Problem Solving." *Synthese* 47:1–27.

Simon, M. 1971. *The Matter of Life*. New Haven: Yale University Press.

Simonsen, M. 1962. "Graft Versus Host Reactions." *Progress in Allergy* 6:349–467.

_____. 1967. "The Clonal Selection Hypothesis Evaluated by Grafted Cells Reacting against their Hosts." *Antibodies*. Cold Spring Harbor Symposia on Quantitative Biology, v. 32, 517–523.

Simpson, G. G. 1964. *This View of Life*. New York: Harcourt, Brace & World.

Sklar, L. 1967. "Types of Inter–Theoretic Reduction." *British Journal for the Philosophy of Science* 18:109–120.

Skyrms, B. 1980. *Causal Necessity*. New Haven: Yale University Press.

Sloep, P. and van der Steen, W. 1987. "The Nature of Evolutionary Theory: The Semantic Challenge." *Biology and Philosophy* 2:1–15.

Small, S. A.; Kandel, E. R.; and Hawkins, R. D. 1989. "Activity-Dependent Enhancement of Presynaptic Inhibition in *Aplysia* Sensory Neurons." *Science* 243:1603–1606.

Smart, J. J. C. 1963. *Philosophy and Scientific Realism*. London: Routledge & Kegan Paul.

_____. 1968. *Between Science and Philosophy*. New York: Random House.

Smith, C. A. B. 1969. *Biomathematics*. 4th ed. vol 2. London: Charles Griffin.

Smith, J. M., ed. 1982. *Evolution Now*. San Francisco: Freeman.

Smith, R. T., and Landy, M., eds. 1975. *Immunobiology of the Tumor-Host Relationship*. New York: Academic Press.

Smith, T. F., and Sadler, J. R. 1971. "The Nature of Lactose Operator Constitutive Mutations." *Journal of Molecular Biology* 59:273.

Smuts, J. 1926. *Holism and Evolution*. New York: Macmillan.

Sneed, J. 1971. *The Logical Structure of Mathematical Physics*. Dordrecht: Reidel.

Sober, E. 1981. "Holism, Individualism, and the Units of Selection." In Asquith and Giere, 1981, 93–121.

_____. 1982. "Frequency–dependent Causation." *Journal of Philosophy* 79:247–253.

_____. 1984a. *Conceptual Issues in Evolutionary Biology*. Cambridge: MIT Press.

_____. 1984b. *The Nature of Selection*. Cambridge: MIT Press.

_____. 1984c. "Fact, Fiction, and Fitness: A Reply to Rosenberg." *Journal of Philosophy* 81:372–383.

_____. 1987. "Explanation and Causation." *British Journal for the Philosophy of Science* 38:243–257.

_____. 1988. *Reconstructing the Past: Parsimony, Evolution, and Inference*. Cambridge: MIT Press.

Sober, E. and Lewontin, R. 1982. "Artifact, Cause, and Genic Selection." *Philosophy of Science* 49:157–180.

Sommerfeld, A. 1964. *Electrodynamics*. New York: Academic Press.

Sommerhoff, G. 1950. *Analytical Biology*. London: Oxford University Press.

Sosa, E., ed. 1975. *Causation and Conditionals*. Oxford: Oxford University Press.

Spemann, H. 1927. "Organizers in Animal Development." *Proceedings of the Royal Society of Edinburgh B* 102:177–187.

_____. 1938. *Embryonic Development and Induction*. New Haven: Yale University Press.

Spirtes, P.; Glymour, C.; and Scheines, R. 1993. *Causality, Prediction, and Search*. New York: Springer-Verlag.

Stebbins, G. L. 1968. "Integration of Development and Evolutionary Progress." In *Population Biology and Evolution*, ed. R. Lewontin, 17–36. Syracuse, N.Y.: Syracuse University Press.

Stefik, M. and Bobrow, D. 1986. "Object-Oriented Programming: Themes and Variations." *The AI Magazine* 6(4): 40–62.

Steen, W. J. van der, and Kamminga, H. 1991. "Laws and Natural History in Biology." *British Journal for the Philosophy of Science* 42:445–467.

Stegmuller, W. 1976. *The Structure and Dynamics of Theories*. Amsterdam: North-Holland.

Stent, G. 1964. "The Operon: On Its Third Anniversary." *Science* 144:816–820.

_____. 1968. "That Was the Molecular Biology That Was." *Science* 160:390–395.

Stewart, C. 1993. "The Powers and Pitfalls of Parsimony." *Nature* 361:603–607.

Stinchcomb, A. 1975. "Merton's Theory of Social Structure." In *The Idea of Social Structure*, ed. R. K. Merton and L. A. Coser, 11–33. New York: Harcourt Brace Jovanovich.

Stitch, S., and Nisbett, R. 1980. "Justification and the Psychology of Human Reasoning." *Philosophy of Science* 47:188–202.

Strickberger, M. W. 1976. *Genetics*. 2d ed. New York: Macmillan.

Suppe, F. 1974a. "Some Philosophical Problems in Biological Speciation and Taxonomy." In *Conceptual Basis of the Classification of Knowledge*, ed. J. A. Wojciechowski, 190–243. Munich: Springer-Verlag.

———. 1974b. "Theories and Phenomena." In *Developments in the Methodology of Social Science*, ed. W. Leinfeller and E. Kohler, 45–97. Dordrecht: Reidel.

———. 1977. *The Structure of Scientific Theories*. 2d ed. Urbana: University of Illinois Press.

———. 1989. *The Semantic Conception of Scientific Theories and Scientific Realism*. Urbana: University of Illinois Press.

Suppes, P. 1957. *Introduction to Logic*. Princeton, N.J.: Van Nostrand.

———. 1962. "Models of Data." In *Logic, Methodology, and Philosophy of Science*, ed. E. Nagel, P. Suppes, and A. Tarski, 252–261. Stanford, Calif.: Stanford University Press.

———. 1967. "What Is a Scientific Theory?" In *Philosophy of Science Today*, ed. S. Morgenbesser, 55–67. New York: Basic Books.

———. 1970. *A Probabilistic Theory of Causality*. Amsterdam: North-Holland.

Szenberg, A.; Warner, N.; Burnet, F. M.; and Lind, P. 1962. "Quantitative Aspects of the Simonsen Phenomena. II. Circumstances Influencing the Focal Counts Obtained on the Chorioallantoic Membrane." *British Journal for Experimental Pathology* 43:129.

Talmage, D. W. 1957. "Allergy and Immunology." *Annual Review of Medicine* 8:239–256.

Taylor, C. 1964. *The Explanation of Behaviour*. London: Routledge and Kegan Paul.

Teller, P. 1973. "Conditionalization and Observation." *Synthese* 26:218–258

———. 1975. "Shimony's A Priori Arguments for Tempered Personalism." In *Induction, Probability, and Confirmation*, ed. G. Maxwell and J. Anderson, 166–203. Minnesota Studies in the Philosophy of Science, vol 6. Minneapolis: University of Minnesota Press.

———. 1976. "Conditionalization, Observation, and Change of Preference." In Harper and Hooker, 1976, vol. 1, 205–253.

Thagard, P. 1988. *Computational Philosophy of Science*. Cambridge: MIT Press.

Thagard, P. and Holyoak, K. J. 1985. "Discovering the Wave Theory of Sound." *Proceedings of the Ninth International Joint Conference on Artificial Intelligence*. Los Altos, Calif.: Kaufmann.

Thompson, P. 1983. "The Structure of Evolutionary Theory: A Semantic Approach." *Studies in History and Philosophy of Science* 14:215–229

_____. 1987. "A Defence of the Semantic Conception of Evolutionary Theory." *Biology and Philosophy* 2:26–32.

_____. 1989. *The Structure of Biological Theories*. Albany: State University of New York Press.

Topley, W. 1930. "The Role of the Spleen in the Production of Antibodies." *Journal of Pathology and Bacteriology*. 33:339–351.

Toulmin, S. 1961. *Foresight and Understanding*. London: Hutchinson.

_____. 1972. *Human Understanding*. Vol. 1. Princeton, N. J.: Princeton University Press.

Touretzky, D. 1986. *The Mathematics of Inheritance Systems*. Los Altos: Morgan Kaufmann.

Touretzky, D. and Hinton, G. 1988. "A Distributed Connectionist Production System." *Cognitive Science* 12:423–466.

Trentin, J., and Fahlberg, W. 1963. "An Experimental Model for Studies of Immunologic Competence in Irradiated Mice Repopulated with Clones of Spleen Cells." In *Conceptual Advances in Immunology and Oncology*, 66–74. New York: Harper and Row. Paper originally presented at Symposium on Fundamental Cancer Research, M. D. Anderson Hospital and Turner Institute, Houston, Texas, 1962.

Tversky, A., and Kahneman, D. 1974. "Judgement under Uncertainty." *Science* 185:1124–1131.

van Fraassen, B. 1970. "On the Extension of Beth's Semantics of Physical Theories." *Philosophy of Science* 37:325–339.

_____. 1977. "The Pragmatics of Explanation." *American Philosophical Quarterly* 14:143–150.

_____. 1980a. *The Scientific Image*. New York: Oxford University Press.

_____. 1980b. "Rational Belief and Probability Kinematics." *Philosophy of Science* 47:165–178.

_____. 1988. "The Problem of Old Evidence." In *Philosophical Analysis: A Defense by Example,* ed. D. Austin, 153–165. Dordrecht: Kluwer.

Vickers, J. 1965. "Some Remarks on Coherence and Subjective Probability." *Philosophy of Science* 32:32–38.

Voeller, B., ed. 1968. *The Chromosome Theory of Inheritance*. New York: Appleton-Century-Crofts.

von Bertalanffy, L. 1933. *Modern Theories of Development*. Trans. J. H. Woodger. Oxford: Oxford University Press.

_____. 1952. *Problems of Life*. London: Watts.

Waddington, C. H. 1968. *Towards a Theoretical Biology*. Vol. 1. Chicago: Aldine Press.

Wade, M. 1976. "Group Selection among Laboratory Populations of Tribolium." *Proceedings of the National Academy of Sciences, USA* 73:4604–4607.

604 \ Bibliography

_____. 1978. "A Critical Review of the Models of Group Selection." *Quarterly Review of Biology* 53:101–114.

Wagner, R. P., and Mitchell, H. K. 1964. *Genetics and Metabolism*. 2d ed. New York: Wiley.

Warner, N., and Szenberg, A. 1964. "The Immunological Function of the Bursa of Fabricius in the Chicken." *Annual Review of Microbiology* 18:253–268.

_____. 1962. "Effect of Neonatal Thymectomy on the Immune Response in the Chicken." *Nature* 196:784–785.

Waters, K. 1990. "Laws, Kinds, and Generalities in Biology." Manuscript.

Watkins, J. 1984. *Science and Skepticism*. Princeton, N.J.: Princeton University Press.

Watson, J. D., and Crick, F. H. C. 1953a. "A Structure for Deoxyribose Nucleic Acid." *Nature* 171:737–738.

_____. 1953b. "Genetical Implications of the Structure of Deoxyribonucleic Acid." *Nature* 171:964–967.

Watson, J.; Hopkins, N.; Roberts, J.; Steitz, J.; and Weiner, A. 1987. *The Molecular Biology of the Gene*. 4th ed. Menlo Park, Calif.: Benjamin/Cummings.

Weiss, P. A. 1962. "From Cell to Molecule." In *The Molecular Control of Cellular Activity*, ed. J. Allen, 1–72. New York: McGraw-Hill.

_____. 1968. *Dynamics of Development: Experiments and Inferences*. New York: Academic Press.

_____. 1969. "The Living System: Determinism Stratified." In *Beyond Reductionism*, ed. A. Koestler and J. Smythies, 3–42. Boston: Beacon Press.

_____. 1973. *The Science of Life*. Mount Kisko: Futura.

Whewell, W. 1968 [1849]. "Mr. Mill's Logic." In *William Whewell's Theory of Scientific Method*, ed. R. E. Butts, 265–308. Pittsburgh: University of Pittsburgh Press.

Whitehouse, H. L. K. 1973. *Towards an Understanding of the Mechanism of Heredity*. 3d ed. London: Edward Arnold.

Wiggins, D. 1967. *Identity and Spatio-Temporal Continuity*. Cambridge: Harvard University Press.

_____. 1980. *Sameness and Substance* Cambridge: Harvard University Press.

Williams, B. 1985. *Ethics and the Limits of Philosophy*. Cambridge: Harvard University Press.

Williams, G. C. 1966. *Adaptation and Natural Selection*. Princeton, N. J.: Princeton University Press.

Williams, J. 1988. "The Role of Diffusible Molecules in Regulating the Cellular Differentiation of *Dictostelium discoideum*." *Development* 103:1–16.

Williams, M. 1970. "Deducing the Consequences of Evolution: A Mathematical Model." *Journal of Theoretical Biology* 29:343–385.

_____. 1981. "Similarities and Differences between Evolutionary Theories and Theories in Physics" In Asquith and Giere, 1980 and 1981, vol. 2, 385–396.

Williams, P. M. 1980. "Bayesian Conditionalization and the Principle of Minimum Information." *British Journal for the Philosophy of Science* 31:131–144.

Wimsatt, W. 1972. "Teleology and the Logical Structure of Function Statements." *Studies in History and Philosophy of Science* 3:1–80.

_____. 1976a. "Reductionism, Levels of Organization, and the Mind–Body Problem." In *Consciousness and the Brain*, ed. G. Globus, G. Maxwell, and I. Savodnik, 205–267. New York: Plenum Press.

_____. 1976b. "Reductive Explanation: A Functional Account." In R. S. Cohen et. al., 1976, 671–710.

_____. 1980. "Reductionistic Research Strategies and Their Biases in the Units of Selection Controversy." In Nickles, 1980b, 213–259.

_____. 1981. "The Units of Selection and the Structure of the Multi-level Genome." In Asquith and Giere, vol. 2, 122–183.

_____. 1985. "Forms of Aggregativity." In *Human Nature and Natural Knowledge*, ed. A. Donagan, N. Perovich, and M. Wedin, M., 259–293. Dordrecht: Reidel.

Winston P. H. 1978. "Learning by Creating and Justifying Transfer Frames." *Artificial Intelligence* 10:147–172.

_____. 1982. "Learning New Principles from Precedents and Exercises." *Artificial Intelligence* 19:321–350.

_____. 1984. *Artificial Intelligence*. 2d ed. Reading, Mass.: Addison-Wesley.

_____. 1986. "Learning by Augmenting Rules and Accumulating Censors." In Michalski, Carbonell, and Mitchell, 1986, 45–61.

Winston, P. H., and Horn, B. 1984. *LISP*. 2d ed. Reading, Mass.: Addison-Wesley.

_____. 1989. *LISP*. 3rd ed. Reading, Mass.: Addison–Wesley.

Wolpert, L. 1978. "Pattern Formation in Biological Development." *Scientific American* 239: 154–164.

Woodbury, M. A.; Clive J.; and Garson, A. 1978. "Mathematical Typology: a Grade of Membership Technique for Obtaining Disease Definition." *Computers in Biomedical Research* 11 (3): 277–298

Woodger, J. H. 1937. *The Axiomatic Method in Biology*. Cambridge: Cambridge University Press.

_____. 1939. *The Technique of Theory Construction*. Chicago: University of Chicago Press.

_____. 1952. *Biology and Language*. Cambridge: Cambridge University Press.

_____. 1959. "Studies in the Foundations of Genetics." In *The Axiomatic Method*, ed. L. Henkin, P. Suppes, and A. Tarski, 408–428. Amsterdam: North-Holland.

Worral, J. 1984. "Review Article: An Unreal Image." *British Journal for the Philosophy of Science* 35:65–80.

Wright, L. 1972. "A Comment on Ruse's Analysis of Function Statements." *Philosophy of Science* 39:512–514.

_____. 1973. "Functions." *Philosophical Review* 82:139–168.

_____. 1976. *Teleological Explanations*. Berkeley: University of California Press.

Wright, S. 1931. "Evolution in Mendelian Populations." *Genetics* 16:97–159.

_____. 1949. "Adaptation and Selection." In *Genetics, Paleontology and Evolution*, ed. G. L. Jepson, G. G. Simpson, and E. Mayr, 365–389. Princeton, N. J.: Princeton University Press.

Zadeh, L. A. 1965. "Fuzzy Sets." *Information and Control* 8:338-353.

Zahar, E. 1973. "Why Did Einstein's Programme Supersede Lorentz's?" Parts 1, 2. *British Journal for the Philosophy of Science* 24:95–123, 223–262.

Index

Abduction
  See Retroduction
Accidentality
  essential, 121–122
  historical, 121
Ad hoc hypothesis, 4, 216, 231, 241–246, 520, 547
Agreement, method of, 143–144
AIDS, 113, 292–293, 477, 491
  See also T (thymus-derived) cells, Antibody formation
Alkon, D., 549
Allison, A. C., 5, 347, 356, 522
AM, 53
Ames, B., 160, 538
Antecedent theoretical meaning, 58, 131–132, 137, 535–536
Antibody formation
  clonal selection theory, 4, 21, 37–38, 40–43, 46–47, 82–84, 87, 90, 117, 130–134, 141–142, 168, 170, 185, 202, 205, 215, 217, 220–228, 231–232, 234, 236, 239–240, 244–246, 249–250, 498, 518, 521, 526, 536, 545, 554
    and subcellular selection, 227, 245
    as an extended theory, 220
    Burnet's 1957 formulation, 526
    main hypotheses of, 222
  instructive theory, 4, 169, 215, 224–225, 229–237, 239–241, 245–246, 249–250, 482, 485–486, 521, 545, 554
    as an extended theory, 224
    main hypotheses of, 224–225
  natural selection theory, 14, 37, 39
Aplysia, 276–278, 283, 285, 291, 293, 296, 403, 495, 549–550
  and parallel processing, 283
  sensitization, long-term, 280–281
  sensitization, short-term, 277

Aptation, 381–382
Arber, A., 70, 88, 124, 530
Archer, O., 85, 531, 538
Aristotle, 12–13, 113, 265, 271–273, 298, 313, 380, 445, 548, 554, 558, 561–562
Arnold, A., 360
Artifact, experimental, 37, 140
Autoimmune diseases, 83–84
Auxiliary hypotheses, 139
Axiomatization
  in biology and medicine, 117

B cells, 86–88
BACON, 50, 53–60, 528
Bacon, F., 9, 20, 48, 143
Balzer, W., 426, 533, 564
Bayes's theorem, 176, 178–179, 181–187, 192, 217–218, 233, 238–243, 246, 250, 514, 541, 545
  and ad hoc hypotheses, 242, 547
  and convergence of personal probabilities, 186
  and novel predictions, 182
  catchall hypothesis, 192–193
  evidence form, 250
  odds form, 178, 182, 185, 187, 239–243, 246, 250, 510–512, 545
Bayes, T., 176–177
Bayesian conditionalization, 179–181, 543, 546
Bayesianism
  and the peripherality thesis of reductionism, 513
  as a framework, 4, 172, 184, 251, 515, 520–521, 541
Beadle, G., 75, 236, 448, 483, 487, 489
Beatty, J., 2, 66, 97, 99, 101, 122, 125, 340, 519–520, 530, 533–535, 555–556
Bechtel, W., 400, 518, 529, 532, 566
Beckner, M., 66, 69–70, 72, 82, 88, 104–105, 124–125, 327–328, 337–338, 340, 350, 358–359, 366–368,

Beckner, M. (*continued*)
  396, 405, 530, 555
  on genetic analysis, 337
  on genetic explanations, 338
Benzer, S., 447–450, 474, 497, 565
Bernal, J. D., 421
Bernard, C., 3, 130, 142, 145, 168, 415, 459, 518, 553
Bertalanffy, L. von,
Bibel, D., 195, 201
Bigelow, J., 365–367
Biomatrix, 285, 490
Biomedical system (BMS), 106, 263–264, 294, 296, 311, 322–323
Birnbaum, A., 189, 543
Blackboard model
  See Selective forgetting, theory of
Blue cone monochromacy, 457
Blum, R., 54
Bohr, N., 200, 217, 384, 505–507
Boyd, R., 354, 535
Branch reduction
  See Reduction, intertheoretic
Brandon, R., 5–6, 328, 353, 355–356, 359–360, 371–373, 379, 391, 397, 522–523, 555–557, 559
  on complete adaptation explanations, 355–356, 372–373, 522, 559
  on function, 372
Brody, B., 272–274, 548
Bromberger, S., 273–274, 318, 549
  flagpole example, 274, 318, 549
Buchanan, B., 22–23, 525, 528
Buckley, C., 229–231, 241, 250
Burian, R., 326, 555–556
Burnet, F. M., 21, 37–48, 51, 58, 82, 87, 131–134, 137, 202, 222–224, 226–230, 234, 236, 245, 249–250, 518, 526–528, 531, 536, 545
Bursa of Fabricius, 85, 362, 388

CADUCEUS, 24, 525
  See also INTERNIST-1
Campbell, N., 66, 558
Cancer, 41–42, 84, 309, 387, 568
Canfield, J., 371, 391, 396, 557
Cartwright, N., 308, 522, 553, 555–556
Causal sequence, 137, 286, 290–291, 297–300, 305–306, 319–320, 369, 428, 459, 468–469, 492, 550, 552–553

Causation
  causal propagation, 286
  epistemology of, 302
  expressed in comparative generalizations, 302
  heterogeneous character, 298
  probabilistic, 264, 307–308, 311, 320, 323, 551
Causey, R., 425, 466–467, 470, 476
Centrality
  extrinsic, 212
  intrinsic, 211
Churchland, P. M., 403, 427, 563
Churchland, P. S., 403, 427, 530, 565
  on the general reduction model, 427
Circumscription, 114
Claman, H., 85
Clarified science, 472–473, 495
Clonal selection theory
  See Antibody formation
Cloner example, 382–383, 389, 558
Cloning, 454
Cognitive science, 2, 518, 528
Cohen, I. B., 150, 538
Cohn, M., 140, 236, 482–483
Cole, J., 544, 566
Collingwood, R. G., 4, 296, 298–299, 303–304, 306, 522, 553
Color coat genes example, 319–321
Comparative experimentation, method of, 3, 145–146, 148–149, 151–152, 459, 518, 553
Concomitant variation, method of, 142, 144–145
Conditionalized realism, 194, 197–200
Connectionism, 62, 529
Constructivist program, 3, 200, 520
Correspondence rules, 3, 100, 131–132, 137, 428, 468–469, 518
Corwin, H., 565
Counterproof, method of, 145
Crick, F., 75–76, 237, 362, 382, 443, 447–449, 503, 509–511, 530, 555
Crow, J., 69, 94, 557
Culp, S., 499–500

DALTON, 53, 57–58
Damuth, J., 360
Darden, L., 82, 285, 440, 491, 518, 528–529, 531–535, 540, 545, 550, 562–563, 565

Darwin, C., 2, 40, 46, 65, 73, 97, 201,
  333–334, 353–354, 356–357, 360,
  370, 373–374, 380, 387, 519, 540,
  555–556
Dawe, C., 426, 564
Deductive, the method, 153
Default logic, 109, 113
DeFinetti, B., 171, 176, 540
Delbruck, M., 15, 325
DENDRAL, 22–23, 25, 49, 525
Descartes, R., 9
Determinism
  causal, 122
Diagnosis, logic of
  See INTERNIST-1
Difference, method of, 3, 144–147,
  149, 154–155, 299, 305, 518, 553
Direct evidence, 3, 130, 144, 156–
  158, 161–168, 170, 195, 198–199,
  241, 519, 538, 545
Discovery, 1–2, 20, 8–14, 17–19, 21–
  25, 35–39, 42–43, 45–54, 58–60,
  62–63, 517–518, 524, 526, 528–529
  context of, 10, 36, 47, 129, 222,
    517
  logic of, 8–9, 17, 22, 37, 48, 52,
    62–63, 182, 190, 222, 517–518
DNA replication, 502–503, 506, 510,
  555
DNA sequencing, 456
Dobzhansky, T., 340, 357
Dorling, J., 171, 539
Dounce, A., 74–75
Driesch, H., 413, 419
Drosophila, 378, 453, 455
Duhem, P., 66, 142, 177, 207, 218,
  241, 273, 289–290, 534, 537
Duhemian thesis, 142, 537
Dutch book argument, 171, 179

Earman, J., 172, 177, 184–185, 203,
  298, 538, 541–542, 551
Edwards, W., 186, 191–193, 542–
  543, 546
Ehrlich, P., 138, 225, 525
Einstein, A., 123, 183, 185, 194, 201,
  203–204, 216–217, 232, 475, 538
Eldredge, N., 360, 556
Elsasser, W. M., 504–507
Embryology, 2, 65, 76, 98, 119, 327,
  329, 336, 338, 519, 555
Emergentism, 413
  See also Reduction, Reductionism

Empirical adequacy, 36, 196, 205,
  216, 219, 232, 234, 238
Enç, B., 397, 466–469, 493
Epistasis, 320
Ethical issues, 6
Eureka experience, 37
Evaluation
  global, 2–3, 169–170, 181, 185,
    193–194, 203–205, 210–211,
    222, 239, 244, 246, 250–251,
    542
  global, a Bayesian logic of, 215
  local, 169–170, 173, 187, 248, 259,
    542
  preliminary, logic of, 18, 20, 25,
    35–36, 47–48, 517–518
  weak evaluation (= preliminary
    evaluation), 22
Evolutionary theory, 5–6, 69–72, 89–
  91, 94, 98, 101, 119, 124, 194, 201,
  265, 324, 326, 329, 331, 340, 350,
  353, 360–361, 363, 373–375, 379–
  380, 382–384, 387–391, 394, 396,
  398, 403, 407–408, 422, 522, 524,
  530, 533–534, 555–557, 560
  as an unrepresentative biological
    theory, 90
  ateleological character of, 373
  metatheoretical function, 90
  more realistic forms approxi-
    mate middle-range theory, 94
  the hierarchical turn in, 360
  use of DNA sequence data in
    testing, 361
  "vulgar" form of, 384
Exaptation, 381–382, 388, 404
Experimental testing
  logic of, 133
Explanation
  causal, 264, 267, 270–271, 273–
    275, 290, 292, 300, 323, 331,
    337–338, 359, 551
  causal/mechanical, 293, 295–
    296, 373
  deductive nomological, 265
  deductive statistical, 267
  epistemic approach, 292, 554
  genetic, 271, 328, 351
  inductive statistical, 265, 267–271
  interlevel, 287, 492
  partial model, 286
  six component model, 263
    the causal component, 264

six component model (*continued*)
the comparative evaluational
inductive component, 265
the ideal explanatory text
background component,
265, 324
the logical component, 264,
287, 323
the semantic (BMS) compo-
nent, 263
the unificatory component,
264, 323
statistical relevance model, 265,
269–270, 274
See also Functional explanation,
Historical explanation

Fahlman, S., 111
Feigenbaum, E., 22–23, 525
Feigl, H., 35
Feyerabend, P. K., 3, 67, 129, 137,
193, 200–202, 205, 216, 426, 520,
544, 562, 567
on incommensurability, 200
Field, H., 180–181
Fikes, R., 110
Fine, A., 203, 544
Fitness, evolutionary, 389
Frame concept, 109–110
Frank-Starling law, 336
Franklin, A., 140, 168, 176, 249, 519
Friedland, P., 60, 110
Friedman, M., 292, 312, 543
Frozen accident
See Accidentality, historical
Full adder, 287–289, 492, 550
Function, biological
most general sense of, 404
primary sense, 388
secondary sense, 389
Functional analysis
and goal-directed behavior, 405
anthropomorphic accounts, 392
containment account (Cummins),
399
etiology and (Wright), 397–398
Hempel on, 392
irreducible to causal analysis, 379
Nagel's account, 368, 370
See also Teleology
Functional explanation
as a heuristic, 390
evolutionary analyses, 370

See also Teleology, Functional
analysis
Fuzzy set theory, 126, 128

Galison, P., 3, 129–130, 157, 167–168,
200, 519
on the stability of experimental
results, 157
Gallie, W., 327–330, 332–336, 338,
358, 555
Gamow, G., 74–75, 530
Garber, D., 180–181, 184, 541
Generality
distinguished from vagueness,
212
three levels of, 212
Generalizations
in biology and medicine, 64
of variable scope, 294
universal, two subtypes, 121
Generalized empiricism, 3, 129, 136,
157, 167, 197, 199, 227, 518
Generalized induction theory, 482,
485–486
GENSIM, 60–61, 115–116
Gilbert, W., 80, 130, 158, 160–164,
168, 170, 455–456, 481, 486, 513,
538
GLAUBER, 53
Glymour, C., 4, 130, 165–168, 176–
177, 182–186, 235–236, 521–522,
538, 541, 546
Goal-directed systems
See Teleology
Good, I. J., 171, 176, 541
Good, R., 84–86, 88, 171, 176, 308,
387, 531, 538, 541, 566
Goudge, T., 66, 326, 328, 330–335,
338, 352, 358, 555
Gould, S., 122, 360–361, 380–382,
398, 404, 558
Graft-versus-host (GVH)
See also Simonson phenomena
Gregg, T., 348, 531
Grene, M., 113, 413
Grobstein, C., 103, 501
Grünbaum, A., 245, 525, 537, 545, 547

Hacking, I., 129, 156–157, 167, 172–
173, 176, 519, 539–540
Hanson, N. R., 1, 11–13, 16–18, 21,
35–36, 67, 137, 155, 193, 200, 314,
517

Hardy-Weinberg law, 91–92, 340
Hart, H. L. A., 4, 160, 296, 298, 302–304, 522, 538, 553
Haurowitz, F., 220–221, 224–227, 229–231, 235–236, 241, 245, 249–250, 545–547
Hempel, C. G., 4–5, 48–50, 52–54, 56–57, 62, 131, 137, 155, 167, 177, 204, 263, 266–269, 271–274, 291, 294, 296, 312–314, 316, 322, 392–394, 407–410, 523, 530, 536, 544, 548–549, 556
   on objections to a logic of scientific discovery, 48
Hesse, M., 176, 180–181, 186–187, 195, 233, 539–542, 546
Heuristic(s), 5, 19, 24, 29–30, 51–54, 56–58, 63, 100, 132, 198, 207, 228–229, 359, 368, 373, 385, 390–391, 404, 406, 409–410, 516, 523–524, 528–529, 536, 558
Hintikka, J., 100
Hinton, G., 62
Historical explanation
   as nonnomological, 328–329, 331
   as nonpredictive, 328, 331
   integrating explanations (Goudge), 331
   narrative explanation (Goudge), 331
   See also Explanation, genetic
HIV disease
   See AIDS
Hofstadter, A., 367
Holism, 416
Holyoak, K., 60, 528
Honoré, A. M., 4, 296, 298, 302–304, 522, 553
Hood, L., 202
Hooker, C., 196, 426–427, 430, 432, 469–474
Horan, B., 328, 353–355, 358, 378, 555–556
   on theoretical models in evolution, 354
Howson, C., 176, 180–181, 183–184, 186, 192, 239, 251, 256, 539–543, 546–548
Hull, D., 6, 66, 70–72, 125, 130, 201–202, 360, 413, 426, 433, 437–440, 443–446, 451–452, 457, 459–465, 474, 481, 493, 523, 530, 533–535, 563–564

on reduction, 438–439
on theories in biology, 71
Human genome project, 567
Hume, D., 296–297, 299, 303, 306, 369, 551, 557
HYPGENE, 60–61, 115–116, 534
Hypothesis testing
   Bayesian approach, 187
   Neyman-Pearson theory, 173–174, 176, 188, 256, 539
   statistical, 3, 182, 193, 215, 248, 251, 256, 520, 547–548
Hypothetical, the method of, 154
Hypothetico-deductive method, 10–11, 16, 35, 55, 155, 165, 167, 177, 257

Ideal explanatory text, 4, 263, 318–319, 322
Identity of indiscernibles, principle of, 470
Immunodeficiency disorders, 88
Immunology
   See Autoimmune diseases, Antibody formation, T cells, Thymus, 83–84
Incommensurability, 200, 203, 205
   and Quinean underdetermination of theory, 205
Indiscernibility of identicals, principle of, 470
Initial conditions
   two types in biology and medicine, 139
Instructive theory,
   See Antibody formation
Interfield connections, 285, 491, 531–532
Intermixture of effects, 143, 153
INTERNIST-1, 24–25, 27–34, 49, 190, 525
   evoking strengths, 28–29
   frequency values, 27
   import values, 27
   nonlinear weighting scheme, 29
   sorting heuristic, 29–30
Interpretive sentences
   See Correspondence rules
inus condition, 301

Jacob, F., 76, 81, 158–161, 164, 317, 431, 445, 481, 483–485, 491, 509, 511–512, 544, 548, 564

612 / Index

Jacquard, A., 69, 91, 93, 341–343, 531, 548, 550, 555–556
Jaynes, E. T., 543
Jeffrey, R., 171, 176, 180–181, 184, 190, 193, 247–248, 540, 543
Jeffreys, H., 176, 233, 235, 259, 543
Jerne, N. K., 13–16, 37, 39–41, 43, 46–48, 224, 228, 518, 526
Judson, H. F., 530
Justification, 1, 8–10, 18, 20–21, 35–37, 47, 67, 129, 171–172, 210, 340
    context of, 10, 36, 47, 129
    logic of, 8–10, 18, 21, 35–37

Kadane, J., 188, 240, 259, 542–543, 546–547
Kandel, E. R., 275–286, 290–291, 293, 296, 302, 317, 403, 413, 548–550, 552
Kant, I., 198, 297, 544
Karp, P., 60–62, 115–116, 529, 533–534
Karush, F., 225, 229, 231
Kauffman, S., 103, 507, 533
KEE, 61–62, 116, 533
Keeton, W. T., 449–450
KEKADA, 60, 528
Kierkegaard, S., 14–15
Kim, J., 461–463, 470, 565
Kimura, M., 69, 94, 557
Kitcher, P., 2, 4, 6, 64–65, 193, 208–210, 263, 274, 292, 295–296, 312–313, 315, 317–318, 322, 356, 360, 378, 424, 427, 433–434, 436, 446–447, 450–451, 474, 477–481, 490, 499–500, 519, 523, 549–551, 556–557, 564–567
    on a practice, 208, 210, 313
    on connectability in reduction, 266, 446, 451, 478, 480, 565
    on derivability in reduction, 266, 478, 481, 564
    on explanation by unification, 312
    on laws in biology, 64
    on laws in reduction, 266, 433, 436, 446, 478, 480, 565
    on reductions as explanatory extensions, 499
Knorr-Cetina, K., 3, 200, 520
Koshland, M., 230–231, 250
Kripke, S., 108, 469, 475–477
Kuffler, S., 276, 311, 549

Kuhn, T. S., 3, 50–51, 53, 59, 62–63, 67, 129, 137, 169, 172, 180, 193, 200–202, 204–207, 216–217, 220, 426, 520, 544, 567
    on a disciplinary matrix, 51–53, 206, 210
    on incommensurability, 200
    on paradigm, 201, 206
Kulkarni, D., 60, 528
Kyburg, H., 176, 180, 539–540

lac operator sequence, 531
lac operon, 3, 76, 80, 90, 98, 104, 115, 117, 161–162, 444, 461, 481, 519
Lakatos, I., 67, 193, 207–208, 210–213, 544
Langley, P., 53, 55, 57–58, 529
Latour, B., 3, 199, 520, 544
Laudan, L., 18, 67, 193, 196, 203–204, 208, 210, 216, 218, 245, 525, 537, 543–545, 547
    on incommensurability, 204
    on a logic of pursuit, 525, 545
Laws
    and reduction in biology, 433
    Mendel's laws, 434, 563
    of working, 122, 287, 306–307
    Smart's argument against in biology, 67–68, 120
Lederberg, J., 22–23, 130, 133–135, 137, 140–141, 168, 170, 224, 226–227, 229, 525–526, 528, 531, 536–537, 540
Leibniz, G. W., 469–470, 473–476
Lennox, J., 555, 557–559
Leplin, J., 543
Level of organization, 103, 337, 385
    level of aggregation, 83, 89, 98, 102–103, 117, 119, 213, 224, 287, 290, 492, 494, 519, 550
Levi, I., 176, 180, 540, 545–546
Levins, R., 89, 95–96, 104, 119, 354
    on theory in biology, 95
Levitan, M., 343–344, 346–347
Lewin, B., 77, 289, 385, 558
Lewis, D., 298, 551
Lewontin, R., 90–91, 340, 360, 373–374, 376–378, 380–383, 387, 393, 398, 410, 532, 557
    on maximization of fitness, 376
Li, C. C., 347–348, 357
Lindley, D., 189, 191, 542–543, 547
Lindley-Savage argument, 189, 191,

542–543
Livingstone, F., 5, 342, 347–349, 354, 356–357, 522
Lloyd, E., 2, 6, 65–66, 99, 101, 350, 360, 519–520, 536, 556
Logic of generation, 19–20, 22–23, 25, 34–36, 43, 48, 517
Logical positivism, 129, 167, 195

Mach, E., 54, 56
Mackie, J., 4, 296–307, 337, 369, 522, 538, 552–553, 555, 558
  chocolate bar machine example, 300, 552
Mäkelä, O., 140–142, 170, 228
Maull, N., 82, 103, 285, 491, 531–532, 550
Maxwell's electromagnetic theory, 74, 138
Mayo, D., 308
Mayr, E., 71, 124, 326–327, 339, 360, 364, 366, 390, 413, 415, 497, 504, 532, 554, 562
  on population thinking, 532
  on the importance of historical narrative, 327
  on unification of science, 124
McGee, V., 249–250
Memory cells, 38–39
Mendelian dominance example
  Bayesian analysis of, 256
  Neyman-Pearson analysis of, 252
Mendelian genetics, 4, 57, 91, 174, 216, 252, 271, 340, 438–440, 463, 480, 521
Mendelian-Morganian genetics, 431, 529
  See also Mendelian genetics
Mental models, 528, 532–533
Merton, R. K., 97, 392, 525, 530–531, 544
Metaphysics
  See Process metaphysics
Methods of experimental inquiry
  See various specific methods
Mettler, L., 348, 531
Mill, J.S., 3, 9, 24, 26–27, 30, 33–34, 62, 84–85, 87, 130, 142–145, 149–151, 153–155, 164–166, 168, 170, 228, 266, 299, 301, 303, 305, 385–387, 389, 408, 415, 420, 513, 518, 525, 537–538, 543, 548, 553, 555

Miller, J. F. A. P., 84–85, 150, 228, 386
Miller, R., 26, 30, 34, 525
Minsky, M., 109
Molecular biology, 3, 60, 62, 64, 66, 73–74, 76, 114, 130, 143, 168, 288–290, 362, 402, 417, 433, 446, 461, 463, 478, 492, 498, 506, 509, 511–513, 518, 533–534, 567
MOLGEN, 60
Monod, J., 76, 81, 158–161, 164, 236, 317, 431, 445, 481–485, 491, 509, 511–512, 544, 548, 564–565
Montague, A., 343–344, 346–347
Moore, G. E., 379, 403, 557
Morgan, T. H., 411–412, 528, 540
Morowitz, H., 2, 285, 490, 504, 519, 549
Muller, H. J., 442, 481, 488–489, 564
Müller-Hill, B., 80, 130, 158, 160–165, 168, 170, 486, 513, 538
Multiple inheritance, 115, 119
Munson, R., 123, 371, 530–531, 534
Muscle stimulation example, 311
Myers, J., 24–26, 29–30, 33–34, 525

Nagel, E., 5, 66, 131, 137, 336, 366–372, 393–394, 399, 405–406, 413, 423–426, 430, 432–433, 438, 446, 461, 472, 477–478, 480, 491, 493, 497, 501, 523, 535, 537, 544, 548, 561–562, 566–567
  on functional analysis, 370
Nathans, J., 457–458
Necessity
  in the circumstances, 299–300, 337, 552, 555
Newell, A., 18–19
Neyman, J., 172–178, 187–190, 215, 252–253, 255–256, 539–540, 542
Nirenberg, M., 76
Nonmonotonic logic, 113–114, 116, 534, 566
Nossal, G., 130, 133–135, 137, 140–141, 168, 170, 226–228, 362, 536–537
Nossal-Lederberg experiment, 130, 134–135, 137, 140–141, 168, 170, 536–537
Null hypothesis, 252, 539

Object-oriented approach, 107

Object-oriented programming
(OOP), 62, 114–115, 215, 452, 550
Observation language, 102, 202, 231
Occam's razor, 227, 236
Olby, R. C., 434–436, 530, 563, 566
Old evidence, 177, 182–185, 192, 316,
541
Oparin, A. I., 414, 420–421, 504
Operator gene, 77, 158, 160, 443, 445,
447, 461, 485, 538
Operon model, 36, 60, 76, 82, 90,
101, 104, 117, 130, 158–159, 164,
167–168, 212, 428, 431, 464, 481–
482, 485–487, 509, 511–513, 530,
534
as an interlevel theory, 82
Oppenheim, P., 266, 291, 423, 425,
530, 548, 562
Optimality arguments
in evolutionary theory, 377–378
Organ transplantation, 84
Orgel, L., 382, 504

"Pajama" experiment (aka Pa-ja-mo
experiment), 464, 483–486, 511,
514
Pap, A., 182, 541
Parastasis, 151–152, 299, 370, 538
Pardee, A., 483–485, 491
Pasteur, L., 195, 483
Pauling, L., 224–225, 229–231, 233,
235, 237, 245
Peirce, C. S., 12–13, 17, 196–197, 538,
543
Peripherality thesis, 6, 509, 511, 513,
515, 524, 567
Perspectival sequence, 290
not necessarily a causal sequence,
291
Phenomenal system, 99, 536–537
Pierce, J., 85, 531
Pittendrigh, C., 364
Plasma cells, 39, 84, 86–87, 132, 202,
223
Plurality of causes, 301, 331
Polanyi, M., 67, 418–419, 501, 503,
505
on antireductionism, 418
Polya, G., 19
Polymerase chain reaction (PCR),
361
Polytypic class
defined, 104

Pople, H., 24, 26, 30, 33–34, 525
Popper, K. R., 10–11, 36, 67, 155, 196,
200, 207, 233, 240, 266, 273, 409,
426, 536, 539, 543
Probabilistic causation
See Causation, probabilistic
Probability
calculus, 170–172, 184, 193, 516,
524, 540
meaning, 171
personal, 171, 265, 323
Problem solving, 18–19, 27, 44–45,
51, 56, 59, 63, 203, 391, 499, 567
Process metaphysics, 299, 307
Progress
See Scientific progress
Ptashne, M., 160, 165, 513
Putnam, H., 67, 107–108, 196–197,
203, 229, 402, 432, 469–470, 472,
475–477, 539

QMR, 24, 525
See also INTERNIST-1
Quine, W. V., 177, 195, 205, 241, 423,
430, 439–440, 473, 476

Raiffa, H., 568
Railton, P., 4, 263, 265, 318–319, 322,
324
Ramsey, F., 171, 176, 475, 540
Realism, scientific, 66, 157, 193
Redhead, M., 245, 547
Reduction
and analogy, 481
connectability, 425, 437, 466
connectability of natural kinds,
437
derivability, 425
General reduction model, 426–
427, 430, 440, 562
General Reduction-Replacement
(GRR) model, 6, 427, 430–431,
481, 488, 491, 493–500, 523, 564
GRR and CM approaches compared, 495, 497–498, 500
identity, meaning of, 469
intertheoretic, 422–423
Kemeny-Oppenheim model, 425
Mendelian-molecular genetics example, 439, 442
multiple levels of analysis in, 487
Nagel model, 423–424, 433
peripherality thesis, 508–510, 516

Suppes-Adams model, 425, 428, 430, 566
synthetic identity in, 379, 425, 430, 437, 440, 462, 468–469, 475, 491, 497–498, 557, 563–564, 566
token-token, 460
type-type, 461
unilevel, 431, 492, 496, 566
Reductionism
defined, 411
different types of approaches, 412
ontological, 413
structural versus ultimate, 503
Regulator genes, 76, 443, 511, 538
Reichenbach, H., 10–12, 131, 176, 270, 296, 305, 307–308, 310, 525, 551
Repressor, 3, 77, 80–82, 84, 101–102, 113, 130, 158–164, 168, 170, 212, 306, 445, 447, 464, 485–486, 490–491, 511–514, 519, 530, 534, 538, 568
Residues, method of, 144–145
Restriction fragment length polymorphisms (RFLPs), 453
Reticularity (in biological theory), 89, 97, 534
Retroduction, 12–13, 16–18, 21, 35
Richardson, R., 518, 529
Rosch, E., 107–108, 532
Rosenberg, A., 2, 6, 64, 66, 72–73, 120, 123–125, 202, 340, 350, 390–391, 400–403, 409, 413, 427, 436, 451–452, 457, 459, 461–463, 474, 497, 519, 523, 530–531, 533–534, 555, 557, 560–562, 565
on biology as a series of case-studies, 73, 533
on connectability in reduction, 451
on intentionality in biology, 401
on Williams's axiomatization of evolution, 72
Rosenbleuth, A., 365–367
Rosenkrantz, R., 172, 176, 191, 233–235, 542–543
Ruse, M., 2, 5, 66, 68–70, 72–73, 120, 123–125, 330, 340, 371–372, 391, 397, 426, 519, 523, 530, 534, 557
on functional analysis, 371
on Smart's arguments about

laws in biology, 68
Rx, 54

Sadler, J., 81, 118
Salmon, W., 4, 134–135, 141, 176, 181, 186, 263, 269–271, 274–275, 291–293, 295–296, 299, 305, 307–308, 311–312, 315–319, 322, 356, 433, 493–494, 500, 525, 527, 536, 539, 541, 546, 548–551, 553–554, 556
Salmonella, 134–135, 141, 536
Savage, L. J., 176, 186, 189–193, 239–240, 251, 259, 521, 542–543, 546
Schaffner, K. F., 34, 73, 131, 181, 245, 286, 425–428, 430, 433, 475, 504, 521, 525, 534, 544, 547, 552, 563, 566
Scheffler, I., 202–203
Scheines, R., 522
Schiller, F. C. S., 9–10
Schwartz, J., 276–277, 279, 285, 403, 475, 548–549, 565
Scientific discovery
See Discovery
Scientific justification
See Justification
Scientific progress, 216–220
criteria of, 232–247
through reductions, 488–489, 495–500
See also Discovery, Evaluation
Scientific realism
See Realism, scientific
See also Conditionalized realism
Screening off, 244, 270, 317, 554
Scriven, M., 66, 267, 270, 318, 328, 353–354, 358, 548–549
barometer example, 267, 270
on predictability in evolutionary theory, 353
paresis example, 318, 549
Seidenfeld, T., 173, 176, 180, 539, 543
Selective forgetting, theory of, 37, 44
Sellars, W., 195–196, 543
Semantic network, 58, 111–112
Sham operation, 147
Shapere, D., 3, 52–53, 67, 129–130, 138, 156–157, 167–168, 193, 205–206, 208, 211, 428, 519, 532, 537
on direct observation, 156
on domain, 52, 138, 211, 532
on Kuhnian relativism, 205

Sheldrake, R., 562
Shimony, A., 171–172, 184, 186, 193, 196, 539–540, 543, 545–546
Sickle-cell anemia
See Sickle-cell disease
Sickle-cell disease, 5, 339
Sickle-cell example, 343–344, 351–354, 357, 398
Sickle-cell trait, 5, 328, 339, 341, 347–348, 350–351
Significance level, 173–175, 191, 253, 259
Silverstein, A., 525, 536, 545–546
Simon, H., 18–19, 37, 43–46, 50, 53, 55–57, 60, 66, 103, 413, 528, 534–535, 539, 557, 559–560
    Tempus and Hora example, 557, 559–560
Simonson, M., 221
Simplicity, 4, 36, 50, 61, 130–131, 165, 167, 196, 206, 216–219, 232–236, 238, 241–242, 244, 373, 386, 459, 478, 520, 535–536, 546
    and sample coverage, 234
Simpson, G. G., 123–124, 326, 413–414, 422, 535, 553, 562
    on compositionist explanation, 422
    on the uniqueness of historical causation, 326
    on unification of science, 123
Skyrms, B., 308, 553–554, 556
Smart, J. J. C., 2, 64, 66–69, 73, 119–121, 123, 479, 519, 530
Smearing out of models
    caused by biological variation, 104
Smith, C. A. B., 191
Smith, J. M., 374
Smith, T., 81, 118
Smolensky, P., 62
Smuts, J., 416
Sober, E., 6, 72, 308, 328, 350, 353–354, 360–361, 553, 555–556, 558
    on evolutionary explanation, 354
    on parsimony in evolutionary theory, 361
Social constructivism, 3, 199–200, 520
Spirtes, P., 522
Stable estimation, principle of, 186, 190, 239
STAHL, 53, 57–58
Steen, W. van der, 2, 122, 519, 530, 534, 556
Stent, G., 160, 212, 448, 538
Stereotypes, 107–108
Strickberger, M., 76–81, 320–321, 441, 530, 548, 554, 563–564
Stryer, L., 401–402, 560
Subjective probability
See Probability, personal
Supervenience, 459, 461–463, 556, 565
Suppe, F., 2, 65–66, 99, 101–102, 127, 520, 532–533, 535–537
Suppes, P., 99, 101, 105–106, 251, 294, 308, 310, 380, 425–426, 428, 430, 536, 566
Szenberg, A., 85, 227
Szilard, L., 226

T (thymus-derived) cells, 84, 86, 88, 409
Tatum, E., 75, 236, 448, 483, 487, 489
Teleology
    cybernetic or systems analyses, 365
    intentional analysis, 364
Teleonomy
See Teleology
Teller, P., 171, 180, 539, 543
Theoretical context sufficiency, 205, 216, 219, 232, 234, 237–238, 241, 244, 526, 540
Theory
    as a polytypic class of models, 105
    as overlapping interlevel temp-oral models, 98
    as prototypes, 98
    extended (diachronic) and the se-mantic conception, 214
    individuation, 4, 211, 220, 474, 487, 520, 545
    integrity, 246
    interfield, 550
    middle-range, 2, 6, 65, 105, 119–121, 125, 519–520, 523, 525, 530
    not universal in biology, 73, 97
    "received"view, 66–67, 174
    semantic conception, 494
    set-theoretic approach (in gener-alized form), 105
    sharpening due to selection pres-sures, 82–83, 170, 188
    state space analysis, 101

structure, 1, 65, 119, 433, 519
    temporally extended, 3, 170,
    211–215, 220-231, 520
Thompson, P., 2, 6, 65–66, 73, 99–
    100, 520, 530, 536, 556
Thymus, immunological function
    of, 85–88, 150, 386
Toulmin, S., 67, 193, 200, 208, 532
Touretzky, D., 62
Trajectory contingency, 122
    See also Accidentality, historical
Triplett, R., 85
Two-component theory (of the im-
    mune response), 86–87, 89–90,
    104, 150, 531
Type I error, 175, 252–253, 255
Type II error, 176

Urbach, P., 176, 180–181, 183–184,
    186, 192, 239, 251, 256, 539–543,
    546–548

van Fraassen, B., 4, 99–102, 180–
    181, 184, 195–196, 263, 265, 270,
    272–273, 296, 313–319, 322, 324,
    537, 541, 548–549, 551, 554, 556
Vitalism, 413, 562
Vrba, E., 380–382, 404, 558

Wade, M., 360
Waksman, B., 85, 387, 531
Warner, N., 85, 227
Waters, K., 66
Watson, J. D., 74–76, 88, 244, 288,
    319, 341, 386–387, 434, 447–449,
    455, 457, 459, 464, 479, 486, 490,
    498, 503–504, 509–511, 526, 530–
    531, 555, 558, 563–564, 567–568
Weiss, P. A., 413, 417–419, 501, 503
Whewell, W., 9
Why-questions, 314, 317
Williams, B., 557–558
Williams, G. C., 374, 404
Williams, M., 72, 340
Wimsatt, W., 2, 5–6, 64–65, 82, 103,
    287, 360, 394–396, 398, 406–409,
    424, 426–427, 433, 470, 490, 492–
    493, 497, 515, 519, 523, 527, 533,
    540, 549, 558–559, 561–562, 564,
    567
    on function and teleological ex-
        planation, 407, 560–561
    on functional analysis, 394
    on mechanisms, 64, 287, 527
Winston, P., 58–59, 109, 529, 533–534
Wolpert, L., 336
Woodfield, A., 364–365, 368
Woodger, J. H., 65, 110, 327, 329,
    333–335, 338, 423, 530, 555
Woolgar, S., 3, 199, 520, 544
Worral, J., 532
Wright model of evolution, 92–94
Wright, L., 396, 406
Wright, S., 340–343, 375, 377, 530
Wrinch, D., 233

Zadeh, L., 126–127
Zahar, E., 547
Zuckerman, H., 544